Calcium in Human Health

NUTRITION ◊ AND ◊ HEALTH

Adrianne Bendich, Series Editor

CALCIUM IN HUMAN HEALTH

Edited by

CONNIE M. WEAVER, PhD

Department of Foods and Nutrition, Purdue University, West Lafayette, IN

and

ROBERT P. HEANEY, MD

John A. Creighton University Professor, Creighton University, Omaha, NE

Foreword by

LAWRENCE G. RAISZ, MD

Division of Endocrinology and Metabolism, University of Connecticut Health Center, Farmington, CT

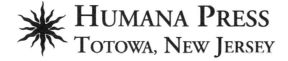

HUMANA PRESS
TOTOWA, NEW JERSEY

© 2006 Humana Press Inc.
999 Riverview Drive, Suite 208
Totowa, New Jersey 07512

www.humanapress.com

Due diligence has been taken by the publishers, editors, and authors of this book to assure the accuracy of the information published and to describe generally accepted practices. The contributors herein have carefully checked to ensure that the drug selections and dosages set forth in this text are accurate and in accord with the standards accepted at the time of publication. Notwithstanding, as new research, changes in government regulations, and knowledge from clinical experience relating to drug therapy and drug reactions constantly occurs, the reader is advised to check the product information provided by the manufacturer of each drug for any change in dosages or for additional warnings and contraindications. This is of utmost importance when the recommended drug herein is a new or infrequently used drug. It is the responsibility of the treating physician to determine dosages and treatment strategies for individual patients. Further it is the responsibility of the health care provider to ascertain the Food and Drug Administration status of each drug or device used in their clinical practice. The publisher, editors, and authors are not responsible for errors or omissions or for any consequences from the application of the information presented in this book and make no warranty, express or implied, with respect to the contents in this publication.

Cover design by Patricia F. Cleary
Production Editor: Robin B. Weisberg

For additional copies, pricing for bulk purchases, and/or information about other Humana titles, contact Humana at the above address or at any of the following numbers: Tel.: 973-256-1699; Fax: 973-256-8341; E-mail: orders@humanapr.com; or visit our Website: www.humanapress.com

This publication is printed on acid-free paper. ∞
ANSI Z39.48-1984 (American National Standards Institute) Permanence of Paper for Printed Library Materials.

Photocopy Authorization Policy:

Printed in the United States of America. 10 9 8 7 6 5 4 3 2 1

eISBN 1-59259-961-3

Library of Congress Cataloging-in-Publication Data

Calcium in human health / [edited by] Connie M. Weaver and Robert P. Heaney
; foreword by Lawrence G. Raisz.
    p. ; cm. -- (Nutrition and health)
  Includes bibliographical references and index.
  ISBN 1-58829-452-8 (alk. paper)
 1. Calcium in the body. 2. Calcium in human nutrition.
  [DNLM: 1. Calcium--metabolism. 2. Calcium--pharmacology. 3. Nutritional
Requirements. QV 276 C14363 2005] I. Weaver, Connie, 1950- II. Heaney,
Robert Proulx, 1927- III. Series: Nutrition and health (Totowa, N.J.)
  QP535.C2C26355 2005
  612.3'924--dc22
                                                                2005006564

Dedication

Calcium in Human Health incorporates many of the main findings of our research careers. It also has chapters written by many of our favorite colleagues and collaborators. Our interest in calcium spans nearly 80 years of work between us. We had more than a decade of collaboration as co-investigators on our long-running bioavailability project. We continue as colleagues and friends, learning from one another still. The wisdom and rich experience that the other brings to our collaborative efforts have shaped much of the basic framework with which we approach research and nutritional policy. We dedicate this book to our wonderful laboratory groups, who work tirelessly, and to the students who continually teach us. We also dedicate this book to our families who have always supported our work (which is more like play to us) with much love, and on occasion even given generously of their time and skills to our research projects.

Connie M. Weaver
Robert P. Heaney

Series Editor's Introduction

The *Nutrition and Health Series* of books have had great success because each volume has the consistent overriding mission of providing health professionals with texts that are essential because each includes (1) a synthesis of the state of the science; (2) timely, in-depth reviews by the leading researchers in their respective fields; (3) extensive, up-to-date fully annotated reference lists; (4) a detailed index; (5) relevant tables and figures; (6) identification of paradigm shifts and the consequences; (7) virtually no overlap of information between chapters, but targeted, interchapter referrals; (8) suggestions of areas for future research; and (9) balanced, data-driven answers to patient/health professionals' questions that are based on the totality of evidence rather than the findings of any single study.

The series volumes are not the outcome of a symposium. Rather, each editor has the potential to examine a chosen area with a broad perspective, both in subject matter as well as in the choice of chapter authors. The international perspective, especially with regard to public health initiatives, is emphasized where appropriate. The editors, whose trainings are both research- and practice-oriented, have the opportunity to develop a primary objective for their book; define the scope and focus, and then invite the leading authorities from around the world to be part of their initiative. The authors are encouraged to provide an overview of the field, discuss their own research, and relate the research findings to potential human health consequences. Because each book is developed *de novo*, the chapters are coordinated so that the resulting volume imparts greater knowledge than the sum of the information contained in the individual chapters.

Calcium in Human Health, edited by Drs. Connie M. Weaver and Robert P. Heaney, is a critical addition to the *Nutrition and Health Series* and fully exemplifies the goals of the series. As an essential mineral that forms the structural components of bones and teeth, calcium is integral to our health and well-being. However, the critical role of calcium in the functioning of nerves and muscles, cellular membrane interactions, the clotting of blood, and even our mood states is less well known. Moreover, there are newer areas of research concerning the importance of calcium in estrogen-related conditions, such as the premenstrual syndrome and the polycystic ovarian syndrome, that may provide clinically relevant options for many women. This volume has been developed to examine the current investigations concerning the importance of calcium in the functioning of the human body and mind, disease prevention, and treatment, and to put these areas of research and medical practice into historic perspective as well as point the way to future research opportunities.

Calcium and Human Health joins three other volumes in the *Nutrition and Health Series* in providing in-depth information about vitamin and mineral nutrients that are essential to bone as well as overall health. Dr. Michael Holick's edited volume, entitled *Vitamin D*, was published in 1999 and is being updated in the Second Edition that is due to be published in 2007. In 2004, both Dr. Holick and Dr. Bess Dawson-Hughes edited the comprehensive volume, *Nutrition and Bone Health*. The editors of this volume on calcium have contributed valuable chapters to the *Nutrition and Bone Health* volume. Dr. Heaney has informative chapters in *Clinical Nutrition of the Essential Trace Elements and Minerals*, edited by Drs. John D. Bogden and Leslie M. Klevay and in the recently published Third Edition of *Preventive Nutrition*, edited by myself and Dr. Richard J. Deckelbaum. Thus, the editors of this volume, Dr. Connie M. Weaver and Dr. Robert P. Heaney, have added greatly to the series and have provided a key volume on calcium that makes the series a place where researchers can look for the best up-to-date information on calcium and other minerals, vitamin D, and bone health.

Both of the editors are internationally recognized leaders in the field of calcium research. Both are excellent communicators and they have worked tirelessly to develop a book that is destined to be the benchmark in the field because of its extensive, in-depth chapters covering the most important aspects of the complex interactions between diet and its nutrient components, bone formation and function, consequences of calcium deficiency as well as potential adverse effects of calcium excess on major body systems. Moreover, the volume includes insightful chapters that review the role of calcium and related nutrients including, but not limited to, vitamin D, in maintaining mental as well as physical health, and an extensive evaluation of its critical importance in the prevention of major disease states. The introductory chapters provide readers with the basics of calcium's biological functions so that the more clinically related chapters can be easily understood. The editors have contributed several chapters and have also chosen 23 of the most well-recognized and respected authors from around the world to contribute the 28 informative chapters in the volume. Key features of this comprehensive volume include the bulleted Key Points that are at the beginning of each chapter, the more than 115 detailed tables and informative figures, the extensive, detailed index, and the more than 1800 up-to-date references that provide the reader with excellent sources of worthwhile information about calcium and human health. To add further value to this benchmark volume, the editors have included five appendices that make this the "go-to" text for useful referenced materials including the detailed tabulation of the Dietary Reference Intake values for calcium across the age span as well as the criteria used to support the intake values; a table that lists the major food sources of calcium and the clinically derived absorption efficiency of calcium from each food source; a detailed dietary assessment tool for calculating daily calcium intakes; and lists of both relevant books and websites where the reader can find further information about calcium.

The book chapters are logically organized in six sections to provide the reader with a basic understanding as well as an appreciation of the development of the field of calcium research, its relationship to organ system functions and the potential for calcium nutriture to affect these variables. The first two sections review basic scientific information on the cellular and metabolic functions of calcium that is essential to understanding the following sections. In these chapters, the reader is introduced to the leading techniques for determining calcium status through both dietary as well as kinetic studies. For every nutrient, there are concerns about the veracity of dietary recall, the actual daily intake requirement and the bioavailability of the nutrient that is consumed in a mixed diet and/or through supplementation or fortification. Each of these factors is crucial in understanding the complexities of the disease states as well as the development of drugs to treat relevant diseases such as osteoporosis. The third section includes chapters that review calcium requirements, tabulate recommendations in the United States compared to 33 other nations, and examine the food sources, supplements, and their bioavailability compared with milk, which is used as the standard. The fourth section examines in depth the body's responses to low calcium intake and its regulation at the molecular level. Figures in this section clearly illustrate the relationships between the internal and external compartments in bone and how these affect bone strength. In addition to internal factors, certain lifestyle choices, such as exercise, smoking, and alcohol consumption can impact on one's calcium status. Moreover, there are data that point to a "calcium appetite," which is discussed in a separate, well-referenced chapter in this section. Equally important is the understanding of the potential for calcium nutriture to affect responses to growth, pubertal changes, and pregnancy and lactation. The fifth section reviews the interactions between the bones, nervous, and endocrine systems and also includes detailed information about the differences in responses between males and females as their bodies undergo maturation.

The sixth and final section of the volume includes 10 chapters that address the interactions between calcium and the major clinical diseases that affect both men and women. The editors have included extensive chapters on calcium's role in the development of osteoporosis in the bones of the central and peripheral skeleton as well as in the oral cavity; the newest research on the potential for calcium to affect the development of, as well as the treatment of, obesity and a separate chapter on the effects of calcium on insulin sensitivity and diabetes; the growing clinical findings of calcium's effects in colon and other cancers; calcium's effects on blood pressure; and a related chapter on the importance of calcium balance in renal disease. Two additional chapters examine the consequences of low calcium status on the development and treatment of the premenstrual and polycystic ovarian syndromes.

This important reference text provides practical, data-driven integrated resources based on the totality of the evidence to help the reader evaluate the critical role of calcium, especially in at-risk populations, in optimizing health and preventing calcium-related chronic illnesses. The overarching goal of the editors is to provide fully referenced information to health professionals so they may have a balanced perspective on the value of foods and nutrients that are routinely consumed and how these help to maintain calcium status to assure both mental as well as physical health.

In conclusion, *Calcium in Human Health*, edited by Weaver and Heaney, provides health professionals in many areas of research and practice with the most up-to-date, well referenced, and easy-to-understand volume on the importance of calcium in reducing the risk of developing chronic diseases and optimizing health. This volume will serve the reader as the benchmark in this complex area of interrelationships between diet, calcium, and other relevant specific nutrients, skeletal, muscle, renal, cardiac, and hormonal functions; environmental factors and their effects on calcium status including exercise, smoking, and alcohol consumption; and calcium's role in obesity, diabetes, cancer, cardiovascular, and kidney disease prevention as well as treatment. The editors are applauded for their efforts to develop the most authoritative resource in the field to date and this excellent text is a very welcome addition to the *Nutrition and Health Series*.

Adrianne Bendich, PhD, FACN
Series Editor

Foreword

In *Calcium in Human Health*, 25 authors have accomplished the daunting task of not only demonstrating the importance of calcium in human health, but also defining its many and complex roles. The roles of calcium in biology became much more complex and critical when animals emerged from the sea, although the fundamental regulatory roles of calcium in cells persisted. The first eukaryotes developed systems for excluding calcium from the intracellular fluid so that nanomolar concentrations could be maintained inside the cell in the face of millimolar concentrations outside, and changes in these concentrations could be used to alter cellular function. Perhaps these primordial organisms developed in an environment of about 1.3 mM calcium, similar to that of our own extracellular fluid. As organisms evolved in the sea, the calcium concentration rose, and new mechanisms for preventing excessive calcium entry developed, which may now be expressed in the limited intestinal absorption of this critical element in mammals. As organisms moved into fresh water and ultimately onto dry land, a new problem needed to be solved. Calcium was no longer abundant in the environment, but scarce. One solution was the development of a calcium-rich skeleton, but the critical functions of calcium in cell regulation and its equally critical role in maintaining a structural framework for the organism now came into conflict.

Calcium in Human Health begins, in Chapters 2 and 3, by setting out the fundamentals of this conflict, not only by indicating the multiple roles of calcium, but also by summarizing the mechanisms by which some of the conflict can be resolved. To understand the role of calcium, it is important to have methods that can accurately measure its bioavailability, absorption, and kinetics. These are described in detail in Chapters 4–6. The next three chapters cover the complex issue of calcium consumption, requirements, and bioavailability. Despite the extremely wide variation in calcium intakes and differences in Recommended Daily Allowances in different countries, it can be concluded that calcium deficiency is a major problem and calcium excess a rare one.

The complex regulation of calcium absorption, distribution, and excretion, as well as the multiple interactions of diet, lifestyle, and physical activity in calcium homeostasis are outlined in Chapters 10–14. Chapter 15 summarizes the evidence for a "calcium appetite" in humans and experimental animals and points out the interesting possibility that our current high intakes of salt and fat may blunt this appetite. This provides a potential explanation for the inadequacy of calcium intake in societies where ample supplies are available. However, another factor may be the decrease in total food intake that has occurred as humans become less physically active in an industrialized society.

Chapters 16–18 cover the special aspects of calcium economy that occur in infancy, childhood, adolescence, and with pregnancy and lactation. These are particularly important areas of public health concern, as emphasized in the recent Surgeon General's report on Bone Health and Osteoporosis.[1]

A unique and exciting aspect of this book is the discussion of specific roles of calcium in a variety of clinical disorders, in the last 10 chapters. Although much has been written about the role of calcium in maintaining the skeleton and of calcium deficiency as a pathogenetic factor in osteoporosis, other interactions have not received as much attention. The chapters on calcium and oral health, obesity, reproductive disorders, and the metabolic syndrome, provide new insights and raise new questions. Much more needs to be learned about the role of calcium in these disorders. Similarly, there is clear evidence that calcium and vitamin D can play a role in cancer, but here again further definition is needed. With the availability of drugs that can alter the function of the extracellular calcium receptor, the complex changes in calcium and phosphate regulation that occur in renal disease and the potential role of calcium in hypertension and vascular disease, which are summarized in the last two chapters, represent additional areas where new studies are both needed and feasible.

Calcium in Human Health might have the subtitle, "Everything You Wanted to Know About Calcium and Needed to Ask." It contains a vast amount of information, but also indicates many gaps in our knowledge. One major gap is the discrepancy between knowledge and practice in the area of public health. Perhaps a companion volume on what must be done to improve the calcium economy of our population and how this can be accomplished could be a next step. Based on present information, this might be a slim volume indeed, but we do have much of the necessary scientific background needed to define both the problems and the opportunities for doing more about calcium in human health.

Lawrence G. Raisz, MD
Division of Endocrinology and Metabolism
University of Connecticut Health Center
Farmington, CT

---

[1]*Bone Health and Osteoporosis: A Report of the Surgeon General* can be accessed on the web at www.surgeongeneral.gov.

Preface

More research is done on calcium with resultant publications than for any other mineral. This interest in calcium is appropriate with its diverse biological functions, the dietary inadequacies in calcium all over the world, and the relationship of calcium status to so many disorders. Calcium serves as a second messenger for nearly every biological process and stabilizes many proteins. It is an unusual nutrient in that the storage reserve of calcium in the skeleton has a biological function. Bone mass predicts risk of fracture. Aside from bone health, calcium insufficiency has been associated with hypertension, cardiovascular health, stroke, polycystic ovary disease, kidney stones, certain types of cancer, weight loss, diabetes, and insulin resistance syndrome.

The aim of *Calcium in Human Health* is to provide students, scientists, and health professionals including physicians, nutritionists, dentists, pharmacists, dietitians, and health educators with up-to-date research on calcium function and its relationship to health. The amount of new information has been almost explosive linking calcium to health in the last decade with the associations to weight loss, diabetes, and insulin resistance syndrome evolving in the last 5 years. Equally exciting are the discoveries coming from molecular biology and genetics. Our basic understanding of calcium absorption and the influence of gene polymorphisms is evolving. Single book chapters cannot do justice to the amount of new information available.

Calcium in Human Health is divided into six parts. Part I discusses calcium function as the main element in bone, as an intracellular messenger, and as a stabilizer of proteins. This section explains why calcium status is part of the etiology of so many disorders. Part II discusses methods for estimating calcium intakes of various populations as well as how to conduct controlled feeding studies. The ability to determine calcium intake sheds light on interpretation of studies of the relationship of calcium intake to disease. The third section discusses calcium intakes, requirements, and dietary sources of calcium. One chapter illustrates how widespread calcium deficiencies are throughout the world. Circumstances that create calcium excesses and the implication of exceeding upper tolerable levels are reviewed. Another chapter discusses calcium bioavailability and food factors that influence calcium absorption. Part IV reviews calcium homeostasis. Molecular mechanisms of calcium absorption and regulators of calcium homeostasis from genetics to lifestyle choices are reviewed in this section. One chapter suggests an interesting role for regulation of intake driven by calcium appetite. The influence of total diet and lifestyle choices on calcium metabolism is also covered in this section. A fifth section covers calcium through development. Various chapters in this section cover infancy and childhood, adolescence, pregnancy, and lactation. The last section covers many of the diseases now associated with calcium intake. Each chapter begins with an overview of the literature, but the emphasis is on recent findings.

We have devoted most of our careers to the study of calcium and its relationship to health. As editors, we hope *Calcium in Human Health* will serve as a critical resource for health professionals to enhance their ability to improve health outcomes of individuals; for researchers who study calcium function and application; for students of health science, nutrition, and medicine; and for those setting dietary requirements and developing disease-prevention programs. This comprehensive coverage of calcium in human health is assembled by the leading researchers in the field of calcium. We believe that *Calcium in Human Health* will serve as a useful text and reference. We invite comments from users of this book about its content and use of various chapters in their investigations and in training.

Connie M. Weaver, PhD
Robert P. Heaney, MD

Contents

Contributors

STEVEN A. ABRAMS, MD • *Pediatrics/Children's Nutrition Research Center, Baylor College of Medicine, Houston, TX*

D. LEE ALEKEL, PhD, RD • *Department of Food Science & Human Nutrition, Iowa State University, Ames, IA*

EMMANUEL M. AWUMEY, PhD • *Cardiovascular Disease Research Program, Julius L. Chambers Biomedical/Biotechnology Research Institute, North Carolina Central University, Durham, NC*

CAROL BOUSHEY, PhD, MPH, RD • *Department of Foods and Nutrition, Purdue University, West Lafayette, IN*

RICHARD D. BUKOSKI, PhD • *(deceased) Cardiovascular Disease Research Program, Julius L. Chambers Biomedical/Biotechnology Research Institute, North Carolina Central University, Durham, NC*

BESS DAWSON-HUGHES, MD • *USDA Human Nutrition Research Center on Aging, Tufts University, Boston, MA*

JAMES C. FLEET, PhD • *Department of Foods and Nutrition, Purdue University, West Lafayette, IN*

KELI M. HAWTHORNE, RD • *Pediatrics/Children's Nutrition Research Center, Baylor College of Medicine, Houston, TX*

ROBERT P. HEANEY, MD • *John A. Creighton University Professor, Creighton University, Omaha, NE*

PETER R. HOLT, MD • *Strang Cancer Research Laboratory, Rockefeller University, Professor of Medicine (Emeritus), Columbia University, New York, NY*

HEIDI J. KALKWARF, PhD • *General & Community Pediatrics, Children's Hospital Medical Center, Cincinnati, OH*

ELIZABETH A. KRALL, PhD, MPH • *Health Policy & Health Services Research, Boston University, Goldman School of Dental Medicine, Boston, MA*

ANNE C. LOOKER, PhD • *Division of Health and Nutrition Examination Statistics, Centers for Disease Control and Prevention, National Center for Health Statistics, Hyattsville, MD*

DAVID S. LUDWIG, PhD • *Division of Endocrinology, Children's Hospital, Boston, MA*

OKSANA MATVIENKO, PhD • *Physical Education, Leisure Services, School of Health, University of Northern Iowa, Cedar Falls, IA*

DAVID A. MCCARRON, MD • *Academic Network, Portland, Oregon; Department of Nutrition, University California at Davis, Davis, CA*

LAWRENCE G. RAISZ, MD • *Center for Osteoporosis, Department of Medicine, University of Connecticut Health Center, Farmington, CT*

ZAMZAM K. (FARIBA) ROUGHEAD, PhD, RD • *Novartis Medical Nutrition, St. Louis Park, MN*

BONNY L. SPECKER, PhD • *E.A. Martin Program in Human Nutrition, South Dakota State University, Brookings, SD*

DOROTHY TEEGARDEN, PhD • *Department of Foods and Nutrition, Purdue University, West Lafayette, IN*

MICHAEL G. TORDOFF, PhD • *Monell Chemical Senses Center, Philadelphia, PA*

SUSAN THYS-JACOBS, MD • *Department of Medicine, St. Luke's-Roosevelt Hospital Center, Columbia University, New York, NY*

MATTHEW VUKOVICH, PhD • *Exercise Physiology Laboratory, South Dakota State University, Brookings, SD*

MERYL E. WASTNEY, PhD • *Metabolic Modeling Service, Dalesford, Hamilton, New Zealand*

CONNIE M. WEAVER, PhD • *Department of Foods and Nutrition, Purdue University, West Lafayette, IN*

YONGDONG ZHAO, MD • *Department of Foods and Nutrition, Purdue University, West Lafayette, IN*

1 Introduction

Connie M. Weaver and Robert P. Heaney

Calcium is one of 21 elements known to be essential to humans. It is one of three minerals required in the diet in relatively large quantities and for which a Dietary Reference Intake (DRI) has been established by the Food and Nutrition Board. At this writing, calcium requirements are set as Adequate Intakes (AI) rather than as Recommended Dietary Allowances (RDA). The decision to set an AI rather than an RDA by the 1997 Food and Nutrition Board related more to the use of a new approach for determining optimal calcium intakes than to the stated paucity of data for determining calcium requirements. Calcium is the most studied of the minerals in relationship to human health. In Spring 2004, a Medline search for articles about minerals published between 1994 and 2004 yielded 62,852 articles about calcium. The next most cited minerals were iron (14,963 articles), zinc (10,399 articles), and magnesium (10,097 articles). The most cited common mineral deficiencies in the world are in iron, iodine, and zinc. Yet, more people are further from their recommended intakes for calcium than for any of these minerals. Inadequate calcium intake has such a long latency period before signs of disease are apparent that its association with health is not adequately appreciated. This book covers the functions of calcium, the approaches for determining calcium intakes for optimal health, and the relationship of calcium status to long-studied and newly identified diseases.

Adequate calcium nutrition has such far-reaching impact because of calcium's unique chemistry. Calcium has an intermediate binding affinity. For example, it is not so tightly bound to proteins—as is zinc—that it cannot readily be removed. Thus, it can serve as an on/off switch in cell regulation. It has only one oxidation state so it is not prone to be toxic at high concentrations or to cause tissue damage under various conditions. As part of hydroxyapatite, it forms a material strong enough to support our bodies for many decades, but light enough to allow mobility. Like other minerals, calcium is immutable, and therefore cannot be synthesized or degraded. This is a huge advantage for analysis, even after long-term storage, so long as samples are protected from contamination from extraneous calcium sources.

Calcium is not efficiently absorbed or retained by the body. It can form complexes that are poorly digested. Much of the small fraction that is absorbed is excreted by obligatory losses or is affected by other dietary constituents. Determining bioavailability of calcium and factors that influence the calcium economy is facilitated by the availability of many useful isotopic tracers of calcium.

From: *Calcium in Human Health*
Edited by: C. M. Weaver and R. P. Heaney © Humana Press Inc., Totowa, NJ

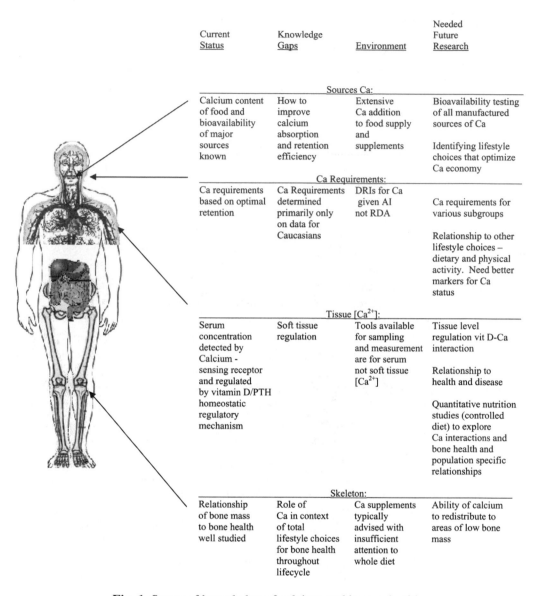

Fig. 1. Status of knowledge of calcium and human health.

Current Status	Knowledge Gaps	Environment	Needed Future Research
Sources Ca:			
Calcium content of food and bioavailability of major sources known	How to improve calcium absorption and retention efficiency	Extensive Ca addition to food supply and supplements	Bioavailability testing of all manufactured sources of Ca Identifying lifestyle choices that optimize Ca economy
Ca Requirements:			
Ca requirements based on optimal retention	Ca Requirements determined primarily only on data for Caucasians	DRIs for Ca given AI not RDA	Ca requirements for various subgroups Relationship to other lifestyle choices – dietary and physical activity. Need better markers for Ca status
Tissue [Ca^{2+}]:			
Serum concentration detected by Calcium - sensing receptor and regulated by vitamin D/PTH homeostatic regulatory mechanism	Soft tissue regulation	Tools available for sampling and measurement are for serum not soft tissue [Ca^{2+}]	Tissue level regulation vit D-Ca interaction Relationship to health and disease Quantitative nutrition studies (controlled diet) to explore Ca interactions and bone health and population specific relationships
Skeleton:			
Relationship of bone mass to bone health well studied	Role of Ca in context of total lifestyle choices for bone health throughout lifecycle	Ca supplements typically advised with insufficient attention to whole diet	Ability of calcium to redistribute to areas of low bone mass

The status of knowledge about calcium and human health is briefly summarized in Fig. 1. Some of the most pressing gaps in our knowledge about calcium and needed research are also included. The interplay of calcium with other environmental factors and its regulation and requirements at the soft-tissue level are the least understood areas, both because they are difficult to measure and because complex research design is required to answer these questions.

Calcium as a nutrient is not useful to health in isolation. For example, utilization of calcium depends on adequate vitamin D status. Dietary sodium greatly influences renal calcium reabsorption. Adequate bone mass requires protein, phosphorus, magnesium, and several trace nutrients as well as nondietary factors including sex steroid hormones and mechanical loading. None of the diseases addressed in this book has as a single etiology calcium deficiency. Nevertheless, it is useful to assemble our knowledge of the broad influence of calcium and its relationship to human health in one book for perspective and convenience.

I   Calcium Functions

2 Bone as the Calcium Nutrient Reserve

Robert P. Heaney

KEY POINTS

- Bone is the body's calcium nutrient reserve.
- This reserve, over the course of evolution, acquired a secondary function—mechanical strength and rigidity—serving to support work against gravity.
- The reserve is added to or drawn upon by net addition or removal of microscopic units of bony tissue, not by simple withdrawal or addition of calcium atoms.
- The size of the reserve is determined by a combination of mechanical loading and net dietary calcium availability.
- Calcium is a threshold nutrient, in that bone mass increases as calcium intake increases up to the point where mechanical needs are met; above that level, no further calcium retention occurs and absorbed calcium is simply excreted.

1. INTRODUCTION

In addition to its obvious structural role, the skeleton is an important reservoir of calcium, serving both to maintain plasma calcium concentrations and to make optimal use of ingested calcium. It serves both functions mainly by adjusting the balance between bone formation (which transfers mineral from blood to bone) and bone resorption (which transfers mineral from bone to blood). It is important to stress at the outset that calcium cannot generally be withdrawn from bone *per se;* instead, it is scavenged from the tearing down of structural bony units. Thus, reduction in skeletal calcium reserves is equivalent to reduction in bone mass, and augmentation of the reserve is equivalent to augmentation of bone mass.

These same processes of formation and resorption are what constitute bone structural remodeling, or turnover. Remodeling of bone continues throughout life, and skeletal tissue is replaced every 10 to 12 yr on average. All bone remodeling occurs at anatomical bone surfaces. Bone-resorbing osteoclasts begin the remodeling process by attaching onto a bone surface, sealing it from the rest of the extracellular fluid (ECF); they then extrude packets of citric, lactic, and carbonic acids to dissolve the bone mineral, and proteolytic enzymes to digest the organic matrix. They thereby remove parcels of bone, leaving behind a cavity, or resorption bay. Later, bone-forming osteoblasts synthesize new bone to fill in the cavity and replace the previously resorbed bone.

From: *Calcium in Human Health*
Edited by: C. M. Weaver and R. P. Heaney © Humana Press Inc., Totowa, NJ

Formation and resorption are coupled both systemically and locally, and when resorption is high, formation is generally high as well. But the coupling is neither continuous nor perfect. Resorption normally exceeds formation during fasting, when no calcium is being absorbed from the intestine, and formation normally exceeds resorption during absorption of calcium from ingested food or supplements. This is how the body adjusts to intermittent intestinal absorptive input. Overall, however, the two processes are about equal when averaged over the day. Continuous net imbalances (i.e., changes in the size of the reserve) do occur in several situations. For example, bone formation exceeds resorption during growth, and resorption exceeds formation during lactation, or in the development of osteoporosis, or in the face of ongoing dietary shortage of calcium.

2. A UNIQUE NUTRIENT

Calcium is a unique nutrient in several respects. It is not the only nutrient with a substantial reserve in healthy individuals, but it is the only one for which the reserve has required an important function in its own right. We use the reserve for structural support (i.e., we literally walk on our calcium nutrient reserve). Calcium is unique also in that our bodies cannot store a continuing surplus, unlike, for example, energy or the fat-soluble vitamins. Calcium is stored not as such but as bone tissue, and the quantity of bone tissue is determined by cellular processes, with the responsible bone cellular apparatus controlled through a feedback loop regulated by mechanical forces, not by calcium intake. In brief, given an adequate calcium intake, we have only as much bone as we need for the mechanical loads we currently experience. Once our skeletons have reached their genetically and mechanically determined mass, unless something intervenes such as pregnancy or pharmacotherapy, we cannot accumulate more bone simply by consuming more calcium.

This feature is the basis for the designation of calcium as a "threshold" nutrient with respect to skeletal status, a term that means that calcium retention rises as intake rises, up to some threshold value that provides optimal bone strength (*see* Fig. 1); then, above that level, increased calcium intake produces no further retention and is simply excreted. This threshold intake is the lowest intake at which retention is maximal, that is, it is the minimum daily requirement (MDR) for skeletal health (*see* Chapter 7). The MDR varies with age, and is currently estimated to be approx 20–25 mmol (800–1000 mg/d) during childhood, 30–40 mmol (1200–1600 mg/d) during adolescence, approx 25 mmol (1000 mg/d) during the mature adult years, and 35–40 mmol (1400–1600 mg/d) in the elderly *(2–4)*. As previously noted, the rise in the published requirement in old age reflects an age-related decline in ability to adapt (i.e., to respond to low intakes with improved absorption and retention).

Calcium is unique in another respect related precisely to the reserve function of the skeleton. The best-attested disease manifestation of calcium deficiency (osteoporosis) is due not to impairment of the metabolic functions of calcium (*see* Chapter 3), which would be the case, for example, with the B vitamins, but instead to a decrease in the size of the reserve. For no other nutrient is this the case. Bone strength is a function of bone mass which, in turn, is equivalent to the size of the calcium nutrient reserve. This reserve is vast relative to the demands of calcium for cell signaling and activation, particularly because these metabolic functions do not actually consume calcium. Hence, nutritional calcium deficiency almost never manifests itself as a shortage of calcium ions in critical cellular or physiological processes. With most other nutrients, the reserve must first be exhausted

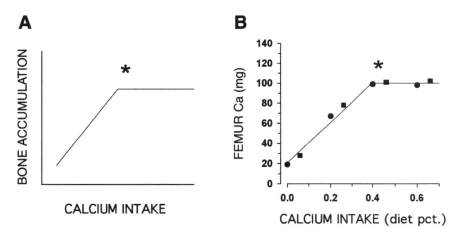

Fig. 1. Threshold behavior of calcium intake. (**A**) Theoretical relationship of bone accumulation to intake. Below a certain value (the threshold, indicated by an asterisk), bone accumulation is a linear function of intake (the ascending line); in other words, the amount of bone that can be accumulated is limited by the amount of calcium ingested. Above the threshold (the horizontal line), bone accumulation is limited by other factors and is no longer related to changes in calcium intake. (**B**) Actual data from two experiments in growing rats showing how bone accumulation does, in fact, exhibit a threshold pattern. (Redrawn from data in Forbes et al. *[1]*. Copyright Robert P. Heaney, 1992. Used with permission.)

before clear manifestations of disease or dysfunction develop. But for calcium, it is the simple reduction in skeletal mass that reduces bone strength and accordingly increases fracture risk. In brief, calcium intake insufficient to offset obligatory losses leads to reduction in bone mass, and is thus one of the causes of osteoporosis.

When excretory and dermal losses exceed absorbed dietary intake, the mechanisms designed to protect ECF $[Ca^{2+}]$ tear down bone to scavenge its calcium. The mechanisms by which the reserves are accessed or augmented are set forth in detail in Chapter 10. Here we note only that parathyroid hormone (PTH) is evoked by a fall in calcium intake. At the same time, PTH is responsible for regulating the prevailing level of bone remodeling. PTH activates remodeling loci, which proceed through an orderly sequence of events consisting of (1) activation, which is manifested morphologically as retraction of lining cells from the bone surface about to undergo remodeling; (2) resorption of bone by osteoclasts; (3) replacement of the osteoclasts by osteoblasts, which lay down new bone to fill the hole created by osteoclastic resorption; and (4) return to the resting state, with the bone surface once again covered by a sheet of lining cells. The destructive, resorptive phase typically takes 3 wk in healthy adults, and the formative, reconstructive phase takes 3–6 mo.

Millions of such remodeling loci, each at different stages of this process, are going through this sequence at any time in the skeleton as a whole, some adding calcium to the blood, and some taking it up into new bone. An acute increase in remodeling activity initially creates an excess of resorption (because the new loci are all in the initial resorptive phase of the cycle). In this way, an increase in remodeling allows bone to contribute calcium to the blood. Conversely, an acute decrease in remodeling initially creates a temporary excess of formation. These imbalances are how the bone accommodates a relative surplus or shortfall of absorbed calcium, hour by hour and day by day.

In providing the calcium needed to maintain critical body fluid concentrations, the reserve is functioning precisely as it should. But sooner or later there has to be payback, or the reserve becomes depleted, with an inescapable weakening of skeletal structures. During growth, on any but the most severely restricted of intakes, some bony accumulation will usually occur, but the result of an insufficient calcium intake is usually failure to achieve the full genetic potential for bone mass. Later in life, the result is failure to maintain the mass achieved. As also noted in Chapter 24, both low bone mass and osteoporotic fractures have many causes other than low calcium intake. Nevertheless, under prevailing conditions in the industrialized nations, at mid-to-high latitudes, the importance of calcium intake is considerable. Calcium-supplementation trials, even those of short duration, have resulted in reductions in fracture in the elderly amounting to 30% or more *(5,6)*.

3. EVIDENCE LINKING CALCIUM INTAKE TO BONE HEALTH

In addition to a large effect size, the evidence for calcium's role is itself very strong. There have been roughly 80 published reports of investigator-controlled increases in calcium intake with skeletal endpoints, most of them randomized, controlled trials and most of them published since 1990 *(7)*. The vast majority demonstrated either greater bone mass gain during growth, reduced bone loss with age, and/or reduced osteoporotic fractures. The exceptions among these studies were, for example, a supplementation trial in men in which the calcium intake of the control group was itself already high (nearly 1200 mg/d) *(8)*, and a study confined to early postmenopausal women *(9)* in whom bone loss is known to be due predominantly to estrogen deficiency.

Complementing this primary evidence are roughly 130 observational studies testing the association of calcium intake with bone mass, bone loss, or fracture *(7)*. It has been shown elsewhere *(10)* that such observational studies are inherently weak, not only for the generally recognized reason that uncontrolled or unrecognized factors may produce or obscure associations between the variables of interest, but because the principal variable in this case, lifetime calcium intake, cannot be directly measured and must be estimated by dietary recall methods. The errors of such estimates are immense and have been abundantly documented *(11,12; see also* Chapter 4). Their effect is to bias all such investigations toward the null. Nevertheless, more than three-fourths of these observational studies reported a significant calcium benefit. Given the insensitivity of the method, the fact that most of these reports are positive emphasizes the strength of the association; at the same time, it provides reassurance that the effects achievable in the artificial context of a clinical trial can be observed in real-world settings as well.

4. CALCIUM INTAKE, BONE REMODELING, AND SKELETAL FRAGILITY

These observations show clearly that variations in calcium intake in the range commonly encountered in the industrialized nations have substantial influences on the osteoporotic fracture burden (when intakes are low) or protect against fracture (when intakes are high). The most obvious explanation is the effect of calcium intake on opti-

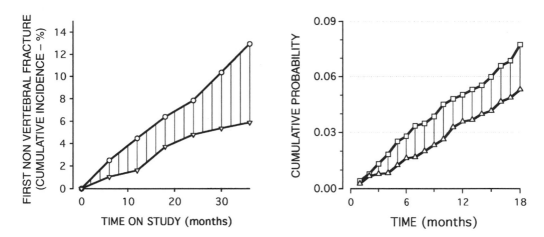

Fig. 2. Plots of the cumulative incidence of fractures, redrawn from the studies of Chapuy et al. *(5)* (right) and Dawson-Hughes et al. *(6)* (left). In both cases, the upper line represents the placebo control subjects, and the lower line represents the calcium and vitamin D-treated subjects. The shaded zones represent the reduction of fracture risk, which, as can be readily seen, starts with the very beginning of treatment. (Copyright Robert P. Heaney, 2004. Used with permission.)

mizing the size of the calcium reserve. But it is likely that there is a second aspect of the reserve involved in bony fragility as well. Examination of the cumulative fracture plots of the calcium intervention trials of Chapuy et al. *(5)* and Dawson-Hughes et al. *(6)* shows that the reduction in fracture risk begins almost immediately after supplementation is started—too soon for there to have been an appreciable effect on bone mass (Fig. 2).

Recent appreciation of the role of bone quality , as distinct from bone quantity , has led to an understanding of the fact that remodeling loci themselves directly contribute to fragility *(13)*, independently of bone mass. Remodeling rate doubles through menopause and continues to rise throughout the remainder of life *(14)*, in part because of inadequate calcium and vitamin D intakes. The immediate effect of calcium and/or vitamin D supplementation in typical postmenopausal women is a reduction of PTH secretion and with it, a corresponding and immediate reduction of bone remodeling. As the data assembled in Fig. 2 show, there is an immediate reduction in bony fragility as well. In brief, not only does low calcium intake contribute to bony fragility by depleting the reserve, but the very process of accessing the reserve itself renders bone fragile. Slowing that process confers an immediate benefit.

Several factors influence the size of the calcium reserve by direct action on bone (rather than by way of the calcium economy). Among these are smoking, alcohol abuse, hormonal status, body weight, exercise, and various medications. Smoking and alcohol abuse exert slow, cumulative effects by uncertain mechanisms that result in reduced bone mass and increased fracture risk. Low estrogen status and hyperthyroidism produce similar net effects, although probably by very different mechanisms. Bone mass rises directly with body weight, again by uncertain mechanisms. Exercise, particularly impact loading, is osteotrophic and is important both for building optimal bone mass during growth and for maintaining it during maturity and senescence.

5. CONCLUSIONS

The body possesses reserve supplies of most nutrients, which it uses to ensure smooth functioning in the face of irregular nutrient intake. Bone is the body's calcium reserve. This reserve is larger than for any other nutrient mainly because it has acquired a secondary, nonnutrient role—internal stiffening and mechanical support of our bodies. The size of the bony reserve is limited at its upper bound by mechanical need, and below that, by net calcium intake. Because the reserve is large, nutritional calcium deficiency virtually never compromises the basic metabolic functions of calcium. Rather, by depleting the reserve, the body weakens bone and jeopardizes its mechanical function. As a consequence and unlike with most other nutrients, reduction in the size of the nutrient reserve has immediate health consequences.

REFERENCES

1. Forbes RM, Weingartner KE, Parker HM, Bell RR, Erdman JW Jr. Bioavailability to rats of zinc, magnesium and calcium in casein-, egg- and soy protein-containing diets. J Nutr 1979;109:1652–1660.
2. NIH Consensus Conference: Optimal Calcium Intake. J Am Med Assoc 1994;272:1942–1948.
3. Dietary Reference Intakes for Calcium, Magnesium, Phosphorus, Vitamin D, and Fluoride. Food and Nutrition Board, Institute of Medicine, National Academy Press, Washington, DC: 1997.
4. Matkovic V, Heaney RP. Calcium balance during human growth. Evidence for threshold behavior. Am J Clin Nutr 1992;55:992–996.
5. Chapuy MC, Arlot ME, Duboeuf F, et al. Vitamin D_3 and calcium to prevent hip fractures in elderly women. N Engl J Med 1992;327:1637–1642.
6. Dawson-Hughes B, Harris SS, Krall EA, Dallal GE. Effect of calcium and vitamin D supplementation on bone density in men and women 65 years of age or older. N Engl J Med 1997;337:670–676.
7. Heaney RP. Calcium, dairy products, and osteoporosis. J Am Coll Nutr 1999;19(2):83S–99S.
8. Orwoll ES, Oviatt SK, McClung MR, Deftos LJ, Sexton G. The rate of bone mineral loss in normal men and the effects of calcium and cholecalciferol supplementation. Ann Int Med 1990;112:29–34.
9. Nilas L, Christiansen C, Rødbro P. Calcium supplementation and postmenopausal bone loss. BMJ 1984;289:1103–1106.
10. Heaney RP. Nutrient effects: Discrepancy between data from controlled trials and observational studies. Bone 1997;21:469-471.
11. Barrett-Connor E. Diet assessment and analysis for epidemiologic studies of osteoporosis, In: Burckhardt P, Heaney RP, eds. Nutritional Aspects of Osteoporosis. Raven, New York, NY: 1991;91–98.
12. Beaton GH, Milner J, Corey P, McGuire V, Cousins M, Stewart E, et al. Sources of variance in 24-hour dietary recall data: implications for nutrition study design and interpretation. Am J Clin Nutr 1979;32:2446–2459
13. Heaney RP. Is the paradigm shifting? Bone 2003;33:457–465.
14. Recker RR, Lappe JM, Davies KM, Heaney RP. Bone remodeling increases substantially in the years after menopause and remains increased in older osteoporosis patients. J Bone Miner Res 2004;19:1628–1633.

3 Cellular Functions and Fluxes of Calcium

Emmanuel M. Awumey and Richard D. Bukoski*

KEY POINTS

- Ionized calcium is an important signaling ion, and its cellular concentration is regulated by the intestine, kidney, bone, and the placenta (during pregnancy).
- The concentrations of Ca^{2+} in extracellular spaces and intracellular compartments are regulated by hormones and through membrane proteins that facilitate transient changes in cellular Ca^{2+} that are vital to cell function.
- Voltage-dependent channels, receptor-operated channels (many coupled to G proteins), and a myriad of transport proteins, all operating by different influx/efflux mechanisms, regulate intracellular Ca^{2+} levels.
- Perturbations in these Ca^{2+} influx/efflux mechanisms lead to various disease states.

1. INTRODUCTION

The divalent cation, or ionized, calcium—Ca^{2+}—is a mineral that is critical to normal human health, playing vital roles in fertilization, metabolism, blood clotting, nerve impulse conduction, muscle contraction, structure of the bony skeleton, and cellular communication. As covered in detail in Chapter 9, the primary dietary sources of calcium in contemporary diets are dairy products and to a lesser extent, leafy green vegetables. Dietary recommendations for calcium vary with age and pregnancy, as discussed in Chapter 8. When considering dietary sources, it is important to recognize the fact that ionized calcium is the biologically active form of the mineral and that bioavailability of calcium varies among different food groups.

Ionized calcium translates external signals into internal signals in the cell, a function facilitated by its small size and its affinity for protein molecules. The Ca^{2+} signal is translated by Ca^{2+}–protein interaction within the secondary and tertiary structure of the peptide. Ca^{2+} is much more suitable as a signaling ion than other prevailing ionic species because of the size of its ionic radius, which is smaller than that of potassium ions (K^+)

*Deceased

From: *Calcium in Human Health*
Edited by: C. M. Weaver and R. P. Heaney © Humana Press Inc., Totowa, NJ

and chloride ions (Cl⁻) but larger than that of magnesium ions (Mg^{2+}) and small enough to fit into intracellular pores, whereas that of sodium ions (Na^+) is too small. In addition to this property, the two positive charges on the Ca^{2+} ion and a coordination number of 6–8 make Ca more flexible in interacting with the polypeptide structure, without constraint, to effect conformational changes necessary for signal transduction.

Cell activity is coordinated and controlled by a variety of signaling mechanisms, many or all of which involve the release of Ca^{2+} from critical intracellular compartments into the cytoplasm.

Furthermore, because the mean path length of Ca^{2+} entering through the plasma membrane is only a fraction of the cell diameter, it has been necessary for cells to evolve an elaborate intracellular calcium storage mechanism, which is activated to release Ca^{2+} into the cytosol in response to appropriate signals. For example, during striated muscle contraction, the initial trigger Ca^{2+} enters the cell from the extracellular space as a result of membrane depolarization. This activates intracellular Ca^{2+} release from internal storage sites into the myoplasm and its subsequent binding to regulatory sites to initiate crossbridge formation. Relaxation follows when Ca^{2+} is removed from the myoplasm.

In view of the critical role that Ca^{2+} plays in the normal health and function of all cells, it is therefore not surprising that elaborate regulatory mechanisms for the transport and storage of Ca^{2+} have evolved at the whole-body and cellular levels. Failure of some or all of these regulatory mechanisms can lead to significant changes in the level of circulating Ca^{2+} that, in some instances, will not be compatible with life.

From this overview, it should be apparent that Ca^{2+} is a critical ion for the maintenance of life. Not surprisingly, elaborate and highly complex mechanisms are involved in maintaining its level within narrow limits in the cell (Fig.1). Calcium homeostasis is complex because it involves the gastrointestinal (GI) tract, kidney, and bones. It is our goal to review these systems with primary emphasis on cellular Ca^{2+} regulation. Where possible, we provide examples of syndromes that are associated with disturbances in Ca^{2+} fluxes.

2. FUNCTIONS OF Ca^{2+} IN CELLS

Activation of excitable cells results in Ca^{2+} influx from extracellular space through voltage-dependent and/or receptor-operated Ca^{2+} channels in the plasma membrane and release from intracellular storage sites to raise the cytosolic Ca^{2+} concentration from nM to μM levels. To return the Ca^{2+} concentration to resting levels, ATP-driven Ca^{2+} transport to the extracellular space and into intracellular stores occurs (1). Ca^{2+} is the main point of intersection for many distinct molecular signaling pathways and in living organisms plays a dual role, both as an ion required for cell survival and as an inducer of cell death. The presence of excess Ca^{2+} in the cytosol or perturbation of intracellular Ca^{2+} compartmentalization leads to Ca^{2+} overload, which triggers apoptotic or necrotic cell death (2). Changes in intracellular Ca^{2+} concentrations are accomplished through modulation of Ca^{2+} influx channels, Ca^{2+} exchange proteins, and various Ca^{2+}-dependent enzymes (3). The loss of regulatory ability of any of these Ca^{2+} influx/efflux mechanisms and the consequent increase in intracellular Ca^{2+} concentration ($[Ca^{2+}]_i$) leads to a wide variety of pathological events such as brain trauma, stroke, and heart failure.

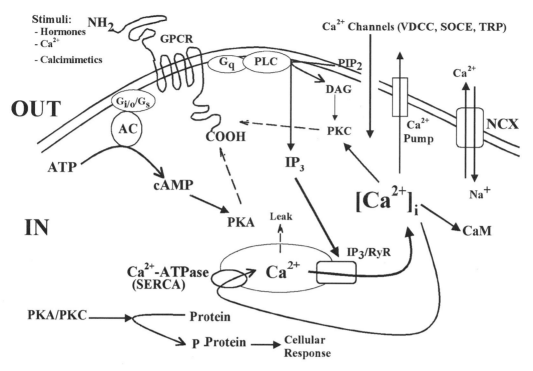

Fig. 1. Cellular Ca^{2+} signal transduction. AC, adenylyl cyclase; ATP, adenosine triphosphate; cAMP, cyclic adenosine monophosphate; Ca^{2+} pump, plasma membrane Ca^{2+}-ATPase; DAG, diacyl glycerol; GPCR, G protein-coupled receptor; $G_{i/o}$, $G\alpha_{i/o}$ G protein subunit; G_q, $G\alpha_q$ G protein subunit; G_s, $G\alpha_s$ G protein subunit; IP$_3$, inositol 1,4,5-trisphosphate; IP$_3$R, inositol 1,4,5-trisphosphate receptor; NCX, sodium-calcium exchanger; PIP$_2$, phosphotidyl-inositol 4,5-bisphosphate; PKA, protein kinase A; PKC, protein kinase C; PLC, phospholipase C; P-protein, phosphorylated protein; RyR, ryanodine receptor; SERCA, sarcoplasmic/endoplasmic reticulum Ca^{2+}-ATPase; SOCE, store-operated Ca^{2+} entry; TRP, transient receptor potential; VDCC, voltage-dependent Ca^{2+} channel.

In nonexcitable cells, changes in [Ca^{2+}]$_i$ are initiated by cellular responses to hormones and growth factors that act through the hydrolysis of membrane-bound inositol phospholipid and that are mediated by at least two second messengers, namely diacyl glycerol (DAG), which activates protein kinase C (PKC), and inositol 1,4,5-trisphosphate (IP$_3$), which binds to the inositol 1,4,5-trisphosphate receptor (IP$_3$R) in the endoplasmic reticulum (ER) membrane to release Ca^{2+} into the cytosol *(4)*. The interaction of cells with their environment occurs through interdependent signals that are mediated by receptors in the plasma membrane, and activation of these receptors by their ligands leads to conformational changes and the transmission of signals across the membrane to trigger a cascade of events in the cell that result in alteration of its function. An increase in the concentration of intracellular Ca^{2+} initiates diffusion, waves, or oscillations of Ca^{2+} that propagate in the nucleus to affect gene transcription or are sequestered by the ER or mitochondria *(5–8)*. These events are regulated by the interplay of multiple counteracting processes in the cell.

3. REGULATION OF CELLULAR Ca^{2+}

Normal [Ca^{2+}]$_i$ is maintained between 20 and 100 nM, relative to the extracellular space calcium concentration ([Ca^{2+}]$_e$) of approx 1.3 mM. In addition to free cytosolic Ca^{2+}, there are storage sites in the cell that can hold Ca^{2+} at a concentration between 10 and 20 mM Ca^{2+} *(9)*. Thus, there are steep Ca^{2+} gradients across the plasma membrane from the interstitial space to the cytoplasm, and across intracellular membranes from storage sites. The main cellular storage sites for Ca^{2+} are the sarcoplasmic reticulum (SR), ER, and mitochondria. As a result of these separate compartments and the fact that [Ca^{2+}]$_i$ can rise to μM levels, systems are in place to regulate it within narrow limits so as to protect the cell from Ca^{2+} overload and subsequent cell death. To achieve this purpose, receptors, transporters, and channels in the cell membrane play important roles. Ca^{2+} movement from the cell to the extracellular space occurs against a Ca^{2+} gradient of 20–100 nM (inside) and 1.3 mM (outside) and is mediated by a Ca^{2+} pump (Ca^{2+}-ATPase) and a Na$^+$/Ca^{2+} exchanger (NCX). The Ca^{2+}-ATPase plays a major role, and the NCX a minor role, in regulating cellular Ca^{2+} fluxes. The Ca^{2+}-ATPase uses ATP to pump Ca^{2+} out of the cell or into ER/SR against concentration and electrical gradients. Many of these Ca^{2+} transport proteins are influenced by 1,25(OH)$_2$D$_3$, which regulates the transcription of genes that code for these proteins.

3.1. Calcium Influx Pathways

Calcium enters the cell from the interstitial space mainly via voltage-dependent or receptor-operated Ca^{2+} channels in the plasma membrane. There are several of these Ca^{2+} entry pathways in mammalian cells, and their characteristics and functions may vary from tissue to tissue. In addition, intracellular Ca^{2+} pumps in organelles rapidly sequester Ca^{2+}, thus restricting its diffusion internally unless it is required. The three main types of Ca^{2+} channels that have been extensively described are voltage-dependent calcium channels (VDCC) *(10)*, receptor-operated calcium channels (ROCC) *(11)*, and store-operated calcium entry (SOCE) or capacitative calcium entry (CCE) channels *(12)*. The CCE mechanism is a very important influx pathway in nonexcitable cells; however, its role in the function of neuronal cells has also been reported *(13)* and may be implicated in some neuropathological conditions *(14–16)*. In addition to these channels, the Ca^{2+}-sensing receptor (CaSR) *(17)* and transient receptor protein (TRP) channels *(18)* also constitute significant Ca^{2+} entry pathways, albeit operating to mediate influx by different mechanisms.

3.1.1. Voltage-Dependent Calcium Channels

VDCC are employed largely by excitable cells (muscle and neurons) to move Ca^{2+} from the extracellular space into the cell. They often exist as multiple isoforms, with tissue-specific expression and different gating characteristics, and are activated by the depolarization of the plasma membrane. Different types of VDCCs have been identified in mammalian tissues and have been shown to mediate specialized cellular functions *(19)*. The voltage-dependent Ca^{2+} channels are important therapeutic targets because of their specific characteristics. The two main types, found in the cardiovascular system, are the L and T type channels, which have distinct electrophysiological properties and may have distinct roles in this tissue. In cardiac and smooth muscle cells, VDCC control excitation–contraction coupling. The L-type Ca^{2+} channel is the best known and characterized among the high voltage-activated calcium channels. It is distinguishable from other voltage-dependent Ca^{2+} channels by its sensitivity to 1,4-dihydropyridine compounds such as nifedipine *(20–22)*. The T-type Ca^{2+} channels, which are also expressed in the cardiovascular system, are prominent in conducting and pacemaking cells but are not normally present in adult myocardium. Although very little is known about the T-type Ca^{2+} channels because of the lack of pharmacological tools for their study, the recent discovery of a selective blocker of this channel with important cardiovascular actions indicates that it, too, may become a useful therapeutic target *(23–25)*. These channels are thought to regulate vascular tone, signal conduction, cardiac pacemaking, and the secretion of certain intercellular transmitters and to play an important role in the tissue remodeling that occurs in pathological processes such as cardiac hypertrophy *(26–28)*. Thus, the availability of novel antagonists that selectively block T-type Ca^{2+} channels will facilitate their future characterization. In recent times, neuron-specific calcium channels have been the subject of intense research and a number of agents that are selective for these channels are being investigated for their potential in the therapy of chronic neuropathic pain *(29)*. These channels are large-conductance, Ca^{2+}-activated potassium channels, which play a major role in the regulation of spike waveform and the temporal pattern of repetitive spike discharge that are important in mature neural circuits *(30)*.

Both type 1 and type 2 diabetes mellitus are associated with disturbances in the regulation of $[Ca^{2+}]_i$. Hyperglycemia leads to acute increases in $[Ca^{2+}]_i$ as a result of influx and release from internal storage sites, secondary to activation of dihydropyridine-sensitive Ca^{2+} channels *(31)*. Spontaneous mutations of VDCC in skeletal muscles lead to malignant hyperthermia and familial hypokalemic periodic paralysis.

3.1.2. RECEPTOR-OPERATED CALCIUM CHANNELS

Receptor-operated Ca^{2+} channels are structurally and functionally diverse and are prevalent on secretory cells and nerve terminals. The nicotinic acetylcholine and *N*-methyl- D-aspartate (NMDA) receptors are classic examples of receptor-operated Ca^{2+} channels. They are activated by agonist binding to the extracellular domain of the channel. In smooth muscles, Ca^{2+} required for contraction comes from both intracellular release from ER and extracellular entry via several ROCC *(32)*. Several hormones and neurotransmitters activate nonselective Ca^{2+} channels in various tissues *(33,34)*. These entry pathways are dependent on activation of pertussis toxin-sensitive, G protein-coupled receptors (GPCRs) and therefore can be considered ROCCs *(35)*. In a human neuroblastoma cell line, carbachol-stimulated Ca^{2+} entry was shown to be mediated by a receptor-operated Ca^{2+} channel that was dependent on IP_3-induced Ca^{2+} release *(36)*; however, in glomerular mesangial cells, it was mediated by epidermal growth factor-activated, SOCE through an IP_3-independent, phospholipase C (PLC)-dependent pathway *(37)*, indicating tissue-specific mechanism of activation of these receptors. In the myocardium, a number of receptor-mediated signaling pathways are activated through PLC and phospholipase D (PLD) *(38)*.

3.1.3. STORE-OPERATED CALCIUM ENTRY CHANNELS

The release of Ca^{2+} from intracellular stores in nonexcitable cells activates Ca^{2+} entry via channels in the plasma membrane, a process known as SOCE or CCE *(12)*. The channels are activated in response to depletion of intracellular Ca^{2+} stores as a result of physiological Ca^{2+} mobilization or by the action of pharmacological agents such as thapsigargin *(39–41)*. Although the precise mechanism of this entry process is the subject of rigorous research in many laboratories, there is a consensus that it involves conformational coupling between Ca^{2+} entry channels in the plasma membrane and Ca^{2+} release channels in the ER membrane *(42)*. It has been proposed that a diffusible calcium influx factor messenger is synthesized by depleted Ca^{2+} stores and that this activates Ca^{2+} entry channels in the plasma membrane. The store-operated Ca^{2+} channels are ubiquitous, having been demonstrated in many different cell types. The electrophysiological characteristics of these channels differ from cell to cell, giving rise to the demonstration of different types of this channel. Although the molecular identity of the channel has not been established unequivocally, TRP proteins have been implicated *(43)*.

Presenilin-1 is one of the genes implicated in the etiology of early-onset autosomal-dominant or familial-onset Alzheimer's disease *(14)*. Mutant *presenilin-1* deregulates neuronal Ca^{2+} homeostasis by direct attenuation of CCE at the cell surface independent of amyloid precursor protein (APP), and by an indirect increase of ER Ca^{2+} stores via processing of APP and generation of amyloid peptides and C-terminal (C99) fragments of APP.

3.1.4. Ca^{2+}-Sensing Receptor-Mediated Ca^{2+} Entry

The CaSR is a seven-transmembrane GPCR that binds Ca^{2+} at the extracellular domain and transduces the signal through cAMP and phospholipases (PLC, PLD, or PLA) depending on the cell type *(17)*. Activation of PLC leads to IP_3 production and release of stored intracellular Ca^{2+} from ER, thus transiently raising the cytoplasmic Ca^{2+} concentration following activation of IP_3R in the ER membrane. Reduction in $[Ca^{2+}]_i$ is rapidly achieved by Ca^{2+} pumps located in the ER and plasma membranes. However, the released Ca^{2+} also opens plasma membrane SOCE or CCE channels that allow influx of Ca^{2+}, resulting in a sustained plateau *(44–47)* or periodic oscillations of $[Ca^{2+}]_i$ that regulate cytosolic as well as nuclear functions of the cell *(4,48)*. A diverse array of signaling mechanisms is implicated in these events, which are linked to membrane channels; however, the molecular mechanisms of these Ca^{2+} signaling pathways are not clear. Studies have shown that stimulation of the CaSR with $[Ca^{2+}]_e$ produces oscillations in $[Ca^{2+}]_i$, the pattern and frequency of which play a key role in signal transduction; but there are conflicting views on the mechanisms involved.

The generally accepted model is based on the negative feedback effects of PKC on the production of IP_3 or on the regulatory properties of $[Ca^{2+}]_i$ on the IP_3R *(49–51)*. Young et al. *(52)* have suggested that negative feedback by PKC could play a role in the generation of $[Ca^{2+}]_e$-evoked $[Ca^{2+}]_i$ oscillations via the CaSR, contradicting the study by Breitwieser and Gama *(8)*, which concluded that the activity of a variety of protein kinases, including PKC, do not influence the pattern of $[Ca^{2+}]_i$ oscillations elicited by activation of the human parathyroid (hPTH) CaSR by Ca^{2+}. It is therefore clear from these reports that the mechanisms of the CaSR-mediated $[Ca^{2+}]_i$ oscillations are yet to be resolved. The CaSR couples, through the intracellular loops and carboxyl terminal chain, to multiple G proteins that mediate its biological actions, and three modes of coupling have been reported: namely, through $G\alpha_i$ to inhibition of adenylate cyclase (AC) and activation of ERK1/2; through $G\alpha_q$ to stimulation of PLC and PLA_2; and through $G\beta\gamma$ to stimulation of PI3-kinase *(53)*. However, $G\beta\gamma$ is also known to activate $PLC\beta$ isoforms, and the expression profile of these isoforms in cells may dictate the ability of the Gβγ to mediate PI and Ca^{2+} signaling. Phosphorylation of PLCβ by PKA and PKC plays an important role in the regulation of this isoform and provides part of a well-recognized negative feedback loop.

It is clear that many GPCRs can simultaneously initiate multiple second messenger pathways by coupling to more than one Gα subunit and influencing the functional properties of Gβγ *(54–56)*. In studies on the human β$_2$-adrenergic receptor, which mediates increases in $[Ca^{2+}]_i$ via cAMP, site-specific mutagenesis indicated that low concentrations of agonist induced receptor phosphorylation at PKA sites, whereas higher concentrations induced phosphorylation at PKC and GPCR kinase (GRK) sites *(57–58)*. Evidence from studies on the metabotropic glutamate receptor (mGluR) indicates that the receptor is regulated by agonist-induced, PKC-dependent feedback inhibition of the IP$_3$ pathway and the agonist-independent, PKA-dependent pathway, which potentiates IP$_3$ signaling *(59)*. Thus, GPCR activation can lead to functional integration of an intricate network of intracellular signaling pathways as well as stimulation of effectors completely independent of G proteins. Calcium mobilization from intracellular stores triggers events that lead to secretion, contraction, and energy generation in the short term and the regulation of proliferation, differentiation, apoptosis, and gene transcription in the long term *(17)*.

Mutations in the hPTH Ca^{2+}-sensing receptor have been linked to disorders of Ca^{2+} homeostasis due to alterations in the set point of parathyroid hormone (PTH) secretion and control of renal Ca^{2+} excretion. Inactivating mutations in the CaSR gene cause familial hypocalciuric hypercalcemia (FHH) and neonatal severe hyperparathyroidism (NSHPT), and activating mutations cause a form of autosomal dominant hypocalcemia *(60–63)*.

3.1.5. TRANSIENT RECEPTOR PROTEIN CHANNELS

TRPs were originally named for the Drosophila transient receptor potential mutant *(64)*, and since the identification of mammalian TRPs, a family of homologs and splice variants has been described *(65,66)*. The mammalian TRPs (also known as TRPCs) belong to the short TRP family of which seven (TRPs 1–7) have been described *(67)*. TRP1 and TRP3 are the most widely studied mammalian TRPs and have been implicated in the mediation of store-depleted Ca^{2+} entry in nonexcitable cells *(68,69)*. As previously discussed, activation of PLC leads to IP$_3$ production and release of stored Ca^{2+} following activation of IP$_3$R in the ER membrane, and a subsequent influx of Ca^{2+} resulting in a sustained plateau *(45,46)* or periodic oscillations of $[Ca^{2+}]_i$ that regulate cytosolic as well as nuclear functions of the cell *(4,48)*.

The identity of the Ca^{2+} entry channels remains a key question, as does the mechanism by which they are activated. Several studies have indicated that SOCE is associated with TRPs, and various lines of evidence support the hypothesis that TRPs can, in certain circumstances, form part of a store-operated, Ca^{2+}-permeable channel in mammalian cells *(43,68)*; but much confusion still exists as to whether SOCE channels are TRP channels, and vigorous investigation is being carried out in many laboratories to definitively identify store-depletion-activated Ca^{2+} channels as TRP channels. Other studies suggest that expression of the hTRP3 in human embryonic kidney (HEK)293 cells forms a nonselective cation channel that opens after activation of PLC but not after store depletion, indicating that TRP3 may be linked to endogenous proteins to form channels that are sensitive to store depletion *(68)*. There is overlap between store-operated and receptor-operated Ca^{2+} entry because the latter is potentiated by the activation of the former, suggesting that both may belong to the same family of mammalian TRP proteins.

3.2. Calcium Release and Reuptake From Internal Storage Sites

The release of Ca^{2+} from intracellular stores is mediated by distinct messenger-activated channels such as the IP_3R and the ryanodine receptor (RyR). These channels provide most of the signal Ca^{2+} in cells *(70)*. The trigger for release is the binding of ligands, such as hormones and growth factors, to specific receptors in the plasma membrane, resulting in the opening of integral Ca^{2+} channels in the ER membrane. Many of these receptors are coupled to G proteins that are linked to PLC activation to cause the release of Ca^{2+} from ER. Stimulation of one type of GPCR can be influenced by the stimulation of a different type, a phenomenon known as cross-talk *(71)*. These interactions may be important in the control of cell function; however, there is no unifying mechanism to explain the many examples of cross-talk among GPCRs that contribute to the control of intracellular Ca^{2+} release. A number of studies indicate that there is direct modulation of PLC activity via $G\beta\gamma$ *(72–74)*; however, regulation of phosphatidylinositol-4,5-bisphosphate (PIP_2) supply *(75–77)* and sensitization of IP_3Rs *(78,79)*, among other processes, have been suggested to play significant roles in these mechanisms.

Reuptake of Ca^{2+} from the cytosol is facilitated mainly by sarcoplasmic/endoplasmic reticulum Ca^{2+}-ATPase (SERCA) pump. Thus, both the IP_3Rs and RyRs are coupled to extracellular signals *(80)*. Studies employing vascular myocytes indicate that activation of IP_3Rs coupled to RyRs releases large quantities of Ca^{2+}, which causes salutatory propagation of $[Ca^{2+}]_i$ waves *(81,82)*. Both the IP_3R and the RyR display considerable amino acid sequence homology and similar channel-opening characteristics *(83–85)*. These systems are controlled by negative feedback mechanisms, which ensure that just enough Ca^{2+} is released to give a meaningful signal, yet avoid Ca^{2+} overload and cytotoxicity.

3.2.1. THE IP_3R

There are at least three isoforms of IP_3Rs, which are coded by different genes and have different characteristics, functions, and tissue distribution patterns *(86–90)*. The IP_3R is activated by the second messenger, IP_3 produced from the hydrolysis of membrane PIP_2, following activation of PLC through GPCRs (91,92). The released IP_3 then binds to the IP_3R in the ER membrane to produce conformational change in the receptor, which leads to the opening of the integral channel allowing Ca^{2+}, at high concentration in the store, to move into the cytoplasm. The opening of the channel is regulated by changes in the cytosolic Ca^{2+} concentration, with modest increases (0.5–1.0 μM) enhancing release, and large increases (>1 μM) leading to inhibition and generation of complex patterns such as waves, sparks, and oscillations *(4,93)*.

Oscillations are spontaneous changes in bulk intracellular Ca^{2+} concentrations, resulting from cycles of release and reuptake of stored Ca^{2+}; they are regulated either by protein kinases or phospholipases *(94–96)*. Intracellular Ca^{2+} oscillations play important roles in cellular signaling to the nucleus. In B lymphocytes, the amplitude and duration of Ca^{2+} oscillations have been shown to control differential activation of the pro-inflammatory transcriptional regulators nuclear factor (NF)κB, c-Jun-N-terminal kinase (JNK), and

NF of activated T-cells (NFAT), which are Ca^{2+}-dependent. Downstream effectors in these pathways can decode information contained in the oscillations, revealing a mechanism by which multifunctional second messengers such as Ca^{2+} can achieve specificity in signaling to the nucleus. Multiple sparks summate to form Ca^{2+} waves in cardiac and skeletal muscles, which propagate along the tissue. Spontaneous mutations in the IP_3R in the central nervous system are linked to Alzheimer's disease *(31)*.

3.2.2. THE RYANODINE RECEPTOR

The RyR is structurally and functionally analogous to the IP_3R, with twice the conductance and molecular mass of the latter. It has a high affinity for the plant alkaloid ryanodine, from which it derives its name. The Ca^{2+} sensitivity of the receptor is between 1 and $10\,\mu M$, and concentrations greater than $10\,\mu M$ inhibit it. Thus, ryanodine acts both as an agonist and an antagonist at the receptor. The receptor also interacts with multiple exogenous ligands such as toxins, xanthines, and anthroquinones *(97)*. Therefore, the receptor constitutes a rich and important pharmacological target for modulating cellular functions because of its role in regulating intracellular Ca^{2+} concentrations and its ability to bind multiple ligands. The receptors are largely present in excitable cells, such as muscle and neurons, where they play significant roles in impulse transmission and are responsible for Ca^{2+}-induced Ca^{2+} release (CICR) from intracellular stores, which amplifies the signal resulting from membrane depolarization.

There are at least three subtypes (RyR1, RyR2, and RyR3) of the RyR, which are coded for by three different genes and expressed in different tissues *(98)*. RyR1 is predominantly expressed in skeletal muscles and can be gated by direct or indirect coupling to dihydropyiridine-sensitive receptors on the T-tubules. RyR2 is the primary isoform in cardiac muscle, where it is involved in excitation, whereas RyR3 is widely expressed in a variety of tissues, including smooth muscles, where it regulates Ca^{2+}sparks and spontaneous outward currents. The RyR3 may also be co-expressed with RyR1 and RyR2 in some tissues *(99–101)*.

The characteristics and functions of RyRs in cardiac, skeletal, and smooth muscles have been well described. In the brain, RyRs are present in presynaptic entities, where they regulate intracellular Ca^{2+}-concentrations, membrane potential, and the activity of a variety of second messengers *(102)* and play significant physiological roles in modulating local Ca^{2+} levels and neurotransmitter release; these functions are important for an understanding of the cellular mechanisms controlling neuronal function. Cyclic adenosine diphosphoribose (cADPR) is a known intracellular Ca^{2+}mobilizing agent in sea urchins, where it is produced together with IP_3 during fertilization and has been shown to play a role as an endogenous modulator of CICR in longitudinal muscle *(103)* and thought to be a modulator of the RyR Ca^{2+}release channels in bone and pancreatic β-cells *(104–107)*.

In skeletal muscles, mutations of the RyR1 isoform are linked to malignant hyperthermia, and the formation of autoantibodies to the receptor is the cause of myasthenia gravis *(31)*. The reduction in RyR2 expression in the heart is associated with cardiomyopathy.

3.2.3. SARCOPLASMIC/ENDOPLASMIC RETICULUM Ca^{2+}-ATPASE (SERCA)

The SERCA pump is structurally and functionally similar to the plasma membrane Ca^{2+}-ATPase. It belongs to a family of highly conserved proteins encoded by three highly homologous genes—*SERCA1*, *SERCA2*, and *SERCA3 (108)*. *SERCA1* gives rise to alternately spliced variants, 1a and 1b, which are expressed in fast-twitch fetal/neonatal and adult muscle, and *SERCA2* gives rise to the variants 2a and 2b. SERCA2a is the primary isoform found in the heart (where it is the critical determinant of Ca^{2+} handling by SR, which is required for excitation–contraction coupling), whereas SERCA2b is expressed ubiquitously in association with IP_3-gated Ca^{2+} stores. The activity of SERCA is modulated by phospholamban, an integral membrane protein *(109)*. Ca^{2+} transients, as well as the activity and expression patterns of Ca^{2+} handling proteins, especially SERCA2a, are altered in the failing heart; thus, the amount of SR Ca^{2+} that is available for contraction is altered *(110)*.

Spontaneous mutations in *SERCA1* in skeletal muscles are associated with Brody Disease, and reduction in the expression of *SERCA2* in the myocardium leads to hypertrophy and heart failure. Mutations in *SERCA3* in pancreatic β-cells have been linked to diabetes mellitus *(31)*.

3.2.4. MITOCHONDRIAL Ca^{2+} REGULATION

The mitochondrion functions in the long-term, large-scale regulation of $[Ca^{2+}]_i$ *(111)*. It protects the cell against large fluctuations in $[Ca^{2+}]_i$, a function achieved by the presence of both a low-affinity, high-capacity Ca^{2+} uniporter (which moves large amounts of Ca^{2+} out of the cytosol into storage in the mitochondria) and the NaCX *(112)*. The mitochondria are able to accumulate large amounts of Ca^{2+} in a relatively slow process and store it, for example, under pathological conditions in which the permeability properties of the SR/ER are altered. This ability is related to the existence of a system for the simultaneous uptake of inorganic phosphate, which then precipitates Ca^{2+} in the mitochondrial matrix in the form of insoluble hydroxyapatite. This mechanism allows for storage of excessive amounts of Ca^{2+} without essential changes in the ionic activity of the mitochondrial matrix. Ca^{2+} transport into the mitochondria from the cytosol is mediated by ruthenium red-sensitive Ca^{2+} uniporters and efflux by a Na^+-dependent and –independent mechanisms *(113)* that play important roles, such as the control of metabolic rate for cellular ATP production, modulation of amplitude and shape of cytosolic Ca^{2+} transients, and induction of apoptosis. In addition, other studies have linked the RyR to the dynamic uptake of Ca^{2+} during $[Ca^{2+}]_i$ oscillations *(114)*, suggesting that the RyR may be responsible for the rapid uptake of Ca^{2+}, a process that may be important in the removal of excess Ca^{2+} from the cytosol.

3.2.5. CALCIUM-BINDING PROTEINS

In addition to the above Ca^{2+} translocation systems, calsequestrin (in SR) and calreticulin (in ER) play significant roles in regulating cellular calcium *(115)*. These hydrophilic, high-capacity and low-affinity proteins are the major Ca^{2+}-binding proteins in muscle and nonmuscle cells, and they achieve this by forming complexes with excess Ca^{2+} in the cytosol. Calsequestrin is an acidic protein which is present in the lumen of the junctional terminal cisternae of the SR and rapidly binds and releases large quantities of Ca^{2+}. It interacts with RyRs, thus ensuring storage of high concentrations of Ca^{2+} near release sites. Calreticulin is present in the ER lumen, where it acts as a chaperone during the synthesis of channel proteins, surface receptors, and transporters and participates in the regulation of intracellular Ca^{2+} homeostasis by modulating ER Ca^{2+} storage and transport *(116)*. Calmodulin is the major Ca^{2+}-binding protein in nonmuscle cells and is the most ubiquitous of intracellular Ca^{2+}binding regulatory proteins. It affects the function of many proteins, enzymes, and ion channels *(117,118)*.

Mutations in cardiac calsequestrin gene (*CSQ2*) are linked to arrhythmias and sudden cardiac death *(119)*.

3.3. Calcium Efflux Pathways

Ca^{2+} extrusion from the cell is carried out mainly by the plasma membrane Ca^{2+}-ATPase and Na^+/Ca^{2+} exchanger.

3.3.1. PLASMA MEMBRANE CA²⁺-ATPASE

The plasma membrane Ca^{2+}-ATPase or Ca^{2+} pump is a high-affinity (K_M: 1 μ*M*), low-capacity transport protein expressed in a tissue-specific manner in both excitable and nonexcitable cells *(120)*. The proteins are encoded by four genes, and alternate mRNA splicing gives rise to multiple isoforms with different regulatory properties *(121,122)*. The plasma membrane Ca^{2+}-ATPase is activated directly by calmodulin to increase its affinity for Ca^{2+} *(120)*. Its role is in the fine-tuning of intracellular free Ca^{2+}, which it achieves by using the energy from the hydrolysis of ATP, in the presence of Ca^{2+} and Mg^{2+} to transport two Ca^{2+} ions from the cytoplasm into the extracellular space. This transport is electroneutral in function, in that two protons (H^+) are exchanged for one Ca^{2+}. Studies by Kip and Stoehler *(123)* show that expression of the plasma membrane Ca^{2+}-ATPase in Madin-Darby canine kidney (MDCK) epithelial cells is upregulated by $1,25(OH)_2D_3$, and this increase correlates with increase in transcellular Ca^{2+} influx from the apical toward the basolateral compartment, supporting the relevance of this hormone in kidney tubular Ca^{2+} absorption. Genetic evidence indicates the existence of mammalian Ca^{2+}-ATPase isoforms generated from a multigene family by alternative RNA splicing with different regulatory properties, probably as a consequence of different tissue specificities and physiological requirements *(120)*.

3.3.2. NA⁺/CA²⁺ EXCHANGER

The NCX is an asymmetric, high-capacity, low-affinity transporter which was initially reported to be abundant in nerve, muscle, and epithelial cells but that has now been identified in a wide range of tissues. Most of the NCXs expressed in other tissues, however, are similar to that found in muscle and neuronal tissue; they are particularly abundant in heart *(124)*. Typically, the NCX moves net Ca^{2+} either out of or into cells depending on the driving electrochemical force, giving rise to "Ca^{2+}-entry" and "Ca^{2+}-exit" modes of exchange. It exchanges two Na^+ ions for every Ca^{2+}. The entry mode is dependent on intracellular Na^+ to drive Ca^{2+} influx and Na^+ efflux, and is insensitive to ouabain *(125)*. The exit mode is dependent on intracellular Ca^{2+} and is sensitive to ouabain but insensitive to tetrodotoxin. Because the affinity of the transporter for intracellular Ca^{2+} is low, under physiological conditions only a small fraction of the exchangers are active at a normal, resting $[Ca^{2+}]_i$ of approx 100 n*M* in most cells. However, at peak activity of excitable and secretory cells, when $[Ca^{2+}]_i$ is in the μ*M* range, the exchanger is fully activated. Thus, this system constitutes a very important mechanism for Ca^{2+} extrusion from excitable and secretory cells, which go through cycles of low- and high-$[Ca^{2+}]_i$. Although cytosolic ATP does not play any role in the extrusion process mediated by the NCX, it substantially alters its kinetics, most likely through phosphorylation at sites in the protein molecule that are important for activity *(126)*. Rosker et al. *(127)* have shown that overexpression of a nonselective TRPC3 cation channel interacts with the NCX in Ca^{2+} signaling, suggesting an association between these transport proteins. A comprehensive review of the properties of the NCX is provided by Blaustein and Lederer *(125)*.

The common abnormalities of heart failure include hypertrophy, contractile dysfunction, and alteration of physiological properties, which contribute to low cardiac output and sudden death *(128)*. Although prolonged NCX currents are implicated in these events, the involvement of Ca^{2+} currents varies. Alterations in inotropy in dilated human cardiomyopathy are associated with impaired intracellular Ca^{2+} handling as a result of the inability to restore basal Ca^{2+} levels leading to Ca^{2+} overload *(129,130)*. The activity of the NCX is apparently reduced in myocardial ischemia, leading to intracellular Ca^{2+} overload which can result in arrhythmia, myocardial stunning, and necrosis *(131)*. On the other hand, congestive heart failure and myocardial hypertrophy are associated with increased NCX activity and decreased inotropic state.

4. OVERVIEW OF WHOLE-BODY CALCIUM HOMEOSTASIS

Under normal conditions, the maintenance of Ca^{2+} balance in the body is the result of the interplay among the intestines, kidney, and bone; the placenta is also involved in the maintenance of this balance during pregnancy. A complex Ca^{2+} traffic occurs among intestines, kidney, and bone and is controlled mainly by the PTH and $1,25(OH)_2D_3$, which is synthesized from $25(OH)D_3$ in the kidney *(132)*. (*See also* Chapter 10, "The Calcium Economy.")

4.1. Calcium Fluxes in the GI Tract

Adequate absorption of Ca^{2+}, Mg^{2+}, and PO_4^{3-} from the GI tract is necessary for normal mineral homeostasis, which in turn is vital to the control of Ca^{2+} levels in blood, skeletal growth during childhood, and the maintenance of bone mass in adulthood. Ca^{2+} absorption in the GI tract occurs mainly in the intestine by a classical epithelial transport mechanism *(9)*. Ca^{2+} is transported across the intestinal epithelium at the brush border or apical membrane into the cell, translocated by a calcium-binding protein (CaBP), calbindin, to the basolateral membrane on the opposite side, and exported via the Ca^{2+}-ATPase pump into the extracellular space. The amount of Ca^{2+} absorbed is dependent on its availability in the diet and the absorption capacity of the intestine, and the absorption process is regulated at least in part by $1,25(OH)_2D_3$. Approximately 200–300 mg/d of total luminal content of 1000 mg (800 mg daily uptake; 200 mg from pancreatic, biliary, and intestinal secretions) is absorbed, giving a gross GI absorption efficiency of 30%. This absorption is influenced by cellular and paracellular transport, systemic modulators of cell function, and intraluminal factors. In addition to the epithelial transport, Ca^{2+} can be transported directly through the gap junctions in the epithelial layer into the extracellular space when the concentration of Ca^{2+} in the lumen is high *(133–135)*. Thus, GI Ca^{2+} absorption is a sum of two transport processes—namely, a saturable, transcellular uptake that is regulated physiologically, and a nonsaturable, paracellular process that is dependent on the concentration of the mineral in the lumen of the intestine.

The transcellular transport of Ca^{2+} involves specific transport systems, which are dependent on an electrical gradient across the mucosal membrane and on Ca^{2+} binding to calbindin intracellulaly for export via the Ca^{2+}-ATPase in the basolateral membrane *(136)*. Thus this process is active, saturable, and unidirectional. Calbindin rapidly binds the free cytosolic Ca^{2+} to maintain the basal level around 100 nM to prevent cellular Ca^{2+} overload (with its associated effects of necrosis and apoptosis) *(135)*. The mucosal transport, intracellular binding, and basolateral extrusion are influenced by $1,25(OH)_2D_3$ via its effect on the synthesis of transport and binding proteins, with maximum effect being exerted on calbindin and ATPase synthesis.

Paracellular Ca^{2+} transport is a passive, nonsaturable, bi-directional process that occurs when luminal Ca^{2+} concentration is high. Although this process may be independent of $1,25(OH)_2D_3$, this hormone is known to increase the permeability of gap junctions and, therefore, can increase Ca^{2+} transport under such conditions *(137)*.

4.2. Calcium Fluxes in the Kidney

An important role of the kidney is the regulation of inorganic ion balance. The kidney filters 10,000 mg of Ca^{2+} per day; approx 99% of this is re-absorbed in the tubules of the nephron and 1% is excreted in the urine *(132)*. To maintain total body balance, the amount excreted is balanced by absorption in the intestine. Reduction in the plasma concentration of Ca^{2+} is counteracted by intestinal re-absorption, renal tubular resorption, and bone resorption. Generally, Ca^{2+} re-absorption in the kidney proceeds in parallel with Na^+ excretion *(138)*. The bulk of the filtered Ca^{2+} is re-absorbed primarily in the proximal tubule, with some re-absorption occurring in the distal and collecting tubules. The mechanisms of re-absorption of Ca^{2+} in the kidney are similar to those in the intestine, because both involve epithelial transport. In the proximal tubule, absorption occurs by two mechanisms—namely, transcellular (20%) and paracellular (80%) processes. The transcellular transport is an active process in which Ca^{2+} diffuses across the apical membrane down an electrochemical gradient and channels, and leaves the cell across the basolateral membrane against its electrochemical gradient, using Ca^{2+}-ATPase and NCX *(139)*. The kinetics of Ca^{2+} transport in the distal luminal membrane indicate the presence of Ca^{2+} channels, which have been shown to be voltage-dependent *(125)*.

4.3. Calcium Fluxes in Bone

Bone is composed of collagen and crystals of hydroxyapatite, $Ca_{10}(OH)(PO_4)_3$, in a ground substance of glycoproteins and proteoglycans *(141)*. This highly anionic environment allows for high cation binding and is thought to play an important role in the calcification of bone after the collagen fibers and ground substance have been laid down during bone formation by osteoblasts. Dietary calcium plays an important role in the growth and development of bone, and intakes below normal (600–800 mg/d) delay the onset of skeletal maturity and may result in deficits in adults. Calcified bone, therefore, constitutes a large reservoir of Ca^{2+}, which is available through bone remodeling, to buffer rises and falls in extracellular fluid (ECF) [Ca^{2+}] *(142)*. Bone remodeling is the algebraic sum of formation by osteoblasts and resorption by osteclasts, and any imbalance in this system results in the preponderance of one over the other.

In order for Ca^{2+} to be released from bone, osteoclasts in contact with the calcified bone surfaces produce and release proteolytic and lysozomal enzymes, as well as hydrogen ions, into the localized area beneath the apical membrane of the cell, creating an acidic environment to dissolve the crystals and expose the matrix. The extrusion of protons requires the presence of ion exchangers, pumps, and channels in the basolateral membrane of the cell to maintain electrochemical balance. Thus, Ca^{2+} transport proteins similar to those found in the epithelium of the intestine and kidney are also present in osteoclastic cells, where they regulate Ca^{2+} fluxes during bone resorption. Osteoblastic and odontoblastic cells have been shown to express splice variants of the NCX, and therefore show high Na^+-dependent Ca^{2+} extrusion activity (143). Studies also indicate that a Ca^{2+}-sensing receptor present on the surface of osteoclasts senses the changes in the Ca^{2+} concentration in the environment and thereby induces signals that are transmitted into the interior of the cell to alter its function (144). The osteoclast Ca^{2+}-sensing receptor is believed to be linked to a plasma membrane RyR receptor (145,146). An interesting observation, however, is that the signaling by the osteoclast Ca^{2+}-sensing receptor is not dependent on coupling to G proteins, unlike the Ca^{2+}-sensing receptors that have been described previously (17).

4.4. Calcium Fluxes in the Placenta

The placenta is the major organ involved in calcium transport from the mother to the developing fetus, a process regulated by a complex array of hormones (147–150). A prerequisite for the reproductive health of the mother and normal fetal development is proper calcium homeostasis, which is regulated by the placental trophoblast epithelium (151–153). Placental calcium transport is an active process that occurs in the syncytiotrophoblastic epithelium, which separates the maternal and fetal circulations, and is developmentally regulated to handle the increasing Ca^{2+} needs of the growing fetus. Under normal conditions, Ca^{2+} and nutrients are translocated in a maternal-to-fetal direction.

A number of Ca^{2+} transport mechanisms have been reported for the placenta; however, there is no consensus on the exact process except that there is a net influx of Ca^{2+} from the maternal side to the fetal side of the placenta (154,155). Ca^{2+} is transported against a concentration gradient because the concentration in fetal plasma is higher than that in maternal plasma, suggesting an active process requiring ATP. Because the trophoblastic layer is an epithelium, it is assumed that its Ca^{2+}-transport machinery consists of components similar to those found in the GI tract—namely, a channel, a pump, and substrate-binding protein. The main transport proteins involved in Ca^{2+} transport in the placenta are the Ca^{2+}-activated ATPase (156–159) and soluble CaBPs such as calbindin-D9K (which is similar to the vitamin D-dependent intestinal protein [160,161]), oncomodulin or parvalbumin (162,163) (whose role in plancental Ca^{2+} transport is unknown), and a high-molecular-weight CaBP expressed exclusively in the placenta and shown to be functionally involved in placental Ca^{2+} uptake (164,165). The expression of these high-affinity Ca^{2+}-binding proteins in the placenta suggest that they play important roles in regulating or shuttling cytosolic Ca^{2+} in the placenta. The exact roles of these proteins in Ca^{2+} uptake in the placenta, however, have not been established. The Ca^{2+}ATPase may function in similar fashion to the plasma membrane transporter that extrudes Ca^{2+} from the cytosol of cells. The Ca^{2+}-activated ATPase has been identified in human placenta and has been shown to be functionally involved in transmembrane Ca^{2+} uptake (156–159).

4.5. Hormonal Regulation of Ca^{2+} Transport

As described in the previous sections (as well as in Chapter 10), the concentration of Ca^{2+} in the blood can be influenced by input from the intestine and kidney and by rapid mobilization from bone remodeling. The two major hormones involved in the regulation of serum Ca^{2+} levels are PTH and $1,25(OH)_2D_3$, the former being the primary, acute controller. When the level of Ca^{2+} in the blood falls, PTH is secreted to restore it to normal levels. This is achieved by the CaSR on parathyroid cells sensing the drop in Ca^{2+} level and transducing this signal into the release of the hormone, which then acts on the kidney to increase Ca^{2+} re-absorption, mainly from the proximal tubule of the nephron, and to increase the activity of vitamin D 1α-hydroxylase *(132)*. The increase in 1α-hydroxylase activity in turn increases the synthesis of $1,25(OH)_2D_3$, which then acts on the intestine to increase Ca^{2+} absorption from the lumen by increasing the synthesis of proteins involved in Ca^{2+} absorption. In addition, increased PTH secretion stimulates osteocytolysis and osteoclastic activity in the bone while decreasing osteoblastic activity. These events combine to return plasma Ca^{2+} to normal. On the other hand, when plasma Ca^{2+} levels rise above normal—for example, as in certain disease states—a second hormone, calcitonin, secreted by C cells in the thyroid gland, acts to decrease this level by stimulating the renal excretion of Ca^{2+} and to inhibit 1α-hydroxylase activity and decrease bone remodeling through inhibition of osteoclastic activity. Thus, PTH and calcitonin exert opposite effects on plasma Ca^{2+} levels. The hormonal regulation of plasma Ca^{2+} level is, therefore, an integrated process, with PTH and $1,25(OH)_2D_3$ playing important roles to maintain the level within narrow limits under normal circumstances. From the foregoing, it is obvious that perturbation in any of these systems is bound to have far reaching effects on whole-body Ca^{2+} homeostasis.

The regulation of Ca^{2+} uptake by the placenta is under the primary control of $1,25(OH)_2D_3$. This conclusion is based on the fact that vitamin D receptors *(166,167)*, $1,25(OH)_2D_3$ synthesis *(168)*, and vitamin D hydroxylase activity *(169)* are all present in the placenta and surgical removal of the kidney, the main source of $1,25(OH)_2D_3$ synthesis, reduces transplacental Ca^{2+} gradient, which is restored by the administration of $1,25(OH)_2D_3$. In humans, regulation of calbindin-D9K expression in the placenta is thought to be under the control of estradiol *(161,170)*, suggesting the involvement of estrogens in the regulation of placental Ca^{2+} transport. Furthermore, the possibility that parathyroid hormone-related peptide (PTHrP) is involved in placental Ca^{2+} metabolism *(171–173)* suggests the participation of multiple endocrine pathways in the regulation of Ca^{2+} transport in this tissue.

5. CONCLUSIONS

Ca^{2+} is an important ion with multiple physiological effects that are vital to survival at all levels of organization. Therefore, plasma Ca^{2+} levels must be maintained within narrow limits for internal harmony, and any disturbance in Ca^{2+} homeostasis is bound to have consequences for multiple body systems. The interplay among the intestine, kidney, and bone serves to ensure that the plasma Ca^{2+} is maintained at optimum levels under normal conditions. There is a steep downward Ca^{2+} gradient from the extracellular space and internal storage sites into the cell cytoplasm. Therefore, mechanisms exist to regulate Ca^{2+} fluxes between these compartments to prevent intracellular Ca^{2+} overload and the associated deleterious effects of apoptosis and necrosis. The changes in intracellular Ca^{2+} concentrations that are necessary for normal functioning of the human body are brought about by cells interacting with their environment by means of receptors, channels, and Ca^{2+} transport proteins to initiate critical events within the cell that lead to contraction, secretion, and transcription of genes.

Calcium influx in cells occurs by means of transport systems such as voltage-dependent Ca^{2+} channels, receptor-operated Ca^{2+} channels, store-operated Ca^{2+}+ entry channels, Ca^{2+}-sensing receptor-mediated Ca^{2+} entry, and transient receptor potential channels. Calcium efflux from cells occurs mainly via plasma membrane Ca^{2+}-ATPase and the NCX. In addition to Ca^{2+} influx and efflux from the cytosol, Ca^{2+} release from internal storage sites into the cytosol plays a central role in cellular signal transduction. This release is part of a mechanism by which cells transmit external stimuli to internal signals to initiate events that lead to activation of ion channels, enzymes, contraction, secretion, and gene transcription. These Ca^{2+}-release mechanisms involve IP_3/IP_3R, ryanodine/RyR, and SERCA. Mitochondria and Ca^{2+}-binding proteins such as calsequestrin, calrecticulin, and calmodulin play important roles in maintaining cytosolic Ca^{2+} level within the limits that are necessary for essential cellular functions. Finally, the various Ca^{2+} transport systems play significant roles in regulating Ca^{2+} movement in the main Ca^{2+}-regulating organs of the body—namely, the intestines, kidneys, and bone. Any event that compromises any of these systems, therefore, leads to disruption of the Ca^{2+} homeostasis of the body.

ACKNOWLEDGMENT

Dr. Richard D. Bukoski passed away during the preparation of this chapter.

REFERENCES

1. Racay P, Kaplan P, Lehotsky J. Control of Ca^{2+} homeostasis in neuronal cells. Gen Physiol Biophys 1996;15:193–210.
2. Orrenius S, Zhivotovsky, Nicotera P. Regulation of cell death: the calcium-apoptosis link. Nature Rev Mol Cell Biol 2003;4:552–565.
3. Ledeen RW, Wu G. Ganglioside function in calcium homeostasis and signaling. Neurochem Res 2002;27:637–647.
4. Berridge MJ. Inositol trisphosphate and calcium signaling. Nature 1993;361:315–325.
5. Jaffe LF. Classes and mechanisms of calcium waves. Cell Calcium 1993;14:736–745.
6. Bootman MD, Lipp P, Berridge MJ. The organization and functions of local Ca^{2+} signals. J Cell Sci 2001;114:2213–2222.
7. Tovey S, de Smet P, Lipp P, et al. Calcium puffs are generic $InsP_3$ activated elementary calcium signals and are downregulated by prolonged hormonal stimulation to inhibit cellular calcium responses. J Cell Sci 2001;114:3979–3989.
8. Breitwieser GE, Gama L. Calcium-sensing receptor activation induces intracellular calcium oscillations. Am J Physiol Cell Physiol 2001;280:C1412–C1421.
9. Kutchai H. Cellular membranes and transmembrane transport of solutes and water. In: Berne RM, Levy MN, eds. Physiology, 4th ed, Mosby, St. Louis: 1998:3–20.
10. Wang MC, Dolphin A, Kitmitto A. L-type voltage-gated calcium channels: understanding function through structure. FEBS Lett 2004;564:245–250.
11. Large WA. Receptor-operated Ca^{2+}-permeable non-selective cation channels in vascular smooth muscle: a physiologic perspective. J Cardiovasc Electrophysiol 2002;13:493–501.
12. Putney JW Jr. Type 3 inositol 1,4,5-trisphosphate receptor and capacitative calcium entry. Cell Calcium 1997;21:257–261.
13. Fagan KA, Graf RA, Tolman S, Schaack J, Cooper MF. Regulation of a Ca^{2+}-sensitive adenylyl cyclase in an excitable cell. Role of voltage-gated versus capacitative Ca^{2+} entry. J Biol Chem 2000;275:40,187–40,194.
14. Herms I, Schneider J, Dewachter I, Caluwaerts N, Kretzshmar H, Van Leuven F. Capacitative calcium entry is directly activated by mutant presenilin-1 independent of the expression of the amyloid precursor protein. J Biol Chem 2003;278:2484–2489.

15. Putney JW Jr. Presenilins, Alzheimer's disease, and capacitative calcium entry. Neuron 2000;27:411–412.
16. Putney JW Jr. Capacitative calcium entry in the nervous system. Cell Calcium 2003;34:339–344.
17. Brown EM, MacLeod RJ Extracellular calcium sensing and extracellular calcium signaling. Physiol Rev 2001;81:239–297.
18. Birnbaumer L, Zhu X, Jiang M, et al On the molecular basis and regulation of cellular capacitative calcium entry: roles for Trp proteins. Proc Natl Acad Sci USA 1996;93:15,195–15,202.
19. Doering CJ, Zamponi GW. Molecular pharmacology of high voltage-activated calcium channels. J Bioenerg Biomembr 2003;35:491–505.
20. Hersel J, Jung S, Mohacsi P, Hullin R. Expression of the L-type calcium channel in human heart failure. Basic Res Cardiol 2002;97:I4–I10.
21. Abernethy DR, Soldatov NM. Structure-functional diversity of human L-type Ca^{2+} channel: perspectives for new pharmacological targets. J Pharmacol Exp Ther 2002;300:724–728.
22. Bourinet E, Mangoni ME, Nargeot J. Dissecting the functional role of different isoforms of the L-type Ca^{2+} channel. J Clin Invest 2004;113:1382–1384.
23. Triggel DJ. The physiological and pharmacological significance of cardiovascular T-type voltage-gated calcium channels. Am J Hypertens 1998;11:80S–87S.
24. Clozel JP, Ertel EA, Ertel SI. Voltage-gated T-type Ca^{2+} channels and heart failure. Proc Assoc Am Physicians 1999;111:429–437.
25. Hermsmeyer K, Mishra S, Miyagawa K, Minshall R. Physiologic and pathophysiologic relevance of T-type calcium channels: potential indications for T-type calcium antagonists. Clin Ther 1997;19:18–26.
26. Furukawa T, Ito H, Nitta J, et al. Endothelin-1 enhances calcium entry through T-type calcium channels in cultured neonatal rat ventricular myocytes. Cir Res 1992;71:1242–1253.
27. Giles TD. Hypertension and pathologic cardiovascular remodeling: a potential therapeutic role for T-type calcium antagonists. Clin Ther 1997;19:27–38.
28. Ertel SI, Ertel EA, Clozel JP. T-type Ca^{2+} channels and pharmacological blockade: potential pathophysiological relevance. Cardiovasc Drugs Ther 1997;11:723–739.
29. Snutch TP, Sutton KG, Zamponi GW. Voltage-dependent calcium channels- beyond dihydropyridine antagonists. Curr Opin Pharmacol 2001;1:11–16.
30. Dryer SE, Lhuillier L, Cameron JS, Martin-Caraballo M. Expression of K_{Ca} channels in identified populations of developing vertebrate neurons: role of neurotrophic factors and activity. J Physiol (Paris) 2003;97:49–58.
31. Missiaen L, Robberecht W, Van Den Bosch L, et al. Abnormal intracellular Ca^{2+} homeostasis and disease. Cell Calcium 2000;28:1–21.
32. McFadzean IM, Gibson A. The developing relationship between receptor-operated and store-operated calcium channels in smooth muscle. Br J Pharmacol 2002;135:1–13.
33. Tsunoda Y. Receptor-operated calcium influx mediated by protein tyrosine kinase pathways. J Recept Signal Transduct Res 1998;18:281–310.
34. Oonuma H, Nakajima T, Nagata T, et al. Endothelin-1 is a potent activator of nonselective cation currents in human bronchial smooth muscle cells. Am J Repir Cell Mol Biol 2000;23:213–221.
35. Wang YX, Kotlikoff MT. Signaling pathway for histamine activation of non-selective cation channels in equine tracheal myocytes. J Physiol 2000;523:131–138
36. Lambert DG, Nahorski SR. Carbachol-stimulated calcium entry in SH-SY5Y human neuroblastoma cells: which route? J Physiol (Paris) 1992;86:77–82.
37. Li WP, Tsiokas L, Sansom SC, Ma R. Epidermal growth factor activates store-operated Ca^{2+} channels through an inositol1,4,5-trisphosphate-independent pathway in human glomerular mesangial cells. J Biol Chem 2004;279:4570–4577.
38. Lamers JM, De Jonge HW, Panagia V, Van Heugten HA. Receptor-mediated signaling pathways acting through hydrolysis of membrane phospholipids in cardiomyocytes. Cardioscience 1993;4:121–131.
39. Flemming R, Cheong A, Dedman AM Beech DJ. Discrete store-operated calcium influx into intracellular compartment in rabbit arteriolar smooth muscle. J Physiol 2002;543:455–464.
40. Ma HT, Venkatachalam K, Parys JB, Gill DL. Modification of store-operated channel coupling and inositol trisphosphate receptor function by 2-aminoethoxydiphenyl borate in DT40 lymphocytes. J Biol Chem 2002;277:6915–6922

41. Ma HT, Venkatachalam K, Rys-Sikora KE, He LP, Zheng F, Gill DL. Modification of phospholipase C-gamma-induced Ca^{2+} signal generation by 2-aminoethoxydiphenyl borate. Biochem J 2003;376:667–676.
42. Putney JW Jr, Broad LM, Braun FJ, Lievremont JP, Bird GSJ. Mechanisms of capacitative calcium entry. J Cell Sci 2001;114:2223–2229.
43. Holfmann T, Schaefer M, Schulz G, Gudermann T. Transient receptor potential channels as molecular substrates of receptor-mediated cation entry. J Mol Med 2000;78:14–25.
44. Takemura H., Hughes AR, Thastrup O, and Putney JW, Jr. Activation of calcium entry by the tumor promoter thapsigargin in parotid acinar cells. Evidence that an intracellular calcium pool and not an inositol phosphate regulate calcium fluxes at the plasma membrane. J Biol Chem 1989;264:12,266–12,271.
45. Putney JW, Jr. Capacitative calcium entry revisited. Cell Calcium 1990;11:611–624.
46. Putney JW, Jr, Bird GSJ. The inositol phosphate-calcium signaling system in no-excitable cells. Endocr Rev 1993;14:610–631.
47. Montero M., Garcia-Sancho, J. and Alvarez J. Inhibition of the calcium store-operated calcium entry pathway by chemotactic peptide and by phorbol ester develops gradually and independently along differentiation of HL60 cells. J Biol Chem 1993;268:13,055–13,061.
48. Clapham DE. Calcium signaling. Cell 1995;80:259–268.
49. Berridge MJ. Calcium oscillations. J Biol Chem 1990;265:9583–9586.
50. Thomas AP, Bird GS, Hajnoczky G, Robb-Gaspers LD Putney JW Jr. Spatial and temporal aspects of cellular calcium signaling. FASEB J 1996;10:1505–1517.
51. Taylor CW, Thorn P. Calcium signaling: IP_3 rises again… and again. Curr Biol. 2001;11:R352–R355.
52. Young SH, Wu SV, Rozengurt E. Ca^{2+}-stimulated Ca^{2+} oscillations produced by the Ca^{2+}-sensing receptor require negative feedback by protein kinase C. J Biol Chem 2002;277:46,871–46,876.
53. Liu KP, Russo AF, Hsiung SC, Adlersberg et al. Calcium receptor-induced serotonin secretion by parafollicular cells: role of phosphatidylinositol 3-kinase-dependent signal transduction pathways. J Neurosci 2003;23, 2049–2057.
54. Gudermann T, Kalkbrenner F, Schultz G. Diversity and selectivity of receptor-G protein interaction. Ann Rev Pharmacol Toxicol 1996;37:429–459.
55. Kuhn B, Christel C, Wieland T, Schultz G, Gudermann T. G protein betagamma-subunits contribute to the coupling specificity of the beta2-adrenergic receptor to G(s). Naunym Schmied Arch Pharmacol 2002;365:231–241.
56. Clapham DF, Neer EJ. G protein beta gamma subunits Ann Rev Pharmacol Toxicol 1997;37:167–203.
57. Hausdorff WP, Bouvier M, O'Dowd BF, Irons GP, Caron MG, Lefkowitz RJ. Phosphorylation sites on two domains of the beta 2-adrenergic recptor are involved in distinct pathways of receptor desensitization. J Biol Chem 1989;264:12,657–12,665.
58. Rockman HA, Koch WJ, Lefkowitz RJ. Seven-transmembrane-spanning receptors and heart function. Nature 2002;415:206–212.
59. Francesconi A, Duvoisin RM. Opposing effects of protein kinase C and protein kinase A on metabotropic glutamate receptor signaling: selective desensitization of the inositol trisphosphate/Ca^{2+} pathway by phosphorylation of the receptor-G protein-coupling domain. Proc Natl Acad Sci USA 2000;97:6185–6190.
60. Bai M, Quinn S, Trivedi S, et al. Expression and characterization of inactivating and activating mutations in the human Ca^{2+}_o-sensing receptor. J Biol Chem 1996;271:19,537–19,545.
61. Bai M, Janicic N, Trivedi S, et al. Markedly reduced activity of mutant calcium-sensing receptor with an inserted Alu element from a kindred with familial hypocalciuric hypercalcemia and neonatal severe hyperparathyroidism. J Clin Invest 1997;99:1917–1925.
62. Watanabe T, Bai M, Lane CR, et al. Familial Hypoparathyroidism: identification of a novel gain of function mutation in transmembrane domain 5 of the calcium-sensing receptor. J Clin Endocrinol Metab 1998;83:2497–2502.
63. D'Souza-Li L, Yang B, Canaff L, et al. Identification and functional characterization of novel calcium-sensing receptor mutations in Familial Hypocalciuric Hypercalcemia and Autosomal Dominant Hypocalcemia. J Clin Endocrinol Metab 2002;87:1309–1318.
64. Hardie RC, Minke B. Novel Ca^{2+} channels underlying transduction in Drosophila photoreceptors: implications for phosphoinositide-mediated Ca^{2+} mobilization. Trends Neurosci 1993;16:371–376.

65. Birnbaumer L, Zhu X, Jiang M, et al. On the molecular basis and regulation of cellular capacitative calcium entry: roles for Trp proteins. Proc Natl Acad Sci USA 1996;93:195–202.

66. Harteneck G, Plant TD, Schultz G. From worm to man: three subfamilies of TRP channels. Trends Neurosci 2000;23:158–166.

67. Elliot AC. Recent developments in non-excitable cell calcium entry. Cell Calcium 2001;30:73–93.

68. Zhu X, Jiang M, Peyton M. Trp, a novel mammalian gene family essential for agonist-activated capacitative Ca^{2+} entry. Cell 1996;85:661–671.

69. Zhu X, Jiang M, Birnbaumer L. Receptor-activated Ca^{2+} influx via human TRP3 stably expressed in Human Embryonic Kidney (HEK) 293 cells. J Biol Chem 1998;273:133–142.

70. Marks AR. Ryanodine receptors/calcium release channels in heart failure and sudden cardiac death. J Mol Cardiol 2001;33:615–624.

71. Werry TD, Wilkinson GF, Willars GB. Mechanisms of cross-talk between G protein-coupled receptors resulting in enhanced release of intracellular Ca^{2+}. Biochem J 2003;374:281–296.

72. Katz A, Wu D, Simon MI. Subunits beta gamma of heterotrimeric G protein activate beta 2 isoform of phospholipase C. Nature (London) 1992;360:686–689.

73. Wu D, Katz A, Simon M. Activation of phospholipase C β_2 by the α and $\beta\gamma$ subunits of trimeric GTP-binding protein. Proc Natl Acad Sci USA 1993;90:5297–5301.

74. Jiang H, Kuang Y, Wu Y, Smrcka A, Simon MI, Wu D. Pertussis toxin-sensitve activation of phospholipase C by the C5a and fMet-Leu-Phe receptors. J Biol Chem 1996;271:13,430–13,434.

75. Stephens L, Jackson TR, Hawkins PT. Activation of phosphatidylinositol 4,5-bisphosphate supply by agonists and non-hydrolysable GTP analogues. Biochem J 1993;296:481–488.

76. Willars GB, Nahorski SR, Challis RA. Differential regulation of muscarinic acetylcholine receptor-sensitive phosphoinositide pools and consequences for signaling in human neuroblastoma cells. J Biol Chem 1998;273:5037–5046.

77. Huang C, Handlogten ME, Miller RT. Parallel activation of phosphatidylinositol 4-kinase and phospholipase C by extracellular Ca^{2+}-sensing receptor. J Biol Chem 2002;277:20,293–20,300.

78. Hajnoczky G, Gao E, Nomura T, Hoek JB, Thomas AP. Multiple mechanisms by which protein kinase A potentiates inositol 1,4,5-trisphosphate-induced Ca^{2+} mobilization in permeabilized hepatocytes. Biochem J 1993;293:413–422.

79. Wojcikiewicz RJH, Luo SG. Phosphorylation of inositol 1,4,5-trisphosphate receptors by cAMP-dependent protein kinase. J Pharmacol Exp Ther 1998;273:5670–5677.

80. MacKrill JJ. Protein-protein interactions in intracellular Ca^{2+}-release channel function. Biochem J 1999;337:345–361.

81. Taylor CW, Marshall IC. Calcium and inositol 1,4,5-trisphosphate receptors: a complex relationship. Trends Biochem Sci 1992;17:403–407.

82. Gordienko DV, Bolton TB. Cross-talk between ryanodine receptors and IP_3 receptors as a factor shaping spontaneous Ca^{2+}-release events in rabbit portal vein myocytes. J Physiol 2002;542:743–762.

83. Taylor CW, Traynor D. Calcium and inositol trisphosphate receptors. J Membr Biol 1995;145:109–118.

84. Gu X, Spitzer NC. Distinct aspects of neuronal differentiation encoded by frequency of spontaneous Ca^{2+} transients. Nature 1995;375:784–787.

85. Spitzer NC, Olson E, Gu X. Spontaneous calcium transients regulate neuronal plasticity in developing neurons. J Neurobiol 1995;26:316–324.

86. Blondel O, Takeda J, Janssen H, Seino S, Bell GI. Sequence and functional characterization of a third inositol trisphosphate receptor subtype, IP_3R-3 expressed in pancreatic islets, kidney, gastrointestinal tract, and other tissues. J Biol Chem 1993;268:11,356–11,363.

87. Ross CA, Danoff SK, Schell MJ, Snyder SH, Ullrich A. Three additional inositol 1,4,5-trisphosphate receptors: molecular cloning and differential localization in brain and peripheral tissues. Proc Natl Acad Sci USA 1992;89:4265–4269.

88. Newton CL, Mignery GA, Sudhof TC. Co-expression in vertebrate tissues and cell lines of multiple inositol-1,4,5-trisphosphate $(InsP_3)$ receptors with distinct affinities for $InsP_3$. J Biol Chem 1994;269:28,613–28,619.

89. Cardy TJA, Traynor D, Taylor CW. Differential regulation of types-1 and -3 inositol trisphosphate receptors by cytosolic Ca^{2+}. Biochem J 1997;328:785–793.

90. Yoneshima H, Miyawaki A, Michikawa T, Furuichi T, Mikoshiba K. Ca^{2+} differentially regulates the ligand-affinity states of type 1 and type 3 inositol-1,4,5-trisphosphate receptors. Biochem J 1997;322:591-596.

91. Pin JP, Duvoisin R. The metabotropic glutamate receptors: structure and functions. Neuropharmacol 1995;34:1–26.

92. Conn PJ, Pin JP. Pharmacology and functions of metabotropic glutamate receptors. Annu Rev Pharmacol 1997;37:205–237.

93. Luo D, Broad LM, Bird GSJ, Putney JW. Signaling pathways underlying muscarinic receptor-induced $[Ca^{2+}]_i$ oscillations in HEK293 cells. J Biol Chem 2001;276:5613–5621.

94. Dolmetsch RE, Lewis RS. Signaling between intracellular Ca^{2+} stores and depletion-activated Ca2+ channels generates $[Ca^{2+}]_i$ oscillations in T lymphocytes. J Gen Physiol 1994;103:365–368.

95. Dolmetsch RE, Lewis RS, Goodnow CC, Healy JI. Differential activation of transcription factors induced by Ca^{2+} response amplitude and duration. Nature 1997;386:855–858.

96. Dolmetsch RE, Pajvani U, Fife K, Spotts JM, Greenberg ME. Signaling to the nucleus by an L-type calcium channel-calmodulin complex through the MAP kinase pathway. Science 2001;294:333–339.

97. Xu L, Tripathy A, Pasek DA, Meissner G. Potential for pharmacology of ryanodine receptor/calcium release channels. Ann NY Acad Sci 1998;853:130–148.

98. Giannini G, Conti A, Mammarella S, Scrobogna M, Sorrentino C. The ryanodine receptor/calcium channel genes are widely and differentially expressed in murine brain and peripheral tissues. J Cell Biol 1995;128:893–904.

99. Ogawa Y, Kurebayashi N, Murayama T. Putative roles of Type 3 ryanodine receptor isoforms. Trends Cardiovasc Med 2000;10:65–70.

100. Lohn M, Jessner W, Furstehau M, et al. Regulation of Ca^{2+} sparks and spontaneous transient outward currents by RyR3 in arterial vascular smooth muscle cells. Circ Res 2001;89:1051–1057.

101. Rossi D, Sorrentino V. Molecular genetics of ryanodine receptors Ca^{2+}-release channels. Cell Calcium 2002;32:307–319.

102. Bouchard R, Pattarini R, Geiger JD. Presence and functional significance of presynaptic ryanodine receptors. Prog Neurobiol 2003;69:391–418.

103. Kuemmerle JF, Makhlouf GM. Agonist-stimulated cyclic ADPribose. Endogenous modulator of Ca^{2+}-induced Ca^{2+} release in intestinal longitudinal muscle. J Biol Chem 1995;270:25,488–25,494.

104. Sun L, Adebanjo OA, Moonga BS, et al. CD38/ADP-ribosyl cyclase: a new role in the regulation of osteoclasic bone resorption. J Cell Biol 1999;146:1161–1172.

105. Okamoto H. The CD38-cyclic ADP-ribose signaling system in insulin secretion. Mol Cell Biochem 1999;193:115–118.

106. Guse AH. Cyclic ADP-ribose (cADPR) and nicotinic acid adenine dinucleotide phoaphate (NAADP): novel regulators of Ca^{2+}-signaling and cell function. Curr Mol Med 2002;2:273–282.

107. Guse AH. Regulation of calcium signaling by the second messenger cyclic adenosine diphosphoribose (cADPR). Curr Mol Med 2004;4:239–248.

108. Misquitta CM, Mack DP, Grover AK. Sarco/endoplasmic reticulum Ca^{2+} (SERCA)-pumps: link to heart beats and calcium waves. Cell Calcium 1999;25:277–290.

109. Frank KF, Bolck B, Erdmann E, Schwinger RHG. Sarcoplasmic reticulum Ca^{2+}-ATPase modulates cardiac contraction and relaxation. Cardiovasc Res 2003;57:20–27.

110. Prestle J, Quinn FR, Smith GI. Ca^{2+}-handling proteins and heart failure: novel molecular targets? Curr Med Chem 2003;10:967–981.

111. Ganitkevich VY. The role of mitochondria in cytoplasmic Ca^{2+} cycling. Expt Physiol 2003;88:91–97.

112. Gunter TE, Buntinas L, Sparagna G, Eliseev R, Gunter K. Mitochondrial calcium transport: mechanisms and functions. Cell Calcium 2000;28:285–296.

113. Huser J, Blatter LA, Sheu SS. Mitochondrial calcium in heart cells: beat to beat oscillations or slow integration of cytosolic transients? J Bioenerg Biomembr 2000;32:27–33.

114. Beutner G, Sharma VK, Giovannucci DR, Yule DI, Sheu SS. Identification of a ryanodine receptor in rat mitochondria. J Biol Chem 2001;276:21,482–21,488.

115. Yano K, Zarain-Herzberg A. Sarcoplasmic reticulum calsequestrins: structural and functional properties. Mol cell Biochem 1994;135:61–70.

116. Michalak M, Corbett EF, Mesaeli N, Nakamura K, Opas M. Calreticulin: one protein, one gene, many functions. Biochem J 1999;344:281–292.

117. Welsby PJ, Wang H, Wolfe JT, Colbran RJ, Johnson ML, Barrett PQ. A mechanism for the direct regulation of T-type calcium channels by Ca^{2+}/calmodulin-dependent kinase II. J Neurosci 2003;23:10,116–10,121.

118. Wu Y, Kimbrough JT, Colbran TJ, Anderson ME. Calmodulin kinase is functionally targeted to the action potential plateau for regulation of L-type Ca^{2+}-current in rabbit cardiomyocytes. J Physiol 2004;554:145–155.

119. Terentyev D, Viatchenko-Karpinski S, Gyyorke I, Volpe P, Williams SC, Gyorke S. Calsequestrin determines the functional size and stability of cardiac intracellular calcium stores: Mechanism for hereditary arrhythmia. Proc Natl Acad Sci USA 2003;100:11,759–11,764.

120. Strehler EE. Plasma membrane Ca^{2+} pumps and Na^+/Ca^{2+} exchangers. Sem Cell Biol 1990;4:283–295.

121. Keeton TP, Burk SE, Shull GE. Alternative splicing of exons encoding the calmodulin-binding domains and C termini of plasma membrane Ca^{2+}-ATPase isoforms 1,2,3 and 4. J Biol Chem 1993;268:2740–2748.

122. Guerini D. The Ca^{2+} pumps and the Na^+/Ca^{2+} exchangers. Biometals 1998;11:19–30.

123. Kip SN, Strehler EE. Vitamin D_3 upregulates plasma membrane Ca^{2+}-ATPase expression and potentiates apico-basal Ca^{2+} flux in MDCK cells. Am J Physiol Renal Physiol 2004;286:F363–F369.

124. Reeves JP, Condrescu M, Chernaya G, Gardner JP. Na^+/Ca^{2+} antiport in the mammalian heart. J Exp Biol 1994;196:375–388.

125. Blaustein MP, Lederer WJ. Sodium/calcium exchange: its physiological implications. Physiol Rev 1999;79:763–854.

126. Smets I, Caplanusi A, Despa S, et al. Ca^{2+} uptake in mitochondria occurs via the reverse action of the Na^+/Ca^{2+} exchanger in metabolically inhibited MDCK cells. Am J Physiol Renal Physiol 2004;286:F784–F794.

127. Rosker C, Graziani A, Lukas M, Eder et al. Ca^{2+} signaling by TRPC3 involves Na^+ entry and local coupling to the Na^+/Ca^{2+} exchanger. J Biol Chem 2004;279:13,696–13,704.

128. Richard S, Leclercq F, Lamaire S, Piot C. Nargeot J. Ca^{2+} currents in compensated hypertrophy and heart failure. Cardiovasc Res 1998;37:300–311.

129. Beucklemann DJ, Nabauer M, Erdmann E. Intracellular calcium handling in isolated ventricular myocytes from patients with terminal heart failure. Circulation 1992;85:1046–1055.

130. Pieske B, Posival H, Minani K, Just H, Hasenfuss G. Alterations in intracellular calcium handling associated with the inverse force-frequency relation in human dilated cardiomyopathy. Circulation 1995;92:1169–1178.

131. Yashar PR, Fransna M, Frishman WH. The sodium-calcium ion membrane exchanger: physiologic significance and pharmacologic implications. J Clin Pharmacol 1998;38:393–401.

132. Stanton BA, Koeppen BM. Potassium, calcium and phosphate homeostasis. In: Berne RM, Levy MN, eds. Physiology, 4th ed, Mosby, St. Louis: 1998; pp. 744–762.

133. Karbach U. Paracellular calcium transport across the small intestine. J Nutr 1992;122:672–677.

134. Wasserman RH, Chandler JS, Meyer SA, et al. Intestinal calcium transport and calcium extrusion processes in the basolateral membrane. J Nutr 1992;122:662–671.

135. Johnson JA, Kumar R. Renal and intestinal calcium transport: roles of vitamin D and vitamin D-dependent calcium binding proteins. Semn Nephrol 1994;14:119–128.

136. Wasserman RH, Chandler JS, Meyer SA. Intestinal calcium transport and calcium extrusion process at the basolateral membrane. J Nutr 1992;122:662–671.

137. Wasserman RH, Fullmer CS. Vitamin D and intestinal calcium transport: facts, speculations and hypothesis. J Nutr 1995;125:1971S–1979S.

138. Friedman PA, Gesek FA. Cellular calcium transport in renal epithelia: measurement, mechanisms and regulation. Physiol Rev;1995;75:429–471.

139. Bindels RJM. Calcium handling by the mammalian kidney. J Exp Biol 1993;184:89–104.

140. Brunette MG, Leclerc M, Couchourel D, Mailloux J, Bourgeois Y. Characterization of three types of calcium channels in the luminal membrane of the distal nephron. Can J Physiol Pharmacol 2004;82:30–37.

141. Genuth S. Endocrine regulation of calcium and phosphate metabolism In: Berne RM, Levy MN, eds. Physiology, 4th ed, Mosby, St. Louis: 1998; pp. 848–871.

142. Meghji S. Bone remodeling. Br Dent J 1992;21:235–242.
143. Lundquist P. Odontoblast phosphate and calcium transport in dentinogenesis. Swd Dent J 2002;154:1–52.
144. Kameda T, Muno H, Yamada Y, et al. Calcium-sensing receptor in mature osteoclasts, which are bone resorbing cells. Biochem Biophys Res Commun 1998;245:419–422.
145. Zaidi M, Moonga BS, Adebanjo OA. Novel mechanisms of calcium handling by the osteoclast: a review-hypothesis. Proc Assoc Am Physicians 1999;111:319–327.
146. Zaidi M, Moonga BS, Huang CL. Calcium sensing and cell signaling processes in the local regulation of osteoclastic bone resorption. Biol Rev Camb Philos Soc 2004;79:79–100.
147. Kamath SG, Smith CH. Na$^+$/Ca^{2+} exchange, Ca^{2+} binding and electrogenic Ca^{2+} transport in plasma membranes of human placental syncytiotrophoblast. Pediatr Res 1994;36:461–467.
148. Kamath SG, Haider N, Smith CH. ATP-dependent calcium transport and binding by plasma membrane of human placenta. Placenta 1994;15:147–155.
149. Hosking DJ. Calcium homeostasis in pregnancy. Clin Endocrinol 1996;45:1–6.
150. Kovacs CS, Lanske B, Hunzelman JL, Guo J, Karaplis AC, Kronenberg HM. Parathyroid hormone-related peptide (PHrP) regulates fetal-placental calcium transport through a receptor distinct from the PTH/PTHrP receptor. Proc Natl Acad Sci USA 1996;93:15,233–15,238.
151. Lafond J, Leclerc M, Brunette MG. Characterization of calcium transport by basal plasma membranes from human placenta syncytiotrophoblast. J Cell Physiol 1991;148:17–23.
152. Brunette MG, Leclerc M. Ca^{2+} transport through the brush border membrane of human placenta syncytiotrophoblasts. Can J Physiol Pharmacol 1992;70:835–842.
153. Kamath SG, Kelley LK, Friedman AF, Smith CH. Transport and binding in calcium uptake by microvillous membrane of human placenta. Am J Physiol 1992;262:C789–C794.
154. Lafond J, Goyer-O'Reilly I, Laramee M, Simoneau L. Hormonal regulation and implication of cell signaling in calcium transfer by placenta. Endocrine 2001;14:285–294.
155. Kovacs CS, Chafe LL, Woodland ML, McDonald KR, Fudge NJ, Wookey PJ. Calcitropic gene expression suggests a role for the intraplacental yolk sac in maternal-fetal calcium exchange. Am J Physiol Endocrinol Metab 2002;282:E721–E732.
156. Kasznica JM, Petcu EB. Placental calcium pump: clinical-based evidence. Pediatr Pathol Mol Med 2003;22:223–227.
157. Moreau R, Simoneau L, Lafond J. Calcium fluxes in human trophoblast (BeWo) cells: calcium channels, calcium-ATPase, and sodium-calcium exchanger. Mol Reprod Dev 2003;64:189–198.
158. Strid H, Powell TL. ATP-Dependent Ca^{2+} transport is up-regulated during third trimester in human syncytiotrophoblast basal membranes. Pediatr Res 2000;48:58–63.
159. Strid H, Care A, Jansson T, Powell T. Parathyroid hormone-related peptide (38-94) amide stimulates ATP-dependent calcium transport in the basal membrane of the human syncytio-trophoblast. J Endocrinol 2002;175:517–524.
160. An BS, Chopi KC, Kang SK, Hwang WS, Jeung EB. Novel Calbindin-D(9k) protein as a useful biomarker for environmental estrogenic compounds in the uterus of immature rats. Reprod Toxicol 2003;17:311–319.
161. Krisenger J, Dann JL, Applegarth O, et al. Calbindin-D9k gene expression during the pereinatal period in the rat: correlation to estrogen receptor expression in uterus. Mol Cell Endocrinol 1993;97:61–69.
162. Henzl MT, Hapak RC, Likos JJ. Interconversion of the ligand arrays in the CD and EF sites of oncomodulin. Influence on Ca^{2+}-binding affinity. Biochem 1998;37:9101–9111.
163. Belkacemi L, Simoneau L, Lafond J. Calcium-binding proteins: distribution and implication in mammalian placenta. Endocrine 2002;19:57–64.
164. Hershberger ME, Tuan RS. Placental 57-kDa Ca^{2+}-binding protein: regulation of expression and function in trophoblast calcium transport. Dev Biol 1998;199:80–92.
165. Derfoul A, Lin FJ, Awumey EM, Kolodzeski T, Hall DJ, Tuan RS. Estrogenic endocrine disruptive components interfere with calcium handling and differentiation of human trophoblast cells. J Cell Biochem 2003;89:755–770.
166. Uerhaeghe J, Bouillon R. Calciotropic hormones during reproduction. J Steroid Biochem Mol Biol 1992;41:469–477.

167. Tanamura A, Nomura S, Kurauchi O, Furui T, Mizutani S, Tomoda Y. Purification and characterization of 1,25(OH)$_2$D$_3$ receptor from human placenta. J Obstet Gynaecol 1995;21:631–639.

168. Hahali A, Diaz L, Sanchez I, Garabedian M, Bourges H, Larrea F. Effects of IGF-I on 1,25-dihydroxyvitamin D$_3$ synthesis by human placenta in culture. Mol Huma Reprod 1999;5:771–776.

169. Diaz L, Sanchez I, Avila E, Halhali A, Vilchis F, Larrea F. Identification of a 25-hydroxyvitamin D$_3$ 1α-hydroxylase gene transcription product in cultures of hyman syncytiotrophoblast cells. J Clin Endocrinol Metab 2000;85:2543–2549.

170. Jeung EB, Leung PC, Krisinger J. The human calbindin-D9k gene. Complete structure and implications on steroid hormone regulation. J Mol Biol 1994;235:1231–1238.

171. Farrugia W, de Gooyer T, Rice GE, Moseley JM, Wlodek ME. Parathyroid hormone (1-34) and parathyroid hormone-related protein (1-34) stimulate calcium release from human syncytiotrophoblast basal membranes via a common receptor. J Endocrinol 2000;166:689–695.

172. Curtis NE, Thomas RJ, Gillespie MT, King RG, Rice GE, Wlodek ME. Parathyroid hormone-related protein (PTHrP) mRNA splicing and parathyroid hormone/PTHrP receptor mRNA expression in human placenta and fetal membrane. J Mol Endocrinol 1998;21:225–234.

173. Laramee M, Simoneau L, Lafond J. Phospholipase C axis is the preferential pathway leading to PKC activation following PTH or PTHrP stimulation in human term placenta. Life Sci 2002;72:215–225.

II Techniques for Studying Calcium Metabolism and Its Relationship to Disease

4 Nutritional Epidemiology

Dietary Assessment Methods

Carol J. Boushey

KEY POINTS

- Estimating dietary exposures is useful for identifying modifiable risk factors for disease.
- Several dietary assessment methods have been developed for use in research.
- Many factors, such as study design and research objectives, must be considered in selecting a dietary assessment method.
- Biomarkers are useful additions to corroborate results from dietary assessment tools.

1. INTRODUCTION

Nutritional epidemiology has developed from an interest in the concept that aspects of diet may influence the occurrence of human diseases. In epidemiology, disease occurrence is measured and related to different characteristics of individuals or their environments. Exposures, or what an individual comes in contact with, may be related to disease risk. The exposure can be a habit such as smoking, which would increase an individual's risk for lung cancer, or the exposure can be an environmental agent such as sun, which may increase an individual's risk for melanoma. In the case of nutritional epidemiology, food and the behaviors surrounding food choices are the exposures. For example, vegetable consumption may reduce an individual's risk for colon cancer, and exposure to television may increase an individual's risk of being overweight secondary to an increased intake of high-energy snack foods.

Measuring dietary intake presents more challenges than other exposures such as smoking. In most cases, the question as to whether an individual smokes can be answered by a simple "never," "yes," or "used to." In addition, smoking is a physiological habit; thus the amount smoked per day is fairly constant. Cigarettes are packaged in uniform amounts, making recall of packs or portions of packs per day fairly straightforward. Most individuals would not be able to tell an interviewer the last time they ate apple pie (unless it was the previous day). On the other hand, an ex-smoker can often tell an interviewer to the month and year, if not the day and hour, when he/she quit smoking.

From: *Calcium in Human Health*
Edited by: C. M. Weaver and R. P. Heaney © Humana Press Inc., Totowa, NJ

Table 1
Suggested Dietary Assessment Methods for Different Study Designs

	Dietary assessment methods			
Study design	Brief methods	24-h dietary recall	Food frequency questionnaire	Food record
Cross-sectional	X	X	X	X
Surveillance	X			
Case–control	X		X	
Cohort	X	X	X	X
Intervention	X	X	X	X

Despite the difficulties encountered in the collection of food intake data, dietary information provides some of the most valuable insights into the occurrence of disease and subsequent approaches for mounting intervention programs for prevention. Food is a universal language. Fortunately, dietary assessment methods continue to evolve to meet the challenge and there is recognition that further improvements will enhance the consistency and strength of the association of diet with disease risk.

The primary purpose of this chapter is to provide readers with information to insure the selection of an appropriate dietary assessment method for a particular need. As with any assessment tool, choosing the right tool for a dietary project is critical to achieving desired results (1,2). The intent is to focus on dietary assessment methods, and not specific sources of calcium, which is covered in Chapter 9. An overview of the four primarily used dietary assessment methods will be discussed and references to more detailed descriptions will be provided. Then the relationship of dietary assessment methods to study designs as shown in Table 1 is emphasized with examples from the literature.

2. DIETARY ASSESSMENT METHODS

2.1. The 24-Hour Dietary Recall

For the 24-h dietary recall, an interviewee is asked by a trained interviewer to remember foods and beverages consumed in the previous 24 h. To assist the interviewee, food models and pictures are often used as prompts for assistance with portion sizes (1). The interviewer uses structured questions and prompts to help the interviewee remember foods eaten. An interviewer conducts the interview, thus the literacy of the respondent is not an issue as it is with some other dietary assessment methods. Because of the immediacy, respondents are generally able to recall most of their dietary intake. The reduced burden on the respondent allows for a sample of participants that may be more representative than individuals completing a more intensive method, such as the keeping of food records. In addition, an unannounced interview takes place after food is consumed; thus, alteration of usual eating habits is unlikely to occur. However, there are circumstances that may prompt the interviewee to alter his/her usual eating pattern, and therefore the amount of food consumed the previous 24 h may be reduced. This could occur when a 24-h dietary recall is prescheduled or occurs after an overnight fast (a common occurrence when recall is scheduled prior to a fasting phlebotomy session).

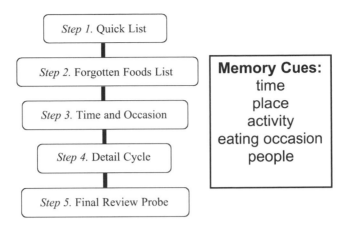

Fig. 1. The sequential steps for the five-step multiple-pass method for conducting a 24-h recall with the topic probes for the memory cues.

The Food Surveys Research Group (FSRG) of the US Department of Agriculture has devoted considerable effort to improving the accuracy of the 24-h recall through development and refinement of the multiple-pass method. The multiple-pass method provides a structured interview format with specific probes. Campbell and Dodds *(3)* found decades ago that interviewees receiving probing while being interviewed reported 25% higher dietary intakes than interviewees without probing. The latest variation of the multiple-pass approach involves five structured sets of probing (*see* Fig. 1) compared with its predecessor, which outlined three passes *(4)*. With this five-step multiple-pass method, the average number of foods reported per day increased by two from the previous triple-pass method, and energy intake increased 17%, suggesting a more complete recall of dietary intake *(5)*. A 24-h recall administered in this style can take 30–60 min.

For the National Health and Nutrition Examination Survey (NHANES), the FSRG uses a computerized version of the five-step multiple-pass method that is not available for public use at this time. However, this technique can be duplicated using the computer-assisted method available from the Nutrient Data System for Research Software developed by the Nutrition Coordinating Center (NCC), University of Minnesota, Minneapolis, MN. The direct coding of the foods saves money in data-entry time, missing values, and standardization. Otherwise, after each interview, the time to enter the dietary information into an appropriate nutrient database must be considered.

The major drawback of the 24-h recall is the issue of underreporting *(6)*. Factors such as obesity, gender, social desirability, restrained eating, hunger, education, literacy, perceived health status, age, and race/ethnicity have been shown to be related to underreporting *(7–10)*. Common forgotten food items include condiments, savory snacks, cake/pie, meat mixtures, white potatoes, fat-type spreads, and regular soft drinks *(11)*. Harnack et al. *(12)* found significant underreporting of large food portions when food models showing recommended serving sizes were used as visual aids for respondents. Larger food portions have been observed over the past 20 to 30 yr *(13,14)*; this may contribute to underreporting, and methods to capture accurate portion sizes are needed. Some work addressing this issue has been reported *(15,16)*.

In studies comparing energy intake estimated from the triple-pass method with energy expenditure estimated from doubly labeled water (DLW) or accelerometers, underreporting of energy intakes ranged from 17% in low-income women *(10)* to 26% in overweight and obese women *(17)*. Comparisons in children under 11 yr of age are mixed. One study showed a 14% greater energy intake than DLW estimated energy expenditure *(18)* and another showed only group estimates of energy intake as being valid *(19)*. Under controlled conditions of weight maintenance, women underestimated energy intake by 13% during a self-selection period, but overestimated by 1.3% under more controlled conditions *(20)*. Men, on the other hand, underestimated 11% and 13% under both conditions. Among African-American women with type 2 diabetes, 58% or 81% of the women underreported energy intake depending on the criteria used for estimating energy expenditure *(21)*.

Two published reports comparing the dietary intake results from the five-step multiple-pass method with actual observed intakes are available at this time *(22,23)*. Conway et al. *(22)* recorded observed intakes in 42 adult men and compared the estimated energy intake from the observations with the energy intake estimated from a five-step multiple-pass 24-h recall. No significant differences were found for energy, protein, carbohydrate, and fat. Further, there was no association of body mass index (BMI) with level of reporting. For women following the same protocol *(23)*, the population was found to have overestimated its energy and carbohydrate intakes by 8–10%. No significant differences between mean observed and recalled intakes of energy and the macronutrients were found. Recalled fat intake was not significantly different from the observed intake across the BMI range studied *(23)*.

The five-step multiple-pass method was one of the dietary assessment methods included in one of the largest, most ambitious studies of biomarkers and dietary intake *(24)*. The Observing Protein and Energy Nutrition (OPEN) Study collected two 24-h dietary recalls approx 3 mo apart, as well as DLW and urinary nitrogen as a protein biomarker, in 484 adults. For men, underreporting of energy intake compared with total energy expenditure was 12–14% and for protein it was 11–12%. For women, these same comparisons indicated underreporting of 16–20% for energy and 11–15% for protein. In general, researchers using the 24-h recall should be aware of the potential for underreporting and be prepared to minimize the factors related to underreporting and, possibly, overreporting in children.

2.2. The Food Record

For the food record, participants are asked to record all food and beverages consumed throughout a 24-h period. To improve the accuracy of the food record, detailed instructions are provided to the participants and tools for measuring or weighing foods and beverages consumed must be provided. Because the food record depends on the individual's ability and desire to record foods eaten, the number of individuals completing records may be limited by motivation and literacy. In addition, the process of recording foods can alter how an individual eats *(25,26)*. Although no staff time is involved with interviewing subjects, as is the case with the 24-h recall, the time required for training subjects, telephoning with reminders to record, reviewing the records for discrepancies, and entering the dietary information into a nutrient database must be considered.

Because the food record does not require dependence on memory, this method is sometimes considered the reference standard with which other dietary assessment methods are compared *(1,2)*. The accuracy of reporting portion sizes can be improved by training the participants prior to starting the recording process *(27)*. Many of the same issues listed for the 24-h dietary recall with regard to underreporting also exist for the food record *(8,9,28–31)*. The food record is especially vulnerable to underreporting because of the complexity of recording food, and also because the process of recording food has been shown to be an effective technique for reducing food consumption *(25,26)*. The range of underreporting for energy intake as compared with energy expenditure as estimated by DLW is between 4 and 37% *(32)*.

The process of reviewing a food record and coding the foods for data entry requires trained individuals and can take a large amount of time. To decrease the burden on staff, some food-record methods provide a list of foods to check-off when consumed. As attractive as this may seem, the restriction in food choices makes this approach similar to a 1-d food frequency method, and limits the ability of investigators to make conclusions based on some foods and food groupings *(33)*.

Most individuals' diets vary greatly from day to day *(34)*. Therefore, it is not appropriate to use data from a single 24-h recall or a single food record to characterize an individual's usual diet. An example of day-to-day variation can be seen in Fig. 2. The figure shows the estimated daily dietary intakes of calcium from 6 d of food records collected from three girls prior to starting a metabolic study. The three girls in Fig. 2 represent the 10th, 50th, and 90th percentiles from 43 girls between the ages of 10 and 14 yr. Had the investigators only collected 1 d, and had that day been day 1 in the figure, the girl at the 10th percentile would have been assessed as having the highest calcium intake among the three, and the girl at the 90th percentile would have had the lowest intake. A single food record or 24-h recall can be used to describe the average dietary intake of a group; however, that single day cannot be used to assess achievement of dietary recommendations without special statistical applications *(34,35)*. Therefore, a minimum of two nonconsecutive days are recommended to make population inferences.

The number of days needed to estimate intake of a particular nutrient depends on the variability of the nutrient being assessed and the degree of accuracy desired for the research question *(2,36–38)*. Most nutrients require more than 4 d for a reliable estimate *(37,38)*. However, most individuals weary of keeping records beyond 4 d, which may decrease the quality of the records *(25)*. Block et al. *(39)* used an interesting approach, collecting 2 d of food records at four different times throughout the year to evaluate a food frequency questionnaire (FFQ). The advantages of this approach are that the collection of multiple days spaced far enough apart prevents record fatigue and captures seasonal variation. In developed countries, the within-person variation of day-to-day dietary intake for any one nutrient is usually greater than between-person variation; thus, collecting an inadequate number of days of intake would jeopardize a study's capacity to accurately describe intake and find important differences between persons *(37)*.

Beaton and colleagues *(38)* have developed guidelines for determining the number of days necessary to estimate an individual's true intake within a specified degree of error. Using the formula developed by Beaton *(38)* and values for the energy-adjusted within-person coefficient of variation from food records completed by US women as published

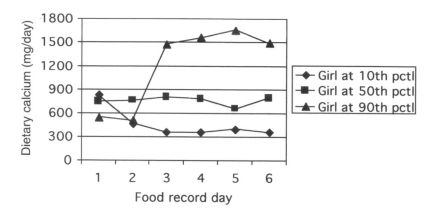

Fig. 2. An example of day-to-day variation in daily dietary intakes of calcium from 6 d of food records collected from three girls between 10 and 14 yr of age. The girls were selected from a larger group and each represented the noted percentile (pctl) in the group for average total dietary calcium intake.

by Willett *(2)*, the number of days needed to estimate a woman's calcium intake to within 20% of her true mean 95% of the time would be 13 d. The nonadjusted estimate would be 17 d. Similar principles by which to obtain the number of days to accurately assess usual intake for a nutrient have been reported by Nelson et al. *(37)* and Liu et al. *(36)*. For this approach *(37)*, the number of days of food records needed to ensure that r ≥ 0.90 for calcium is 4 for toddlers and male children (5–17 yr of age). The number of days for adult males is 5, and for adult females is 8. The largest number of days needed, secondary to having the largest within-person variation, is 12 days for female children (5–17 yr of age). All of the estimates described here were derived from data collected prior to the 1990s, before fortification of the food supply with calcium became common. If the calcium-fortified foods are consumed only occasionally, then the number of days to accurately estimate calcium intake would increase (as within-person variability would increase). If these fortified foods are consumed regularly, then the estimates above would most likely still be valid.

2.3. Food Frequency Questionnaires

The FFQ estimates usual frequency of consumption of foods from a list for a specific period of time. Depending on the questionnaire used, estimates can be made for total diet or a specific nutrient or food. There are three basic types of FFQs: qualitative, semi-quantitative, and quantitative (*see* Fig. 3) *(40)*. Each style has its advantages and disadvantages based on the foods or nutrients being assessed, the objectives of the research, and the population being assessed. Some widely used and available FFQs are the "Block" FFQ, which is a quantitative FFQ, and the "Willett" or "Harvard" FFQ, which is a semi-quantitative FFQ *(41)*. Newly developed and available from the Risk Factor Monitoring and Methods Branch of the National Cancer Institute is the Diet History Questionnaire (DHQ), which is a quantitative FFQ. The performance of these three FFQ tools has been compared and found to be similar *(41)*. The qualitative FFQ, which attempts to classify individuals according to nutrient intake on the basis of frequency of consumption alone,

Qualitative	Semi-quantitative	Quantitative	
How often do you eat the following vegetables?	How often do you eat the following vegetables?	How often do you eat the following vegetables?	
Green beans or peas	Green beans or peas (1/2 cup)	Green beans or peas (1/2 cup)	How much each time
O Never	O Never	O Never	
O A few times per year	O A few times per year	O A few times per year	
O Once per month	O Once per month	O Once per month	O ¼ cup
O 2-3 times per month	O 2-3 times per month	O 2-3 times per month	O ½ cup
O Once per week	O Once per week	O Once per week	O 1 cup
O 2 times per week	O 2 times per week	O 2 times per week	O 2 cups
O 3-4 times per week	O 3-4 times per week	O 3-4 times per week	
O 5-6 times per week	O 5-6 times per week	O 5-6 times per week	
O Everyday	O Everyday	O Everyday	
Frequency only	Frequency plus addition of reference portion size	Frequency plus selection of usual portion size	

Fig. 3. Examples of the three types of food frequency questionnaires.

has not been used routinely since the mid-1980s *(42)*. Recently, the qualitative FFQ was resurrected as a "food propensity questionnaire" to help derive usual intake over time from the 24-h dietary recalls collected in the NHANES *(43)*.

The FFQ estimates usual intake of foods and nutrients over a specified period of time, e.g., 1 wk, 1 mo, 1 yr. The FFQ is unique in that one can also specify a period of reference to recall, such as 5 yr ago or 10 yr ago. Like the 24-h dietary recall, the FFQ does not influence the eating behaviors of respondents. To complete the FFQ, there is a low burden on respondents. Almost all are optically scannable for easy data entry, some are available as interactive multi-media *(44)*, and some are moving to a Worldwide Web platform.

The FFQ is intended to rank or compare dietary intakes (e.g., foods or nutrients) among individuals *(45)*. In particular, the FFQ separates the "highs" from the "lows" with respect to intake of the specific foods in the FFQ and, to some extent, the nutrients in those foods. Because of the constraints imposed on the respondent with regard to food choices and portion sizes, the FFQ should not be used to assess the adequacy of dietary intakes of individuals or groups *(46)*. The foods in an FFQ are limited to foods representing the major contributors to a specific nutrient *(46)*, bioactive compound *(47)*, or food groups *(48)*, and rely heavily on differences in frequency of intake vs portion sizes. Foods are grouped together, thus limiting specificity if a respondent only eats one food in a group. As a result, the dietary estimates from an FFQ are not quantifiably precise and have a larger measurement error than the food record or 24-h dietary recall *(33)*. In addition, the use of an FFQ is limited to the populations for which the instrument was designed; thus, whole groups of foods central to a particular eating pattern may be missing from a particular FFQ *(49)*. Despite these limitations, the probability approach to estimate the prevalence of inadequate nutrient intakes in a regional population was successfully used with an FFQ developed to estimate total diet *(50)*.

Most FFQs have been designed to be self-administered and require 30–60 min to complete, depending on the instrument and the respondent. The process of completing an FFQ, although not burdensome, can be a high-level cognitive process. Subar et al. *(51)* attempted to address many of the cognitive processes involved with completing an FFQ when redesigning the DHQ. However, the mathematical and conceptual burden of calculating usual intake may be a particular challenge to individuals with lower education levels. As a result, a proportion of respondents report intakes that are implausible—either too high or too low. For example, the same interactive multimedia FFQ *(44,52)* was administered to middle- and upper-income adults, high-school seniors, and graduate equivalency diploma (GED) enrollees *(53)*. The prevalence of erroneous results (e.g., <600 kcal or ≥5000 kcal) ranged from 2.5%, 9%, to 19%, respectively. Low-literacy audiences are especially prone to difficulties with the FFQ that can be attenuated by using an interviewer as opposed to self-administration *(54)*.

The studies that have used a self-administered semi-quantitative FFQ most successfully include the Nurses' Health Study and the Health Professional Follow-Up study *(2,55)*. All of the respondents in these cohorts are well-educated, which likely contributes to more valid dietary estimates from the FFQ, compared with other study samples. This may explain the ability of the researchers affiliated with these cohorts to detect strong associations between FFQ dietary estimates and disease *(56)*, because dietary measurement error would be attenuated. When the estimated energy intake from the "Willett" FFQ was compared with total energy expenditure based on DLW in 10 young women (mean age 25.2 yr) and 10 older women (mean age 75.0 yr), the FFQ gave significantly lower values for the young women, but not the older women *(9)*. On the other hand, the OPEN Study recruited highly educated subjects and found underreporting in men to be 31–36% for estimated energy intake from the DHQ compared with total energy expenditure as measured by DLW *(24)*. The equivalent comparison for women was underreporting of 34–38%. This is of great concern because underreporting in an FFQ contributes to severe attenuation in estimating disease relative risks. Schatzkin *(57)* and Kipnis and colleagues *(58)* provide excellent discussions of this problem.

3. MANAGING IMPLAUSIBLE DIETARY ESTIMATES

Because it is impossible to monitor the energy expenditure (EE) of every subject in a study, methods to evaluate under- and overreporters become necessary. Goldberg and colleagues *(59)* proposed a cutoff based on energy intake (EI) as estimated by a dietary assessment method, and EE as estimated by available formulas that include age, weight, height, and gender. Underreporters are considered to be those individuals in whom the EI is less than 0.76 of the EE. Acceptable levels are 0.76–1.24. Overreporters are considered to be those with an EI to EE of more than 1.24. The original formula assumes that everyone has a sedentary lifestyle, and this has been improved with the addition of physical activity level *(60,61)*. Several researchers have examined alternatives to identifying inaccurate dietary reports *(7,62)*. Although these cutoffs are based on energy, it is important to realize that underreporting and overreporting are selective, and not all nutrients or foods may be underreported or overreported the same way. Another approach is to identify absolute levels of energy intake that are improbable given the FFQ instrument used. Commonly used cut-offs are less than 600 kcal and 5000 kcal or more *(2)*. It is important to check that any individuals identified with implausible values do not differ from the entire sample, especially with respect to any parameters directly related to the study's objective. Completing data analysis with and without the extreme values can strengthen any conclusions made.

4. BRIEF DIETARY ASSESSMENT METHODS

The questionnaires for brief dietary assessment methods are developed specifically for measuring a single food group or nutrient *(63)*, or behaviors such as removing skin from chicken before eating or using low-fat salad dressing *(64)*. If an FFQ is shortened to 15–30 foods, then it is considered a brief dietary assessment method *(32)*. For example, to develop a brief "fat screener," Block identified 13 foods that accounted for most of the intake of fat of American women *(65)*, and used the same technique to develop a "fruit and vegetable screener" *(65)*. In the fruit and vegetable module for the Behavioral Risk Factor Surveillance System (BRFSS), two questions assess fruit intake, and four questions assess vegetable intake for a total of seven questions *(66)*. By reducing a 31-item FFQ to a seven-item questionnaire, a brief assessment method to estimate fruit, juice, and vegetable intake in an African-American population was created *(67)*.

Neuhouser and colleagues *(68)* developed and validated a useful brief dietary assessment tool blending features of the 24-h dietary recall and the FFQ, and coined the term *focused recall*. The focused recall is intended to produce detailed information that is focused on a specific group of foods eaten during the previous 24 h. The investigators' purpose in developing the tool was to target the co-consumption of carotenoid-containing fruits and vegetables with savory snacks; however, the approach can be generalized to any specific group of foods, such as dairy or milk products. As a brief method, the tool holds promise when recent intake of a limited class of foods is relevant to a research project.

As with any dietary assessment method, the brief assessment method needs to be evaluated against some other measure of truth; as was done by Neuhouser et al (68). The advantages of the brief methods are their inherent ease in completion by the respondent and their ease of analysis by the investigators. The method's advantage is also its disadvantage—the narrow focus may be limiting for many studies.

5. TYPES OF EPIDEMIOLOGIC STUDIES AND DIETARY ASSESSMENT METHODS

Other dietary assessment methods do exist, and traditional methods are being adapted; however, the four previously covered represent the major methods in use today. An excellent overview of available tools can be found in the comprehensive review done by Thompson and Byer (1) and later adapted (32). Keeping in mind the primary principles of each method, their uses in different study designs are covered next.

5.1. Cross-Sectional Study Design and Surveillance Systems

One of the most common study designs is the cross-sectional study that provides a "snapshot" of the dietary practices of a population at a particular point in time as outlined in Fig. 4. In population study designs, one first determines the target population for which the conclusions of the study will be drawn. This will comprise the source population. Because it is nearly impossible to collect dietary and health information on a complete census, a sample from the source population is selected following recognized sampling techniques.

The source population can be the entire noninstitutionalized population in the country, as is the case with the sample drawn for the NHANES, or the residents of a state, as in the BRFSS, or targeted residents of a state, as in the Massachusetts Hispanic Elders Study (MAHES) (69). For these types of studies, the investigators would assess the subjects' dietary characteristics, then, for analysis purposes, the individuals would be classified as either exposed to a dietary factor and "diseased," exposed to a factor and not "diseased," not exposed to a factor and "diseased," or not exposed to a factor or not "diseased."

This study design has its limitations when examining the association of diet and its role in the etiology of a disease. Any disease that has a long latency period, such as cancer or osteoporosis, would not work for this design. This design cannot be used with diseases that alter the exposure. For example, individuals diagnosed with osteoporosis may increase their dietary and supplemental calcium intake secondary to physician orders, thus leading to the false conclusion that high calcium intake is associated with osteoporosis. In these cases, results cannot distinguish if diet was a result of the disease or if the diet preceded the disease. Nonetheless, this is a valuable study design that can address many research questions using the appropriate dietary assessment methods and research questions for this design.

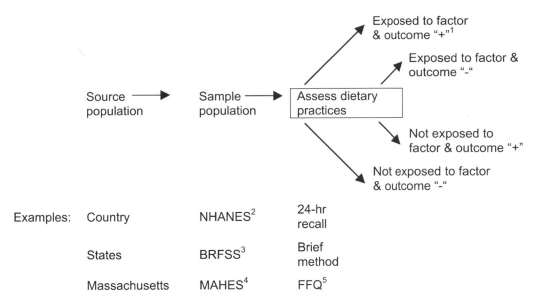

Fig. 4. Cross-sectional study and surveillance system basic design with examples of studies and dietary assessment methods used to assess dietary exposures for health outcomes (*see* text for references).

[1]"+" is positive, "−" is negative. Traditionally, outcomes have been disease-present or disease-absent, such as high blood pressure. However, outcomes can also be risk factors or measures of nutritional status, such as overweight, level of nutrient stores, hyperlipidemia.

[2]National Health and Nutrition Examination Survey, United States.

[3]Behavioral Risk Factor Surveillance System, United States.

[4]Massachusetts Hispanic Elders Study, a statewide survey conducted between 1993 and 1997 that included a representative sample of elderly Hispanics and a neighborhood control group of non-Hispanic whites.

[5]Food frequency questionnaire.

For the cross-sectional study, both the 24-h recall and the food record have the advantage of providing dietary intake information about actual foods eaten during the specified period of time of the cross-sectional analysis. The detail of foods consumed can be used for analysis according to nutrients and portion sizes, as well as dietary and food patterns. On the other hand, if the period of recall desired is months prior to the interview, the FFQ may be the more appropriate choice, as long as relative differences between groups is appropriate to answer the primary research question. The FFQ almost becomes the instrument of choice when study population size becomes large and/or if resources are limited. If the subjects are at remote sites in relation to the research center, the FFQ may be favored because it can be mailed to subjects. Alternatively, the 24-h dietary recall has been shown to work equally well in-person as well as over the telephone, allowing access to distant subjects (70).

5.1.1. USING THE 24-HOUR DIETARY RECALL IN A CROSS-SECTIONAL STUDY

A study by Novotny et al. (71) had as its primary purpose to identify contributors to differences in calcium intakes among Asian, Hispanic, and non-Hispanic White adolescents. In selecting a dietary assessment method, the investigators considered the potential differences in dietary intakes secondary to cultural food practices; thus a method that allowed for specific foods to be recorded was necessary. Another factor was the age of the subjects. With ages between 11 and 19 yr, the investigators questioned the ability of the younger subjects to thoroughly complete food records. Based on these concerns and given that sufficient trained staff were available, the decision was made to use the 24-h dietary recall. Ideally, more than 2 d were desired; however, resources limited the final decision to two nonconsecutive days at least 1 wk apart, with the completion of approx 75% of the 24-h dietary recalls on weekdays and 25% on weekends. In the end, two 24-h dietary recalls were collected from 176 children of Asian, Hispanic, or non-Hispanic White background using the triple-pass method for the 24-h dietary recall. The multiple-pass method added the advantage of being a well-documented method with specific procedures that worked well, as the study sites encompassed five different states and identical procedures could be implemented.

After compiling the dietary data, Novotny and colleagues were able to ascertain that milk consumption was the most powerful indicator of calcium intake among each group of children despite their varied intakes. Further, the detail of the 24-h recall allowed for the observation that milk portion size was significantly associated with soda consumption, especially among the Hispanic adolescents, whereas the Asian children tended to consume higher-fat dairy foods with lower calcium content (e.g., ice cream and milk shakes). Thus, the detail of the two 24-h dietary recalls allowed the investigators to conclude that displacement of milk by soda among the Hispanic adolescents and filling-up on higher-fat milk products for the Asian adolescents may contribute to their lower calcium intakes than the non-Hispanic White adolescents, thus providing direction for targeted messages to youth concerning inadequate calcium intakes.

5.1.2. Using a Food Frequency Questionnaire in a Cross-Sectional Study

Application of an FFQ is limited to the populations for which the FFQ was designed. This becomes especially important with regard to cultural or regionally based foods. The MAHES is a cross-sectional study that was initiated to study issues of diet and health among Hispanic adults living in the northeastern United States (69). To estimate dietary intake, the investigators adapted a version of the "Block" FFQ by modifying the food list and portion sizes based on data from the Hispanic Health and Nutrition Examination Survey and the Second NHANES. The revised FFQ was evaluated by comparing nutrient intakes between the FFQ and 24-h dietary recalls. Added foods included plantains, avocado, mango, cassava, empanadas, and custard. One of the published manuscripts from this cross-sectional study using the FFQ assessed fruit and vegetable intake and its association with total homocysteine (Hcy) and C-reactive protein (CRP) (72). Significant dose–response relationships for both plasma CRP and Hcy concentrations with frequency of fruits and vegetable intake were observed. Had the investigators not made the initial investment to revise and test the FFQ, this significant relationship may not have been found in this cross-sectional analysis.

5.1.3. Using a Brief Dietary Assessment Method in Surveillance

The BRFSS is a telephone-based surveillance program conducted by the Centers for Disease Control and Prevention. As mentioned earlier, the fruit and vegetable brief dietary assessment questionnaire used by BRFSS has seven questions that have been

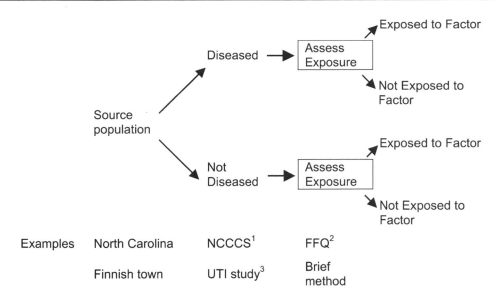

Fig. 5. Case–control study basic design with examples of studies and dietary assessment methods used to assess dietary exposures by disease outcome (*see* text for references).
[1]North Carolina Colon Cancer Study.
[2]Food frequency questionnaire.
[3]Urinary tract infection.

evaluated against other measures *(73)*. This questionnaire works well for the surveillance system because of its brevity especially in the context of other modules covered in one telephone interview. Keeping the interview within a reasonable amount of time improves participation. Each state uses the same set of questions, thus allowing comparisons of fruit and vegetable intake across states. The same questionnaire is used between years so that the achievement of five servings of fruits and vegetables daily over time can be monitored.

5.2. Case–Control Study Design

The case–control study design is often the study design of first choice when the disease of interest is a relatively rare event, such as cancer. Either all individuals with the disease of interest are recruited as being in the study population as "cases," or a random sample of individuals with disease are recruited as "cases." The comparison group or "controls" are selected as a random sample of the study population that represents the same community from which the "cases" were derived, as shown in Fig. 5. In matched case–control studies, each "case" is matched with one or more "controls" of the same age, gender, and possibly other factors that may confound the relationship of dietary exposure to disease.

Because the cases already have disease, the period of exposure of interest is the time before the onset of disease. Given this situation, the food record and 24-h recall, which reflect recent intake, are not applicable to this study design, because intakes are often altered by treatment regimens and the primary exposure may be in the distant past. That leaves the FFQ as the method of choice for a case–control study, with the reference period for food recall usually being 1 yr prior to the diagnosis of disease. Because the cases generally are recruited fairly quickly after diagnosis of disease, the period of dietary recall reference for controls is often the year preceding the interview. Although there is the possibility of recall bias on the part of the cases having more at stake in remembering past events, there is otherwise no reason to think that the cases' and controls' abilities to recall over a past year would systematically vary. For some diseases, an individual's long-term dietary profile (e.g., the last 10 yr) would be an ideal time frame for dietary exposure; however, the ability of an individual to recall diet decreases when asked to recall 5 or 10 yr back (1,74,75).

5.2.1. USING A FOOD FREQUENCY QUESTIONNAIRE IN A CASE–CONTROL STUDY

The North Carolina Colon Cancer Study (NCCCS) examines risks for colon cancer in African Americans and whites (76). The investigators of this study modified the "Block" FFQ to accommodate commonly eaten foods in North Carolina. For the analyses of the association of micronutrients to colon cancer risk (76), only those nutrients that are reasonably captured by FFQs were included. These were identified as β-carotene, lutein, vitamins C and E, folate, and calcium. Supplement use was assessed with separate closed-ended questions. The researchers observed that in whites, the highest quartiles of β-carotene, vitamin C, and calcium intakes were associated with 40–60% reductions in colon cancer risk compared with the lowest quartiles. In African Americans, vitamins C and E were strongly inversely associated with a reduced risk for colon cancer. Despite the findings being consistent with previous research, the difference in risk by nutrients between the two groups was puzzling to the authors. Such observations could potentially result from errors in the measurement of diet by the FFQ and justifies further examination of diet and disease relationships and investigation of improved long-term recall methods.

5.2.2. USING A BRIEF DIETARY ASSESSMENT METHOD IN A CASE–CONTROL STUDY

A brief dietary assessment method was implemented very cleverly by Finnish investigators examining the role of diet as a risk factor for urinary tract infection (UTI) with a case–control study design (77). Because UTIs are believed to be caused by bacteria in the stool, dietary factors may affect the risk of contracting a UTI by altering the properties of the fecal bacterial flora. Women of an average age of 31 yr with a diagnosis of UTI were case-matched with women with no episode of UTI in the past 5 yr. A total of 107 case–control pairs were recruited. The investigators used a remarkably simple brief dietary assessment questionnaire that included 18 questions on milk and other dairy products, berries and berry juices, soft drinks, and coffee. For example, women were asked their frequency of consumption during the past month of milk (fresh or fermented with probiotics) and responses were never, less than one time per week, one to three times per week, and three or more times per week. Another question asked their average consumption during the past month of certain products, including milk, sour milk, and yogurt, as glasses (2 dL/d). The results showed an inverse association between mean daily use of fresh juice (fruit or berry, dL) and onset of UTI, odds ratio: 0.66 (95% confidence interval: 0.48, 0.92). For probiotic milk products, a significant inverse association was observed between frequency of consumption and occurrence of UTI. This particular tool was short and identified very specific dietary patterns; however, it performed its purpose of identifying possible mediators of UTI in this sample of women.

5.3. The Cohort or Prospective Study Design

The cohort study design starts with a healthy group exposed to varying extents to a given nutrient, and follows the group prospectively, counting the members who develop disease. It may be either concurrent (i.e., the observation is concurrent with the exposure) or nonconcurrent (i.e., the exposure precedes much or all of the observation). An example of the enrollment of participants that will be followed over a period of time is shown in Fig. 6. Closed cohort studies with fixed membership often include some type of dietary assessment. For a closed cohort, a source population is identified, then a sampling frame is created and only those individuals at risk for the disease or diseases under investigation are included at baseline. For example, the Nurses' Health Study was initiated to investigate the potential long-term consequences of the use of oral contraceptives *(78)*. So even though no single disease was identified, one needed to be a woman to be at risk for consequences due to oral contraceptives. The investigators selected nurses to follow, because they would provide a motivated population-base of women capable of completing detailed health questionnaires. The selection process was further narrowed to married registered nurses between 30 and 55 yr of age, who lived in the 11 most populous states and whose nursing boards agreed to supply their members' names and addresses. The final baseline cohort members were those women that responded to the initial questionnaire.

Once the members of a cohort have been established, baseline characteristics and risk factors of interest are measured, and then the members of the cohort are followed for onset of disease. There is a profound advantage with the cohort approach. Dietary intake is recorded prior to occurrence of any disease; therefore the dietary information is not biased by the diagnosis of disease. On the other hand, if the follow-up of the cohort members is a long period prior to the onset of disease, the diet may not appropriately reflect the average intake of the cohort members over time. Many cohorts in existence today have addressed this issue by collecting dietary intake at periodic intervals.

Because the purpose of the dietary assessment at baseline for a cohort is to estimate their current intake, almost every dietary assessment method can be considered. Recall that most nutrients have large day-to-day variation; thus, if a 24-h dietary recall or food record were selected, two or more days of each would have to be collected *(36,38)*. Given that cohorts must be large in order to detect any significant differences between exposed groups, the collection and analysis of 24-h dietary recalls and food records would prove to be expensive and impractical. The Nurses' Health Study previously described enrolled 122,000 women *(78)*—that would be too great a number of food records or 24-h dietary recalls to collect over the telephone. For this reason, the dietary assessment method of first choice in a cohort study is the FFQ. As an alternative, investigators can collect more detailed dietary information via multiple food records from a smaller sample of cohort members to assist with evaluation of the FFQ (if it had not been previously validated) and correction of possible measurement error in the FFQ *(79)*. However, sample selection from the cohort is not a trivial task, if one wants to ensure unbiased correlations between the two intake methods *(80)*. Some of the earlier initiated cohorts, such as the Framingham Heart Study *(81)* and the Honolulu Heart Study *(82)*, initially used a single 24-h dietary recall and later adopted study-specific FFQs.

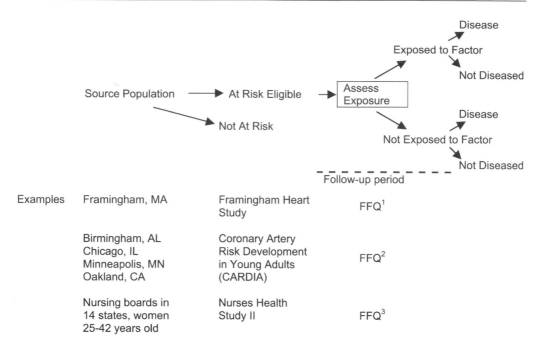

Fig. 6. Cohort or prospective basic design with examples of studies and dietary assessment methods used to assess dietary exposures prior to health outcomes (*see* text for references).
[1]Framingham Heart Study originally used a 24-h dietary recall to collect dietary information and switched to a semi-quantitative food frequency.
[2]A quantitative food frequency questionnaire is used.
[3]A semi-quantitative food frequency is used.

Another form of the cohort or prospective study design is the randomized trial. This is set apart from the observational cohort study in that the eligible subjects are randomized to receive an exposure of interest (e.g., vitamin A supplements or intensive dietary intervention). Figure 6 can be used to depict a randomized trial by replacing "Assess Exposure" with "Allocate Exposure at Random." Whichever dietary assessment method is used to measure effectiveness of an intervention, the subjects, in providing their responses, are more prone to social desirability, especially the treatment subjects *(83)*. Some approaches to counteracting this phenomenon include using more than one dietary assessment measure, using grocery shopping receipts, or using a biomarker. Much less work has been done on developing valid methods for measuring dietary change in population-based randomized trials than for any other study design *(83–85)*.

Another modification of the cohort method or prospective method is to use the prerecorded disease rates in a national or regional population for control purposes, rather than selecting a specially selected control group. This approach is appropriate when the exposure to the risk factor in the general population is negligible. Goulding and colleagues *(86,87)* adopted this approach using a nonconcurrent cohort design for 50 children 3–10 yr of age who had a history of avoiding the consumption of cow milk for less than 4 mo at some stage in their lives. Assuming that the exposure in the general population is minimal with regard to long-term avoidance of cow milk, the number of fractures in this group of 50 children was compared with the fracture rates in a pre-existing birth cohort

(87). In this analysis, the number of fractures in the avoidance group was compared with the numbers that would have been expected if subjects had experienced the same fracture rates specific for age and sex as the birth cohort (representing the general population). Although the exposure of cow milk avoidance was gathered retrospectively, this type of dietary exposure is not subject to the same recall bias as the detailed consumption of specific foods. In addition, among this young age group, the assumption that few children avoid cow milk for long periods of time is probably valid, thus allowing this approach of using the birth cohort as a general community control group.

5.3.1. USING A SEMI-QUANTITATIVE FOOD FREQUENCY QUESTIONNAIRE IN A COHORT STUDY

In 1980, the Nurses' Health Study started measuring dietary exposures with the addition of a semi-quantitative food frequency questionnaire to its battery of questionnaires (http://www.nurseshealthstudy.org/). The decision to use a self-administered FFQ worked well for this cohort because the questionnaire could be mailed to the respondents residing in 11 different states and easily returned upon completion with the other questionnaires. Because the members of this cohort are well-educated, they are in a position to appropriately calculate some of the mathematical problems posed by having one reference portion size. For example, the frequency would need to be increased if the usual portion size was double the portion size noted in the questionnaire.

The contribution of portion size to the ranking of individuals for vitamin A intake was examined by Samet et al. *(88)*. They compared the ranking of individuals by frequency alone and by "usual" portion sizes based on an in-person interview. The correlations between the methods were 0.86 for controls and 0.91 for cases. These results suggested that portion size questions provided little additional information and supported their decision to use the semi-quantitative FFQ with the cohort of nurses. Another decision was the period of recall. Women were asked to recall food intake for over the past year. An extensive evaluation was conducted by Willet and colleagues among a sub-sample of the cohort population *(89)*. The FFQ was completed followed by 28 d of food records spread out over 1 yr. At the end of the year, another FFQ was completed. The average nutrient intakes from the food records were compared to the estimated nutrient intakes from the FFQ. The correlation coefficients ranged between 0.5 and 0.7, indicating a satisfactory comparison between the two dietary assessment methods.

5.3.2. USING A QUANTITATIVE FOOD FREQUENCY QUESTIONNAIRE IN A COHORT STUDY

The Coronary Artery Risk Development in Young Adults (CARDIA) Study was initiated to study the evolution of cardiovascular disease risk factors *(90)*. This is a multicenter population-based prospective study of black and non-Hispanic white young adults using four study centers in Birmingham, AL, Chicago, IL, Minneapolis, MN, and Oakland, CA. The goal for the dietary assessment measure was to assess patterns of food and nutrient intake relating to the development of coronary heart disease. The food frequency approach was appealing because it does not bias intakes and a minimum level of education is needed to complete the questionnaire. The investigators modified the 28-d dietary history used with the Western Electric study because this method had adequately defined intakes of saturated fat and cholesterol, which were found to be significantly associated with coronary heart disease *(79)*. Modifications included identifying foods frequently consumed from results of the NHANES II to reflect the current food supply (at the time) and the intakes of a younger and more diverse population. The final format consisted of three parts: (1) questions about usual dietary patterns, (2) an assessment of sodium intake, and (3) a quantitative FFQ. The period of recall was set to the previous 28 d because this time-frame was found to be compatible with an achievable recall period and the period would correlate well with serum measures influenced by diet within this period of time. Rather than allow it to be self-administered, the decision was made to administer the questionnaire by interview, thus further minimizing the issue of differences in comprehension among study participants. The investigators recognized in advance that a 28-d recall period would not reflect seasonal changes in food intake. However, interviews were scheduled throughout the year so that seasonal intakes would be determined for the group. The relative validity of the final dietary assessment tool was evaluated by comparison with food records *(79)*. Even after 15 yr of follow-up, the detail incorporated into the questionnaire allowed the investigators to identify the frequency of dairy foods consumed by the subjects *(91)*. In overweight adults, the exposure to dairy foods was found to be inversely associated with insulin resistance syndrome, a risk factor for type 2 diabetes and cardiovascular disease.

6. CALCIUM-SPECIFIC FOOD QUESTIONNAIRES

There is a unique tool called the "Dietary Assessment Calibration/Evaluation Register" available on-line that catalogs the evaluation of dietary assessment methods. When selecting a dietary assessment method, this may be a useful first stop (http://www-dacv.ims.nci.nih.gov/) *(92)*. The comprehensive review by McPherson and colleagues in 2000 *(93)*, which evaluated dietary assessment methods among children 5–18 yr of age, would be useful for planning projects with children. Many calcium-specific FFQs have been evaluated among a variety of adult populations in the United States *(94–99)* with correlation coefficients ranging between 0.33 and 0.85. For Asian, Hispanic, and non-Hispanic white adolescents in the United States, a semi-quantitative FFQ has been extensively evaluated *(46,100)*. Calcium-specific FFQs have been developed and evaluated for use with adults in Sweden *(101)*, Italy *(102)*, Australia *(103)*, Malaysia *(104)*, and Mexico *(105)*, as well as children in New Zealand *(106)*. If one were to adopt one of these tools, it would be important to evaluate the tool if the populations differ dramatically. In addition, with the current level of calcium fortification in the food supply, tools developed in the distant past may not reflect these new sources of calcium.

7. EVALUATING DIETARY ASSESSMENT METHODS

The examples previously described highlight that the final choice of a dietary assessment method is driven not only by the study design, but by the target population, the study objectives, the outcome of interest, and the available resources *(45)*. The other issue alluded to throughout this chapter is the validity of any method for measuring the nutrient, food or food patterns of interest. Before closing this chapter, this issue will briefly be addressed. More detailed discussions can be found elsewhere *(2,24,26,32,107–110)*.

As with any measure, there is a desire to insure that the measure is reliable or reproducible and valid. With dietary assessment methods, this presents a challenge because the opportunities to directly observe and record what individuals eat over an extended period of time are limited (e.g., feeding studies). As a result, a common approach to evaluating a dietary assessment method is to compare one method with a different type of method. For example, a food frequency may be compared with multiple food records; an advantage of comparing an FFQ to food records is that the records would not have the same memory bias as the food frequency. Because this type of comparison is basically relating one method to another, some have referred to this as "calibration" *(111)*. However, this may be confusing because calibration implies a resetting to a standard, which is not the intention of "calibration" with regard to dietary assessment. Thus, a recommendation has been made to refer to all aspects of testing the reliability and validity of dietary assessment methods as "evaluation" *(112)*. In general, correlation coefficients range between 0.4 and 0.7 for comparison between dietary assessment methods *(2,45)*. These coefficient ranges highlight the existence of measurement error in all dietary assessment methods, and thus various methods of energy adjustment *(2)*, methods of correcting for measurement error *(113)*, and investigations to better understand measurement error have been employed *(24)*.

It may be tempting to use a method previously evaluated as reliable and valid; however, one must recognize that a method validated with one group may not be applicable to another *(45,114)*. For example, Jensen et al. *(46)* evaluated a semi-quantitative food frequency among Asian, Hispanic, and non-Hispanic white adolescents primarily in the Western United States. The tool may not work as well with African-American adolescents in the southern United States, and an effort to evaluate the tool with this group would be prudent prior to adopting its use in a research study. All dietary assessment methods have some degree of measurement error *(115)*; therefore, efforts to keep these errors to a minimum must be implemented *(116)*.

The real challenge is comparing the results of the dietary assessment method with some measure of "truth." This is best achieved by identifying a biomarker of a nutrient or dietary factor *(26,117)*. The underlying assumption of a biomarker is that it responds to intake in a dose-dependent relationship *(2)*. The method that has widest consensus as a valid biomarker is DLW for energy *(26,118)*. Because DLW provides an accurate measure of total energy expenditure in free-living subjects, it has been successfully used to compare energy expenditure to estimated energy intake as determined by a dietary assessment tool. A biomarker does not rely on a self-report of food intake, thus theoretically the measurement errors of the biomarker are not likely to be correlated with those of the dietary assessment method. Another proposed biomarker is analysis of nitrogen from 24-h urine collections as an indicator for protein intake *(29,119)*. Other biomarkers collected from urine samples include potassium and sodium *(29)*. Plasma or serum biomarkers that have been explored are levels of ascorbic acid for vitamin C intake *(29,120)*, β-carotene for fruits and vegetables or antioxidants *(85,120,121)*. These latter markers are widely influenced by factors such as smoking status and supplement use, thus their interpretation as measures of absolute intake is limited.

Whereas a biomarker for a nutrient makes sense, a biomarker for an identified "healthy food pattern" may be unrealistic. Some nutrients are lacking in biologically valid biomarkers, such as calcium for adults. On the other hand, bone mineral content (BMC) as measured by dual-energy X-ray absorptiometry in young non-Hispanic white girls may be considered a cumulative historic marker. When comparing the estimated calcium intake from a semi-quantitative FFQ to bone measures in 14 non-Hispanic white females between 10 and 14 yr of age, a significant correlation coefficient ($r = 0.638$, $p = 0.014$) between total body BMC and calcium intake was observed *(100)*. However, this was not found to be the case in African-American girls representing the same age group and following the same study protocol. The correlation coefficient was $r = -0.116$ ($p = 0.680$). This discrepancy could be due to differences in reporting, the FFQ not being appropriate for the African-American girls, and/or the BMC not being a biomarker for African-American girls. This highlights that any biomarker must be fully evaluated prior to its adoption in a particular study. Biomarkers cannot substitute for the dietary information collected from recalls, records, FFQs, or brief dietary assessment methods. Biomarkers can be used to validate the dietary information; however, the foods that contribute to a nutrient's presence can only be found by asking individuals what they eat.

8. CONCLUSIONS

Nutritional epidemiology is concerned with quantifying dietary exposures and their association with disease risk. There is no one dietary method that is considered a "gold standard." The choice of an appropriate dietary assessment method is dependent on the study design, the research objectives, the target population, and resources. Improved methods of collecting more accurate dietary information continue to be developed and refined. To corroborate results from dietary intake data, biological markers of nutritional exposures and nutritional status (referred to as biomarkers) are being developed to be used in tandem with dietary assessment methods. This chapter has described the reasons for adopting a particular dietary assessment method given a specific study design. Examples from the literature aid in outlining the decisions that investigators make to select or adapt a dietary assessment tool.

REFERENCES

1. Thompson FE, Byers T. Dietary assessment resource manual. J Nutr 1994;124 (Supplement)(11S): 2245S–2317S.
2. Willett W. Nutritional Epidemiology, 2 ed. Oxford University Press, New York: 1998.
3. Campbell VA, Dodds ML. Collecting dietary information from groups of older people. J Am Diet Assoc 1967;51:29–33.
4. Moshfegh AJ. The national nutrition monitoring and related research program: Progress and activities. J Nutr 1994;124(Supplement):1843S–1845S.
5. Moshfegh A, Borrud L, Perloff B, LaComb R. Improved method for the 24-hour dietary recall for use in national surveys. FASEB J 13(4), A603. 1999.
6. Klesges RC, Eck LH, Ray JW. Who underreports dietary intake in a dietary recall? Evidence from the Second National Health and Nutrition Examination Survey. J Consult Clin Psychol 1995;63:438–444.
7. Tooze JA, Subar AF, Thompson FE, Troiano RP, Schatzkin A, Kipnis V. Psychosocial predictors of energy underreporting in a large doubly labeled water study. Am J Clin Nutr 2004;79:795–804.
8. Bathalon GP, Tucker KL, Hays NP, Vinken AG, Greenberg AS, McCrory MA et al. Psychological measures of eating behavior and the accuracy of 3 common dietary assessment methods in healthy postmenopausal women. Am J Clin Nutr 2000;71:739–745.
9. Sawaya AL, Tucker K, Tsay R, et al. Evaluation of four methods for determining energy intake in young and older women: comparison with doubly labeled water measurements of total energy expenditure. Am J Clin Nutr 1996;63:491–499.
10. Johnson RK, Soultanakis RP, Matthews DE. Literacy and body fatness are associated with underreporting of energy intake in US low-income women using the multiple-pass 24-hour recall: a doubly labeled water study. J Am Diet Assoc 1998;98(10):1136–1140.
11. Krebs-Smith SM, Graubard BI, Kahle LL, Subar AF, Cleveland LE, Ballard-Barbash R. Low energy reporters vs others: a comparison of reported food intakes. Eur J Clin Nutr 2000;54(4):281–287.
12. Harnack L, Steffen L, Arnett DK, Gao S, Luepker RV. Accuracy of estimation of large food portions. J Am Diet Assoc 2004;104:804–806.

13. Nielsen SJ, Popkin BM. Patterns and trends in food portion sizes, 1977–1998. JAMA 2003;289(4):450–453.

14. Young LR, Nestle M. The contribution of expanding portion sizes to the US obesity epidemic. Am J Public Health 2002;92(2):246–249.

15. McGuire B, Chambers E4, Godwin S, Brenner S. Size categories most effective for estimating portion size of muffins. J Am Diet Assoc 2001;101(4):470–472.

16. Matheson DM, Hanson KA, McDonald TE, Robinson TN. Validity of children's food portion estimates. Arch Pediatr Adolesc Med 2002;156:867–871.

17. McKenzie DC, Johnson RK, Harvey-Berino J, Gold BC. Impact of interviewer's body mass index on underreporting energy intake in overweight and obese women. Obes Res 2002;10(6):471–477.

18. Fisher JO, Johnson RK, Lindquist C, Birch LL, Goran MI. Influence of body composition on the accuracy of reported energy intake of children. Obes Res 2000;8(8):597–603.

19. Johnson RK, Driscoll P, Goran MI. Comparison of multiple-pass 24-hour recall estimates of energy intake with total energy expenditure determined by the doubly labeled water method in young children. J Am Diet Assoc 1996;96(11):1140–1144.

20. Jonnalagadda SS, Mitchell DC, Smiciklas-Wright H, et al. Accuracy of energy intake data estimated by a multiple-pass, 24 hour dietary recall technique. J Am Diet Assoc 2000;100(3):303–308.

21. Samuel-Hodge CD, Fernandez LM, Henriquez-Roldan CF, Johnston LF, Keyserling TC. A comparison of self-reported energy intake with total energy expenditure estimated by accelerometer and basal metabolic rate in African-American women with type 2 diabetes. Diabetes Care 2004;27(3):663–669.

22. Conway JM, Ingwersen LA, Vinyard BT, Moshfegh AJ. Effectiveness of the US Department of Agriculture 5-step multiple-pass method in assessing food intake in obese and nonobese women. Am J Clin Nutr 2003;77(5):1171–1178.

23. Conway JM, Ingwersen LA, Moshfegh AJ. Accuracy of dietary recall using the USDA five-step multiple-pass method in men: an observational validation study. J Am Diet Assoc 2004;104(4):595–603.

24. Subar AF, Kipnis V, Troiano R, et al. Using intake biomarkers to evaluate the extent of dietary misreporting in a large sample of adults: The OPEN Study. Am J Epidemiol 2003;158(1):1–13.

25. Rebro SM, Patterson RE, Kristal AR, Cheney CL. The effect of keeping food records on eating patterns. J Am Diet Assoc 1998;98(10):1163–1165.

26. Trabulsi J, Schoeller DA. Evaluation of dietary assessment instruments against doubly labeled water, a biomarker of habitual energy intake. Am J Physiol Endocrinol Metab 2001;281:E891–E899.

27. Bolland JE, Ward JY, Bolland TW. Improved accuracy of estimating food quantities up to 4 weeks after training. J Am Diet Assoc 1990;90(10):1402–1407.

28. Johnson RK, Goran MI, Poehlman ET. Correlates of over- and underreporting of energy intake in healthy older men and women. Am J Clin Nutr 1994;59(6):1286–1290.

29. McKeown NM, Day NE, Welch AA, et al. Use of biological markers to validate self-reported dietary intake in a random sample of the European Prospective Investigation into Cancer United Kingdom Norfolk cohort. Am J Clin Nutr 2001;74:188–196.

30. Craig MR, Kristal AR, Cheney CL, Shattuck AL. The prevalence and impact of 'atypical' days in 4-day food records. J Am Diet Assoc 2000;100(4):421–527.

31. Hebert JR, Ebbeling CB, Matthews CE, et al. Systematic errors in middle-aged women's estimates of energy intake: Comparing three self-report measures to total energy expenditure from doubly labeled water. Ann Epidemiol 2002;12:577–586.

32. Thompson FE, Subar AF. Dietary Assessment Methodology. In: Coulston AM, Rock CL, Monsen ER, eds. Nutrition in the Prevention and Treatment of Disease. Academic, San Diego: 2001; pp. 3–30.

33. Institute of Medicine National Academy of Sciences. *Dietary Reference Intakes Applications in Dietary Assessment*. National Academy Press, Washington, DC: 2001.

34. Palaniappan U, Cue RI, Payette H, Gray-Donald K. Implications of day-to-day variability on measurements of usual food and nutrient intakes. J Nutr 2003;133(1):232–235.

35. Nusser SM, Carriquiry AL, Dodd KW, Fuller WA. A semiparametric transformation approach to estimating usual daily intake distribution. J Am Stat Assoc 1996;91:1440–1449.

36. Liu K, Stamler J, Dyer A, McKeever J, McKeever P. Statistical methods to assess and minimize the role of intra-individual variability in obscuring the relationship between dietary lipids and serum cholesterol. J Chron Dis 1978;31:399–418.

37. Nelson M, Black AE, Morris JA, Cole TJ. Between- and within-subject variation in nutrient intake from infancy to old age: estimating the number of days required to rank dietary intakes with desired precision. Am J Clin Nutr 1989;50:155–167.

38. Beaton GH, Milner J, Corey P, et al. Sources of variance in 24-hour dietary recall data: Implications for nutrition study design and interpretation. Am J Clin Nutr 1979;32:2546–2549.

39. Block G, Thompson FE, Hartman AM, Larkin FA, Guire KE. Comparison of two dietary questionnaires validated against multiple dietary records collected during a 1-year period. J Am Diet Assoc 1992;92:686–693.

40. Nelson M, Margetts BM, Black AE. Checklist for the methods section of dietary investigations (Letters to the Editors). Br J Nutr 1993;69:935–940.

41. Subar AF, Thompson FE, Kipnis V, et al. Comparative validation of the Block, Willett, and National Cancer Institute food frequency questionnaires. Am J Epidemiol 2001;154:1089–1099.

42. Chu SY, Kolonel LN, Hankin JH, Lee J. A comparison of frequency and quantitative dietary methods for epidemiologic studies of diet and disease. Am J Epidemiol 1984;119:323–334.

43. Krebs-Smith SM, Subar AF, Guenther P, et al. Food propensity questionnaires (FPQs) in the National Health and Nutrition Examination Survey (NHANES): a step in the evolution of usual dietary intake estimation. Paper presented at: Experimental Biology;April 19; 2004;Washington, DC.

44. Block G, Miller M, Harnack L, Kayman S, Mandel S, Cristofar S. An interactive CD-ROM for nutrition screening and counseling. Am J Public Health 2000;90(5):781–785.

45. Subar AF. Developing dietary assessment tools. J Am Diet Assoc 2004;104(5):769–770.

46. Jensen JK, Gustafson D, Boushey CJ, et al. Development of a food frequency questionnaire to measure calcium intake of Asian, Hispanic, and white youth. J Am Diet Assoc 2004;104(5):762–769.

47. Kirk P, Patterson RE, Lampe J. Development of a soy food freuqency questionnaire to estimate isoflavone consumption in US adults. J Am Diet Assoc 1999;99(5):558–563.

48. Khani BR, Ye W, Terry P, Wolk A. Reproducibility and validity of major dietary patterns among Swedish women assessed with a food-frequency questionnaire. J Nutr 2004;134(6):1541–1545.

49. Hankin JH. 23rd Lenna Frances Cooper Memorial Lecture: a diet history method for research, clinical, and community use. J Am Diet Assoc 1986;86(7):868–875.

50. Cid-Ruzafa J, Caulfield LE, Barron Y, West SK. Nutrient intakes and adequacy among an older population on the eastern shore of Maryland: The Salisbury Eye Evaluation. J Am Diet Assoc 1999;99(5):564–571.

51. Subar AF, Thompson FE, Smith AF, et al. Improving food frequency questionnaires: A qualitative approach using cognitive interviewing. J Am Diet Assoc 1995;95(7):781–788.

52. Kolasa KM, Miller MG. New developments in nutrition education using computer technology. J Nutr Educ 1996;28:7–14.

53. Machtan A. *Stages of change for nutrition behaviors among GED enrollees and high school seniors.* [master's thesis]. Purdue University, 2002.

54. Slattery ML, Caan BJ, Duncan D, Berry TD, Coates A, Kerber R. A computerized diet history questionnaire for epidemiologic studies. J Am Diet Assoc 1994;94(7):761–766.

55. Wei EK, Giovannucci E, Wu K, et al. Comparison of risk factors for colon and rectal cancer. Int J Cancer 2004;108(3):433–442.

56. Rimm EB, Willett WC, Hu FB, et al. Folate and vitamin B_6 from diet and supplements in relation to risk of coronary heart disease among women. JAMA 1998;279:359–364.

57. Schatzkin A, Kipnis V, Carroll RJ, et al. A comparison of a food frequency questionnaire with a 24-hour recall for use in an epidemiological cohort study: results from the biojarker-based Observing Protein and Energy Nutrition (OPEN) study. Int J Epidemiol 2003;32:1054–1063.

58. Kipnis V, Subar AF, Midthune D, et al. Structure of dietary measurement error: Results of the OPEN study. Am J Epidemiol 2003;158:14–21.

59. Goldberg GR, Black AE, Jebb SA, et al. Critical evaluation of energy intake data using fundamental principles of energy physiology: 1. Derivation of cut-off limits to identify under-recording. Eur J Clin Nutr 1991;45:569–581.

60. Black AE. The sensitivity and specificity of the Goldberg cut-off for EI:BMR for identifying diet reports of poor validity. Eur J Clin Nutr 2000;54:395–404.

61. Livingstone MBE, Robson PJ, Black AE, et al. An evaluation of the sensitivity and specificity of energy expenditure measured by heart rate and the Goldberg cut-off for energy intake: basal metabolic rate for

indentifying mis-reporting of energy intake by adults and children: a retrospective analysis. Eur J Clin Nutr 2003;57:455–463.

62. McCrory MA, McCrory MA, Hajduk CL, Roberts SB. Procedures for screening out inaccurate reports of dietary energy intake. Public Health Nutr 2002;5(6A):873–882.

63. Prochaska JJ, Sallis JF, Rupp J. Screening measure for assessing dietary fat intake among adolescents. Prev Med 2001;33:699–706.

64. Kristal AR, Abrams BF, Thornquist MD, et al. Development and validation of a food use checklist for evaluation of community nutrition interventions. Am J Public Health 1990;80:1318–1322.

65. Block G, Gillespie C, Rosenbaum EH, Jenson C. A rapid food screener to assess fat and fruit and vegetable intake. Am J Prev Med 2000;18(4):284–288.

66. Nelson DE, Holtzman D, Bolen J, Stanwyck CA, Mack KA. Reliability and validity of measures from the Behavioral Risk Factor Surveillance System (BRFSS). Soz Praventivmed 2001;26(Suppl 1):S3–S42.

67. Warneke C, Davis M, De Moor C, Baranowski T. A 7-item versus a 31-item food frequency questionnaire for measuring fruit, juice, and vegetable intake among a predominantly African-American population. J Am Diet Assoc 2001;101(7):774–779.

68. Neuhouser ML, Patterson RE, Kristal AR, Eldridge AL, Vizenor NC. A brief dietary assessment instrument for assessing target foods, nutrients and eating patterns. Public Health Nutr 2000;4(1):73–78.

69. Tucker KL, Bermudez OI, Castaneda C. Type 2 diabetes is prevalent and poorly controlled among Hispanic elders of Caribbean origin. Am J Public Health 2000;90:1288–1293.

70. Tran KM, Johnson RK, Soultanakis RP, Matthews DE. In-person vs telephone-administered multiple-pass 24-hour recalls in women: validation with doubly labeled water. J Am Diet Assoc 2000;100(7):775–776.

71. Novotny R, Boushey C, Bock MA, et al. Calcium intake of Asian, Hispanic and White youth. J Am Coll Nutr 2003;22(1):64–70.

72. Gao X, Bermudez OI, Tucker KL. Plasma C-reactive protein and homocysteine concentrations are related to frequent fruit and vegetable intake in Hispanic and non-Hispanic White elders. J Nutr 2004;134:913–918.

73. Field AE, Colditz GA, Fox MK, et al. Comparison of 4 questionnaires for assessment of fruit and vegetable intake. Am J Public Health 1998;88:1216–1218.

74. Sobell J, Block G, Koslowe P, Tobin J, Anders R. Validation of a retrospective questionnaire assessing diet 10–15 years ago. Am J Epidemiol 1989;130:173–187.

75. Willett WC, Sampson L, Browne ML, et al. The use of a self-administered questionnaire to assess diet four years in the past. Am J Epidemiol 1988;127(1):188–199.

76. Satia-Abouta J, Galanko JA, Martin CF, Potter JD, Ammerman A, Sandler RS. Associations of micronutrients with colon cancer risk in African Americans and Whites: Results from the North Carolina Colon Cancer Study. Cancer Epidemiol Biomarkers Prev 2003;12:747–754.

77. Kontiokari T, Laitinen J, Jarvi L, Pokka T, Sundqvist KUM. Dietary factors protecting women from urinary tract infection. Am J Clin Nutr 2004;77(3):600–604.

78. Buring JE, Hennekens CH, Lipnick RJ, et al. A prospective cohort study of postmenopausal hormone use and risk of breast cancer in US women. Am J Epidemiol 1987;125(6):939–947.

79. Liu K, Slattery M, Jacobs D, et al. A study of the reliability and comparative validity of the Cardia dietary history. Ethn Dis 1994;4(15):27.

80. Wang CY, Anderson GL, Prentice RL. Estimation of the correlation between nutrient intake measures under restricted sampling. Biometrics 1999;55(3):711–717.

81. Feinleib M, Kannel WB, Garrison RJ, McNamara PM, Castelli WP. The Framingham Offspring Study. Design and preliminary data. Prev Med 1975;4(4):518–525.

82. Worth RM, Kagan A. Ascertainment of men of Japanese ancestry in Hawaii through World War II selective service registration. J Chron Dis 1970;23:389–397.

83. Caan B, Ballard-Barbash R, Slattery ML, et al. Low energy reporting may increase in intervention participants enrolled in dietary intervention trials. J Am Diet Assoc 2004;104(3):357–366.

84. Bogers RP, van Assema P, Kester ADM, Westerterp KR, Dagnelie PC. Reproducibility, validity, and responsiveness to change of a short questionnaire for measuring fruit and vegetable intake. Am J Epidemiol 2004;159:900–909.

85. Townsend MS, Kaiser LL, Allen LH, Joy AB, Murphy SP. Selecting items for a food behavior checklist for a limited-resource audience. J Nutr Educ Behav 20043;35(2):69–77.

86. Black RE, Williams SM, Jones IE, Goulding A. Children who avoid drinking cow milk have low dietary calcium intakes and poor bone health. Am J Clin Nutr 2002;76:675–680.

87. Goulding A, Rockell JEP, Black RE, Grant AM, Jones IE, Williams SM. Children who avoid drinking cow's milk are at increased risk for prepubertal bone fractures. J Am Diet Assoc 2004;104:250–253.

88. Samet JM, Humble CG, Skipper BE. Alternatives in the collection and analysis of food frequency interview data. Am J Epidemiol 1984;120:572–581.

89. Willett WC, Reynolds RD, Cotrell-Hoehner MS, Sampson L, Browne ML. Validation of a semi-quantitative food freuqency questionnaire: comparison with a 1-year diet record. J Am Diet Assoc 1987;87(1):43–47.

90. McDonald A, Van Horn L, Slattery M, et al. The CARDIA dietary history: development, implementation, and evaluation. J Am Diet Assoc 1991;91(9):1104–1112.

91. Pereira MA, Jacobs DR, Jr., Van Horn L, Slattery ML, Kartashov AI, Ludwig DS. Dairy consumption, obesity, and the Insulin Resistance Syndrome in young adults. JAMA 2002;287(16):2081–2089.

92. Thompson FE, Moler JE, Freedman LS, Clifford CK, Stables GJ, Willett WC. Register of dietary assessment calibration-validation studies: A status report. Am J Clin Nutr 1997;65 (Supplement):1142S–1147S.

93. McPherson RS, Hoelscher D, Alexander M, Scanlon KS, Serdula MK. Dietary assessment methods among school-aged children: validity and reliability. Prev Med 2000;31:S11–S33.

94. Cummings SR, Block G, McHenry K, Baron RB. Evaluation of two food frequency methods of measuring dietary calcium intake. Am J Epidemiol 1987;126:796–802.

95. Blalock SJ, Currey SS, DeVellis RF, Anderson JJB, Gold DT, Dooley MA. Using a short food frequency questionnaire to estimate dietary calcium consumption: a tool for patient education. Arthritis Care and Research 1998;11(6):479–484.

96. Hertzler AA, Frary RB. A dietary calcium rapid assessment method (RAM). Top Clin Nutr 1994;9(3):76–85.

97. Taitano RT, Novotny R, Davis JW, Ross PD, Wasnich RD. Validity of a food frequency questionnaire for estimating calcium intake among Japanese and white women. J Am Diet Assoc 1995;95:804–806.

98. Brown JL, Griebler R. Reliability of a short and long version of the Block food frequency form for assessing changes in calcium intake. J Am Diet Assoc 1993;93(7):784–789.

99. Musgrave KO, Giambalvo L, Leclerc HL, Cook RA, Rosen CJ. Validation of a quantitative food frequency questionnaire for rapid assessment of dietary calcium intake. J Am Diet Assoc 1989;89(10):1484–1488.

100. Boushey CJ, Liesmann JM, Yang J, Martin BR, Weaver CM. Validation of a semi-quantitative food frequency questionnaire for assessing calcium intake of youth in the United States. Paper presented at the Fifth International Conference on Dietary Assessment Mehtods; January 27, 2003; Chiang Rai, Thailand.

101. Angbratt M, Moller M. Questionnaires about calcium intake: can we trust the answers? Osteoporos Int 1999;9:220–225.

102. Montomoli M, Gonnelli S, Giacchi M, et al. Validation of a food frequency questionnaire for nutritional calcium intake assessment in Italian women. Eur J Clin Nutr 2002;**56**:21–30.

103. Angus RM, Sambrook PN, Pocock NA, Eisman JA. A simple method for assessing calcium intake in Caucasian women. J Am Diet Assoc 1989;89(2):209–214.

104. Chee WSS, Suriah AR, Zaitun Y, Chan SP, Yap SL, Chan YM. Dietary calcium intake in postmenopausal Malaysian women: comparison between the food frequency questionnaire and three-day food records. Asia Pac J Clin Nutr 2002;11(2):142–146.

105. Hernandez-Avila M, Romieu I, Parra S, hernandez-Avila J, Madrigal H, Willett W. Validity and reproducibility of a food frequency questionniare to assess dietary intake of women living in Mexico City. Salud Publica Mex 1998;39(40):133–140.

106. Taylor RW, Goulding A. Validation of a short food frequency questionnaire to assess calcium intake in children aged 3 to 6 years. Eur J Clin Nutr 1998;52(6):464–465.

107. Margetts BM, Nelson M (eds.). *Design Concepts in Nutritional Epidemiology*. 2nd ed. Oxford University Press, Oxford: 1997.

108. Johnson RK, Hankin JH. Dietary assessment methods and validation. In: Monsen ER, editor. Research: Successful Approaches. Chicago, IL: American Dietetic Association, 2003: 227–242.

109. Schoeller DA. Recent advances from application of doubly labeled water to measurement of human energy expenditure. J Nutr 1999;129:1765–1768.
110. Schoeller DA. Validation of habitual energy intake. Public Health Nutr 2002;5(6A):883–888.
111. Buzzard IM, Sievert YA. Research priorities and recommendations for dietary assessment methodology. Am J Clin Nutr 1994;59(suppl):275S–280S.
112. Kipnis V. Looking at dietary assessment with an OPEN mind: Lessons learned from biomarker studies. Paper presented at: The Fifth International Conference on Dietary Assessment Methods;January 27;2003;Chiang Rai, Thailand.
113. Freedman LS, Midthune D, Carroll RJ, et al. Adjustments to improve the estimation of usual dietary intake distributions in the population. J Nutr 2004;134:1836–1843.
114. Hankin JH, Wilkens LR. Development and validation of dietary assessment methods for culturally diverse populations. Am J Clin Nutr 1994;59(1 Suppl):198S–200S.
115. Kipnis V, Midthune D, Freedman LS, et al. Empirical evidence of correlated biases in dietary assessment instruments and its implications. Am J Epidemiol 2001;153(4):394–403.
116. Byers T. Food frequency dietary assessment: how bad is good enough? Am J Epidemiol 2004;154(12): 1087–1088.
117. Freudenheim JGE. Biomarkers of nutritional exposure and nutritional status. J Nutr 2003;133 (Supplement)(3S):871S–973S.
118. Black AE, Prentice AM, Goldberg GR, Jebb SABSA, Livingstone MB, Coward WA. Measurments of total energy expenditure provide insights into the validity of dietary measurements of energy intake. J Am Diet Assoc 1993;93(5):572–579.
119. Bingham SA. Urine nitrogen as a biomarker for the validation of dietary protein intake. J Nutr 2003;133:921S–924S.
120. Mayne ST. Antioxidant nutrients and chronic disease: Use of biomarkers of exposure and oxidative stress status in epidemiologic research. J Nutr 2003;133:933S–940S.
121. Murphy SP, Kaiser LL, Townsend MS, Allen LH. Evaluation of validity of items for a food behavior checklist. J Am Diet Assoc 2001;101(751):761.

5 Clinical Approaches for Studying Calcium Metabolism and Its Relationship to Disease

Connie M. Weaver

KEY POINTS

- Metabolic balance plus kinetic studies can pinpoint how calcium metabolism is perturbed (i.e., at the gut, kidney, or bone).
- Isotopic tracers can be used to quantitate calcium absorption efficiency and the bioavailability of calcium sources.
- Randomized, controlled trials are effective for showing the relationship of calcium intake to health outcomes.

1. INTRODUCTION

This chapter describes several types of clinical studies for studying the relationship of dietary calcium to health. Fractional calcium absorption studies are used to evaluate bioavailability from various sources or intrinsic calcium absorption capacity. The latter is an important risk factor for osteoporosis and possibly other disorders associated with low calcium status. The accuracy of different methods commonly used to determine fractional calcium absorption varies widely. Calcium retention measurements are useful to determine influences on bone mass in short-term studies. Randomized, controlled trials (RCTs) are the inferentially strongest approach to understanding the relationship between calcium intake and outcome measures of disease.

2. WHEN TO USE VARIOUS CLINICAL NUTRITION APPROACHES

Controlled feeding studies can provide valuable insights on how well calcium is absorbed and utilized from various sources by different individuals and under different conditions. They also may be used to determine the relationship between intake and risk for disease. Whereas the epidemiological approach to study the relationship between indices of health or disease risk (described in Chapter 4) can enroll large numbers of subjects, controlled feeding studies are typically more labor-intensive and necessitate smaller sample sizes. Well-done epidemiological studies can be representative of the

From: *Calcium in Human Health*
Edited by: C. M. Weaver and R. P. Heaney © Humana Press Inc., Totowa, NJ

general population and utilize the best outcome measures including disease endpoints. However, their ability to estimate calcium intake is imprecise and multiple confounding variables are not controlled, although better understood factors can be accounted for in the analysis. In contrast, the best-done clinical feeding studies can precisely control calcium intake and other dietary confounders. Some even control physical activity and use a crossover design to eliminate unforeseen confounders inherent in individuals. The more that diet and other variables are controlled, the more resources are required. This leads to reduced sample sizes and costs, and runs a risk of not representing the general population. Although the independent variable can be precisely controlled, the typical clinical study is too short to determine disease endpoints. With calcium, bone health is a frequent dependent variable of interest. Even changes in the best biomarkers for bone health, using bone densitometry or imaging, require longer periods than is feasible for a controlled diet study.

Clinical feeding studies are useful when quantitative information about calcium intake and an outcome is desired. The study design of choice depends on the particular outcome information sought. For any design, it is important to perform power calculations and to recruit sufficient subjects to ensure that meaningful effects are found.

In this chapter, various methods for determining calcium absorption are reviewed. Metabolic balance studies, which can provide quantitative data on calcium excretion and retention, are described. When calcium isotopic tracers are used in combination with metabolic balance studies, kinetic analysis, which provides information on rates of transfer among body compartments (*see* Chapter 6), can be performed. RCTs are also described briefly in this chapter. They represent an intermediate level of control between epidemiological studies and quantitative, controlled diet studies, and consequently require an intermediate number of subjects to determine the relationship between calcium intake and an index of health. The level of certainty of the diet–health relationships from cause-and-effect to associational usually also parallels types of studies from controlled, diet studies →RCTs → epidemiological studies. However, even changes observed in controlled feeding studies using a randomized-order, crossover design may not represent a cause-and-effect relationship if residual treatment effects remain because of an insufficient washout period.

3. METHODS FOR STUDYING CALCIUM ABSORPTION

Fractional calcium absorption from a fixed load is useful for determining physiological absorptive capacity or for determining bioavailability of calcium sources. There are many study designs that have been used to determine fractional calcium absorption. Most do not adapt subjects to a controlled diet, especially if calcium absorption is the only metabolic parameter of interest. When the question relates to calcium bioavailability from a particular source, the strongest design is to compare calcium absorption from that source with a referent source, such as milk or calcium carbonate, in a crossover design. This allows relative bioavailability to be determined with minimal influence of individual subject characteristics. Approximately 60% of the variance in cross sectional measures of calcium absorption can be accounted for by intrasubject absorption efficiency *(1)*. For menstruating women, this means studying each source at the same phase of the menstrual cycle, typically days 4–11 of the follicular cycle. When the calcium source is the focus of interest, a controlled diet is often not necessary. The gastrointestinal environment should be similar between study phases, which is usually accomplished by an overnight fast. Similar results were found for bioavailability of calcium from tofu after an overnight fast or when the test meal was given in the middle a of the 4-d controlled diet period *(2)*. Longer feeding studies are required for measuring the influence of adaptation to the calcium source , level of calcium in the diet, or other dietary constituents on calcium absorption.

Examples of factors that are thought to alter calcium absorption through adaptation are nondigestible carbohydrates, which may influence lower gut bacterial fermentation or intestinal microvillar surface area (*see* Chapter 12), vitamin D and estrogen status (*see* Chapter 11), and chronically low calcium intakes.

3.1. Metabolic Balance Studies

On a controlled diet, net calcium absorption can be determined as

$$I - F,$$

where I = calcium intake and F = fecal calcium and each parameter is expressed in the same units (mg or mmol) and measured over the same time period (24 h, 1 wk, etc.). Net calcium absorption efficiency is determined as

$$(I \quad F)/I.$$

Balance studies are rarely the method of choice for determining calcium absorption for a number of reasons. Measured calcium in excreta from a test food cannot be distinguished from calcium in the rest of the diet nor from endogenous secretions. The former leads to uncertainty about bioavailability of calcium from the test source. The latter leads to underestimation of true bioavailability or absorption capacity. Furthermore, the large variability in fecal calcium even on controlled diets results in poor ability of the balance approach to discriminate between different sources. Further description of the conduct of metabolic balance studies and associated errors are discussed under Subheading 4.1. Even fecal markers, although necessary, are insufficient to deal adequately with the variability in daily fecal calcium excretion.

The metabolic balance approach for determining calcium absorption more often provides satisfactory results in animal models than in humans. Use of semi-purified diets enables all of the calcium to be provided by the test source of calcium. Use of inbred animals housed in metabolic cages under controlled conditions can reduce sources of variation. Calcium bioavailability in animal models has been shown to give similar rank order to humans and, dependent on the calcium load of the test meal, similar absolute values *(3)*. However, results from animal models (typically rats) can differ from those obtained using humans because the animals practice coprophagy, have intestinal phytases, and have substantially lower urinary calcium excretion, among other differences.

3.2. Calcium Isotopic Tracer Absorption

Isotopic tracer data are less variable than balance data. Thus, although fractional absorption determined by tracer studies results in conclusions similar to net calcium

Table 1
Calcium Isotopic Tracers

| Atomic number | Symbol and mass number | Radioisotopes | | | Stable isotopes |
| | | Half-life | Maximum radiation energies | | Natural abundance (%) |
			β (Mev)	E (Mev)	
20	^{41}Ca	10^5y	–	–	10^{-15}
	^{42}Ca	–	–	–	0.646
	^{43}Ca	–	–	–	0.135
	^{44}Ca	–	–	–	2.083
	^{45}Ca	164d	0.255	–	–
	^{46}Ca	–	–	–	0.0033
	^{47}Ca	4.53d	1.98	1.29	–
	^{48}Ca	–	–	–	0.18

absorption determined by balance studies (4), more subtle differences can be discriminated with isotopic tracer studies, and sample sizes can be much smaller. Fractional calcium absorption and total absorbed calcium determined from kinetic modeling using data collected in metabolic balance and tracer studies is described in Chapter 6 and is not covered in this section. When the whole spectrum of calcium metabolism parameters is not needed, there are several approaches available for determining calcium absorption using isotopic tracers that require substantially fewer resources. However, caution must be exercised when only absorption is determined because a dietary component being tested may have an impact on another aspect of calcium metabolism that can either augment or minimize an apparent effect on absorption (see Chapter 9).

A list of isotopic tracers of calcium appears in Table 1. Useful radiotracers of calcium are ^{47}Ca and ^{45}Ca. ^{47}Ca is a γ- emitter, and therefore can be used for whole-body counting in studies of calcium absorption and retention in animals or humans in facilities where animal or human γ-counters are available. Its short half-life limits the length of the experiment and is a reason for its scarcity and relatively high expense. A limitation of whole-body counting is that mechanisms cannot be investigated because the organs affected (i.e., gut, kidney, or bone) cannot be inferred from whole-body retention curves. Another limitation is how long it takes the oral isotope to clear the gut. If the study is too short, unabsorbed calcium tracer in the colon will appear as if it were retained calcium. As a β-emitter, ^{45}Ca is measured in a liquid scintillation counter and is appropriate for biological fluids or samples that can be converted to fluids. Although ^{47}Ca can also be measured in biological fluids, the lower costs and longer half-life typically make ^{45}Ca the preferred radioisotope for tracer studies. Precision of analysis with radioisotopes depends on the counting rate, but samples can usually be counted to 1–2% precision.

There are many more nonradioactive (stable) isotopes of calcium than radioisotopes. These isotopes, of heavier mass than ^{40}Ca—which represents almost 97% of calcium in nature—are measured as isotopic ratios by mass spectroscopy. The methods of choice currently are high-resolution, inductively coupled plasma mass spectrometry (HR-ICPMS) (5) and thermal ionization mass spectrometry (TIMS) (6). The former has the advantage of greater sample throughput and the latter has the advantage of greater precision (<0.1–0.2% vs 1–2%). Stable isotopic tracers offer the advantage of not exposing subjects to radioactivity and not having to time experiments around a short half life tracer. They have the disadvantage of being more expensive to purchase and analyze. Use of calcium stable isotopes for clinical studies of calcium metabolism was first proposed in 1983 *(7)*.

The long-lived radioisotope ^{41}Ca can be used in such small doses (≤ 100 nCi) that it can be considered to be radiologically benign. A single dose of this size labels the skeleton for life, which poses a lifetime radiation exposure of <0.1 mre. The benefits of this tracer are that the tracer can be monitored for long experiments in contrast with the upper limit of approx 2 wk with other isotopes. Urinary appearance of ^{41}Ca after 100 d from dosing, when the ^{41}Ca can be considered to be coming from the skeleton, provides a direct, sensitive measure of bone resorption. Changes in bone loss can be accurately measured following an intervention. The disadvantage of this approach is that ^{41}Ca is measured with an accelerator mass spectrometer (AMS), which is not available in most research centers. There are two in the United States—one at Purdue University and one at Lawrence Livermore National Laboratory. Opportunities involving AMS in nutrition have been recently reviewed *(8)*.

The design of the study using calcium isotopic tracers depends on available resources and capacity of the laboratory to measure and administer isotopic tracers in humans. The ideal approach (short of full kinetic modeling, described in Chapter 6) is the use of double isotope tracers described by de Grazia et al. *(9)*. One isotope is administered orally to label dietary calcium and the other intravenously to measure calcium removal from the blood. Oral isotopes take longer to enter the plasma pool than intravenous doses, so we give the oral isotope 1–2 h prior to giving the intravenous isotope. The two isotopes track identically after 20 h *(10)* *(see* Fig. 1). Precise timing sequence of the oral and intravenous tracers is not important if total urinary recovery is measured, as is necessary for a single collection timepoint. Ratios of the oral to intravenous tracers can be made in the first 24-h urine sample postdose, or in a single sample of urine or serum after 20 h, although the later may be less accurate *(11)*. When adjusted for dose, this represents fractional calcium absorption as:

Fractional true absorption:

$$\frac{\int_0^t T_{OR}\,dt}{\int_0^t T_{IV}\,dt} \bullet \frac{DOSE_{IV}}{DOSE_{OR}}$$

$$\cong \frac{T_{OR}}{T_{IV}} \bullet \frac{DOSE_{IV}}{DOSE_{OR}}$$

where T = tracer concentration in serum or urine calcium.

A variation of this method uses a single oral calcium isotopic tracer to label the diet without the intravenous tracer. This method is most reliable when used in a crossover design to compare relative bioavailability, as it is more likely that calcium clearance, a product of body pool size and turnover rate, would be similar between two test phases in the same individual. The most common application of this method is to measure the oral tracer in a single blood draw 5 h postdose. This method has been highly correlated with the double-isotope tracer technique *(12,13)*.

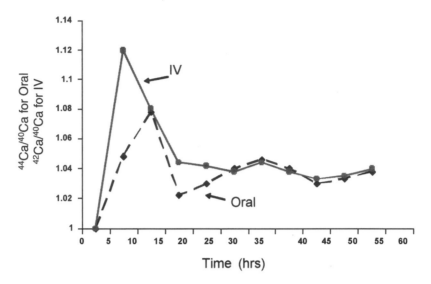

Fig 1. Enrichment of tracer isotopes in urine after a 77-kg male received 13 mg of ^{44}Ca orally and 4 mg of ^{42}Ca intravenously. (Adapted from ref. *10*.)

Using the single tracer method in adults, fractional calcium absorption can be calculated by adjusting for body size area as:

$$FxAbs = (SA_5^{\ 0.92373})\ \mu\ [BSC\ \mu\ (H_t^{\ 0.52847})\ \mu\ (W_t^{\ 0.37213})]$$

where Fx Abs = fractional absorption, SA_5 = 5-h serum calcium specific radioactivity, Ht= height in meters, Wt = weight in Kg. BSC is body size correction, and has a value of 0.3537 in women and 0.3845 in men.

This method was used to determine calcium bioavailability of most of the sources reported in Chapter 9. A 5% difference in fractional calcium absorption can usually be detected with 10–15 subjects using a crossover design. Other investigators have used a 1-h *(14)* or 3-h *(15)* blood draw. However, these shorter sample times do not correlate as well with true calcium absorption as does the 5-h timepoint *(12)*. Any single point in time poses the risk of a shifting serum profile, which could alter apparent bioavailability from one test period to the next. Consequently, some investigators prefer to measure total tracer appearance in the urine *(16)* or feces *(17)*. The accuracy of these approaches depends on completeness of collection, unlike single point sampling. A further problem with the 1-h *(14)* approach is the use of a very small test load (e.g., 20 mg). Such small test loads may provide insights on the active absorption component, but do not provide otherwise nutritionally relevant information.

Good agreement has also been reported between the double tracer method and the fecal recovery method from a single isotope *(9)*. When absorption is calculated from unabsorbed tracer appearing in the stools, the diet must be controlled long enough to encompass the transit time of the tracer *(18)*. When tracer appearance in blood or urine is used to monitor fractional calcium absorption, often the tracer is given at breakfast following an overnight fast. Typically, the diet is not controlled except for the breakfast, when blood is collected or for just 1 d when urine is collected *(19)*. A 24-h urine collection may be sufficient, but when a response delay is expected, as occurs in the presence of nondigestible fiber (20), urine might need to be collected for several days. In this example, a sufficient prefeeding period is also needed to allow microbial gut adaptation.

When determining physiological absorption capacity, important considerations are the size of the calcium load and the chemical form of calcium to be administered. As fractional absorption is inversely related to load, all comparisons should be made using the same load. Frequently, loads of between 100 and 300 mg calcium are tested. Some choose the load equivalent to one-third of the daily intake. When fractional absorption is being compared across experiments, it is better to include a common source as a reference. Radioisotopes typically are purchased as $CaCl_2$. This soluble isotope can be mixed with milk or juice for consumption or converted to another salt. It is not recommended to give pure $CaCl_2$, as it is a stomach irritant. Alternatively, a capsule of a preweighed calcium salt containing the tracer can serve as the oral dose. This is common with stable isotopes of calcium that are purchased as calcium carbonate.

The method chosen to incorporate an isotope into the food being tested for bioavailability deserves thoughtful consideration. Intrinsic labeling techniques (which incorporate isotopes during growth of plants or animals as previously described [21] or during the synthesis of a supplement [22]), attempt to prepare the label in the same physical and chemical form as the native calcium of the tested source. Extrinsic labeling of calcium sources is simpler and frequently, but not always, allows a good approximation of calcium absorption from intrinsically labeled sources (23). This approach involves premixing a soluble form of the calcium isotope with the food to be tested prior to consumption. It assumes that the tracer has adequately exchanged with endogenous calcium, a point that generally must be validated before proceeding.

Calcium isotopic tracer absorption can also be determined from whole-body ^{47}Ca retention curves. An example of this approach is shown in Fig. 2 of Chapter 12. This is an excellent method for determining calcium absorption, but few laboratories have the capacity to administer ^{47}Ca to humans and to measure subsequent whole-body retention. The use of this special method and exposure to radioactivity from a γ-emitter is better justified for more complicated problems that measuring fractional absorption.

3.3. Serum Profiles of Calcium, Parathyroid Hormone, and Vitamin D Metabolites

Calcium bioavailability from a number of sources has been estimated from areas under the curve (AUC) of profiles of total or ionized serum calcium or its regulators, that is, parathyroid hormone (PTH) or vitamin D metabolites following an oral load after an overnight fast. This approach is useful for determining calcium absorption from preformulated commercial products, where intrinsic labeling cannot be used. Some examples of this approach comparing calcium salts to a blank are shown in Fig. 2. This approach may be more easily achievable for many laboratories in that isotopic tracers are not required. However, the method is crude compared with isotopic tracer approaches. Changes in serum calcium are small, as serum calcium is tightly regulated so that subtle changes would likely be missed. Note that there is only an approx 5% rise in serum calcium on a 500-mg load (Fig. 2A). Similarly, changes in regulators of calcium absorption are difficult to observe (Fig. 2B).

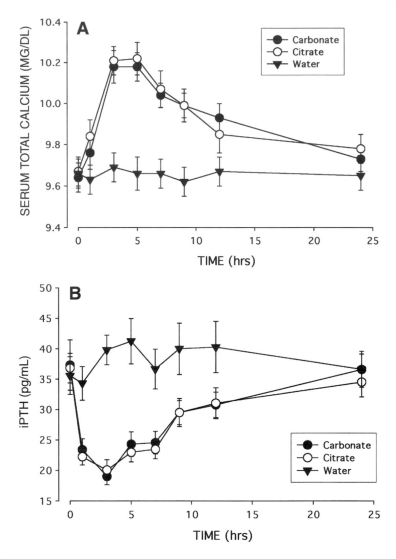

Fig 2. (A) Time course of the total serum calcium, both as absolute values for two calcium sources and for the blank load. Error bars are 1 SEM. **(B)** Time course of serum iPTH following ingestion of two calcium sources and for the blank load, both as absolute values. Error bars are 1 SEM. (Copyright Robert P. Heaney, 2004. Used with permission.)

AUCs have been successfully used to determine responses in large doses, i.e., a 500-mg calcium supplement vs placebo *(24)* (Fig. 2A) or fractional calcium absorption efficiency differences in vitamin D-deficient and -sufficient individuals *(25)*. The acute PTH suppression method *(26)* can be made more sensitive by adapting subjects to a low calcium diet the week before they receive the test meal. Using this approach, AUC for serum PTH was significantly altered for test meals containing 500 mg Ca as milk, $CaCO_3$, or fortified orange juice, but not for serum Ca *(27)*. If serum AUC for any measured variable is used to estimate calcium absorption, it is important to collect data points long enough to avoid misclassification.

3.4. Urinary Calcium

Urinary calcium excretion following a bolus dose has been used to estimate calcium absorption, but this method is plagued with even more uncertainties than serum calcium profiles. As for observing changes in serum AUC (discussed in the previous section), test loads must be large. Following a 500-mg Ca load, the postprandial increase in urinary calcium excretion was only approx 5% of the load over a 5- to 8-h period in elderly men and women (27). Postprandial increments in urinary calcium excretion were approximately twice as variable as for serum calcium in a study comparing calcium carbonate and calcium citrate in postmenopausal women (77–99% vs 38–60% CV, respectively) (24). In addition to reflecting absorbed calcium spilled over into the urine, urinary calcium is influenced by diuretics, the prior day's salt intake, and size and turnover of the exchangeable pool. That makes use of a crossover design and standard conditions especially important for this method.

Urinary calcium can derive from diet or bone, and without tracers the source cannot be distinguished. This may explain why relative calcium absorbability estimated from urinary calcium excretion does not always agree with calcium tracer data. For example, urinary calcium excretion was greater for calcium citrate than for calcium carbonate (28), whereas the calcium tracer approach showed no difference in fractional calcium absorption between these salts (29). Suppressed serum ionized calcium with calcium carbonate suggests a slight alkalosis, which would be expected to reduce urinary calcium excretion compared to calcium citrate (24). The increased urinary calcium from calcium citrate likely comes from bone rather than increased absorption from the diet. Other studies reporting enhanced calcium absorption that have utilized urinary calcium increments, such as for coral calcium (30), must be repeated using isotopic tracer methods.

Use of urinary calcium excretion to estimate calcium absorption would be especially problematic for growing animals and children because of the low correlation between calcium intake and urinary excretion. In adolescent girls, only 6% of the variation in urinary calcium was explained by calcium intake (31).

4. METHODS FOR DETERMINING CALCIUM RETENTION

Cumulative calcium retention can be determined from total body calcium content measured by bone densitometry. This is a reasonable index of calcium status. Shorter term calcium retention studies while subjects are fed controlled diets can be used to quantify factors that can offset calcium retention. Two such methods are metabolic balance and whole-body ^{47}Ca retention.

4.1. Metabolic Balance

Balance studies calculate net retention as intake minus excretion:

$$\text{Calcium retention} = I - (F + U)$$

where I = intake, F = feces, and U = urinary calcium.

Balance studies are sufficiently sensitive, when rigorously controlled, to distinguish differences when large effects are expected as exists when comparing pubertal growth with that of adults (32), lactating state with nonlactating state (33) racial differences (34), the effects of skeletal unloading (35), and some diet effects such as calcium intake (36).

The treatment differences in these examples can exceed 200 mg calcium retention per day. Power calculations show that sample sizes of five to six subjects per group are sufficient to find significant differences of this magnitude at an α of 0.05 with 80% power even though the variances were large. The ability to determine smaller effects of diet depends on the magnitude of the effect and the specific population. We have been able to show treatment effects on calcium retention of 40 mg/d with 10–15 adolescent subjects in crossover studies. However, for treatment differences in calcium retention of approx 40 mg/d in postmenopausal women using the variance that we observed in a recent study, power calculations suggest 180 subjects would be needed to show significance using a crossover design.

Balance studies can also be used to determine calcium requirements as the response of calcium retention to calcium intake reaches a plateau when calcium intake is no longer limiting maximal calcium retention, that is, bone accrual (*see* Chapter 7). The errors associated with measuring balance are not symmetrically distributed. Errors associated with incomplete consumption of the diet or collection of urine and fecal excretion and failure to measure other, including cutaneous, losses are often cited limitations, because they often bias results toward more positive retention values. However, useful information about the role of other dietary factors or lifestyle choices in shifting the location of the inflection point of the maximal retention curve (which, thus, shifts calcium requirements higher or lower) can be determined. This application has the advantage of not depending on actual values of calcium retention. The maximal retention approach seeks the intake where a plateau occurs rather than focusing on absolute retention. Finally, analytical procedures typically have a CV of 5% or more.

Metabolic balance studies involve feeding a controlled diet, collecting excreta, and measuring calcium input and output. Intake cannot be estimated from food composition tables. All foods and beverages containing calcium must be prepared by weighing ingredients to the nearest 0.1 g. Prepared commercial foods can be used if their composition is homogeneous. Duplicate collections of all of the foods and beverages consumed in a 24-h period are analyzed for calcium and other constituents that influence calcium balance, including protein, phosphorus, fiber, and electrolytes. Diets should be designed to be constant in these constituents throughout the study period. Foods, beverages, and oral health care products, including tap water, which contain calcium, inhibitors of calcium absorption such as tea, which contains oxalate, or hypercalciuric ingredients such as salt cannot be allowed to vary from day to day.

If the metabolic study is not conducted in all subjects simultaneously, but rather as a rolling enrollment, it may not be practical to analyze a duplicate sample of each day. In that case, dietary composites representing each cycle day from a dietary intervention should be prepared in intervals throughout a study period to track the variability that occurs over time and the variability between the daily diets. Dietary composites should be measured for calcium and those nutrients that could potentially affect calcium metabolism, e.g., protein, sodium, potassium, and phosphorus. Dietary homogenates representing each day of the menu cycle, for example, 7 d for a 7-d menu cycle, should be freeze-dried and aliquoted in triplicate for all nutrient analysis. Variation among these triplicate samples is an indication of homogeneity in the sample and analytical precision. Replicate analysis of dietary composites prepared over the entire study period demonstrates variation owing to variability in food items, dietary preparation, and laboratory analysis. Analysis across cycle menus represents daily variability within the diet.

Analysis of dietary composites from a metabolic balance study in our laboratory, which used a 7-d menu cycle over a 19-mo period, demonstrated 3% variation in calcium from triplicate analysis of dietary samples. The variation in calcium from the replicate analysis of dietary composites, which were collected at quarterly intervals over the 19-mo study period, was 5%. Daily variation in calcium across the 7-d cycle menus was 6%.

Urine and feces are collected in acid-washed containers for later analysis of total calcium by atomic absorption or ICPMS. In adolescents, a 1-d lag is used when calculating intake minus fecal excretion to account for the approx 19-h transit time in the gut. (That transit time can rise to 11–12 d in mature or older adults.) Menstrual losses of calcium can generally be ignored. Cutaneous losses are often ignored but can be measured by extracting acid-washed clothing worn for 24 h in addition to whole-body washdown procedures before and after the collection. Using this method, we have determined cutaneous losses of approx 52 mg/d in adolescents. Cutaneous losses determined by patches overestimated calcium losses by almost eightfold (37). These approaches do not measure losses from hair and nails. Cutaneous losses in adults have been estimated to be 60 mg/d by the difference between whole-body retention of ^{47}Ca and excretion in urine and feces (38).

To determine the effect of a variable on calcium retention within a population, the best approach is the use of a crossover design in the same subjects to minimize confounding effects that are constant within an individual, such as hormonal status, gastrointestinal and kidney function, mucosal mass, transit time, and vitamin D status. Randomized-order assignments of treatment can minimize seasonal effects of vitamin D status. Nevertheless, the presence or absence of an order effect should be tested statistically. Subjects can also be pretreated with vitamin D supplements before and throughout the study period to ensure normal vitamin D status.

The length of the run-in period needed for a subject to adapt to the study diet and the length of the balance period once steady state is reached must be carefully considered. Misinterpretations have occurred when subjects have been switched from high to low calcium intake periods without an appropriate adaptation period, as the higher calcium intakes spill into the feces during the lower calcium period for several days. When a nonabsorbable fecal marker such as polyethylene glycol (PEG) is given at every meal, the fecal calcium:PEG ratio can be used to determine when steady state is achieved. We have found that the Ca:PEG ratio becomes constant after 6 d in adolescents and most adults (Table 2, adapted from ref. 39 as well as unpublished data). Similarly, when adult black and white women were switched from a diet containing 2000 mg/d for 3 wk to 300 mg/d for 8 wk, whole-body retention of ^{47}Ca varied from week 1 to week 2, but not from week 2 to week 8 (40). Thus, determining balance during the run-in period can give useful information about when steady state is achieved in calcium balance or another dietary constituent being tested for its effect on calcium retention. Subjects cannot adapt to a low calcium intake, that is, cannot come into balance, as the homeostatic control mechanisms is inefficient. Malm (41) studied prisoners for up to 2 yr and found continued negative calcium balances on low intakes.

Balance periods should be sufficiently long to evaluate trends over multiple periods. Some investigators make collections in several day pools and monitor multiple periods. We typically make collections in 24-h periods for 2 to 3 wk after a 1-wk adaptation period. Calculating daily balances for multiple periods allows an error term to be determined so that differences from zero balance can be determined for each individual. In pubertal

Table 2
Fecal Calcium:Polyethylene Glycol Ratios (mg/mg) During a 3-wk Balance Period*

Group	Calcium Intake (mg/d)	Week 1	Week 2	Week 3
Adolescent girls				
	800	0.25 ± 0.13^a	0.21 ± 0.06^b	0.19 ± 0.04^b
	1300	0.82 ± 2.20^a	$0.32 \pm 0.06b$	0.38 ± 0.72^b
	1800	0.53 ± 0.08^a	0.48 ± 0.09^b	0.48 ± 0.07^b
Adults				
	1300	1.49 ± 5.20^a	0.36 ± 0.09^b	0.36 ± 0.08^b

*Different letter superscripts within rows indicate means are significantly different for each level of calcium intake at $p < 0.05$. (Data from ref. *39* and unpublished data.)

children, balance periods should not exceed rapid hormonal shifts, which can outweigh the influence of diet on calcium retention *(42)*.

Methods to assess compliance of urine and fecal collections and to adjust for discrete 24-h periods are helpful in reducing variation in balance data and in interpreting the quality of data. However, errors can be made in measuring compliance markers so that corrected data may be less accurate than uncorrected data for any given day. Thus, all components of any calculation should be carefully inspected. Especially troublesome is the apparent overcorrection of fecal calcium when using a marker to adjust for low compliance.

Adjustment of urine is usually made with creatinine. Subjects excrete a rather constant level of creatinine proportional to lean body mass. The mean daily creatinine excretion of a subject over the study period can be used to adjust each day to a more precise 24-h period, as it is difficult to completely empty one's bladder at precise regular time periods, especially for children. Twenty-four-hour pools with creatinine values less than 11 mg/kg should be discarded as substantially incomplete (except, perhaps, in emaciated individuals).

Daily fecal calcium output is highly variable despite constant conditions, as a result of variable gut transit times that do not segregate into discrete periods and because calcium flows forward and backward in the intestine *(43)*. A number of nonabsorbable fecal markers have been employed to evaluate compliance and transit time, and to convert individual stools collected at irregular intervals to daily fecal calcium output. We use PEG 4000 as a continuously administered, nonabsorbable marker as developed by Wilkinson *(44)*, who demonstrated clearly a reduction in daily variation by correcting stool samples by recovery of this marker. Capsules are prepared containing PEG weighed to the nearest mg and consumed at each meal throughout the study. The ratio of Ca to PEG in each 24-h pool is multiplied by the amount of PEG consumed during 24 h in order to determine daily fecal calcium. PEG excretion can also be used to estimate fecal lag (or intestinal transit) time. In the first few days after starting a PEG-labeled balance study, fecal PEG may be negligible, reflecting the fact that current fecal collections reflect prestudy diet residue. The time required for PEG excretion to approximate PEG input is the fecal lag time. The week 1 data in Table 2 show the effect of fecal lag clearly.

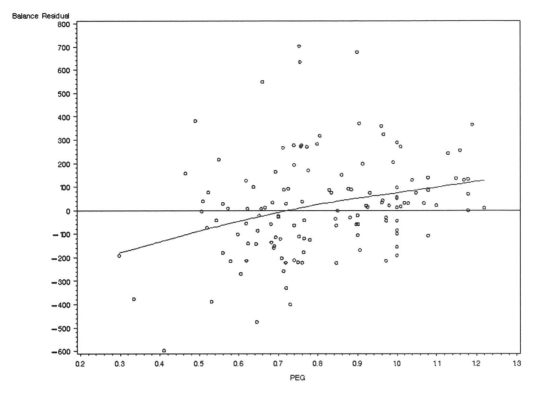

Fig 3. Calcium balance residuals vs fractional polyethylene glycol recovery in one study of postmenopausal women *(46)*.

The week 1 fecal collections were dominated by prestudy food (prevailing calcium plus zero PEG). It is important to measure fecal lag when performing kinetic studies (*see* Chapter 6), in order to time the fecal recovery of the intravenous tracer correctly.

Dissolved minerals and minerals as part of particulates do not move through the gut at the same rate. For water-soluble dietary constituents such as calcium, PEG is superior to previously used markers which more closely match the insoluble materials, such as Cr_2O_3 and barium sulphate, although recovery of all three markers was 98–100% *(44)*. It should be noted that PEG analysis is a tedious and difficult method.

Adjusting fecal calcium as described above supposedly corrects for incomplete stool collections. However, Eastell et al. *(45)* reported a PEG recovery of only 81% compared with 95% using ^{51}Cr in the same experiment. Therefore, we suspect that adjusting fecal calcium with PEG may overcorrect, which becomes worse with decreasing compliance. To examine this issue, we used data from one of our studies in which we calculated calcium balance using the PEG adjustment. Each group was studied three times, and we computed residuals for calcium balance by subtracting the group mean from each individual observation. A plot of these residuals vs PEG is given in Fig. 3. The plot includes a center line at zero (the mean of the residuals) as well as a smooth fit to the data. There appears to be a positive association between the PEG value and the residual. This means that observations with low values of PEG tend to be associated with balance values that are low relative to the group mean and, similarly, high PEG values are associated with balance values that are high relative to the group mean. This association is consistent with a scenario in which the PEG overcorrects the fecal calcium values: when the PEG is low, the corrected fecal values are too high and, therefore, the balance values are too low. The effect of compliancy on treatment effect can be determined by examining the F statistic when data are evaluated by using various cutoffs for % PEG recovery as inclusion criteria.

4.2. Whole-Body ^{47}Ca Retention

Whole-body retention of the γ-emitter ^{47}Ca can be determined with a precision of 2.6% of the administered dose *(47)*. With doses of 1–4 μCi ^{47}Ca, whole-body retention has been followed for 1 wk *(38;* Chapter 24, Fig. 2, this volume) to 4 wk *(48;* Chapter 12, Fig. 2, this volume).

Whole-body ^{47}Ca retention is more precise than retention determined by metabolic balance. However, it lacks the ability to determine the mechanism of the impact of an intervention (i.e., gut, kidney, or bone). Mechanisms are best understood by kinetic modeling *(see* Chapter 6).

5. RANDOMIZED, CONTROLLED TRIALS

An RCT is a strong study design for determining the relationship between calcium supplementation and a health outcome measure. Typically, subjects are randomized to the test calcium source or placebo. Ideally, the RCT is double-blinded to the subject and researcher. This requires the placebo to be indistinguishable from the calcium source. This is not always possible—for example, when the trial is milk or another source for which there is no feasible placebo.

The length of the trial and number of subjects depends on the outcome measures of interest. For changes in bone density, power calculations typically show that to detect a mean change of 0.7 to 1.1% or a group difference of 1.0 to 1.5% in bone mineral density of the spine or total hip in adults, 50 subjects per group is necessary for 80% power. Shorter time periods may be acceptable in growing children. For other outcome measures such as insulin resistance or body weight changes, a few weeks may be satisfactory *(see* Chapters 20 and 26).

RCTs can directly assess response to changes in diet that might be confounded in epidemiological approaches. A classic example of this was recently reported *(49)*. Cross-sectional analysis of the relationship between dairy calcium intake and total hip bone mineral density showed a positive relationship for elderly men, but not women. Others have also shown no relationship between calcium intake and bone measures in postmenopausal women *(50)*. However, an RCT of 750 Ca/d in the same individuals showed a similar positive response in men and women *(51)*. Perhaps women's self-reports underestimated dietary calcium intakes more than did men's. Regardless, this shows the need to confirm hypotheses generated by epidemiological approaches with controlled feeding experiments or RCTs.

6. CONCLUSIONS

Controlled feeding studies are important to establish cause-and-effect relationships between calcium intake and health outcome measures. Studies of fractional calcium absorption also are used to determine bioavailability of calcium from various food sources. Calcium retention studies are useful for setting calcium requirements.

Accurate information depends on careful consideration of study design and measurement methods. Mechanistic information can be obtained with controlled diets and isotopic tracers. This requires a dedicated laboratory and special attention to ethical issues. As we learn more about health outcomes that are related to calcium intakes, the nature of clinical studies expands.

REFERENCES

1. Heaney RP, Weaver CM, Fitzsimmons ML, Recker RR. Calcium absorption consistency. J Bone Miner Res 1990;5:1139–1142.
2. Weaver CM, Heaney RP, Connor L, Martin BR, Smith DL, Nielsen S. Bioavailability of calcium from tofu as compared with milk in premenopausal women. J Food Sci 2002;67(8):3144–3147.
3. Weaver CM, Martin B, Ebner J, Krueger C. Oxalic acid decreases calcium absorption in rats. J Nutr 1987;117:1903–1906.
4. Abrams SA, Yergey AL, Heaney RP. Relationship between balance and dual tracer isotopic measurements of calcium absorption and excretion. J Clin Endocrinol Metab 1994;79:965–969.
5. Stürup S, Hansen M, Mølgaard C. Measurements of ^{44}Ca: ^{43}Ca and ^{42}Ca: ^{43}Ca isotopic ratios in urine using high resolution inductively coupled plasma mass spectrometry. J Anal At Spectrom 1997;12:919–923.
6. Kastenmayer P. Thermal ionization mass spectrometry (TIMS). In: Mellon, FA, Sandström B, eds. Stable isotopes in human nutrition. Academic, London: 1996; pp. 81–86.
7. Smith DL. Determination of stable isotopes of calcium in biological fluids by fast atom bombardment mass spectrometry. Anal Chem 1983; 55:2391–2393.
8. Jackson GS, Weaver C, Elmore D. Use of accelerator mass spectrometry for studies in nutrition. Nutr Res Rev 2001;14:317–334.
9. DeGrazia JA, Ivanovich P, Fellows H, Rich C. A double isotope method for measurement of intestinal absorption of calcium in man. J Lab Clin Med 1965;66:822–829.
10. Smith DL, Atkin C, Westenfelder C. Stable isotopes of calcium as tracers: methodology. Clin Chim Acta 1985;146:97.
11. Yergey AL, Abrams SA, Viera NE, Aldreribi A, Marini J, Sidbury JE. Determination of fractional absorption of dietary calcium in humans. J Nutr 1994;124:674–682.
12. Heaney RP, Recker RR. Estimation of true calcium absorption. Ann Intern Med 1985;103:516–521.
13. Heaney RP, Recker RR. Estimating true fractional calcium absorption. Ann Intern Med 1988;108:905–906.
14. Marshall DH, Nordin BEC. A comparison of radioactive calcium tests with net calcium absorption. Clin Sci 1981;61:477–481.
15. Kung AWC, Luk KDK, Chu LW, Chin PKY. Age-related osteoporosis in Chinese: an evaluation of the response of intestinal calcium absorption and calcitropic hormones to dietary calcium deprivation. Am J Clin Nutr 1998;68:1291–1297.
16. Schulze KJ, O'Brien KO, Germain-Lee EL, Baer DJ, Leonard A, Rosenstein BJ. Effeciency of calcium absorption is not compromised in clinically stable prepubertal and pubertal girls with cystic fibrosis. Am J Clin Nutr 2003;78:110–116.
17. Nickel KP, Martin BR, Smith DL, Smith JB, Miller GD, and Weaver CM. Calcium bioavailability from bovine milk and dairy products in premenopausal women using intrinsic and extrinsic labeling techniques. J Nutr 1996;126:1406–1411.
18. Martin BR, Weaver CM, Heaney RP, Packard PT, Smith DL. Calcium absorption from three salts and $CaSO_4$-fortified bread in premenopausal women. J Agric Food Chem 2002;50(13):3874–3876.
19. O'Brien KO, Abrams SA. Effects of development on techniques for calcium stable isotope studies in children. Biol Mass Spec 1994;23:357–361.
20. van den Heuvel EG, Mays T, van Dokkum W, Schaafsma G. Oligofructose stimulates calcium absorption in adolescents. Am J Clin Nutr 1999;69:544–548.
21. Weaver CM. Intrinsic mineral labeling of edible plants: Methods and Uses. CRC Critical Reviews in Food Science and Nutrition 1985;23:75–101.
22. Weaver CM, Martin BR, Costa NMB, Saleeb FZ, Huth PJ. Absorption of calcium fumarate salts is equivalent to other calcium salts when measured in the rat model. J Agric Food Chem 2002; 50:4974–4975.

23. Weaver CM, Proulx WR, Heaney R. Choices for achieving adequate dietary calcium with a vegetarian diet. Am J Clin Nutr 1999; 70:543S–548S.
24. Heaney RP, Dowell MS, Bierman J, Hale CA, Bendich A. Absorbability and cost effectiveness in calcium supplementation. J Am Coll Nutr 2001;20:239–246.
25. Heaney RP, Dowell S, Hale CA, Bendich A. Calcium absorption varies within the reference range for serum 25-hydroxyvitamin D. J Am Col Nutr 2003;22:142–146.
26. Guillemant J, Guillemant S. Comparison of the suppressive effect of two doses (500 kg vs. 1500 mg) of oral calcium on parathyroid hormone secretion and on urinary cyclic AMP. Calcif Tissue Int 1993;53:304–306.
27. Martini L, Wood RJ. Relative bioavailability of calcium-rich dietary sources in the elderly. Am J Clin Nutr 2002;76:1345–1350.
28. Heller HJ, Greer LG, Haynes SD, Poindexter JR, Pak CYC. Pharmacokinetic and pharmacodynamic comparison of two calcium supplement in postmenopausal women. J Clin Pharmacol 2000;40:1237–1244.
29. Heaney RP, Dowell MS, Barger-Lux MJ. Absorption of calcium as the carbonate and citrate salts, with some observations on method. Osteoporosis Int 1999;9:19–23.
30. Ishitani K, Itakura E, Goto S, Esashi T. Calcium absorption from the ingestion of coral-derived calcium by humans. J Nutr Sci Vitaminol 1999;45:509–517.
31. Jackman LA, Millane SS, Martin BR, Wood OB, McCabe GP, Peacock M, Weaver CM. Calcium retention in relation to calcium intake and postmenarcheal age in adolescent females. Am J Clin Nutr 1997;327–333.
32. Weaver CM, Martin BR, Plawecki KL, et al. Differences in calcium metabolism between adolescent and adult females. Am J Clin Nutr 1995;61:577–581.
33. DeSantiago S, Alonso L, Halkali A, Larrea F, Isoard F, Bourges H. Negative calcium balance during lactation in rural Mexican women. Am J Clin Nutr 2002;76:845–851.
34. Bryant RJ, Wastney ME, Martin BR, et al. Racial differences in bone turnover and calcium metabolism in adolescent females. J Clin Endocrinol Metab 2003;88(3):1043–1047.
35. Rambaut PC, Leach CS, Whedon GD. A study of metabolic balance in crewmembers of Skylab W. Acta Astronautica 1979;6:1313–1322.
36. Wastney ME, Martin BR, Peacock M, Smith D, Jiang X-Y, Jackman LA, Weaver CM. Changes in calcium kinetics in adolescent girls induced by high calcium intake. J Clin Endocrinol Metab 2000;85:4470–4475.
37. Palacios C, Wigertz K, Martin BR, Weaver CM. Sweat mineral loss from whole body, patch and arm bag in white and black girls. Nutr Res 2003;23:401–411.
38. Charles P, Jensen FT, Mosekilde L, Hanson HH. Calcium metabolism evaluated by [47]Ca kinetics estimation of dermal calcium loss. Clin Sci 1983;65:415–422.
39. Heaney RP, Weaver CM, and Barger-Lux MJ. Food Factors Influencing Calcium Availability. Challenges of Modern Med. In: Burckhardt P. and Heaney RP, ed. Nutritional Aspects of Osteoporosis '94 (Proceedings of 2nd International Symposium on Osteoporosis, Lausanne, May 1994). Ares-Serono Symposia, Rome: 1995;229–241.
40. Dawson-Hughes B, Harris S, Kramiek C, Dallal G, Rasmussen HM. Calcium retention and hormone levels in black and white woman on high- and low- calcium diets. J Bone Miner Metab 1993;8:779–787.
41. Malm OJ. Calcium requirement and adaptation in adult men. Scand J Clin Lab Invest 1958;10(Suppl 36):1–280.
42. Weaver CM, Martin BR, Peacock M. Calcium metabolism in adolescent girls. Challenges of Modern Medicine. Burckhardt P, Heaney RP, eds. In: Nutritional Aspects of Osteoporosis '94. Ares-Serono Symposium Publications 1995;7:123–128.
43. Isaksson B, Lindholm B, Sjögren B. A critical evaluation of the calcium balance technic. II Dermal calcium losses. Metabolism 1967;16:303–313.
44. Wilkinson R. Polyethylene glycol 4000 as a continuously administered non-absorbable fecal marker for metabolic balance studies in human subjects. Gut 1971;12:654–660.
45. Eastell R, Dewanjee MK, Riggs BL. Comparison of polyethylene glycol and chromium-51 chloride as nonabsorbable stool markers in calcium balance studies. Bone Miner 1989;6:95–105.
46. Weaver CM, Wastney M, Spence LA. Quantitative clinical nutrition approaches to the study of calcium and bone metabolism. Clin Rev Bone Miner Metab 2003;1:219–232.

47. Shipp CC, Maletskos CJ, Dawson-Hughes B. Measurement of [47]Ca retention with a whole-body counter. Calcif Tissue Int 1987;41:307–312.

48. Roughead ZK, Johnson LK, Lykken GI, Hunt JR. Controlled high meat diets do not affect calcium retention or indices of bone status in healthy postmenopausal women. J Nutr 2003;13:1020–1026.

49. McCabe LD, Martin BR, McCabe GP, Johnston CC, Weaver CM and Peacock M. Dairy intake impacts bone density in the elderly, Am J Clin Nutr In press.

50. Feskanich D, Willett WC, Colditz GA. Calcium, vitamin D, milk consumption, and hip fractures: a prospective study among postmenopausal women. Am J Clin Nutr 2003;77:504–11.

51. Peacock M, Liu G, Carey M, et al. Bone mass and structure at the hip in men and women over the age of 50. Osteoporosis Int 1998;85:231–239.

6 Kinetic Studies

Meryl E. Wastney, Yongdong Zhao,
and Connie M. Weaver

KEY POINTS

- Kinetic studies employing tracers can be used to calculate rates of calcium metabolism at sites not accessible for direct measurement.
- The design of a tracer study must take into account the question being addressed, because this will influence the tracer dose, sampling sites, and length of the study.
- Different mathematical approaches can be used to analyze the data. Compartmental analysis uses pools and pathways that are analogous to physiological processes and can therefore be used to investigate sites where metabolism changes during different nutritional or disease states.
- Short-term kinetic studies (days–weeks) provide a snapshot on calcium and bone metabolism at one point of time. Multiple kinetic studies over the course of a therapeutic intervention can tell us the continuing effect on calcium metabolism.
- With increased computing power, and dedicated modeling software, we can now measure dynamic properties of calcium metabolism to increase our understanding of calcium homeostasis.

1. INTRODUCTION

Kinetic studies have been used to calculate changes in rates of calcium absorption, excretion, and bone turnover in children, adolescents, and adults. The studies have shown how absorption and bone turnover change with intake. For example, adolescents absorb more calcium on higher calcium intakes, sparing bone resorption. Different approaches to analyzing kinetic data have been compared, and in the future, linking kinetics with biochemical and endocrine indices may be necessary in order to understand dynamic changes in calcium homeostasis during health and in disease.

2. TRACER STUDIES: WHAT THEY CAN TELL US

For many in vivo studies, it is not possible to access pathways of metabolic interest, so we need to rely on indirect measures. Tracers provide such a window into metabolism. By literally "tracing" an element or compound and applying mathematical techniques,

From: *Calcium in Human Health*
Edited by: C. M. Weaver and R. P. Heaney © Humana Press Inc., Totowa, NJ

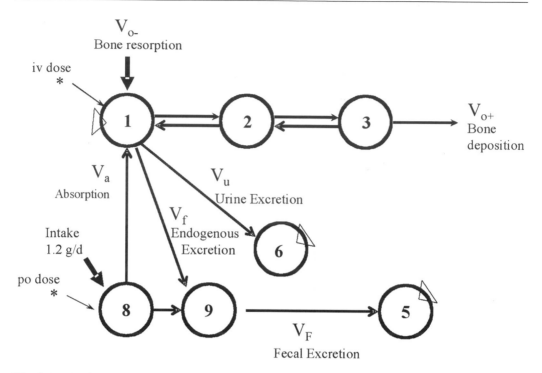

Fig.1. Model for calcium metabolism. Circles represent compartments; numbers in circles represent compartment number; arrows represent movement between compartments; thick arrows represent entry of calcium via the diet, or bone resorption (Vo-). Asterisks indicate entry of tracer and triangles identify sampled compartments. Compartment 1 contains blood, compartment 2, soft tissue, and compartment 3, exchangeable calcium on bone. (Adapted from Wastney et al., 1996 *[1]*.)

we can deduce how the compound moves through the body without actual direct measurements (Fig. 1).

Examples of body processes not susceptible to direct measurement, but which readily yield their secrets to kinetics methods, include measurement of rates of calcium deposition in and removal from bone, rate of entry of calcium into the gut through digestive secretions, exchange rates between cellular and extracellular calcium, and many other, similar variables.

Use of tracers implies making assumptions, an important one being that the tracer exactly follows the path of the compound being traced, while itself not perturbing the system.

3. EXPERIMENTAL CONSIDERATIONS

The adage that you "can't get something for nothing" certainly applies to tracer kinetics. The tissues sampled, the length of the study, and the frequency of sampling will determine the type of information that can be obtained from a study. The more data collected, the more information obtained and the more reliable the results. It is sometimes said that one well-designed kinetic study is more valuable than a large number of studies with limited data per subject. That is because a large amount of data, collected from different sites, on one (representative) subject provides a more comprehensive view of the system working as an integrated whole, and ensures that the calculated model parameter values are well-determined, with low associated error.

3.1. Type, Dose, and Site of Tracer Administration

The type of isotope selected is usually determined by the cost of the isotope and the analytical capability for detection of the tracer in samples. Some of these issues are discussed in more detail in Wastney et al. *(2)*. Tracers of calcium may be radioactive (e.g., ^{41}Ca, ^{45}Ca, ^{47}Ca) or stable (^{42}Ca, ^{43}Ca, ^{44}Ca, ^{46}Ca, ^{48}Ca) (*see* Chapter 5). The dose administered must be small, so the added tracer does not contribute sufficient mass to perturb the system. Multiple doses can be given if the system is to be traced for a long period, or an isotope such as ^{41}Ca (which can be measured with high sensitivity) can be used to trace bone resorption for years.

The questions to be addressed influence the site of tracer administration. If the interest is absorption, doses are given orally, whereas if the interest is bone turnover, intravenous (iv) administration is preferable because it circumvents absorptive variability. Often, two tracers are administered, one orally and one intravenously. This enables both absorption and bone turnover to be determined simultaneously, assuming, as always, that both isotopes, once in the system, are handled in the same way.

3.2. Tissues Sampled

Generally, serum, urine, and feces are sampled, although saliva can also be useful in representing serum, because the calcium tracer in saliva reflects that of serum *(4)*. With γ-emitting tracers, such as ^{47}Ca, even whole-body regions, such as an arm or a leg, can be measured.

3.3. Length of Study

When kinetic modeling is used to investigate bone turnover, the length of a study may influence the results. For adolescents, sampling for 14 d vs 7 d provided more reliable estimates of bone turnover, whereas continuing sampling for 21 d did not provide more information than 14 d (Fig. 2 and Table 1) *(3)*. However, for adults, in whom bone turnover is slower, it was determined that studies of 20 d were necessary to define rate of bone resorption *(5)*. On the other hand, sampling beyond 7 d did not improve calcium absorption measures (Table 1) *(3)*.

When a tracer is used to follow the changes in bone resorption due to therapeutic interventions, kinetic studies can be extended for years with the long-lived ^{41}Ca and sensitive detection using accelerator mass spectrometry (AMS) (*see* Table 1 in Chapter 5).

3.4. Frequency of Sampling

The sampling frequency depends on the purpose of the study. The serum tracer concentration drops very rapidly during the few hours following an intravenous introduction of a tracer, which makes early collection time points important in determining initial compartment sizes. On the other hand, after an oral dose, serum tracer concentration usually reaches the peak around 5 h postdose, which has been proven to be the most relevant time for sampling to estimate calcium absorption. Thus, serum collection has to be at least 5 h long in most calcium absorption studies. When bone turnover is the primary

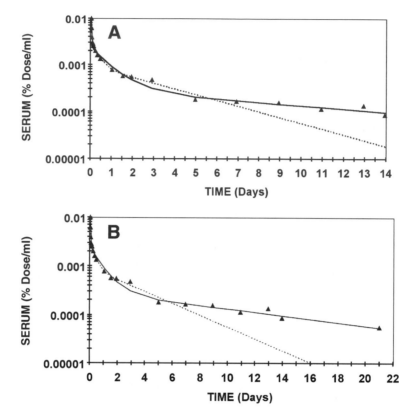

Fig. 2. The effects of length of study on serum disappearance curves of intravenous stable calcium isotopic tracer in an adolescent girl. Symbols are observed data, lines are values calculated by the model shown in Fig. 1 for 7 d (dotted line) compared with (**A**) data collected for 14 d and (**B**) 21 d. (From Weaver et al., 2003 [3].)

Table 1
Results of 7-, 14-, and 21-d Study in Teenaged Girl (1300 mg Ca/d intake)

	7 d	*14 d*	*21 d*
L(0,3) fract/day	0.355	0.090	0.085
Absorption (%)	52	49	49
Vo$^+$ (mg/d)	2282	1583	1557
Vo$^-$ (mg/d)	2273	1472	1447
Balance (mg/d)	9	111	110
V$_u$ (mg/d)	113	113	113

Parameters refer to the model in Fig 1. L(0,3) is the fraction of the calcium in compartment 3 (Fig. 1) that is incorporated into bone each day. Vo$^+$ is bone formation rate; Vo$^-$ is bone resorption rate; V$_u$ is urinary calcium excretion rate.

Table 2
Informational Content of Serum Samples After Tracer Administration as Calculated by WinSAAM

	IV					Oral				
Sample priority	Information content	Sample time			Sample priority	Information content	Sample time		
		Days	Hours	Min			Days	Hours	Min
1	0.455	14	336	20160	1	0.954	0.125	3	180
2	0.230	3	72	4320	2	0.471	0.042	1	60
3	0.226	1	24	1440	3	0.162	3	72	4320
4	0.214	13	312	18720	4	0.160	0.045	1.08	65
5	0.198	11	264	15840	5	0.157	0.049	1.17	70
6	0.183	5	120	7200	6	0.154	1	24	1440
7	0.154	1.5	36	2160	7	0.134	0.055	1.33	80
8	0.142	9	216	12960	8	0.067	2	48	2880
9	0.128	7	168	10080	9	0.066	5	120	7200
10	0.126	2	48	2880	10	0.065	1.5	36	2160
11	0.121	0.417	10	600	11	0.061	0.417	10	600
12	0.100	0.333	8	480	12	0.029	0.333	8	480
13	0.073	0.146	3.5	210	13	0.018	0.250	6	360
14	0.070	0.208	5	300	14	0.011	0.208	5	300
15	0.064	0.250	6	360	15	0.009	0.083	2	120
16	0.062	0.167	4	240	16	0.005	0.167	4	240
17	0.058	0.104	2.5	150	17	0.004	0.146	3.5	210
18	0.056	0.125	3	180	18	0.004	0.104	2.5	150
19	0.046	0.083	2	120					
20	0.034	0.055	1.33	80					
21	0.020	0.049	1.17	70					
22	0.007	0.045	1.08	65					

Information content is a relative value (with no units).

focus of the study, serum collection points after the first week become critical, as shown in Table 1. Experience provides an empirical basis for decisions regarding collection points. However, once a model is established with preliminary data, there are formal ways to quantify the timepoints at which it is more important to satisfy the research purpose (6). One of these approaches is informational analysis (using the INFO command) in WinSAAM (6). An example is shown in Table 2. Parameter values for young women (1) were used to determine the information content of serum samples taken following iv or oral tracer administration. The program determines the relative contribution of each sample. In Table 2, these values have been prioritised according to their informational content. Because sampling was extended over a wide time range, the times are shown as days, hours, and minutes after tracer administration for clarity.

The prioritization of samples according to informational content differed depending on whether the tracer was administered intravenously or orally, i.e., whether the research purpose related to bone or to absorption. It can be seen that following iv dosing, samples with the highest information are those taken 1–3 d and 11–14 d after dosing; whereas after oral dosing, the samples with the most information are those taken within 1–3 h. Using this approach, an investigator can design a sampling schedule to maximize the information obtained from a study.

Although it is apparent that, in measuring absorption, samples taken during actual absorption will be more useful than samples taken days later, and that in measuring bone mineralization, it would be best to allow sufficient time for tracer to exchange with the various exchangeable compartments, these facts can prove invaluable to the investigator for determining which points within the respective time windows are most useful. For absorption, is a 3-h value better than a 5-h value? For bone mineralization, how long should a study go? When is the earliest timepoint that provides useful information? And so forth.

4. DATA ANALYSIS AND MODELING

Modeling is the process of representing pathways of metabolism by mathematical equations. A number of studies have been analyzed using kinetic models with time-invariant rate constants. The review by Heaney *(8)* describing principles of tracer kinetics is still highly relevant. What has changed is the software and computing power available to analyze kinetic data *(9)*.

Both compartmental and noncompartmental approaches have been applied, with the power-function the most common of the latter category. By contrast, compartmental models are expressed as a series of differential equations. Comparison of compartmental vs noncompartmental analysis has been reported by Jung et al. *(5)*. The noncompartmental approach does not provide insight into the underlying biological processes of calcium deposition into bone *(8)*. The compartmental approach has evolved, based on more extensive sampling, from a single compartment up to five compartments *(10)*. The differences among and pitfalls of these models have been extensively discussed elsewhere *(8)*. The description of an approach for analyzing calcium kinetic data by compartmental analysis using WinSAAM is provided in Wastney et al. *(2)*.

4.1. Absorption

Methods for measuring calcium absorption have been discussed in Chapter 5. Here, we will elaborate on tracer-based methods. Each of the methods for determining calcium absorption has limitations and involves assumptions, but generally with more data it becomes possible to test the assumptions. Fecal recovery of an oral tracer is the least invasive method. However, this method can only determine apparent calcium absorption, not true calcium absorption. Fecal tracer consists both of unabsorbed tracer and tracer absorbed and then excreted in the digestive secretions. Unless the endogenous component of the total fecal tracer can be measured (usually requiring a different tracer, given intravenously), true absorption will be underestimated. By contrast, the double-tracer method can determine true absorption, but it requires two tracers, and an intravenous injection.

In the double-tracer method, the ratio of the two tracers at 24 or 48 h postdose is used to estimate the absorption fraction, because the iv tracer parallels the oral tracer closely after 20 h. In an outpatient setting, a much easier method is the single-tracer, single-sample, 5-h specific activity method, developed and validated in women by Heaney and Recker *(11)*. Following a practical calcium load (e.g., approximately one-third of daily calcium intake), serum tracer specific activity peaks around 5 h postdose. This value, after adjustment for height and weight, explains 93% of the variance of calcium absorption measured by the double-tracer method. An even more accurate, but resource-demanding, method uses kinetic modeling with a series of serum, urine, and fecal samples postdose. Serum profiles of iv and oral tracers can be integrated to determine true calcium absorption.

The research purpose dictates the best method. The various purposes for measuring absorption include: (1) determining relative bioavailability of foods and supplements; (2) measuring active calcium absorption to identify malabsorbers or to study mechanisms; and (3) characterizing absorption as a component of calcium metabolism. If comparative bioavailability is the goal, reproducibility of the absorption test within subjects is more critical than the accuracy of the method. In contrast, when the vitamin D-mediated, active component of calcium absorption is the desired information, a small calcium dose is preferable so as not to saturate the first order kinetics of the absorptive apparatus. In this type of assessment, early serum samples (i.e., 1-h or 3-h) must be taken rather than a 5-h serum sample because, with a small load, calcium absorption would have finished by 3-h. But results using this method do not correlate well with *total* calcium absorption. Finally, when calcium absorption is assessed as one of the principal components of whole-person calcium metabolism, as for comparing treatments or defining different populations, or when actual quantities absorbed are needed (as in nutrition studies), absolute values are critically important.

Several approaches to determining calcium absorption have been compared from data collected in a double-tracer study in which serum samples were collected from 1 h postdose up to 12 h on 23 subjects *(12)*. Serum data were fitted to calculate calcium absorption by deconvolution, a type of kinetic modeling. A 24-h urine and a spot urine were also collected and used to calculate calcium absorption. Yergey et al. *(12)* found no difference between absorption determined from the ratio of tracers excreted in urine after 24 h and deconvolution, whereas the value determined from a spot urine sample differed significantly. We have compared values determined from our own data sets for young women (Table 3). Calcium absorption was estimated by determining the ratio of oral and iv tracers in urine collections, oral tracer in 5-h serum sample, and kinetic analysis by compartmental modeling *(1)*. The estimate of absorption from the double-isotope ratio in urine collections increased with the length of collection period, with the increase being larger in some subjects than in others (e.g., Subject Xb vs Xa, Table 3). This is a result of differing kinetics between subjects. The 5-h serum value was not different from the values determined from 24- or 48-h urine samples. The absorption determined from the breakfast test meal (44%) was higher than from dietary calcium (22%, not shown in Table 3) because the latter reflects the effect of different bioavailabilities of the various calcium sources making up a mixed diet as compared with a sole calcium source (usually a drink or tablet) in a test meal *(1)*.

4.2. Bone Deposition and Bone Resorption

With tracer kinetics, bone deposition is determined from the final slope of the exponential curve, which is influenced mainly by movement of calcium in and out of bone. If we can assume that the system is in steady state (pool sizes, apart from bone, remain constant), we can multiply the fractional loss by the mass of the slowest exchangeable

Table 3
Values Calculated for Absorption Following Tracer Administration

| | Fractional Ca Absorption | | | | |
| | Double isotope (urine) | | | Oral isotope specific activity (serum) | Kinetics (serum, urine, feces) |
Subject	24-h	48-h	14-d	5-h	Model from 14-d
Xa	0.255	0.269	0.257	0.252	0.481
Xb	0.106	0.178	0.335	0.244	0.447
Xd	0.193	0.201	0.291	0.255	0.364
Xe	0.236	0.247	0.364	0.274	0.456
Xf	0.313	0.338	0.429	0.260	0.486
Xg	0.285	0.296	0.309	0.261	0.431
Xh	0.319	0.427	0.355	0.291	0.588
Xi	0.255	0.263	0.321	0.243	0.355
Xj	0.241	0.295	0.350	0.247	0.374
Xk	0.290	0.344	0.388	0.276	0.385
Xl	0.183	0.174	0.203	0.241	0.452
Average	0.243^a	0.276^b	0.327^c	0.259^{ab}	0.438^d
Std Dev.	0.063	0.077	0.062	0.016	0.068

Paired t-test was used for statistics. Different letters indicate significant differences ($p < 0.05$).

pool to determine the rate of bone deposition termed "A" (for accretion) by Heaney (8), or "Vo+" in SAAM. Bone resorption is the rate of calcium release from bone termed "R" or "Vo−", and it represents the calcium required to enter blood from bone to maintain a constant pool size.

Most calcium tracers can only be followed for days or weeks, either because, if radioactive, they decay, or, if stable, they cannot be given in large enough quantity without perturbing the system. Thus, multiple times of introducing tracers are required for studying bone resorption over a long period. In contrast, [41]Ca can be tracked for years mainly because of the sensitivity of its detection using AMS. From [41]Ca studies, urinary [41]Ca specific activity decreases by a single exponential after approx 100 d (13). This is considered to reflect skeletal calcium loss. In addition to acting as a clinically useful tool for assessing anti-resorptive therapy, [41]Ca, after prolonged periods, may also provide useful insights into bone metabolism, such as the sizes and interactions of intraskeletal compartments.

Changes in bone resorption and deposition from short-term studies may not accurately reflect long-term changes in bone balance. Because bone is constantly being remodeled (areas of bone are resorbed and then replaced with new bone), any intervention that slows down remodeling will first appear as a decrease in resorption. There is a delay before deposition will slow to match the reduced resorption rate. Heaney (14) has described this phenomenon as the "remodeling transient." Kinetic studies are essential for defining, delimiting, and characterizing the processes that underlie this transient. In studies that do not involve a treatment intervention, short-term kinetic studies may accurately predict long term changes in bone turnover and balance because the remodeling transient is not present. Heaney *(14)* cites studies in which conclusions on the magnitude of the effects of treatment (estrogen) on bone loss would differ if the study had ceased after 1 yr vs 2 yr vs 3 yr, even though any of those time points would have demonstrated the overall protective effect of estrogen on bone. Short-term kinetic studies at several time points could have characterized these dynamic changes.

4.3. Excretion: Urinary, Fecal, and Endogenous

Urinary and fecal excretion of calcium can be measured. Endogenous excretion, by contrast, can only be determined from the amount of iv tracer excreted in feces, adjusted for the time delay in fecal calcium excretion. The appearance of iv tracer in feces is a function of tracer concentration in serum calcium, and this in turn is determined by how rapidly serum calcium turns over. Therefore, either a compartmental approach that accounts for fecal, urine, and serum data simultaneously *(15)*, or calculation of the integral of serum- or urine-specific activity values *(16,17)* must be used. In any event, adjusting for fecal lag time so as to match the fecal collection to the corresponding serum interval that governs tracer appearance in feces is also necessary. In compartment modeling, this is achieved by adding a fecal delay compartment.

4.4. Retention

Retention, the difference between calcium absorbed and calcium excreted, can be determined by balance studies or by the difference between bone deposition and bone resorption from kinetic analysis. The value obtained for retention from kinetic studies is underestimated from shorter kinetic studies (7 d vs 14 and 21 d) (Table 1)

5. USING MODELS TO EXPLORE METABOLISM: RELATIONSHIP OF KINETICS TO OTHER MEASURES OF CALCIUM METABOLISM

Models can be used to explore metabolism by comparing kinetics in a healthy (or treated condition) with those in a disease (or untreated state) *(18)*.

The degree to which kinetic parameters relate to other measures of calcium metabolism has been investigated in a number of studies. Lauffenburger et al. *(19)* compared histomorphometry, kinetics, and biochemical parameters in patients with either low (osteoporosis) or high (Paget's disease) bone turnover. They found high correlation between the results of the different approaches *(19)*. O'Brien et al. *(20)* studied differences between generations of females in families with or without histories of osteoporosis using compartmental modeling analysis. Bone turnover rates were determined from stable calcium isotopic tracer kinetics. Although exact values for bone resorption cannot be determined with confidence in this study, which did not control diet or collect feces, bone formation rates can be estimated from serum tracer profiles. Bone turnover increased more in families with a history of osteoporosis in response to higher calcium intakes than in healthy families. This is an example of the kind of question that can be addressed with tracer kinetics.

6. CONCLUSIONS: THE NEXT GENERATION OF MODELS

Calcium kinetic models will be expanded in the future to represent dynamics, and the homeostatic mechanisms *(21)*. This means linking models for parathyroid hormone, vitamin D, and other calcitropic hormones to calcium metabolism. Several dynamic models have been proposed for humans *(22,23)*. Most have been theoretical and compared only with limited, if any, data. With the additional computing power, more powerful software packages and accumulated data now available for calcium and bone metabolism, there is a need for a dynamic model to integrate knowledge on calcium regulation. Results from kinetic studies could be combined with data from balance studies, bone scans, biomarkers, biochemical indices, and hormonal regulators of calcium to aid our understanding of the temporal and quantitative relationships.

REFERENCES

1. Wastney ME, Ng J, Smith D, Martin BR, Peacock M, Weaver CM. Differences in calcium kinetics between adolescent girls and young women. Am J Physiol 1996;271:R208–R216.
2. Wastney ME, Patterson BH, Linares OA, Greif PC, Boston RC. Investigating Biological Systems Using Modeling: Strategies and Software. Academic, New York: 1998; p. 395.
3. Weaver CM, Wastney M, Spence LA. Quantitative clinical nutrition approaches to the study of calcium and bone metabolism. In: Holick MF, Dawson-Hughes B, eds. Nutrition and Bone Health. Humana, Totowa, NJ: 2003; pp. 133–151.
4. Smith SM, Wastney ME, Nyquist LE, et al. Calcium kinetics with microgram stable isotope doses and saliva sampling. J Mass Spectrom 1996;31:1265–1270.
5. Jung A, Bartholdi P, Mermillod B, Reeve J, Neer R. Critical analysis of methods for analysing human calcium kinetics. J Theor Biol 1978;73:131–157.
6. Berman M, Van Eerdewegh P. Information content of data with respect to models. Am J Physiol 1983; 245:R620–R623.
7. Berman M, Beltz WF, Greif PC, Chabay R, Boston RC. CONSAM User's Guide. DHEW Publication No 1983-421-132:3279. US Govt Printing Office, Washington, DC: 1983.
8. Heaney R. Calcium kinetics in plasma: as they apply to the measurements of bone formation and resorption rates. In: Bourne G, ed. The Biochemistry and Physiology of Bone. Vol. 4. Academic, New York: 1976; pp. 105–133.
9. Stefanovski D, Moate PJ, Boston RC. WinSAAM: A Windows-based compartmental modeling system. Metabolism 2003;52:1153–1166.
10. Wajchenberg BL, Leme PR, Ferreira MNL, Modesto Filho J, Pieroni RR, Berman M. Analysis of 47Ca kinetics in normal subjects by means of a compartmental model with a non-exchangeable plasma calcium fraction. Clin Sci 1979;56:523–532.
11. Heaney RP, Recker RR. Estimation of true calcium absorption. Ann Int Med 1985;103:516–521.
12. Yergey AL, Abrams SA, Vieira NE, Aldroubi A, Marini J, Sidbury JB. Determination of fractional absorption of dietary calcium in humans. J Nutr 1994;124:674–682.
13. Freeman SPHT, Beck B, Bierman JM, et al. The study of skeletal calcium metabolism with [41]Ca and [45]Ca. Nucl Instr Meth Phys Res 2000;172:930–933.
14. Heaney RP. The bone remodeling transient: interpreting interventions involving bone-related nutrients. Nutr Rev 2001;59:327–334.
15. Neer R, Berman M, Fisher L, Rosenberg LE. Multicompartmental analysis of calcium kinetics in normal adult males. J Clin Invest 1967;46:1364–1379.
16. Heaney RP. Calcium tracers in the study of vertebrate calcium metabolism. In: Zipkin I, ed. Biological Mineralization: Wiley, NY: 1973.
17. Abrams SA, Vieira NE, Yergey AL. Interpretation of stable isotope studies of calcium absorption and kinetics. In: Siva Subramanian KN, Wastney ME, eds. Kinetic Models of Trace Element and Mineral Metabolism during Development. CRC, Boca Raton: 1995; pp. 283–290.
18. Wastney ME, Martin BR, Bryant RJ, Weaver CM. Calcium utilization in young women: New insights from modelling. Adv Exp Biol Med 2003;537:193–205.
19. Lauffenburger T, Olah AJ, Dambacher MA, Guncaga J, Lentner C, Haas HG. Bone remodeling and calcium metabolism: A correlated histomorphometric, calcium kinetic, and biochemical study in patients with osteoporosis and Paget's Disease. Metab Clin Exp 1977;26:589–605.

20. O'Brien KO, Abrams SA, Liang LK, Ellis KJ, Gagel RF. Bone turnover response to changes in calcium intake is altered in girls and adult women in families with histories of osteoporosis. J Bone Miner Res 1998;13:491–499.

21. Wastney ME, Zhao Y, Smith SM. Modelling human calcium dynamics as a mechanism for exploring changes in calcium homeostasis during space flight. In: Hargrove J, Berdanier C, eds. Mathematical Modelling in Nutrition and Toxicology. Mathematical Biology Press, Athens, GA; 2005, pp. 157–170.

22. Doty SE, Seagrave RC. Human water, sodium, and calcium regulation during space flight and exercise. Acta Astronaut 2000;46:591–604.

23. Jaros GG, Coleman TG, Guyton AC. Model of short-term regulation of calcium-ion concentration. Simulation 1979;32:193–204.

III   CALCIUM CONSUMPTION, REQUIREMENTS, AND BIOAVAILABILITY

7 Requirements for What Endpoint?

Robert P. Heaney and Connie M. Weaver

KEY POINTS

- The official calcium intake requirement is pegged to a bony endpoint.
- Adequate calcium intake supports many health outcomes in addition to bone.
- For some ethnic groups and for some life stages in all groups, optimal calcium intake may relate to nonskeletal endpoints.
- Hence, current recommendations, although generally satisfactory for bone, may not be adequate for optimal total body health.

1. INTRODUCTION

In Chapter 2, we noted that calcium was a threshold nutrient and we introduced the term "minimum daily requirement" (MDR), defined as the intake just sufficient to get an individual up to the bone retention threshold, i.e., the point at which no further increase in bone mass will occur despite further increases in calcium intake. The concept of an MDR has been largely abandoned for many other nutrients, but it remains apt for calcium, as Fig. 1 in Chapter 2 shows graphically.

In defining the calcium intake requirement, the Calcium and Related Nutrients panel of the Food and Nutrition Board used the notion of maximal calcium retention, that is, the retention plateau at or above the threshold intake (1). In doing so, they explicitly chose bone mass as the functional indicator for calcium nutritional adequacy. It was recognized then that calcium plays a role in other disorders (see Part VI of this book), but information was insufficient to allow the panel to peg the requirement to the optimal functioning of systems other than bone. Much information has been accumulated since the recommendations of the Calcium and Related Nutrients panel were submitted to the Food and Nutrition Board, and we discuss some of that new information in Part VI. Here, we review the considerations that went into setting the calcium requirement, show how the MDR may itself not be optimal, even for bone, and set forth the physiology that undergirds the fact that, for certain disease endpoints, the calcium intake requirement may be substantially higher than that needed for skeletal health.

From: *Calcium in Human Health*
Edited by: C. M. Weaver and R. P. Heaney © Humana Press Inc., Totowa, NJ

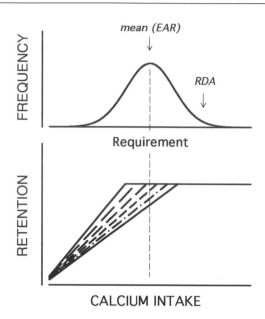

Fig. 1. Schematic depiction of varying utilization efficiencies for calcium (lower panel) and the distribution of such efficiencies (upper panel). For each of the utilization efficiencies, the maximal retention value is the same, but some individuals reach maximal retention at a lower calcium intake than others, while still others require more. The upper panel schematically presents the distribution of such individual intake requirements. The mean of that distribution is the Estimated Average Requirement (EAR), and the Recommended Dietary Allowance (RDA) for calcium would, accordingly, be set roughly two standard deviations above that mean value. (Copyright Robert P. Heaney, 2004. Used with permission.)

2. SETTING THE REQUIREMENT

For most or all nutrients, the published requirement represents the least intake an individual can get by on and still attain some desired health outcome or reach some target value for a functional indicator of nutritional status. Because of differences in absorption or utilization efficiency from individual to individual, there will be a range of requirements, with some individuals able to achieve the desired outcome at lower intakes and others requiring more to produce the same effect. This concept is illustrated for calcium in Fig. 1. In the bottom panel are depicted what a range of requirements means in terms of individual threshold diagrams. Individuals reach their particular bone retention thresholds at various intakes. The top panel presents, schematically, what the distribution of such individual requirement values might look like. The mean value of this distribution is the Dietary Reference Intake (DRI) called an "Estimated Average Requirement" (EAR). By contrast, a "Recommended Dietary Allowance" (RDA) is an intake sufficient to meet the needs of roughly 97% of the population, a value that would be located about two standard deviations to the right of the EAR in the top panel of Fig. 1.

The currently recommended intake values *(1)* for calcium are the so-called "Adequate Intakes" (AI). These happen to be identical to the EAR for calcium, and hence represent an intake that is below the threshold for roughly half the population.

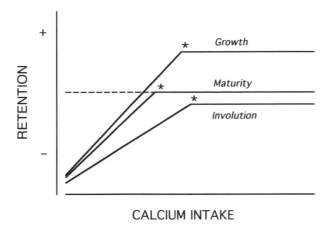

Fig. 2. Retention curves for three life stages. The dashed horizontal line represents zero retention and hence maintenance of bone mass, whereas during growth one would expect positive retention, and during involution, some degree of bone loss, irrespective of calcium intake. For each curve, the asterisks indicate the minimum daily requirement (MDR). (Copyright Robert P. Heaney, 1998. Used with permission.)

Taking the "least to get by on" approach to nutritional recommendations inevitably leads to different recommendations for different ages and physiological states. For example, during a woman's reproductive years, when she has high circulating estrogen levels (and correspondingly better conservation of calcium), she can "get by on" a lower calcium intake than is possible in a postmenopausal, estrogen-deprived state. At least, her bones can get by on less calcium (discussed later).

These age- and state-specific differences in the requirement are illustrated in Fig. 2, once again schematically, but for three age-states: growth, maturity, and involution. There are three key features about each of the retention diagrams in Fig. 2: (1) the steepness of the ascending limb of the retention curve; (2) the location of the threshold point along the range of calcium intakes (horizontal axis); and (3) the location of the plateau region along the range of retention values (vertical axis). The *steepness* of the ascending limbs of the curves is a reflection of the efficiency with which the organism uses dietary calcium; the threshold *intake* is the MDR; and the threshold *retention* is the desired physiological state, that is, bone accumulation during growth, bone maintenance during maturity, and minimization of bone loss during involution.

The desired retention values for growth and maturity are intuitively obvious, but the negative value for retention in the involutional phase of life deserves comment. It reflects the fact that there are other factors operating in the body during involution which lead to diminution in bone mass. These factors cannot be countered by calcium, because they are not caused by insufficient calcium intake. They include decreased physical activity, declines in the production of various hormones that are trophic for bone, and intercurrent illnesses and infections, among others. From the standpoint of nutrition during this phase of life, the goal is to achieve a calcium intake during involution that minimizes bone loss and ensures that nutritional inadequacy is not contributing to whatever decline in bone mass may otherwise be occurring.

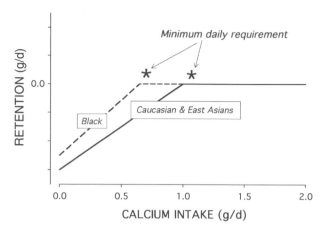

Fig. 3. Calcium retention curves for blacks, as contrasted with Caucasians and east Asians, with an approximate estimate of the quantitative differences in minimum daily requirement (MDR). (Copyright Robert P. Heaney, 2001. Used with permission.)

3. ETHNICITY AND THE REQUIREMENT

In animals, it is possible to perform dose–response experiments, controlling calcium intake at various life stages for long enough to determine the location of the intake thresholds. An example is the work of Forbes et al. *(2)* depicted in Fig. 1 in Chapter 2. For the most part, comparable studies have not been done in humans of any ethnic or racial background. Partial exceptions can be found in the work of Matkovic and Heaney *(3)* and of Jackman et al. *(4)*. Using calcium balances measured across a range of intakes, these investigators have provided estimates of the location of the intake thresholds. However, these data have been accumulated mainly in Caucasians. From the limited evidence that is available, it appears that East Asians have approximately the same requirements as do Caucasians, particularly when diet calcium is corrected for differences in body size. However, two lines of evidence indicate that blacks have a lower requirement for the skeletal endpoint, as illustrated schematically in Fig. 3. The evidence comes from two sources: adult bone mass values are higher in African Americans than in Caucasians, and at the same time, the distribution of their calcium intakes is shifted to the left of that for Caucasians. This means that, despite a lower calcium intake, they acquire more bone than Caucasians or East Asians. The second line of evidence, discussed briefly in Chapter 10, lies in the fact that the bony resorptive apparatus of blacks is relatively resistant to parathyroid hormone (PTH). This means that, in order to maintain extracellular fluid (ECF) [Ca^{2+}] in the face of lower intake, they must secrete more PTH and maintain higher levels of 1,25 dihydroxyvitamin D (1,25[OH]$_2$D), which, in fact, is found to be the case *(5)*. As a consequence, they make better use of dietary calcium: through most of life by reduced urinary calcium loss, and, at some stages, by more efficient intestinal absorption as well. It is as a consequence of these adjustments that the slope of the ascending limb of the retention curve is steeper in blacks, and the retention maximum is reached at a lower calcium intake. The precise value of the difference in the requirement between blacks on the one hand and whites and East Asians on the other can only be roughly estimated, but is probably on the order of 300 mg/d, as Fig. 3 suggests.

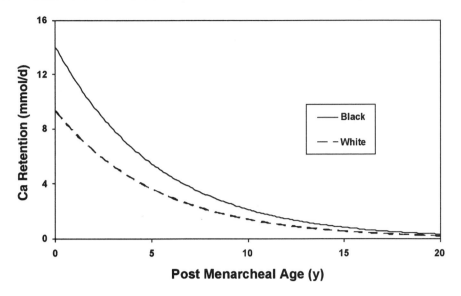

Fig. 4. Model fit for calcium retention, as a function of postmenarcheal age, in black and white females. The cumulative racial difference in bone mass, based on calcium accretion from onset of menarche to 20 yr postmenarche, is predicted to be 12%. (Reprinted from ref. *6.*)

Evidence of more efficient calcium absorption and suppressed bone resorption in black compared with white pubertal girls is shown in Chapter 17. The racial difference in calcium retention during formation of peak bone mass appears to be greatest at onset of menses and diminishes as peak bone mass is reached. Figure 4 *(6)* shows calcium retention as a function of postmenarcheal age in black and white women. The model was developed using data from whites that spanned the whole age range. The curve for blacks was created using data from adolescent black girls projected using the model developed on white women. An estimate of the cumulative difference in retained calcium from the area between the two curves converted to bone mass is 12%, consistent with the 10 and 13% higher femoral neck bone mineral content and density, respectively, observed in black compared with white women from National Health and Nutrition Examination Survey (NHANES) III 1990–1994 *(7)*. Thus, much of the difference in adult mass can be accounted for by the differences in calcium handling during growth. Accordingly, one would expect that the racial differences in calcium retention depicted in Fig. 3 would be most pronounced during adolescence and diminish after peak bone mass has been achieved. Consistent with this expectation are the similar whole-body [47]Ca retention curves for adult black and white women in Fig. 2 in Chapter 19.

4. IS THE MDR OPTIMAL?

As Fig. 2 makes clear schematically, and as the very name MDR suggests, this intake is "the least one can get by on." Simply expressing the requirement in this way suggests automatically that the MDR may not be optimal, even for the bony endpoint which currently serves as the functional indicator for calcium nutrition. There is, in fact, a body of evidence suggesting that somewhat higher intakes would be optimal.

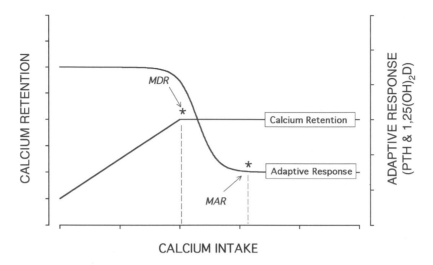

Fig. 5. A curve for the adaptive response to insufficient calcium intake, superimposed on the calcium retention curve, showing that the minimal adaptive response (MAR) is not achieved until an intake somewhat in excess of the minimum daily requirement (MDR). (Copyright Robert P. Heaney, 2004. Used with permission.)

As is evident from an understanding of the physiology involved (*see* Chapters 10 and 11), any intake located along the ascending limb of the retention curve will tend to evoke an adaptive response from the organism (i.e., increased PTH secretion) with its cascade of effects. But simply getting up to the threshold itself requires continuing adaptation. Although increasing intake beyond the threshold point will not lead to higher bone mass, it will lead to decreased adaptation because, as the diet becomes richer and richer in calcium, less and less compensation will be required to permit obtaining all the calcium that might be needed both for growth and to offset obligatory losses (i.e., to remain on the plateau of the retention curve). Thus, there is a phase lag between calcium retention and the adaptive response, depicted schematically in Fig. 5.

There are two implications for optimal calcium nutrition that flow from this insight. The first relates to the bony endpoint and the second to nonskeletal disease. For bone, even though maximal calcium retention may be achieved, the still somewhat elevated PTH levels would be expected to elevate the level of bone remodeling which, as discussed in Chapter 2, is a fragility factor in its own right. This is shown, for example, in the fracture experience of patients with untreated, mild primary hyperparathyroidism *(8)* in whom, despite no appreciable difference in bone mass, fracture risk is approximately threefold greater than in age-matched normal controls. Thus, one would predict that fracture risk would decline somewhat as calcium intake increases past the threshold intake. The precise amount required to produce this level is unclear, and probably rises with age. For example, McKane et al. *(9)* were able to reduce PTH levels in healthy women over age 65 yr to young adult normal values at an intake of 2400 mg Ca/d, a value well above the current AI. Importantly, this seemingly high intake did not depress PTH levels below the young adult normal range. Such an intake, although high by contemporary standards, would probably be in the mid range of calcium intakes for hunter–gatherer populations (adjusted for differences between primitive and contemporary body sizes) *(10)*, and hence may be close to the intake for which human physiology has been adapted over the course of evolution. Additional evidence supporting this conclusion is seen in the calcium homeostatic response to a challenge such as sodium-induced hypercalciuria (*see* Chapter 10). This behavior illustrates beautifully how the fine-tuning of the calcium economy presumes an intake such as that employed by McKane et al.

The second facet of this phase lag of Fig. 5 relates to the calcium paradox diseases discussed in Part VI, and introduced briefly in Chapter 19. There we note that diseases such as hypertension may be aggravated or initiated as a consequence of high circulating levels of $1,25(OH)_2D$. Thus, to the extent that a threshold intake may still be associated with some elevation of serum $1,25(OH)_2D$, susceptibility to the calcium paradox diseases will be aggravated. This is probably most clearly seen in the case of blacks who, as noted above, have lower calcium intakes than whites, higher circulating levels of PTH and $1,25(OH)_2D$ (5), and a lower bone threshold intake than whites or East Asians. At the same time, African Americans are known to be at increased risk of hypertension and cardiovascular disease, and they have been shown to respond with significant blood pressure reductions to a diet high in calcium and fruits and vegetables (*see* Chapter 28) (11). The calcium intake that produced this benefit was approx 1200 mg/d, well above the bony retention threshold for blacks illustrated in Fig. 3. Thus, although the Food and Nutrition Board selected bone calcium retention as the functional indicator of calcium nutrient adequacy for all persons, newer evidence indicates that, for at least some population groups (e.g., African Americans) blood pressure and/or cardiovascular status is a more appropriate functional indicator.

The evidence supporting use of a non-bony functional indicator is clearest for hypertension, particularly in blacks, and much work needs to be done in order to clarify the optimal calcium intake for the remaining nonskeletal health outcomes. However, it can be noted that the calcium intakes associated in observational studies with minimizing the expression of the nonskeletal diseases related to low calcium intake are all in the range of 1100–1800 mg/d. These values are above the AI for all individuals up to age 50 yr, and at or above the AI for older individuals. Hence, when the requisite data are finally accumulated and the calcium requirement is once again revisited by the Food and Nutrition Board, it would not be surprising to see intake recommendations which may be higher than those required simply for the bony endpoint.

5. CONCLUSIONS

An adequate calcium intake is necessary to ensure optimal functioning of many body systems. Yet current intake recommendations were pegged exclusively to a skeletal endpoint and represent the lowest intake an individual can ingest without compromising the mechanical function of the skeleton. Available evidence indicates that, for certain physiological states and certain ethnic groups, nonskeletal functions of calcium may be more sensitive indicators of the requirement and thus, the optimal *total body* requirement may be higher than the current, bone-related DRIs.

REFERENCES

1. Dietary Reference Intakes for Calcium, Magnesium, Phosphorus, Vitamin D, and Fluoride. Food and Nutrition Board, Institute of Medicine. National Academy Press, Washington, DC: 1997.

2. Forbes RM, Weingartner KE, Parker HM, Bell RR, Erdman JW Jr. Bioavailability to rats of zinc, magnesium and calcium in casein-, egg- and soy protein-containing diets. J Nutr 1979;109:1652–1660.
3. Matkovic V, Heaney RP. Calcium balance during human growth. Evidence for threshold behavior. Am J Clin Nutr 1992;55:992–996.
4. Jackman LA, Millane SS, Martin BR, et al. Calcium retention in relation to calcium intake and postmenarcheal age in adolescent females. Am J Clin Nutr 1997;66:327–333.
5. Heaney RP. Ethnicity, bone status, and the calcium requirement. Nutr Res 2002;22:(1–2):153–178.
6. Bryant RJ, Wastney ME, Martin BR, et al. Racial differences in bone turnover and calcium metabolism in adolescent females. J Clin Endocrinol Metab 2003;88(3):1043–1047.
7. Looker AC, Wahner HW, Dunn WL, et al. Updated data on proximal femur bone mineral levels of US adults. Osteoporos Int 1998;8:468–489.
8. Khosla S, Melton LJ III, Wermers RA, Crowson CS, O'Fallon WM, Riggs BL. Primary hyperparathyroidism and the risk of fracture: a population-based study. J Bone Miner Res 1999;14(10):1700–1707
9. McKane WR, Khosla S, Egan KS, Robins SP, Burritt MF, Riggs BL. Role of calcium intake in modulating age-related increases in parathyroid function and bone resorption. J Clin Endocrinol Metab 1996;81:1699–1703.
10. Eaton B, Nelson DA. Calcium in evolutionary perspective. Am J Clin Nutr 1991;54:281S–287S.
11. Appel LJ, Moore TJ, Obarzanek E, et al. A clinical trial of the effects of dietary patterns on blood pressure. N Engl J Med 1997;336:1117–1124.

8 Dietary Calcium

Recommendations and Intakes Around the World

Anne C. Looker

KEY POINTS

- Many countries have published calcium intake recommendations since 1988. These recommendations vary by as much as 900 mg/d.
- Calcium recommendations published after 1997 tend to be higher than those published during 1988–1996.
- Data on calcium intakes in children are too scanty to draw conclusions about adequacy.
- Young men are the only group among adolescents and adults that appears unlikely to have inadequate calcium intakes.
- Data on calcium intakes above the upper limit of 2500 mg/d are too scanty to draw firm conclusions; nonetheless, the risk of inadequate intakes is likely much higher than the risk of excessive intakes.

1. INTRODUCTION

The critical role of calcium in human health has been recognized for many years, as reflected by a long history of calcium intake recommendations (*1*). Although the need for an appropriate intake of calcium is well recognized among health authorities, data on calcium intakes suggest that a large percentage of the population in most countries does not consume recommended amounts. The objective of the present chapter is to review calcium recommendations and intakes in various countries to provide a current snapshot of calcium nutrition around the world.

To meet this goal, several methods were used to locate published information on calcium recommendations and dietary intake data collected in the 15-yr period from 1988 to 2003. These included a Medline search and use of several Internet search engines to identify papers or other relevant sources of information. The International Reference Guide on Health Data (*2*) was used to identify 13 countries that conduct national surveys that include some type of dietary information. Internet websites of several regional and national health agencies were also searched. Finally, reference lists and professional contacts were used to identify additional sources of information. Nonetheless, this chap-

From: *Calcium in Human Health*
Edited by: C. M. Weaver and R. P. Heaney © Humana Press Inc., Totowa, NJ

ter is not meant to be an exhaustive list of all existing recommendations or datasets on calcium intakes worldwide, but rather to provide selected examples that can illustrate the variability in recommendations and intakes around the world.

2. CALCIUM RECOMMENDATIONS

2.1. Recent Calcium Recommendations in Different Countries

Calcium recommendations published since 1988 were located for 33 countries or organizations using the methods described in the Introduction. A detailed summary of these recommendations is given in Table 1 (for summaries of recommendations published prior to 1988, see refs. 3 and 4). Approximate age groupings have been used to summarize the recommendations, because the exact definitions of the age categories differ between countries. As illustrated in Fig. 1, the absolute amounts of recommended calcium vary widely between the different countries. For example, 75% of the recommended intakes for adolescent males fall between 850 and 1200 mg/d, but the range varies from a low of 500 mg/d (recommended in Sri Lanka) to a high of 1300 mg/d (recommended in the United States and Venezuela and by the Food and Agriculture Organization [FAO] of the World Health Organization [WHO]). In general, the range of recommended values in these 33 countries tended to be narrower in infants, toddlers and younger children than in older children, adolescents and adults: the average difference between the highest and lowest amount recommended was 537 mg/d in the younger groups versus 820 mg/d in the older groups, respectively.

The recommendations also vary depending on how recently they were developed. An upward trend in calcium recommendations has been noted in the past 15 years in some European and North American countries (5–9). This trend is illustrated in Fig. 2, which shows that recommendations shown in Table 1 for adults published after 1997 are significantly higher than those published in 1989–1996. Recommendations for older children and adolescents published after 1997 also tended to be higher than those published earlier, but the differences were not statistically significant.

Possible reasons for the variability in calcium recommendations include differences in their conceptual basis (e.g., avoidance of deficiency vs prevention of chronic disease), the endpoint being used (calcium balance vs bone mineral density), assumptions about the percent of ingested calcium that is absorbed, inclusion of insensible loss of calcium via skin, hair, or nails, and the possibility that the calcium requirement itself may vary from culture to culture for dietary, genetic, body size, lifestyle, and geographical reasons (10). Recommendations may also vary as a result of different interpretations of the same data (3). Some recommendations are based solely on review of original research, others are based solely on a review of other recommendations, while still others may use a combination of both approaches (3).

Some countries choose to adopt recommendations from other countries or from authoritative bodies (such as FAO/WHO or European Community [EC]) rather than developing their own unique recommendations (11,12). There is a growing trend toward harmonization of recommendations across countries, as witnessed by the joint development of recommendations for the Nordic countries (13), and the D-A-CH 2000 (Austria, Germany, and Switzerland) (14). The European Union has compiled a set of recommendations for use across the EC (15). Canada and the United States have collaborated recently to develop Dietary Reference Intakes for use in both countries *(9)*. Other regions, such as Southeast Asia, are also moving toward greater harmonization *(16,17)*. Reasons to consider harmonization include similarities between populations in some countries, expense and lack of resources to undertake nutrition research, reduction in consumer confusion, increase in world trade, and creation of a global food supply *(12)*.

2.1.1. UPPER AND LOWER LIMITS FOR CALCIUM INTAKES

In addition to identifying a target amount of calcium to consume, calcium recommendations from some countries also include a tolerable upper limit (UL) and a lowest acceptable level for calcium intake. The UL is defined as "the highest average daily nutrient intake level likely to pose no risk of adverse health effects for almost all individuals in the general population" *(9)*. Intakes that rise above the UL are believed to carry an increasing risk of adverse effects. Several countries or organizations have identified an upper limit for calcium of 2500 mg/d; examples among those listed in Table 1 include Belgium, EC, Japan, the Netherlands, the Nordic countries (Denmark, Finland, Iceland, Norway, and Sweden), Taiwan, and the United States *(9,13,15,18–23)*.

The lowest acceptable level for calcium has been defined as "the intake below which there may be cause for concern for a substantial section of the population" *(15)*, or an amount of the nutrient that is enough for only the few people in a group who have low needs *(24)*. As these definitions imply, the lowest acceptable level is intended to be used for assessment of results from dietary surveys, rather than in assessing an individual's diet *(13)*. Selected examples of countries that have set a lowest acceptable level for calcium include the Nordic countries and the EC *(13,15)*. Both groups defined 400 mg/d as the lowest level for males and females, but the EC indicated that this value applied to adults only *(15)*, whereas the Nordic recommendation covers ages 15–50 yr *(13)*. The United Kingdom has defined a Lower Reference Nutrient Intake (LRNI) for calcium, equal to two standard deviations below the Estimated Average Requirement (EAR), for several age groups: 200–275 mg/d for infants and young children, 325 mg/d for older children, 450–480 mg/d for adolescents, and 400 mg/d for adults *(24)*. Ireland has defined a Lowest Threshold Intake for adults as 430 mg/d *(25)*.

3. CALCIUM INTAKES

3.1. Calcium Intakes in Different Countries

Calcium intake from food in 20 selected countries around the globe are summarized in Table 2. National data have been included whenever possible; however many countries either do not routinely collect dietary data from a nationally representative sample, have not collected it recently, or do not report individual intake data *(2,26,27)*. To provide a more complete picture of calcium intakes, Table 2 also includes regional data for selected countries for which nationally representative data could not be located. Because data were located for only 20 (10%) of the 192 independent states in the world *(28)*, the information on calcium intakes is not intended to be an exhaustive review, but rather to illustrate the variability in calcium intake that exists in different countries. It should also be noted that these data do not include calcium intake from nonfood sources, such as vitamin-mineral supplements, antacids, hard water, or medicines that contain calcium as an excipient or inert ingredient.

Table 1

Recommended Calcium Intakes (mg/d)[a] From Selected Countries Published Since 1988

Country/organization	Infants	Toddlers	Young children	Older children	Adolescents	Young adult	Middle-aged adult	Older adult	Pregnant	Lactating
Australia (1991) (65)										
Male	300–550	700	800	800	1000–1200	800	800	800	–	–
Female	300–550	700	800	900	800–1000	800	800	1000	+300	+400
Austria[b] (2000) (14)										
Male & Female	220–400	600	700	900	1100–1200	1000–1200	1000	1000	1000	1000
Belgium (2000) (18)										
Male & Female	400–600	800	800	800	1000–1200	900	900	1200[c]	1200	1200
Canada[d] (1997) (9)										
Male	250–500	550	600	700	900–1100	800	800	800	–	–
Female	250–500	550	600	700	700–1100	700	800	800	+500	+500
China (2001) (66)										
Male & Female	300–400	600	800	800	1000	800	800	1000	800–1200[e]	1200
Colombia (1992) (67)										
Male & Female	400–550	450	450	450	550–650	500	500	500	+300	+400
European Community (1993) (15)										
Male	400	400	450	550	1000	700	700	700	–	–
Female	400	400	450	550	800	700	700	700	700	1200
Denmark[f] (1996) (13)										
Male & Female	360–540	600	600	700	900	800	800	800	900	1200
FAO/WHO (2002) (10)										
Male & Female	300–400	500	600	700	1300	1000	1000	1300[c]	1200	1000
Finland (1998) (13,68)										
Male & Female	360–540	600	600	700	900	800[g]	800	800	900	900
France (2000) (69,70)										
Male & Female	–	500	700–900	1200	1200	900	900[h]	1200	1000	1000
Germany[b] (2000) (14)										
Male & Female	220–400	600	700	900	1100–1200	1000–1200	1000	1000	1000	1000

Country (year) (ref), Sex										
Iceland[f] (1996) (13)										
Male & Female	360–540	600	700	900	800	800		800	900	1200
Indonesia (1994) (71,72)										
Male & Female	400–600	500	500–700[i]	600–700	500		500	500	+400	+400
Ireland (1999) (25)										
Male & Female	800	800	1200	800	800		1200	1200	1200	
Italy (1996) (73)										
Male	600	800	1000	1200	1000	1000	800	1000	–	–
Female	600	800	1000	1200	1000	1000	1200–1500/1000[j]	1200–1500/1000[j]	1200	1200
Japan (2002) (19)										
Male	200–500	500	600–700	800–900	600–700	600	600	600	–	–
Female	200–500	500	600–700	700	600	600	600	600	+300	+500
Mexico (1994) (74)										
Male & Female	450–600	800	800	1200	800–1200	800	800	800	1200	1200
The Netherlands (2000) (20)										
Male	210–450	500	1200	1200	1000	1000–1100	1200	800	–	–
Female	210–450	500	1100	1100	1000	1000–1100	1200	800	1000	1000
Norway[f] (1996) (13)										
Male & Female	360–540	600	700	900	800	800	800	800	900	1200
The Phillipines (2002) (75)										
Male	200–400	500	700	1000	750	750	750	800	–	–
Female	200–400	500	700	1000	750	750	800	800	800	750
Poland (1998) (76)										
Male & Female	–	–	1000	1100–1200	1000	1000	1000	1000	1500	2000
Singapore (2002) (77)										
Male & Female	300–400	500	700	1000	800	800	800	1000	1000	1000
Spain (1994) (78)										
Male	500	600	650	800–850	850	600	600	700	1200	1300
Female	500	600	650	500–600	850	600	600	700	1200	1300
Sri Lanka (1998) (79)										
Male & Female	500	400	400	500–600	400	400	400	400	1000	1000
Sweden (1996) (21)										
Male & Female	360–540	600	700	900	800	800	800	800[k]	900	1200

(continued)

Table 1 (Continued)

Country/organization	Infants	Toddlers	Young children	Older children	Adolescents	Young adult	Middle-aged adult	Older adult	Pregnant	Lactating
Switzerland[b] (2000) (14)										
Male & Female	220–400	600	700	900	1100–1200	1000–1200	1000	1000	1000	1000
Thailand (1989) (80)										
Male & Female	360–480	800	800	800–1200	1200	800	800	–	1200	1200
Taiwan (2002) (23)										
Male & Female	200–400	500–600	800–1000	1200	1000	1000	1000	1000	+0	+0
United Kingdom (1991) (24)										
Male	525	350	450	550	1000	700	700	700	–	–
Female	525	350	450	550	800	700	700	700	–	+550
United States[d] (1997) (9)										
Male & Female	210–270	500	800	1300	1300	1000	1200	1200	1000–1300[l]	1000–1300[l]
Venezuela (2000) (81)										
Male	210–270	500	500	800	1300	1000	1000	1200	–	–
Female	210–270	500	500	800	1300	1000	1000	1300	1300	1300
Vietnam (1996) (82)										
Male & Female	300–500	500	500	500	700[m]	500	500	500	1000	1000

FAO, Food and Agriculture Organization; WHO, World Health Organization.

[a]Calcium intake ranges reflect different recommendations for age subgroups within an age category except where noted. For infants, range may also reflect different recommendations for breast-vs bottle-fed infants.

[b]Austria, Germany, and Switzerland share the same recommended intakes (DACH 2000).

[c]Applies to postmenopausal women.

[d]Canada and the United States share the same recommendations (IOM, 1997).

[e]Amount depends on trimester.

[f]The Nordic Countries (Denmark, Iceland, Norway, and Sweden) share the same recommended intakes.

[g]900 mg/d recommended for 19- to 20-yr-old individuals.

[h]1200 mg/d recommended for women age 55+ yr.

[i]600–700 mg/d recommended for 10- to 12-yr-old individuals.

[j]Higher amount (1200–1500 mg/d) recommended for postmenopausal women who do not use estrogen therapy.

[k]A supplement of 500–1000 mg/d may, to a certain extent, delay bone loss.

[l]1300 mg/d recommended for girls ≤ 18 yr.

[m]600 mg/d recommended for 16- to 19-yr-old girls.

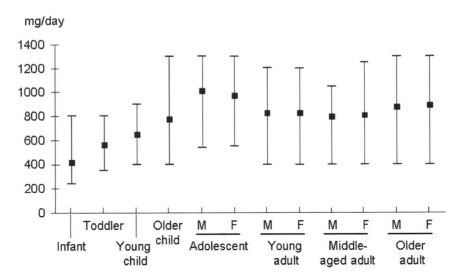

Fig. 1. Range of calcium recommendations from 33 countries. Highest value is at the top of each bar; black box indicates mean value; lowest value is at the bottom of each bar.

Some additional caveats arise when comparing calcium intakes in Table 2 between world regions or individual countries. The small number of countries for which calcium data were obtained limits regional comparisons because some regions either are not represented or are represented by a few countries only. Use of different dietary methods in the different studies may also affect comparisons: mean intakes are generally similar when based on questionnaires vs diet records, but one study found a difference of 125 mg between the two methods *(29–34)*. Finally, differences in the presentation of the data in the different published reports (e.g., use of different age groups, means vs medians, or combined vs sex-specific estimates) also complicate a comparison of the data from different countries.

With these caveats in mind, some general trends emerge. For example, mean intakes among adolescents and adults vary considerably in the different countries, with the highest versus lowest mean intakes differing by as much as 900 mg/d in some age groups (Fig. 3; data for younger age groups are not included in Figs. 3 and 4 because there were less than 10 observations for these ages). When world regions for which there were data for at least two countries in the sample were compared, calcium intakes generally appeared highest in Scandinavian countries, lowest in Asian countries, and intermediate in western European, Oceania (Australia/New Zealand), and North American countries (data not shown).

3.1.1. ADEQUACY OF CALCIUM INTAKES

Published estimates of the prevalence of inadequate calcium intake in different countries suggest that in many countries, a large proportion of the population fails to consume a sufficient amount of this mineral *(35–49)*. However, precise estimates of inadequacy are difficult to define because of the complicated nature of assessing dietary adequacy. This complexity results from several factors, but a major difficulty stems from the conceptual basis that underlies the recommended intakes. For example, a Recommended Dietary Allowance (RDA) is typically defined as the amount of a nutrient that covers the

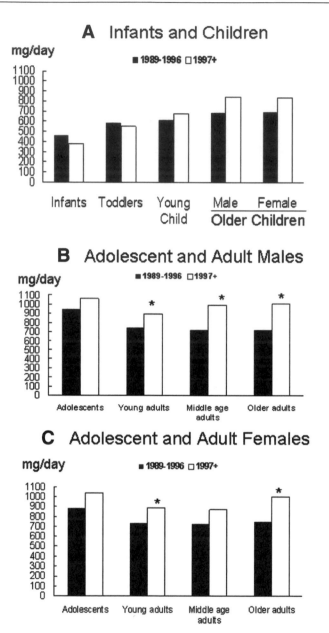

Fig. 2. Time trends in calcium recommendations in the United States. *$p < 0.05$. (From refs. 6–9.)

needs of 97–98% of healthy individuals (9), so failure to consume the full RDA does not necessarily mean that intakes are deficient in that nutrient. One approach to addressing this issue has been to calculate the percentage of the group that consumes some proportion of the RDA, generally ranging from 50 to 77% (35–37,50). Another approach has been to calculate the prevalence with intakes that fall below an EAR, e.g., the amount of nutrient that is estimated as the requirement, as defined by a specified indicator of adequacy, in 50% of the individuals in a particular group (9). Unfortunately, EARs for calcium are not available for many countries.

Table 2
Calcium Intake Data

Country	Children	Adolescents	Young adults	Middle-aged adults	Older adults
Australia: national data	√	√	√	√	
Austria: national	√	√	√	√	√
Britain: national data	√	√	√	√	
Canada: regional data	√	√	√		
Denmark: national data	√	√	√	√	√
Finland: national data	√	√			
France: national data	√	√	√	√	√
Germany: national data	√	√			
Hong Kong: regional data	√	√			
Hungary: regional data	√	√	√	√	
Iceland: national data	√	√	√	√	
Ireland: national data	√	√			
Italy: national data	√	√	√	√	√
The Netherlands: national data	√	√	√	√	√
New Zealand: national data	√	√	√	√	
Norway: national data	√	√	√		√
Singapore: national data	√	√	√		
Spain: regional data	√	√	√	√	√
Sweden: national data	√	√	√		
United States: national data	√	√	√	√	√

Mean or median calcium intake (mg/d) in selected countries collected since 1988

Community/country	Survey name and/or areas covered	Sample size[a]	Year of data collection	Dietary method used	Age (yr)	Calcium intake Both sexes	Male	Female
I. National data								
Australia (83)	National Nutrition Survey	3399[b] (61.4%)	1995	24-h recall	10–15	–	1054	794
					25–64	–	983	760
Australia (41)	National Nutrition Survey	13,858 (61.4%)	1995	24-h recall	4–7	–	800[c]	675[c]
					12–15	–	1006[c]	732[c]
					19–24	–	1005[c]	691[c]
					19+	–	866[c]	688[c]
Austria (42)	Vienna and lower Austria	3590	1998	Weighed 7	4–6	1095	–	–

(continued)

113

Table 2 (Continued)

Community/country	Survey name and/or areas covered	Sample size[a]	Year of data collection	Dietary method used	Age (yr)	Calcium intake		
						Both sexes	Male	Female
	(Austrian Study on Nutritional Status)			day records	7–9	770	—	—
					10–12	747	—	—
					13–14	726	—	—
					15–19	743	—	—
					20–25	870	—	—
					26–35	867	—	—
					36–45	840	—	—
					46–55	804	—	—
					56–65	774	—	—
					>65	734	—	—
Britain (43,84)	National Diet and Nutrition Survey	1640	1992–1993	4 weighed food records	1.5–2.5	—	682	643
					2.5–3.5	—	642	628
					3.5–4.5	—	625	595
		1724 (47%)	2000–2001	7 weighed food records	19–24	—	867	706
					25–34	—	(825)[c]	(669)[c]
						—	1030	736
					35–49	—	(951)[c]	(718)[c]
						—	1049	814
					50–64	—	(1017)[c]	(789)[c]
						—	1035	903
						—	(1002)[c]	(850)[c]
		1687	1994–1995	4 weighed food records	65–74, free living	—	852	704
					75–84, free living	—	813	680
					65–84, institutionalized	—	935	900
					85+, free living	—	764	647
					85+, institutionalized	—	981	828

Country	Survey	n (%)	Year	Method	Age			
Denmark (85)	Danskernes Kostvaner 1995	3098 (66%)	1995	7-d dietary record	1–3	996	910	—
						(886)c	(886)c	
					4–6	890	1053	—
						(874)c	(957)c	
					7–10	1093	1224	—
						(1056)c	(1177)c	
					11–14	1061	1266	—
						(1007)c	(1196)c	
					15–18	1121	1362	—
						(983)c	(1423)c	
					19–24	1100	1379	—
						(958)c	(1151)c	
					25–34	1015	1121	—
						(935)c	(1162)c	
					35–44	901	1027	—
						(927)c	(993)c	
					45–54	947	983	—
						(916)c	(978)c	
					55–64	885	1051	—
						(844)c	(901)c	
					65–74	912	954	—
						(904)c	(977)c	
					75–80	864	822	—
						(861)c	(834)c	
Finland (86)	National FINNDIET 2002	2007 (63% of invited)	2002	Two 24-h recalls	25–34	1001	1391	—
					35–44	986	1203	—
					45–54	954	1137	—
					55–64	946	1075	—
France (87)	L'enquête INCA, 1999	3003	1998–1999	7-d dietary records	3–5	—	—	790
					6–8	—	—	836
					9–11	—	—	833
					12–14	—	—	835
					15–24	—	—	817
					25–44	—	—	884
					45–64	—	—	856
					65+	—	—	857

(continued)

Table 2 (Continued)

Community/country covered	Survey name and/or areas covered	Sample size[a]	Year of data collection	Dietary method used	Age (yr)	Calcium intake		
						Both sexes	Male	Female
Germany (88)	German Nutrition Survey	4030 (56% of invited)	1998	Dietary History	18–24	—	1395[c]	1129[c]
					25–34	—	1319[c]	1118[c]
					35–44		1189[c]	1116[c]
					45–54	—	1211[c]	1114[c]
					55–64		1117[c]	1066[c]
					65–79	—	949[c]	973[c]
Iceland (45)	Dietary Survey of The Icelandic Nutrition Council 2002	1366 (70.6%)	2002	24-h recall	15–19	—	1355	1004
					20–39	—	1377	1034
					40–59	—	1133	871
					60–80	—	1032	835
Ireland (89)	North/South Ireland Food Consumption Survey (63%)	1379	1997–1999	7-d food record	18–35	—	996[d] (957)[cd]	682[d] (673)[cd]
					36–50		962[d] (928)[cd]	742[d] (713)[cd]
					51–64	—	840[d] (803)[cd]	722[d] (666)[cd]
Italy (44)	Nationwide Nutritional Survey of Food Behaviour INN-CA 1994–1996	2734 (47% of contacted households; 72% of surveyed individuals)	1994–1996	7-d food diary	1–9	797	826	742
					10–14	862	933	780
					18–64	893	946	850
					>64	845	936	795
The Netherlands (90,91)	Dutch National Food Consumption Survey DNFCS-3	5958 (71%)	1997–1998	2-d diet record	1–4	—	846	790
					4–7	—	872	858
					7–10	—	914	901
					10–13	—	1006	912
					13–16	—	1045	904
					16–19	—	1095	908
					19–22	—	1114	865
					22–50	—	1068	963
					50–65	—	1112	995
					65+	—	1024	959

Country (ref)	Survey	Year	Method	n (response)	Age			
New Zealand (46,92)	National Nutrition Survey	1997	24-h recall	4636 (50% of originally selected; 85% of invited)	15–18	—	957 (894)[c]	783 (740)[c]
					19–24	—	938	760 (713)[c]
					25–44	—	(875)[c] 998	759
					45–64	—	(908)[c] 864	(714)[c] 712
					65+	—	(809)[c] 799	(676)[c] 670
							(751)[c]	(636)[c]
Norway (93)	Kosthold blant 4-åringer Ungkost 2000 (National dietary survey of 4-yr-old children)	2000		391 (52%)	4	—	673	687
Norway (94)	Ungkost-2000 (National dietary survey of 9- and 13-yr-old pupils)	2000		Age 9: 815 (80%) Age 13: 1009 (85%)	9	—	914	751
					13	—	933	785
Norway (95)	Nationwide study on dietary behavior of adolescents	1993	Food frequency	1564 (88%)	18	—	1626[c]	1048[c]
Norway (96)	NORKOST 1997	1997	Food frequency	2672 (54%)	16–19	—	1400	1000
					20–29	—	1300	900
					30–39	—	1100	800
					40–49	—	1000	800
					50–59	—	900	800
					60–69	—	800	800
					70–79	—	900	800
Singapore (37)	National Nutrition Survey 1998	1998	24-h recall	2400	18–29	480 (420)[c]	510 (443)[c]	455 (390)[c]
					30–39	480 (430)[c]	523 (475)[c]	446 (402)[c]
					40–49	486 (418)[c]	513 (471)[c]	462 (389)[c]
					50–59	506 (455)[c]	509 (473)[c]	503 (444)[c]
					60–69	447 (386)[c]	445 (395)[c]	448 (371)[c]

(continued)

117

Table 2 (Continued)

Community/country	Survey name and/or areas covered	Sample size[a]	Year of data collection	Dietary method used	Age (yr)	Calcium intake		
						Both sexes	Male	Female
Sweden (97)	Riksmaten	1215	1997–1998	7-d food record	17+	—	1069	927
							(1010)c	(904)c
					17–24	—	1201	937
							(1163)c	(886)c
					25–34	—	1090	973
							(1035)c	(970)c
					35–44	—	1029	888
							(977)c	(872)c
					45–54	—	1041	901
							(999)c	(868)c
					55–64	—	1035	927
							(1013)c	(904)c
					65+	—	1064	937
							(962)c	(912)c
United States (98)	National Health and Nutrition Examination Survey	8604 (71% of originally selected sample; 93% of examined)	1999–2000	24-h recall	<6	853	916	785
						(768)c	(809)c	(708)c
					6–11	889	915	860
						(821)c	(843)c	(812)c
					12–19	938	1081	793
						(787)c	(956)c	(661)c
					20–39	909	1025	797
						(762)c	(856)c	(684)c
					40–59	853	969	744
						(720)c	(834)c	(621)c
					60+	721	797	660
						(619)c	(716)c	(563)c
II. Regional data								
Canada (99)	Nova Scotia (Nova Scotia Nutrition Survey)	2200 (80%)	1990	24-h recall	18–34	—	1161	738
					35–49	—	913	624
					50–64	—	822	582
					65–74	—	776	595

Country (ref)	Survey	Year (response rate)[a]	Method	Age (y)			
Canada (47)	Prince Edward Island (Prince Edward Island Nutrition Survey)	1995 (80%)	24-h recall	18–34	—	1151 (969)[c]	714 (621)[c]
				35–49	—	838 (771)[c]	637 (581)[c]
				50–64	—	791 (706)[c]	600 (530)[c]
				65–74	—	785 (691)[c]	547 (496)[c]
Canada (100)	Québec (Québec Nutrition Survey)	1995 (69%)	24-h recall	18–34	—	1114	788
				35–49	—	922	658
				50–64	—	736	622
				65–74	—	771	574
Canada (101)	Saskatchewan (Saskatchewan Nutrition Survey)	1993 (46%)[e]	24-h recall	18–34	—	1251	822
				35–49	—	994	761
				50–64	—	793	651
				65–74	—	812	633
Hong Kong (48)	Hong Kong Chinese	1995–1996 (40%)	Food frequency	34–55	—	605	570
Hungary (102)	Budapest and 7 other counties	1992–1994	Dietary record, 24-h recall, food frequency	18–34	—	868	630
				35–54/59	—	659	579
				≥55/60	—	699	613
Spain (38)	Canary Islands (Encuesta de Nutrición de Canarias)	1997–1998 (69%)	Two 24-h recalls	6–10	1019	1093	959
				11–17	1027	1092	952
				18–24	922	987	859
				25–34	900	996	810
				35–44	974	1101	874
				45–54	938	936	940
				55–64	926	956	901
				65–75	936	930	940

[a]Response rate given in parentheses when available.
[b]Subset of total sample created to be comparable with 1983 survey sample.
[c]Median.
[d]Food sources only.
[e]Not considered representative of the population (47).
h, hour; d, day.

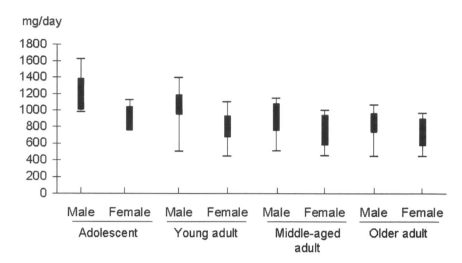

Fig. 3. Range of mean calcium intakes from 20 countries. Highest value is at the top of each bar; black box indicates range in which 75% of mean values fall; lowest value is at the bottom of each bar.

A third, more indirect approach to evaluating calcium adequacy is to assess whether the population or group has a mean or median intake at or above the recommended intake; if so, it is likely there is a low prevalence of inadequate intakes *(51)*. This approach is used in Fig. 4, which summarizes the percent of adolescent and adult population subgroups with a mean or median intake that meets or exceeds country-specific recommendations in 20 selected countries. Only young adult men appeared highly likely to have a low prevalence of inadequate intakes: mean intakes in this age group in approx 94% of the 20 countries met or exceeded the country-specific calcium recommendation. The percent with mean intakes at or above recommended levels ranged from roughly 50 to 71% in the other age and sex groups. The exact extent of inadequate calcium intakes in these groups may be uncertain, but it is probably reasonable to assume that their risk is not negligible.

3.1.1.1. EXCESSIVE CALCIUM CONSUMPTION

Excessive calcium intake can also have detrimental effects on health. The UL of 2500 mg/d for calcium described earlier was suggested primarily to avoid these effects. The most extensively studied adverse effects include nephrolithiasis, hypercalcemia, and renal insufficiency (milk-alkali syndrome) *(9,52)*. The possibility that calcium may have negative effects on the metabolism of other minerals, such as iron, magnesium, or zinc, has also been studied *(53–58)*. Results from these studies have been inconclusive. For example, high calcium intake has been linked to poorer magnesium status in rats *(53)* but not in humans *(54)*. Likewise, high calcium intakes in single meal studies reduce iron absorption, but the effect is diminished when the total diet is studied, and up to 12 wk of calcium supplementation did not produce changes in iron status *(58)*.

Estimates of calcium intakes that reach or exceed the UL of 2500 mg/d were only located for a few countries. For example, according to the 1994 Continuing Survey of Food Intakes of Individuals, approx 1% of adolescent boys aged 14–18 yr in the United States consumed more than 2500 mg/d from food alone; no other age or sex group had

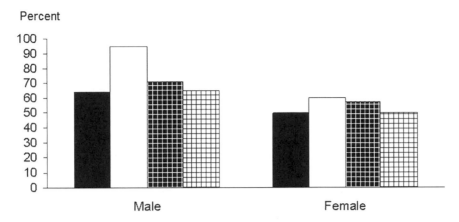

Fig. 4. Percent of adolescents and adults in 20 countries meeting country-specific calcium recommendations. ■ Adolescent; □ Young adult; ▦ Middle-aged adult; ▦ Older adult.

intakes that exceeded the UL *(9)*. Data from the 1997–1998 Food Habits of Canadians Survey indicated that the prevalence with calcium intakes above the UL in the total population of Canadian men aged 18–65 yr was 1.4% when based on food alone and 2.1% when supplements were included *(59)*. Comparable figures for Canadian women were less than 1% regardless of whether supplement intake was considered or not. Interestingly, if supplement users were considered exclusively, the prevalence with intakes above the UL rose to 7% among Canadian men and 2% among Canadian women *(59)*. A greater prevalence of high intakes from food alone was found among adult Finnish men: data from the 1992 FINDIET indicated that approx 10% had calcium intakes that were 2300 mg/d or higher *(60)*. These data are too scanty to draw any firm conclusions about the possibility of excess calcium intakes worldwide. But the likelihood of potentially excessive calcium intakes appeared to be low in two of the three countries for which relevant data were located. Young adult and adolescent males appeared to be most likely to exceed the UL.

Nonetheless, concerns about possible excessive calcium intakes exist in light of the increasing number of calcium-fortified food products that are available. For example, informal market surveys in the United States found that availability of calcium fortified foods increased between 1994 and 1996 *(61)*, and nearly four times more foods and beverages with added calcium were introduced in 1999 than in 1995 *(62)*. Policies regarding calcium fortification (e.g., amounts, food vehicles, voluntary vs mandatory) vary in different countries; for example, calcium fortification is currently voluntary in the United States, whereas fortification of flour with calcium is mandatory in Britain *(63)*. The amount of calcium that can be added to foods is not controlled in the United States, whereas discussions are ongoing among members of the European Commission regarding controls on the amounts of vitamins and minerals in supplements and fortified foods *(63,64)*.

A few studies have assessed the potential ability of these calcium-fortified products to contribute to excessive calcium intakes. For example, Whiting and Wood *(52)* illustrated how calcium intake by a hypothetical 25-yr-old man could increase from 2000 mg/d to 3800 mg/d if some currently available calcium-fortified foods were substituted for their unfortified versions. Johnson-Down et al. *(59)* performed simulations using different fortification scenarios and found that any scenario sufficient to increase the mean intake of Canadian women close to recommended levels led to 6–7% of men having calcium intakes above the UL. Suojanen et al. *(60)* found that calcium intakes would reach the UL of 2500 mg/d among approx 10% of Finnish women and exceed 3000 mg/d among 10% of Finnish men if all unfortified foodstuffs were replaced by their counterparts that were either already calcium-fortified or for which an application to fortify had been submitted. It should be noted that the UL was judged to be conservative by the Dietary Reference Intake (DRI) panel, and that "for the majority of the general population, intakes of calcium from food substantially above the UL are probably safe" *(9)*. Nonetheless, these findings lend support to the recommendation made by the Food and Nutrition Board *(9)* regarding the need to maintain surveillance of calcium-fortified products in the market place and monitor their impact on calcium intake.

4. CONCLUSIONS

Several countries have published recommendations for calcium intake since 1988. These recommendations vary by as much as 900 mg/d, with differences being greater for older children, adolescents, and adults than for infants, toddlers, and younger children. Recommendations published in 1997 or later tend to be higher than those published in 1988–1996. Among adults and adolescents in the 20 countries considered, only young men appeared to be highly likely to be at low risk for inadequate calcium intake. Data for younger age groups were too scanty to draw conclusions about adequacy. Published data on calcium intake above the UL of 2500 mg/d are scanty for all age groups, so firm conclusions on the prevalence of excess calcium intakes are not possible. More data on the prevalence with intakes above the UL are needed, given the increased number of calcium-fortified products in the food supply of many countries. At present, however, the risk of inadequate intakes is probably much higher than the risk of excessive intakes.

ACKNOWLEDGMENTS

The author gratefully acknowledges the invaluable assistance of several individuals in writing this chapter. For providing information on calcium recommendations and/or dietary calcium data, along with translations when necessary, she would like to thank Dr. Juliana Boros (Hungary), Dr. Monika Eichholzer (Switzerland), Dr. Sisse Fagt (Denmark), Dr. Jan Hales (New Zealand), the staff of the Health Promotion Board in Singapore, Dr. Karin Hulshof (The Netherlands), Dr. Lars Johansson (Norway), Dr. GBM Mensink (Germany), Dr. Åsa Moberg (Sweden), Dr. Jan Pokorny (Poland), Dr. Laufey Steimgrímsdóttir (Iceland), Dr. Aida Turrini (Italy), Dr. Jean-Luc Volatier (France), and Dr. Susan Whiting (Canada). For translations of articles and reports, she would like to thank the following colleagues at the National Center for Health Statistics: Dr. Yinong Chong (Chinese and Japanese), Dr. Yelena Gorina (Russian), and Mr. Rubén Montes de Oca (Spanish and Portuguese).

REFERENCES

1. Mertz W. Three decades of dietary recommendations. Nutr Rev 2000;58:324–331.
2. National Center for Health Statistics. International Health Data Reference Guide, 1999. US Department of Health and Human Services, Centers for Disease Control and Prevention. DHHS Publication No. (PHS) 2000-1007. National Center for Health Statistics: Hyattsville MD 2000. Available at http://www.cdc.gov/nchs/data/misc/ihdrg99.pdf.
3. Trichopoulou A, Vassilakou T. Recommended dietary intakes in the European community member states: an overview. Eur J Clinical Nutrition 1990;44 (Suppl 2):51–126.
4. Truswell AS, Irwin T, Beaton GH, et al. Recommended dietary intakes around the world. A report by Committee 1/5 of the International Union of Nutritional Sciences (1982). Nutr Abstracts and Reviews 53:939–1016 and 1075–1119.
5. Scientific Committee on Food. Opinion of the Scientific Committee on Food on the revision of reference values for nutrition labeling (expressed on 5 March 2003). European Commission, Health & Consumer Protection Directorate-Generals. Brussels, Belgium, 2003. Available at http//europa.eu.int/comm./food/fs/sc/scf/out171_en.pdf. Accessed on 10/27/03.
6. Committee on Dietary Allowances, Food and Nutrition Board. Recommended Dietary Allowances, 8th edition. National Academy of Sciences, Washington, DC: 1974.
7. Committee on Dietary Allowances, Food and Nutrition Board. Recommended Dietary Allowances, 9th edition. National Academy of Sciences, Washington, DC: 1980.
8. Subcommittee on Tenth Edition of the RDAs, Food and Nutrition Board. Recommended Dietary Allowances, 9th edition. National Academy Press, Washington, DC: 1989.
9. Food and Nutrition Board, Institute of Medicine, Standing Committee on the Scientific Evaluation of Dietary Reference Intakes,. Dietary Reference Intakes for Calcium, Phosphorus, Magnesium, Vitamin D and Fluoride. National Academy Press, Washington, DC: 1997.
10. Food and Agriculture Organization. Human vitamin and mineral requirements. Report of a joint FAO/WHO expert consultation, Bangkok, Thailand. World Health Organization, Rome, 2002. Available at http://www.fao.org/docrep/004/y2809e/y2809e00.htm. Accessed 08/14/03.
11. U.S. National Committee to the International Union for Nutritional Sciences. Global Survey. Available at http://www.iuns.org/features/global-survey.htm . Accessed 10/30/03.
12. Cobiac L, Dreosti I, Baghurst K. Recommended Dietary Intakes: is it time for a change? Commonwealth of Australia, Canberra ACT, 1998. Available at http://www.health.gov.au/pubhlth/publicat/document/dietary.pdf. Accessed 08/04/03.
13. Anonymous. Nordic nutrition recommendations 1996. Scand J Nutrition 1996;40:161–165.
14. German Nutrition Society, Austrian Nutrition Society, Swiss Society for Nutrition Research and Swiss Nutrition Association. Reference values for nutrient intake (D-A-CH Reference Values). Frankfurt, Germany, 2000. Available in English at: http://www.dge-medienservice.de. Accessed 08/07/03.
15. Scientific Committee for Food. Nutrient and energy intakes for the European Community. Reports of the Scientific Committee for Food (Thirty first series). Commission of the European Communities, Luxembourg, 1993. Available at http://www.europa.eu.int/comm/food/fs/sc/scf/out89.pdf
16. Lam SL. Opening address: Recommended Dietary Allowances: Scientific Basis and Future Directions. Nutrition Reviews 1998;56:S1.
17. Tee ES. Southeast Asian perspectives on nutrition needs for the new millennium. Biomedical Environ Sciences 2001;14:75–81
18. Conseil Supérieur d'Hygiène. Recommadations nutritionnelles pour la Belgique. Révision 2000. Ministère des Affaires Sociales de la Santé publique et de l'Environment. Bruxelles Belgium. Available at http://www.health.fgov.be/CSH_HGR/Francais/Brochures/recommandations%20nutritionnelles.htm. Accessed 08/07/03. (In French).
19. Kobayashi S. Recommended dietary allowances for Japanese—6th revision. Nippon Rinsho 2002;60 (suppl 10):761–769. (In Japanese).
20. Hart W. Recommendations on calcium and vitamin D in the report 'Nutritional standards' of the Netherlands Health Council Ned Tijdschr Geneeskd 2000;144:1991–1994. (In Dutch with English abstract).

21. Swedish Food Administration (Livsmedelsverket). Svenska Naringsrekommendationer 1997. Statens Livsmedelsverket, Uppsala, 1997. (In Swedish).

22. Scientific Committee on Food. Opinion of the Scientific Committee on Food on the Tolerable Upper Intake Level of Calcium. (expressed on 4 April 2003). Brussels: European Commision. 2003. Available at http://europa.eu.int/comm/food/fs/sc/scf/out194_en.pdf Accessed 11/07/03

23. Department of Health. Taiwan Dietary Reference Intakes (DRI's). Taiwain: Department of Health, 2002.

24. COMA (Committee on Medical Aspects of Food and Nutrition Policy). Department of Health. Dietary Reference Values for Food Energy and Nutrients for the United Kingdom. Report of the Panel on Dietary Reference Values of the Committee on Medical Aspects of Food. London: HMSO. (Report on Health and Social Subjects; 41). 1991.

25. Food Safety Authority of Ireland. Recommended dietary allowances for Ireland 1999. Food Safety Authority of Ireland, Dublin. 1999. Available at. http://193.120.54.7/publications/reports/recommended _dietary_allowances_ireland_1999.pdf Accessed 08/14/03.

26. Eichholzer M. Micronutrient deficiencies in Switzerland: causes and consequences. J Food Engineering 2003;56:171–179.

27. Food and Nutrition Research Institute. Phillipine Nutrition Facts and Figures. Department of Science & Technology, Manila, 2002. Available at http://www.fnri.dost.gov.ph/facts/mainpn.html. Accessed on 10/16/03.

28. Office of The Geographer and Global Issues. The number of countries in the world. Washington, DC: U.S. Department of State 2002. Available at http://www.countrywatch.com/@school/number_ countries.htm. Accessed 11/06/03.

29. Wilson P, Horwath C. Validation of a short food frequency questionnaire for assessment of dietary calcium in women. Eur J Clin Nutr 1996;50:220–228.

30. Nelson M, Hague GF, Cooper C, Bunker VW. Calcium intake in the elderly: validation of a dietary questionnaire. J Hum Nutr Dietetics 1988;1:115–127.

31. Rómieu I, Hernandez-Avila M, Rivera JA, Ruel MT, Parra S. Dietary studies in countries experiencing a health transition: Mexico and Central America. Am J Clin Nutr 1997;65(suppl):1159S–1165S.

32. Cummings SR, Block G, McHenry K, Baron RB. Evaluation of two food frequency methods of measuring dietary calcium intake. Am J Epidemiol 1987;126:796–802.

33. Musgrave KA, Giambalvo L, Leclerc HL, Cook RA, Rosen CJ. Validation of a quantitative food frequency questionnaire for rapid assessment of dietary calcium intake. J Am Diet Assoc 1989;89:1484– 1488.

34. Angus RM, Sambrook PN, Pocock NA, Eisman JA. A simple method for assessing calcium intake in Caucasian women. J Am Diet Asooc 1989;89:209–214.

35. Ge KY, Chang SY. Dietary intake of some essential micronutrients in China. Biomed Environ Sci 2001;14:318–324.

36. Flores M, Melgar H, Cortés C, Rivera M, Rivera J, Sepúlveda J. Consumo de energía y nutrimentos en mujeres mexicanas en edad reproductiva. Salud Pública Mex 1998;40:161–171

37. Health Promotion Board, Singapore. National Nutrition Survey 1998. 110. Calcium intakes. Personal communication, August 6, 2003.

38. Serra Majem L (ed). 1999. Encuesta de Nutrición de Canarias. ENCA 1997–1998. Vol 3. Consumo de Energía y Nutrientes y Riesgo de Ingestas Inadecuadas. Las Palmas de Gran Canaria: Servicio Canaria de Salud. Available at http://www.gobiernodecanarias.org/psc/enca/index.html. (In Spanish). Accessed 08/01/2003.

39. Monge-Rojas R. Marginal vitamin and mineral intake of Costa Rican adolescents. Arch Med Res 2001;32:70–78.

40. Boclè JC, Vanrullen I, Touvier M, Lioret S (eds). Cahier des charges pour le choix d'un couple Nutriment-Aliment Vecteur. Agence Française de Securite Sanitaire des Aliments, Paris: 2003

41. Marks GC, Rutishauser IHE, Webb K, Picton P. 2001. Key food and nutrition data for Australia 1990– 1999. Canberra Australia: Australian Food and Nutrition Monitoring Unit, Commonwealth Department of Health and Aged Care. Available at http://www.health.gov.au/pubhlth/strateg/food/pdf/keydata.pdf. Accessed 08/04/2003.

42. Koenig J, Elmadfa I. Status of calcium and vitamin D of different population groups in Austria. Int J Vitam Nutr Res 2000;70:214–220.

43. Henderson L, Irving K, Gregory J, et al. The National Diet & Nutrition Survey: adults aged 19 to 64 years. Vitamin and mineral intake and urinary analytes. Volume 3 National Diet and Nutrition Survey. 2003. The Stationery Office, London: Available at http://www.statistics.gov.uk/downloads/theme_health/ NDNS_V3.pdf. Accessed 11/20/2003.

44. Turrini A, Saba A, Perrone D, Cialfa E and D Amicis A. Food consumption patterns in Italy: the INN-CA Study 1994–96. Eur J Clin Nutr 2001;55:571–588.

45. Steimgrímsdóttir L, fiorgeirsdóttir H, Ólafsdóttir AS. The Diet of Icelanders. Dietary Survey of The Icelandic Nutrition Council 2002. Main findings. (In Icelandic with English summary). Summary information available at http://www.manneldi.is. Accessed 11/19/03.

46. Russell D, Parnell W, Wilson N and the principal investigators of the 1997 National Nutrition Survey. 1999. NZ Food: NZ People. Key results of the 1997 National Nutrition Survey. Wellington, New Zealand: Ministry of Health. Available at http://www.moh.govt.nz

47. Taylor J, Van Til L, MacLellan D. Prince Edward Island Nutrition Survey. Prince Edward Island Health and Social Services and University of Prince Edward Island. Charlottetown PE. 2002.

48. Woo J, Leung SSF, Ho SC, Lam TH, Janus ED. Dietary intake and practices in the Hong Kong Chinese population. J Epidemiol Community Health 1998;52:631–637.

49. U.S. Department of Health and Human Services. Healthy People 2010 2nd ed. With Understanding and Improving Health and Objectives for Improving Health. 2 vols. U.S. Government Printing Office, Washington DC: 2000 (Also available at http://www.health.gov/healthypeople). Accessed 12/01/03

50. Federation of American Societies for Experimental Biology, Life Sciences Research Office. Third Report on Nutrition Monitoring in the United States. Volume 1. U.S. Government Printing Office, Washington, DC:. 1995; p 105.

51. Subcommittee on Interpretation and Uses of Dietary Reference Intakes and Upper Reference Levels of Nutrients. Dietary Reference Intakes: Applications in Dietary Assessment. National Academy Press, Washington DC: 2000.

52. Whiting SJ, Wood RJ. Adverse effects of high-calcium diets in humans. Nutrition Reviews 1997;55:1–9.

53. Evans GE, Weaver CM, Harrington DD, Babbs CF. Association of magnesium deficiency with blood pressure lowering effects of calcium. J Hypertension 1990;8:327–337.

54. Andon MB, Ilich JZ, Tzagournio MA, Matkovic V. Magnesium balance in adolescent females consuming a low- or high-calcium diet. Am J Clin Nutr 1996;63:950–953.

55. Wood RJ, Zheng JJ. High dietary calcium intake reduces zinc absorption and balance in humans. Am J Clin Nutr 1997;65:1803–1809.

56. Gleerup A, Rossander-Hulten L, Gramatkovski E, Hallberg L. Iron absorption from the whole diet: comparing the effects of two different distributions of daily calcium intake. Am J Clin Nutr 1995;61:97–104.

57. Whiting SJ. The inhibitory effect of dietary calcium on iron bioavailability: a cause for concern? Nutr Rev 1995;53:77–80.

58. Ilich-Ernst JZ, McKenna AA, Badenhop NE, et al. Iron status, menarche and calcium supplementation in adolescent girls. Am J Clin Nutr 1998;68:880–887.

59. Johnson-Down L, L'Abbé, Lee NS, Gray-Donald K. Appropriate calcium fortification of the food supply presents a challenge. J Nutrition 2003;133:2232–2238.

60. Suojanen A, Raulio S, Ovaskainen ML. Liberal fortification of foods: the risk. A study relating to Finland. J Epidemiol Community Health 2002;56:259–264.

61. Park YK, Yetley EA, Calvo MS. Calcium intake levels in the United States: issues and considerations. Food, Nutrition and Agriculture 1997;20: 34–43. Available at http://www.fao.org/docrep/W7336T/ w7336t00.htm. Accessed 10/29/03.

62. Parker-Pope T. Health Journal. Flood of new products may push some to get too much calcium. Wall Street Journal, May 19, 2000.

63. Expert Group on Vitamins and Minerals. Safe upper levels for vitamins and minerals. Available at http:/ /www.food.gov.uk/multimedia/pdfs/vitmin2003.pdf. Accessed 10/29/03.

64. Oldreive S. Safe intakes of vitamins and minerals: recommendations from the Expert Group on Vitamins and Minerals. Nutrition Bulletin 2003;28:199–202.

65. National Health and Medical Research Council. Recommended dietary intakes for use in Australia. Commonwealth of Australia, 1991, Reprinted 1998. Available at http://www.health.gov.au/nhmrc/publications/diet/n6index.htm. Accessed 08/04/03.

66. Chinese Nutrition Society. Chinese Dietary Reference Intakes. Institute of Nutrition and Food Hygiene, Chinese Academy of Preventive Medicine. China Light Industry Press, Beijing: 2001.

67. Ministerio de Salud, Instituto Colombiano de Bienestar Familiar. Recomendaciones de Consumo Diario de Calorias y Nutrientes para la Población Colombiano, ICBF, Bogotá, 1992.

68. National Nutrition Council, Nutrition Recommendation Section. Committee Report 1998:7. Finnish nutrition recommendations. Ministry of Agriculture and Forestry, Helsinki 1999. Available at http://www.ktl.fi/nutrition/finnutrec98.pdf Accessed 10/30/03.

69. Martin A. Nutritional recommendations for the French population. The Apports nutritionnels conseillés. (English condensed version). Sciences des Aliments 2001;21:315–458.

70. ANC 2001 : Apports nutritionnels conseillés pour la population française. 3e édition CNRS/CNERNA/AFSSA. Tec et Doc Lavoisier, Paris 2001. (In French). Available at http://www.afssa.fr/ouvrage/fiche_apports_en_calcium.html. Accessed 08/07/2003.

71. Tee ES. Current status of recommended dietary allowances in Southeast Asia: a regional overview. Nutrition Reviews 1998;56:S10–S18.

72. Ministry of Health Indonesia. 1994. Recommended daily dietary allowances for Indonesians. Jakarta: Ministry of Health Indonesia.

73. Societá Italianna di Nutrizione Umana. Livelli de assunzione giornalieri raccomandati di nutrienti per la popolazione italiana (LARN). Revisione 1996. Milano, EDRA srl, 1998. Available at http://sinu.it/larn.asp. (In Italian)

74. Chavez A, Ledesma JA. Recomendaciones de Nutrimento para México. Available at http://www.nutripac.com.mx/software/rec-mex.pdf Accessed 08/14/03. (In Spanish).

75. RENI Committee, Task Forces, and the FNRI-DOST Secretariat. Recommended Energy and Nutrient Intakes (RENI). Phillipines, 2002 Edition. Available at http://www.fnri.dost.gov.ph/reni/reni.htm. Accessed 10/16/2003.

76. Ziemlanski S, Bulhak-Jachymczyk B, Budzynska-Topolowska J, Paneczko-Kresowska B, Wartanowicz M. Recommended dietary allowances for the Polish population (energy, protein, fats, vitamins and minerals). New Medicine 1998;1:1–27.

77. Health Promotion Board. Recommended Daily Dietary Allowances for Normal Healthy Persons in Singapore. 2002. Available at http://www.hpb.gov/sg/hpb/adu/adu010101.asp. Accessed 08/06/03.

78. Sociedad Española de Dietética y Ciencias de la Alimentación (SEDCA). Ingesta Recommendada de Nutrientes (I.R.) ó R.D.A. Madrid, 1994. (In Spanish) Available at http://nutricion.org/RDA.htm

79. Department of Nutrition. Recommended dietary allowances for Sri Lankans. Colombo: Medical Research Institute, 1998.

80. Department of Health. Recommended daily dietary allowances and dietary guidelines for Thais. Bangkok: Ministry of Public Health, 1989.

81. National Institute of Nutrition and the CAVENDES Foundation. Energy and nutrient reference values for the Venezuelan population. Caracas: National Institute of Nutrition, 2000.

82. Lien DTK, Giay T, Khoi HH. Development of Vietnamese Recommended Dietary Allowances and their use for the National Plan of Action for Nutrition. Nutrition Reviews 1998;56:S25–S28.

83. Cook T, Rutishauser IHE, Allsopp R. 2001. The bridging study - comparing results from the 1983, 1985 and 1995 Australian national nutrition surveys. Canberra Australia: Australian Food and Nutrition Monitoring Unit, Commonwealth Department of Health and Aged Care. Available at http://www.health.gov.au/pubhlth/strateg/food/pdf/bridging.htm. Accessed 08/04/2003.

84. Subgroup on Bone Health, Working Group on the Nutritional Status of the Population of the Committee on Medical Aspects of Food and Nutrition Policy. 49. Nutrition and Bone Health: with particular reference to calcium and vitamin D. The Stationery Office, London: 1998.

85. Andersen NL, Fagt S, Groth MV, et al. Danskernes Kostvaner 1995. Copenhagen: National Food Agency. 1996. (In Danish, English summary).

86. Mannisto S, Ovaskainen ML, Valsta L. 2003. Finravinto 2002-tutkimus. The National FINNDIET 2002. Helsinki: National Public Health Institute. (In Finnish and English). Available at http://www.ktl.fi/ravitsemus/fr2002/fr2002.html. Accessed 07/18/2003.

87. Volatier JL. Enquête INCA (Individuelle et Nationale sur les Consummations Alimentaires). TEC & DOC, Paris: 2000.

88. Mensink G. Beiträge zur Gesundheitsberichterstattung des Bundes. Was essen wir heute? (What do we eat today?). Ernährungsverhalten in Deutschland. Robert Koch Institut, Berlin: 2002.

89. Kiely M. North/South Ireland Food Consumption Survey. Summary report on food and nutrient intakes, anthropometry, attitudinal data and physical activity patterns. Dublin: Irish Universities Nutrition Alliance, 2001. Available at http://www.iuna.net/survey2000.htm. Accessed 11/07/03.

90. Anonymous. Zo eet Nederland, 1998. Resultaten van de Voedselconsumptiepeiling 1997–1998. Netherlands Nutrition Centre, The Hague: 1998.

91. Hulshof KFAM, Brussaard JH, Kruizinga AG, Telman J, Löwik MRH. Socio-economic status, dietary intake and 10 y trends: the Dutch National Food Consumption Survey. Eur J Clin Nutr 2003;57:128–137.

92. Horwath C, Parnell W, Wilson NC, Russell DG. Attaining optimal bone status: lessons from the 1997 National Nutrition Survey. New Zealand Medical J 2001:114:138–141.

93. Pollestad ML, Øverby NC, Andersen LF. Kosthold blant 4-åringer. Landsomfattende kostholdsundersøkelse. UNGKOST-2000. (In Norwegian). Oslo: Instiutt for ernaeringsforskning UiO, 2002. Available at http://www.sef.no

94. Øverby NC, Andersen LF. UNGKOST-2000. Landsomfattende kostholdsundersøkelse blant elever I 4.-og 8. klasse i Norge. (In Norwegian) Oslo: Instiutt for ernaeringsforskning UiO, 2002. Available at http://www.sef.no

95. Andersen LF, Nes M, Sandstad B, Bjøneboe G-EAa, Drevon CA. Dietary intake among Norwegian adolescents. Eur J Clin Nutr 1995;49:555–564.

96. Johansson L, Sovoll K. NORKOST 1997. National dietary survey among men and women 16–79 years of age. Report 3/1999. (In Norwegian) Oslo: National Council on Nutrition and Physical Activity, 1999. Available at http://www.sef.no

97. Becker W, Pearson M. Riksmaten 1997–98. Dietary habits and nutrient intake in Sweden. The second national food consumption survey. Uppsala: Livsmedelsverket, 2003. Summary available at http://www.slv.se/default.asp Accessed 11/07/03.

98. Wright JD, Wang CY, Kennedy-Stephenson J, Ervin RB. Dietary intake of ten key nutrients for public health, United States: 1999–2000. Advance data from vital and health statistics; no. 334. Hyattsville, MD: Natioanl Center for Health Statistics, 2003. Available at http://www.cdc.gov/nchs/data/ad/ad334.pdf

99. Nova Scotia Department of Health. Report of the Nova Scotia Nutrition Survey. Nova Scotia Heart Health Program. Nova Scotia Department of Health, Halifax: 1993.

100. Santé Québec. Les Québécois-mangent-ils-mieux? Rapport de l'Enquête québécoise sur la nutrition. 1990. Montréal: Ministère se la Santé et des Services sociauz, gouvernement de Québéc. 1995.

101. Stephen AM, Reeder BA. Saskatchewan Nutrition Survey. Report of a survey in the province of Saskatchewan, 1993–94. University of Saskatchewan, Saskatoon, 2001.

102. Biró G, Antal M, Zajkás G. Nutrition survey of the Hungarian population in a randomized trial between 1992–1994. Eur J Clin Nutr 1996;50:201–208.

9 Food Sources, Supplements, and Bioavailability

Connie M. Weaver and Robert P. Heaney

KEY POINTS

- Most of the calcium in the American diet comes from dairy products.
- Calcium intake is a marker for diet quality.
- Without adequate dairy products, calcium requirements can only practically be met by consuming fortified foods or supplements.
- Calcium absorption is inversely related to the calcium load of the meal.
- Calcium bioavailability is influenced by the presence of inhibitors and enhancers of calcium absorption in the food or meal.
- Calcium absorption from various salts has at most only a weak relationship to solubility.

1. INTRODUCTION

Early humans are thought to have consumed a diet rich in calcium from a wide range of plant sources (1). With cultivation of plants, a few staple cereal crops became the major source of energy for modern man. Botanically speaking, cereal grains are the fruit of the plant, which is the part of the plant that accumulates the least amount of calcium. Since the agricultural revolution, the main food source of calcium in the diet of most populations is dairy products. Calcium adequacy in the diet became directly related to dairy consumption. In the last few years, an enormous increase in diversity of food sources of calcium has become available in North America through extensive fortification. Now, calcium requirements can be met through consumption of dairy products (primarily milk); through fortified foods; or through supplements.

The choice of source or combination of sources to meet the calcium needs of an individual depends on many factors and has implications for overall health. Some individuals do not consume sufficient milk to meet their calcium needs because of health reasons such as milk protein allergies or perceived milk intolerance, taste preferences, or philosophies. Others simply never acquired a habit of drinking milk as the beverage of choice. Milk-drinking habits track from early age and are related to milk-drinking habits of the mother (2,3). Habits, once formed, are difficult to change. Fortification of foods already being consumed has the advantage of probable compliance if the indi-

From: *Calcium in Human Health*
Edited by: C. M. Weaver and R. P. Heaney © Humana Press Inc., Totowa, NJ

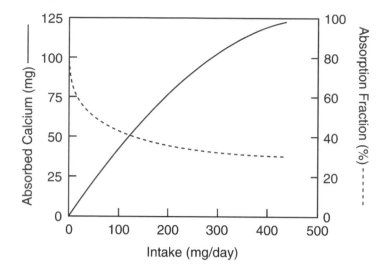

Fig. 1. Theoretical relationship between calcium intake and net calcium absorbed (solid line) and absorption efficiency (dashed line). (Reproduced from ref. *52*, with permission from ILSI Press.)

viduals whose intakes are most inadequate are actually being targeted. Using calcium-fortified foods to meet calcium requirements requires more attention to ensure adequacy because of the varied levels of fortification among sources and the generally lower frequency of consumption of any one fortified food in contrast with milk as the beverage of choice among milk drinkers. Supplements may be effective for meeting calcium needs on an individual basis, but reliance on supplements has limited effectiveness for a whole population because of issues with adherence.

The choice of calcium source influences not only the amount of consumed calcium but also of that of other nutrients. Furthermore, the source of calcium can vary in cost and bioavailability or absorbability. The rest of this chapter focuses on these issues. Dietary factors that influence postabsorptive retention of calcium are discussed in Chapter 12.

2. PHYSIOLOGICAL FACTORS AFFECTING CALCIUM ABSORPTION

Regardless of the source of calcium, calcium absorption efficiency decreases with increasing intake, as depicted in Fig. 1. However, total calcium absorbed keeps increasing with load. Consequently, calcium absorption efficiency is greater if calcium is ingested in divided doses throughout the day. However, with a high enough intake at one time, the calcium need for the day can be met from an increasing proportion of paracellular absorption. This is the concept used by General Mills for manufacturing Total® cereal, which supplies 100% of the recommended daily intake of calcium per serving.

Calcium status of the individual, as determined by habitual calcium intake, influences calcium absorption efficiency. Girls on low calcium intakes had higher calcium absorption efficiencies *(4)*. Figure 2 illustrates the adaptive efficiency based on low compared with adequate calcium intakes in adult women. The ability to adapt to chronically low calcium intake is insufficient to protect bones in most individuals of Caucasian or East Asian origin.

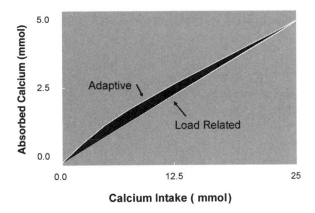

Fig 2. Relationship between calcium intake and absorbed calcium in women tested on their usual calcium intakes (adaptive) and in women tested with no prior exposure to the test load (load-related, a physiochemical effect). (Reproduced from ref. *53*, with permission from Raven Press.)

Life stage is another physiological factor that influences calcium absorption from a given source. This topic is discussed in detail in Part V of this book. Briefly, noteworthy stages that affect calcium absorption efficiency are adolescence, pregnancy, and aging. The high calcium absorption that occurs with rapid bone accretion during puberty is little affected by calcium load. Calcium absorption efficiency is also upregulated in the third trimester of pregnancy. Age-related declines in calcium absorption efficiency are the basis for increased requirements of older individuals. Disorders that influence calcium absorption include hyperparathyroidism and diseases of the kidney, which compromise active calcium absorption. Achlorhydria does not lead to a decrease in calcium absorption if calcium is consumed with food *(5)*.

Assuming an obligatory calcium loss of the average adult of 5 mmol (200 mg)/d, net calcium absorption (intake minus fecal output), with no consideration for bone accretion, must be at least this amount to prevent negative calcium balance. The calcium intake to produce this level of net calcium absorption at various calcium absorption efficiencies is given in Fig. 3. Zero active calcium absorption represents only passive absorption. In this state, with zero active calcium absorption, a calcium intake greater than 60 mmol (2400 mg) is required to prevent negative calcium balance.

Lactose intolerance is a reason given by many individuals for avoiding dairy foods. In many individuals, levels of functioning intestinal lactase declines in childhood. However, lactose nonpersistence is not a reliable indicator of lactose intolerance symptoms associated with consuming large quantities of lactose. Even those individuals with verified lactose intolerance can digest lactose-containing foods without evidence of intolerance by consuming up to 2 cups of milk or equivalent amounts of lactose together with food at a meal *(6)*.

3. FOOD SOURCES OF CALCIUM

Milk and other dairy foods provided 84% of the calcium from foods in the United States in 1989–1993 *(7)*. Unfortunately, milk is being displaced as a beverage of choice

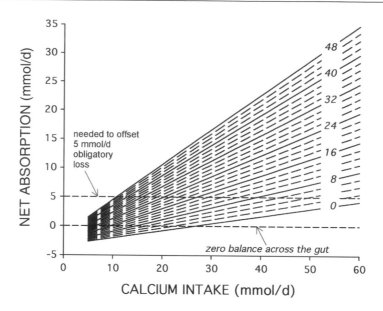

Fig. 3. Relationship between calcium intake and net absorption for varying levels of active absorption (indicated at the right of the contour lines). Net absorption is defined as the difference between oral intake and fecal output. The various contour lines are plots of the equation: NetAbs = (Intake + 3.75) × (PassAbs + ActAbs) − 3.75, where PassAbs = passive absorption fraction (=[0.125], and ActAbs = active absorption fraction). (Copyright Robert P. Heaney, 1999; with permission.)

by sweetened soft drinks and juices (Fig. 4). Americans drank more than four times as much milk as carbonated soft drinks in 1945; in 2001, they drank nearly 2.5 times more soda than milk. Table 1 shows the nutrient contribution of 1 c of milk to the diet. Milk is a nutrient-dense food in that it supplies concentrated nutrients relative to calories. Clearly, milk is a rich package of nutrients, and drinking milk is the most economical strategy for achieving sufficiency of a broad range of nutrients. Limiting milk in the diet necessitates dietary adjustments beyond meeting calcium needs. This often is not accomplished in the general population. Low calcium intakes from limiting milk in the diet have been associated with low intakes of magnesium, riboflavin, vitamins B_6 and B_{12}, and thiamin. The degree to which calcium intakes serve as a marker for total diet quality from one study (8) is shown in Fig. 5. Using 7-d diet records in 272 healthy Caucasian premenopausal women, scores were assigned for 9 nutrients: 0, if the nutrient was consumed in quantitites less than two-thirds of recommended intakes for that nutrient, and 1 if intake exceeded that level. A maximum possible score for each women was 9, and scores of 4 or below were considered poor diets. Of the women who had calcium scores of 0, 53% had poor overall diet quality, that is, five or more nutrients ingested at less than two-thirds recommended levels. Only 10% of women with calcium scores of 1 had overall poor quality diets.

The effectiveness of a particular source depends on the calcium content in a serving and its absorbability. Generally, calcium content varies more widely than bioavailability. Table 2 (expanded from Weaver et al. [9]) gives both these parameters for a variety of foods in addition to a comparison of how many servings are needed to supply the same amount of absorbable calcium as a glass of milk. Figure 6 demonstrates graphically the

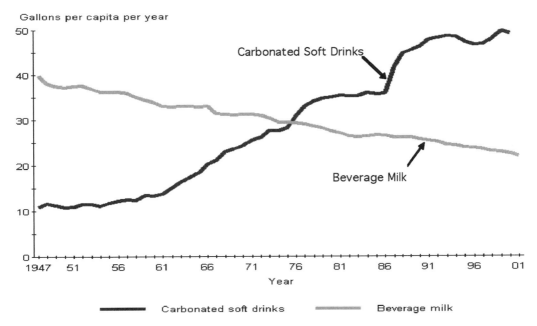

Fig. 4. Trends in milk and carbonated soft drink consumption from 1945 to 2001. (From US Department of Agriculture/Economic Research Service, courtesy of Patricia Britton.)

wide range of calcium absorbed per serving. Calcium absorption from dairy, milk, yogurt, and cheddar cheese is similar and is not affected by flavorings such as chocolate, fat content, or removal of lactose *(12,24)*.

Bioavailability of calcium from the foods in Table 2 was determined using foods intrinsically labeled with either stable or radioactive isotopic tracers. Intrinsic labeling of milk was accomplished by intravenously injecting a stable calcium isotope into the jugular vein of a cow and collecting the milk over 3 d. The milk was pasteurized, homogenized, and aseptically packaged. A portion of the labeled milk was processed into cheese or yogurt at Kraft, Inc. Plant foods were labeled with isotopes of calcium through their administration into the nutrient solution of hydroponically grown plants or direct insertion, i.e., into the petioles of wheat. Calcium fractional absorption was determined in humans using either a single 5-h blood sample (which has been shown to correlate highly with the double isotope technique, as described in Chapter 5) or fecal recovery of unabsorbed isotope.

In order to estimate the amount of calcium from a standard serving in Table 2, the calcium load has to be adjusted from the actual test dose to the level in a typical serving. This is because absorption efficiency is inversely related to load (Fig 1). The equation for adjusting the load is given in a footnote in Table 2. In most of our studies of calcium bioavailability from foods, our reference food was milk. Thus, once absorption efficiency was adjusted to the load in a serving, the ratio of efficiency of the test food compared with milk could be used to determine absorption efficiency at that load. Failure to adjust for calcium load has led to nonsensical reports on the literature *(25)*, such as the same absorption fraction for fresh and frozen broccoli, when frozen broccoli has twice the calcium content per half-cup serving.

Table 1
Nutrient Contributions of 1 Cup of 1% Milk

Nutrient	Amount[a]	% AI/RDA[b]
Calcium	290 mg	29
Phosphorus	231 mg	33
Protein	8.2 g	18
Potassium	366 mg	9
Magnesium	27 mg	8
Riboflavin	0.45 mg	10
Vitamin D (fortified)	127 IU	32
Energy	102 kcal	

[a]Source: ARS Nutrient Data Base for Standard Reference, Release 16-1.
[b]For adult female aged 31–50 yr.

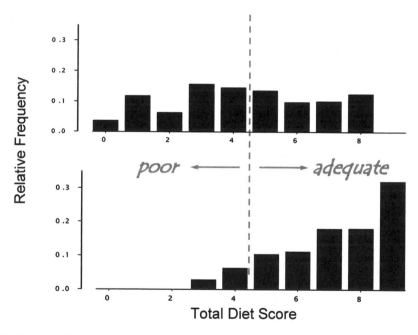

Fig. 5. Distribution of diet scores for nine total nutrients (calcium, iron, magnesium, vitamins A, C, B$_6$, thiamin, and riboflavin) for 151 premenopausal women with calcium intake less than two-thirds of the recommended dietary allowances (RDA) (top panel) and 121 premenopausal women with calcium intakes greater than two-thirds of the RDA (bottom panel). (Adapted from ref. *8.*)

A few foods that contain appreciable amounts of calcium have not been tested for calcium absorption. These include small fish with bones and some ethnic foods.

Differences in calcium absorption between sources, once load is accounted for, relate to the food matrix. The matrix may contain enhancers or inhibitors of calcium absorption. Although solubility at neutral pH has little effect on calcium absorption except at extreme limits outside 0.14 m*M*/L for calcium carbonate to 7.3 m*M*/L for calcium citrate *(26)*, some enhancers and inhibitors to calcium absorption work by affecting calcium solubility, and therefore, availability to the enterocyte, within the gut.

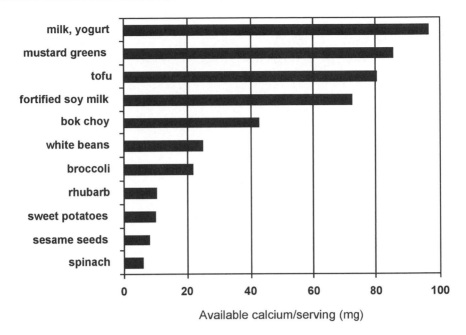

Fig. 6. Total calcium absorbed from various food sources. The value for calcium-fortified soymilk is only true if the calcium is well suspended. (Copyright Robert P. Heaney, 2004; with permission.)

3.1. Calcium Absorption Inhibitors

The most potent inhibitor to calcium absorption is oxalic acid. Oxalic acid forms an extremely insoluble salt with calcium (0.04 mM/L). Its presence in foods usually reduces calcium bioavailability considerably. Vegetables in the Brassica family have more calcium than other vegetables and the calcium is highly absorbable, because they do not accumulate oxalate. Spinach calcium is the least bioavailable of the calcium sources. The oxalic acid content of spinach is more than sufficient to bind all the calcium present. However, a small amount of calcium in spinach is exchangeable with an externally added isotope tracer *(27)* in contrast with the calcium in the pure salt of calcium oxalate *(28)*. Spinach as a matrix is more complex than the simple salt. Some matrices nearly neutralize the effect of the oxalate present in the food. This is the case with soybeans that have similar calcium bioavailability to milk *(29)*. Common beans are of intermediate bioavailability, and they too contain sufficient oxalate to bind all the bean calcium. Thus, for any given source, bioavailability has to be measured because it cannot be predicted.

Another inhibitor to calcium absorption is phytic acid, but it is considerably less potent than oxalic acid. Phytic acid is the storage form of phosphorus in seeds. The negative charges of the phosphate groups bind divalent cations such as calcium, as well as positively charged groups on amino acids and proteins. These phytins are poorly digested and absorbed, but calcium is bound less tightly than other cations such as zinc, thus lessening the effect. Therefore, phytic acid only appreciably affects calcium absorption when present in large amounts. High-phytate bran cereal had reduced calcium absorption, but calcium absorption from cookies and bread made from whole wheat was as high or higher than that from milk *(18)*. Phytases in yeast reduce the inhibitory effects in leavened breads and fermented products even further. A threefold increase in phytic acid reduced calcium absorption 25% *(29)*. Fiber was once considered to reduce the bioavailability of calcium in whole-wheat bread *(30)*. However, purified fibers have little effect on calcium bioavailability and the fibers in low-oxalate vegetables do not reduce calcium absorption relative to milk. Thus, the negative calcium balance associated with high fiber diets is likely the result of the phytate associated with the fiber. High-phytate bran cereals can physically absorb great quantities of calcium and reduce absorbability in this way. The ingestion of psyllium fiber used as a laxative has no significant detrimental effect on calcium absorption *(31)*. Vegetable sources which are low in oxalate and phytate frequently have greater calcium bioavailability than milk. The reason for this is unclear. We have evaluated the effects of isolated constituents from kale, without identifying an enhancer of calcium absorption. Regardless, the concentration of calcium is so low in most of these plants that an impractical quantity would have to be consumed to meet calcium requirements, as shown by the number of servings required to replace one glass of milk in terms of absorbable calcium (*see* Table 2).

3.2. Calcium Absorption Enhancers

Although it is easier to increase the quantity of calcium absorbed simply by consuming more calcium, there is much interest in increasing calcium absorption efficiency. This is a tempting strategy given the inefficiency of calcium absorption from a typical diet. However, enhancers of calcium absorption typically would have to be present in higher concentrations than normally found in foods.

The main absorption enhancers that have been investigated for potential as additives to foods to enhance calcium absorption are selected protein products, amino acids (notably lysine), and nondigestible oligosaccharides (NDOs) *(32–34)*. Proteins such as casein phosphopeptides (CPPs) are thought to work by solubilizing calcium and thus preventing its precipitation by phosphates in the gut. The efficiency of CPPs has been modest, and in humans, a benefit was found only in those who had poor calcium absorption efficiency *(33)*. NDOs are thought to increase calcium absorption in the lower gut and to increase mucosal mass. In the lower gut, bacteria ferment the fiber, producing volatile fatty acids and lactic acid that could solubilize calcium and stimulate transcellular calcium absorption. Studies that are too short can miss the effect. because it can take more than 2 d for these adaptive changes to affect calcium absorption. The effects of fructo-oligosaccharides, especially inulin, have been mixed and possibly related to such factors as type of NDO and physiology of the host, including life stage, dietary calcium, intestinal microflora, and so on. More research is required to clarify the role of NDOs on calcium bioavailability. Complicating the picture of the effect of calcium absorption enhancers is the possibility that some putative enhancement is merely because of the presence of food in the stomach, which is known to enhance calcium absorption *(5)*. Thus, it is important not to design a test with the source ingested without food.

4. CALCIUM-FORTIFIED FOODS

Many calcium-fortified foods have been developed in an attempt to close the gap between calcium intakes and calcium recommendations. Fortification of commonly consumed foods can lead to consumption of intakes above the upper levels by some, especially men *(35)*. Fortified-food consumption by those vulnerable to low calcium

Table 2
Comparing Sources for Absorbable Calcium

Source	Serving size[1] (g)	Calcium content[b] (mg/serving)	Estimated absorption efficiency[c] (%)	Absorbable Ca/serving[d] (mg)	Servings needed to = 1 cup milk	Reference
Foods:						
Milk	240	290	32.1		1.0	12
Beans, pinto	86	44.7	26.7	11.9	8.1	13
Beans, red	172	40.5	24.4	9.9	9.7	13
Beans, white	110	113	21.8	24.7	3.9	13
Bok choy	85	79	53.8	42.5	2.3	14
Broccoli	71	35	61.3	21.5	4.5	4
Cheddar cheese	42	303	32.1	97.2	1.0	12
Cheese food	42	241	32.1	77.4	1.2	12
Chinese Cabbage Flower leaves	85	239	39.6	94.7	1.0	15
Chinese Mustard green	85	212	40.2	85.3	1.1	15
Chinese Spinach	85	347	8.36	29	3.3	15
Kale	85	61	49.3	30.1	3.2	16
Spinach	85	115	5.1	5.9	16.3	17
Sugar cookies	15	3	91.9	2.76	34.9	18
Sweet Potatoes	164	44	22.2	9.8	9.8	15
Rhubarb	120	174	8.54	10.1	9.5	15
Whole wheat bread	28	20	82.0	16.6	5.8	18
Wheat bran cereal	28	20	38.0	7.54	12.8	18
Yogurt	240	300	32.1	96.3	1.0	12
Fortified foods:						
Tofu, calcium set	126	258	31.0	80.0	1.2	19
Orange juice with Ca citrate malate	240	300	36.3	109	0.88	20
Soy milk with tricalcium phosphate	240	300	24	72	1.3	21
Bread with calcium sulfate	16.8	300	43.0	129	0.74	22

[a]Based on a one-half cup serving size (~85 g for green leafy vegetables) except for milk and fruit punch (1 c or 240 mL) and cheese (1.5 oz).

[b]Taken from refs. 10 and 11 (averaged for beans and broccoli processed in different ways) except for the Chinese vegetables which were analyzed in our laboratory.

[c]Adjusted for load using the equation for milk (fractional absorption = 0.889–0.0964 ln load [23]) then adjusting for the ratio of calcium absorption of the test food relative to milk tested at the same load, the absorptive index.

[d]Calculated as calcium content × fractional absorption.

Table 3
Percent Calcium in Common Salts

	%
Calcium carbonate	40
Tricalcium phosphate	38
Dicalcium phosphate, dihydrate	29
Bone meal	31
Oyster shell	28
Dolomite	22
Calcium citrate	21
Calcium citrate malate	13
Calcium lactate	13
Calcium gluconate	9
Calcium glubionate	6.5

intakes can be very helpful. However, few calcium-fortified foods have been tested for bioavailability. Some are shown in Table 2. The choice of the calcium salt used as a fortificant depends on compatibility with the food and processing considerations for texture and stability as well as cost. When calcium carbonate is heated in the presence of food acids, carbon dioxide is released, which is undesirable for many products. Anions may influence flavor. Citrate and malate anions are compatible with fruit juice. The bulk of the total salt required to fortify a food depends on the proportion of calcium in the salt (Table 3).

Most pure salts have similar calcium absorption, but the food matrix can affect absorption substantially so they must be tested. For example, calcium absorption from tricalcium phosphate-fortified soy milk was lower than that of cow's milk [21], even though the pure salt is similarly absorbed to milk calcium [26]. This would not have been predicted from other studies using similar products i.e., calcium absorption from calcium-set tofu was not significantly different than that from milk [19]. Calcium as calcium sulfate in high-calcium water is also similarly absorbed [36], but few waters have been tested for absorbability. When calcium citrate malate (CCM) has been used as the fortificant, absorption has been reported to be approx 5–10% higher in some studies [20,37] but not others [20,38], nor was postprandial parathyroid hormone (PTH) suppression different between orange juice fortified with CCM and milk in elderly subjects [39]. Calcium absorption from $CaSO_4$-fortified bread and cereal was also found to be comparable with milk [22]. Calcium-fortified breakfast cereal was a good delivery vehicle for children [40]. Although few fortified foods have been tested for calcium bioavailability, even fewer have been tested for their benefits on bone. One randomized, controlled trial in 149 prepubertal girls, using food products fortified with 850 mg calcium from milk extracts daily for 1 yr, showed a significant gain in bone mass and bone size in six skeletal sites as well as height due with the fortified products [41], compared to control foods.

5. SUPPLEMENTS

Calcium supplements are usually prescribed to prevent, or treat patients with, osteoporosis. It is considered easier to prescribe supplements than to work with a patient to meet their calcium needs through diet. Supplements vary considerably in characteristics and cost.

The ability to chew, swallow, and tolerate a supplement will influence compliance. Supplements with heavy metal contaminants should be avoided.

Most salts of calcium have similar absorbability, as shown by isotopic tracer studies, so long as the dose size is similar. Moreover, supplement calcium absorbability is comparable with that of milk (Table 4). Milk calcium, calcium citrate, and CCM have been compared with calcium carbonate by PTH suppression and found similar as well *(39,43)*. Calcium oxalate is poorly absorbed because it is extremely insoluble.

Our work with calcium oxalate demonstrated that an external calcium tracer is not exchangeable with the calcium in the salt *(28)*. Furthermore, although absorption is poor, the salt is absorbed intact, that is, without dissociation *(44)*. Small molecules like calcium oxalate and calcium carbonate can be absorbed to some extent in the lower gut without being dissociated in the presence of acid in the stomach and without requiring vitamin D-enhanced saturable absorption *(45)*.

Several calcium salts have been extensively marketed as superior sources, often based on solubility. Sometimes the evidence is based on crude methods of calcium absorption, as for coral calcium *(46)* and algal calcium (produced by heating oyster shell calcium and seaweed *[47]*). When sensitive isotopic tracer methods are used to assess calcium absorption, controversy over comparison of salts can be clarified as was done for calcium citrate. Calcium carbonate and calcium citrate salts have comparable bioavailability (Table 4). A rather new series of salts, calcium fumarate and calcium malate fumarate, are also absorbed similarly to calcium carbonate, calcium citrate, and CCM in rats *(38)*. Calcium ascorbate has unusually high absorbability, at least in the rat model *(48,49)*.

Absorbability of calcium from pharmaceutical preparations can fall short of what would be expected from studies of the pure salts. The presence of binding agents and other ingredients in the formulation can affect calcium absorption appreciably. One such supplement provided one-half of the bioavailable calcium as the pure salt *(50)*. Furthermore, the cost of supplements can vary fivefold *(43)*. Calcium carbonate supplements tend to be the least expensive supplemental source of calcium *(25)*. Supplement use is more prevalent in individuals with a higher education and higher incomes *(51)*.

The best source of calcium is food, because good health is dependent on a good diet, not adequacy of a single nutrient. Dairy products provide not only calcium, but a rich source of many nutrients and functional components. Milk and yogurt are the best and most economical way to obtain the whole package of nutrients important to bone health. Sometimes, fortified foods or supplements are important for an individual's meeting of their calcium requirements. Choices may be influenced by preference, convenience, cost, tolerability, the presence of other nutrients, and the absence of undesirable contaminants. It is important that the calcium bioavailability of the selected form of these manufactured sources of calcium be established.

6. CONCLUSIONS

Dairy products provide nearly three-fourths of dietary calcium in the Western diet. Individuals who do not consume approximately three servings of dairy products daily are likely to have inadequate calcium intakes unless they select calcium-fortified foods or supplements. They are also more likely to be deficient in other micronutrients. The various sources of calcium in the diet should be evaluated for total calcium content and bioavailability. Exogenous and endogenous factors that influence calcium absorption also influence calcium nutrition.

Table 4
Calcium Absorption From Salts

Source	Load (mg)	Population	Absorption efficiency (%)	Estimated absorbable calcium (mg)	Normalized to milk	Normalized to $CaCO_3$	Ref.
Calcium sulfate	250	Premenopausal women	41 ± 7	102.5			21
Calcium lactate	250	Premenopausal women	47 ± 8	117.5			21
Calcium glubionate	200	Postmenopausal women	36.8	73.6		0.75	Unpublished
Calcium glycerophosphate	300	Premenopausal women	27.1	81.3	0.868	0.712	Unpublished
Calcium oxalate	200	Premenopausal women	10.2 ± 4.0	20.4			27
Tricalcium phosphate	200	Premenopausal women	25.2 ± 13.0	50.4			19
$CaH PO_4$	300	Premenopausal women	24.8	74.4	0.919		Unpublished
$CaH PO_4 \cdot 2 H_2O$	300	Premenopausal women	27.4	82.1	1.012		Unpublished
Calcium citrate malate	250	Premenopausal women	37.3 ± 2.0	93.3			26
	250	Adolescents	36.2 ± 2.7	90.5		1.37	37
Calcium citrate	300	Adult men, premenopausal women	37.9 ± 10.4	113.7		1.1	42
	1000	Adult men, premenopausal women	26.8 ± 6.9	26.8	0.975	0.89	
Calcium carbonate	200	Premenopausal women	41.2	82.6	1.117		Unpublished
	250	Premenopausal women	39 ± 7				21
	300	Adult men, postmenopausal women	34.2 ± 10.1	102.6			42
	1000	Adult men, postmenopausal women	30.1 ± 5.4	301			

REFERENCES

1. Eaton B, Nelson DA. Calcium in evolutionary perspective. Am J Clin Nutr 1991;54:281S–287S.
2. Teegarden D, Lyle RM, Proulx WR, Johnston CC, Weaver CM. Previous milk consumption is associated with greater bone density in young women. Am J Clin Nutr 1999;69:1014–1017.
3. Skinner JD, Bound W, Carruth BR, Ziegler P. Longitudinal calcium intake is negatively related to children's body fat indices. J Am Diet Assoc 2003;103:162–163.
4. Abrams S, Griffin J, Hicks PD, Gunn SK. Pubertal girls only partially adapt to low calcium intakes. JBMR 2004;19:759–763.
5. Recker RR. Calcium absorption and achlorhydia. N Engl J Med 1985; 313:70–73.
6. Suarez FL, Savaiano DA, Arbisi P, Levitt MD. Tolerance to the daily ingestion of two cups of milk by individuals claiming lactose intolerance. Am J Clin Nutr 1997;65:1502–1506.
7. Huang KS. How economic factors influence the nutrient content of diets. Food and Rural Economics Division, Economics Research Service, U.S. Department of Agriculture Technical Bulletin NO. 1864. 1997; p. 20.
8. Barger-Lux MJ, Heaney RP, Packard PT, Lappe JM, Recker RR. Nutritional correlates of low calcium intake. Clin Appl Nutr 1992; 2:39–44.
9. Weaver CM, Proulx WR, Heaney RP. Choices for achieving adequate dietary calcium with a vegetarian diet. Am J Clin Nutr 1999;70:543S–548S.
10. Pennington JAT. Bowes and Church's Food Values of Portions Commonly Ued. 15th ed. Harper & Row, New York: 1989.
11. U.S. Department of Agriculture. Composition of foods: vegetables and vegetable products (Agriculture Handbook No. 8-11). US Government Printing Office, Washington, DC: 1989.
12. Nickel KP, Martin BR, Smith DL, Smith JB, Miller GD, Weaver CM. Calcium bioavailability from bovine milk and dairy products in premenopausal women using intrinsic and extrinsic labeling techniques. J Nutr 1996;126:1406–1411.
13. Weaver CM, Heaney RP, Proulx WR, Hinders SM, Packard PT. Absorbability of calcium from common beans. J Food Sci 1993;58(6):1401–1403.
14. Heaney RP, Weaver CM, Hinders SM, Martin B, Packard PT. Absorbability of calcium from Brassica vegetables: broccoli, bok choy, and kale. J Food Sci 1993;58(6):1378–1380.
15. Weaver CM, Heaney RP, Nickel KP, Packard PT. Calcium bioavailability from high oxalate vegetables: Chinese vegetables, sweet potatoes, and rhubarb. J Food Sci 1997;62(3):524–525.
16. Heaney RP, Weaver CM. Calcium absorption from kale. Am J Clin Nutr 1990;51:656–657.
17. Heaney RP, Weaver CM, Recker RR. Calcium absorbability from spinach. Am J Clin Nutr 1988;47:707–709.
18. Weaver CM, Heaney RP, Martin BR, Fitzsimmons ML. Human calcium absorption from whole-wheat products. J Nutr 1991;121:1769–1775.
19. Weaver CM, Heaney RP, Connor L, Martin BR, Smith DL, Nielsen S. Bioavailability of calcium from tofu as compared with milk in premenopausal women. J Food Sci 2002;67(8):3144–3147.
20. Smith KT, Heaney RP, Flora L, Hinders SM. Calcium absorption from a new calcium delivery system (CCM). Calcif Tissue Int 1987;41:351–352.
21. Heaney RP, Dowell MS, Rafferty K, Bierman J. Bioavailability of the calcium in fortified imitation milk with some observations on method. Am J Clin Nutr 2000;71:116–119.
22. Martin BR, Weaver CM, Heaney RP, Packard PT, Smith DL. Calcium absorption from three salts and CaSO$_4$-fortified bread in premenopausal women. J Ag Food Chem 2002;50(13):3874–3876.
23. Heaney RP, Weaver CM, Fitzsimmons ML. Influence of calcium load on absorption fraction. J Bone Miner Res 1990;5:1135–1138.
24. Recker RR, Bammi A, Barger-Lux MJ, Heaney RP. Calcium absorbability from milk products, an imitation milk and calcium carbonate. Am J Clin Nutr 1988;47:93–95.
25. Keller JL, Lanou AJ, Barnard ND. The consumer cost of calcium from food and supplements. J Am Diet Assoc 2002;102:1669–1671.
26. Heaney RP, Recker RR, Weaver CM. Absorbability of calcium sources. The limited role of solubility. Calcif Tissue Int 1990;46:300–304.
27. Weaver CM, Heaney RP. Isotopic exchange of ingested calcium between labeled sources. Evidence that ingested calcium does not form a common absorptive pool. Calcif Tissue Int 1991;49:244–247.

28. Heaney RP, Weaver CM. Oxalate: Effect on calcium absorbability. Am J Clin Nutr 1989;50:830–832.
29. Heaney RP, Weaver CM, Fitzsimmons ML. Soybean phytate content: effect on calcium absorption. Am J Clin Nutr 1991;53:745–747.
30. McCance RA, Widdowson EM. Mineral metabolism of healthy adults on white and brown bread dietaries. J Physiol 1942;101:44–85.
31. Heaney RP, Weaver CM. Effect of psyllium on absorption of co-ingested calcium. J Am Geriatr Soc 1995;43:1–3.
32. Mykkanen HM, Wasserman RH. Enhanced absorption of calcium by casein phosphopeptides in rachitic and normal chicken. J Nutr 1980;110:2141–2148.
33. Heaney RP, Saito Y, Orimo H. Effect of caseinphosphopeptide on absorbability of co-ingested calcium in normal postmenopausal women. J Bone Miner Met 1994;12:77–81.
34. Cashman K. Prebiotics and calcium bioavailability. Am Cum Issues Intest Microbiol 2003;4:21–32.
35. Johnson-Down L, L'Abbé MR, Lee NS, Gray-Donald K. Appropriate calcium fortification of the food supply presents a challenge. J Nutr 2003; 1333:2232–2238.
36. Couzy F, Kastenmayer P, Vigo M, Clough J, Munoz BR, Barclay DV. Calcium bioavailability from a calcium and sulfate-rich mineral water, compared with milk in young adult women. Am J Clin Nutr 1995;62:1239–1244.
37. Miller JZ, Smith DL, Flora L, Slemenda C, Jiang X, Johnston CC Jr. Calcium absorption from calcium carbonate and a new form of calcium (CCM) in healthy male and female adolescents. Am J Clin Nutr 1998;48:1291–1294.
38. Weaver CM, Martin BR, Costa NMB, Saleeb FZ, Huth PJ. Absorption of calcium fumarate salts is equivalent to other calcium salts when measured in the rat model. J Ag Food Chem 2002;50:4974–4975.
39. Martini L, Wood RJ. Relative bioavailability of calcium-rich dairy sources in the elderly. Am J Clin Nutr 2002;76:1345–1350.
40. Abrams SA, Griffin IJ, Davila P, Liang L. Calcium fortification of breakfast cereal enhances calcium absorption in children without affecting iron absorption. J Pediatrics 2001;139:522–526.
41. Bonjour RP, Carrie Al, Ferrari S, et al. Calcium-enriched foods and bone mass growth in prepubertal girls—a randomized, double-blind, placebo-controlled trial. J Clin Invest 1997;99:1287–1294.
42. Heaney RP, Dowell MS, Barger-Lux MJ. Absorption of calcium as the carbonate and citrate salts, with some observations on method. Osteoporos Int 1999;9:19–23.
43. Heaney RP, Dowell S, Bierman J, Hale CA, Bendich A. Absorbability and cost effectiveness in calcium supplementation. J Am Coll Nutr 2001;20:239–246.
44. Hanes DA, Weaver CM, Heaney RP, Wastney ME. Absorption of calcium oxalate does not require dissociation in rats. J Nutr 1999;129:170–173.
45. Kanerva RL, Webb DR, Andon MB, Smith KT. Intraduodenal delivery of intrinsically and extrinsically labeled $CaCO_3$ in the rat: effect of solubilization on calcium bioavailability. J Pharm Pharmacol 1993;45:75–77.
46. Ishitani K, Itakura E, Goto S, Esashi T. Calcium absorption from the ingestion of coral-derived calcium by humans. J Nutr Sci Vitaminol 1999;45:509–517.
47. Fuhuda S. Effects of active amino acid calcium. Its bioavailability on intestinal absorption, osteoporosis and removal of plutonium in animals. J Bone Miner Met 1993;11:S23–S32.
48. Tsugawa N, Yamabe T, Takenchi A, et al. Intestinal absorption of calcium from calcium ascorbate in rats. J Bone Miner Metab 1999;17:30–36.
49. Cai J, Zhang Q, Wastney ME, Weaver CM. Calcium bioavailability and kinetics of calcium ascorbate and calcium acetate in rats. Exp Biol Med 2004;229:40–45.
50. Heaney RP, Barger-Lux MJ. Not all calcium carbonate supplements are equally absorbable. J Bone Miner Res 2002;17:S371.
51. Berner LA, Clydesdale FM, Douglass JS. Fortification contributed greatly to vitamin and mineral intakes in the United States. 1989–1991. J Nutr 2001;131:2177–2183.

IV CALCIUM HOMEOSTASIS

10 The Calcium Economy

Robert P. Heaney

KEY POINTS

- Calcium ion concentration in extracellular fluid (ECF [Ca^{2+}]) is the central, controlled quantity in the operation of the calcium economy.
- ECF [Ca^{2+}] is sustained by three independent control loops, involving bone resorption, renal clearance, and intestinal absorption.
- Parathyroid hormone (PTH) acts on all three effector systems to protect against hypocalcemia.
- Differences in calcium intake requirements in different ethnic groups and at different life stages are due to differences in relative responsiveness to PTH of the three effector loops.
- This system functions optimally when dietary calcium intakes are at or above currently recommended values, i.e., *both* ECF [Ca^{2+}] and bone mass are protected. At lower calcium intakes, ECF [Ca^{2+}] is sustained, but decreased calcium intake or altered calcium demands reduce bone mass.

1. CALCIUM IN THE BIOSPHERE

Calcium is the fifth most abundant element in the biosphere (after iron, aluminum, silicon, and oxygen). It is the stuff of limestone and marble, coral and pearls, seashells and eggshells, antlers and bones. Because calcium salts exhibit intermediate solubility, calcium is found both in solid form (rocks) and in solution. It was probably present in abundance in the watery environment in which life first appeared. Today, seawater contains approx 10 mmol calcium per liter (approximately eight times higher than the calcium concentration in the extracellular water of higher vertebrates). Even fresh waters, if they support an abundant biota, typically contain calcium at concentrations of 1–2 mmol (in the range of vertebrate extracellular fluid [ECF] calcium levels). In most soils, calcium exists as an exchangeable cation in the soil colloids. It is taken up by plants, whose parts typically contain from 0.1 to as much as 8% calcium. Generally, calcium concentrations are highest in the leaves, lower in the stems and roots, and lowest in the seeds (a fact that has important consequences for the shift to seed-based foods at the time of the agricultural revolution).

From: *Calcium in Human Health*
Edited by: C. M. Weaver and R. P. Heaney © Humana Press Inc., Totowa, NJ

2. CALCIUM IN THE HUMAN BODY

In land-living mammals, calcium accounts for 2–4% of gross body weight. A 60 kg adult human female typically contains approx 1000–1200 g (25–30 mol) of calcium in her body. More than 99% of that total is in the bones and teeth. Approximately 1 g (25 mmol) is in the plasma and ECF bathing the cells, and 6–8 g (150–200 mmol) in the tissues themselves (mostly sequestered in calcium storage vesicles inside of cells (*see* Chapter 3).

In the circulating blood, calcium concentration is typically 2.25–2.5 mmol (9–10 mg/dL). Approximately 40–45% of this quantity is bound to plasma proteins, approx 8–10% is complexed with ions such as citrate, and 45–50% is dissociated as free ions. In the ECF outside of the blood vessels, total calcium is on the order of 1.25 mmol (5 mg/dL). It is the ionic calcium concentration ($[Ca^{2+}]$) in the ECF which the cells see, and which is tightly regulated by the parathyroid, calcitonin (CT), and vitamin D hormonal control systems (discussed later; *see also* Chapter 11).

ECF $[Ca^{2+}]$ is one of nature's great physiological constants, extending across the vertebrate phylum (at least in healthy individuals of the species concerned). When elevations of serum calcium occur in different physiological situations (such as during egg laying in reptiles and birds), the elevation is almost always in the protein-bound fraction, not in the ionized calcium concentration.

The ECF calcium serves two major groups of functions. It is the source of the calcium that pours into the cells of many tissues at the point of their activation, thereby triggering the specific cascade that produces tissue-specific cellular responses (*see* Chapter 3). Here, ECF concentration is critically important, and clinicians have long recognized that hyper- and hypocalcemia are each associated with neuromuscular symptoms such as hypo- and hypertonia, conduction defects on electrocardiograms, and overt clinical symptoms such as constipation or muscular spasms and rigidity.

The second role of ECF calcium is that its ions constitute the multidirectional calcium "traffic," that is, calcium entering the circulation through absorption of dietary calcium or resorption of bone calcium, and calcium leaving the blood in the process of bone mineralization, or through excretory or cutaneous losses. Both sets of processes are closely integrated in many complex ways, one of the more obvious of which is the fact that the physiological apparatus regulating ECF $[Ca^{2+}]$ also affects the fluxes in and out of the ECF.

Figure 1 depicts the principal routes of entry into and exit from the ECF, and includes typical values for transfer rates in a woman approx 5 yr postmenopause. It is necessary to stress, however, that the indicated values of these transfer rates are highly interdependent. The individual processes are considered briefly in the sections that follow, but their interrelationships can be briefly summarized with some examples.

When absorptive input from the diet falls, bony resorption rises to offset the absorptive shortfall. This effect is produced by an increased secretion of parathyroid hormone (PTH). The immediate consequences are maintenance of the extracellular $[Ca^{2+}]$ and an offsetting reduction (however small) of the bony reserves of calcium. Similarly, vigorous physical exercise leads to sweat losses that can be 10–20 times the level of resting losses shown in Fig. 1 *(1)*. Also, various nutrient–nutrient interactions may alter either calcium absorption efficiency or obligatory urinary calcium losses. Sodium, (in the form of sodium chloride), for example, can increase urinary calcium by approx 1 mmol per 100 mmol

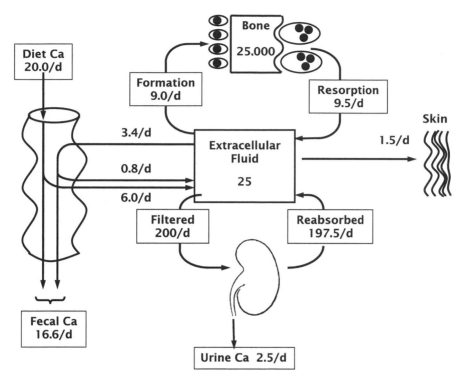

Fig. 1. Principal routes of calcium entry into and exit from the extracelluar fluid (ECF) of an adult human. The values for bone and ECF are total masses; transfer rates are given in mmol/d and represent typical values. *See also* Fig. 4 for expanded detail of endogenous calcium entry into the gut. Total body balance in this illustration is –0.5 mmol/d. (Copyright Robert P. Heaney, 1996, 2004. Used with permission.)

ingested salt *(2,3)*. These nutrient influences, together with great variability in food choices and hence, dietary calcium intake, constitute unregulated stresses on the system (i.e., they are perturbations to which the control mechanisms must respond).

In brief, the system depicted in Fig. 1 operates as an integrated whole: change in the size of one movement evokes opposite changes in one or more of the others. For most stresses, bone resorption is the factor that is regulated up or down to compensate.

The examples just cited represent influences that, if not countered would result in a lowering of ECF [Ca^{2+}]. But the opposite stress, that is, a trend toward hypercalcemia, can be equally important and/or threatening. This half of the regulatory control environment is rarely encountered in adult human physiology, largely because contemporary diets are relatively low in calcium, and hypercalcemic stresses, accordingly, uncommon. However, animals with naturally high calcium intakes, subjected to thyro-parathyroidectomy but given thyroid replacement (i.e., deprived only of PTH and CT) tend to exhibit not so much *hypo*calcemia as wildly fluctuating levels of ECF calcium—sometimes low, sometimes high—depending almost totally on absorptive inputs from the gut.

These examples are intended simply to introduce the "push–pull" character of the regulatory system and the way it responds to unregulated inputs. More detailed description of system operation follows.

3. CONTROL MECHANISMS

The concentration of calcium in the ECF is maintained in two distinct ways: (1) by a combination of adjustments to the inputs and outputs in Fig. 1, and (2) by controlling the level of the renal calcium threshold. This latter function, though very well established, is commonly underappreciated, and is at least as important as the control of inputs. A threshold, in the context of excretion, functions much like a dam at the downstream end of a pond. Inputs serve to elevate the level of the pond until that level reaches the height of the dam. Then further inputs spill out of the pond, over the dam. Because the threshold is the point at which blood calcium begins to spill into the urine, it is clear why raising that point is a first line defense against renal calcium loss. PTH, by augmenting tubular reabsorption of filtered calcium, is the principal regulator of the renal calcium threshold. The importance of the threshold in the regulation of ECF [Ca^{2+}] is clearly evidenced in the common clinical experience of the difficulty of elevating serum calcium in patients with hypoparathyroidism, even with sometimes heroic inputs of calcium into the system.

The physiological effects of PTH are complex and are diagrammed schematically in Fig. 2. These hormonal actions, in approximately the order in which they occur, can be described briefly as follows: (1) decreased renal tubular reabsorption of serum inorganic phosphate (P_i); (2) increased resorptive efficiency of osteoclasts already working on bone surfaces; (3) increased renal 1α-hydroxylation of circulating 25 hydroxyvitamin D (25[OH]D) to produce calcitriol, the chemically most active form of vitamin D; (4) increased renal tubular reabsorption of calcium (the mechanism behind elevation of the renal threshold); and (5) activation of new bone remodeling loci. These effects interact and reinforce one another in important ways, indicated by the connections between the loops of Fig. 2. For example, the reduced ECF P_i caused by the immediate fall in tubular reabsorption of phosphate is a potent stimulus to the synthesis of 1,25 dihydroxyvitamin D (1,25[OH]$_2$D), and it also increases the resorptive efficiency of osteoclasts already in place and working in bone. 1,25(OH)$_2$D directly increases intestinal absorption of both ingested calcium and the endogenous calcium contained in the digestive secretions. It also is necessary for the full expression of PTH effects in bone, particularly the maturation of cells in the myelomonocytic line that produce new osteoclasts, and ultimately for an efficient resorptive response to PTH.

The three arms of Fig. 2 make graphic the fact that the system uses three independent end-organs to regulate ECF [Ca^{2+}]—what Chapter 11 refers to as a "tri-axial system". Their actions are to reduce losses through the kidneys, to improve utilization of dietary calcium, and to draw down calcium from the bony reserves. The aggregate effect of them all, as Fig. 2 indicates, is to prevent or reverse a fall in ECF [Ca^{2+}]. Importantly, PTH secretion is inversely related to the amount of calcium made available by the aggregate effect of *all three mechanisms*, not to the response of one or the other of them.

Although hypocalcemia is a much more common risk in contemporary adults than is hypercalcemia, in infants and small children both deviations would be a physiological threat. The principal defense against hypercalcemia is release of CT by the *C* cells of the thyroid gland. CT is a peptide hormone with binding sites in the kidney, bone, and central nervous system. Absorption of calcium from an 8-oz feeding in a 6-mo-old infant dumps 150– 220 mg calcium into the ECF. This is enough, given the small size of the ECF compartment at that age (1.5–2 L), to produce near-fatal hypercalcemia if other adjustments are not made. What happens is that CT is released, in part in response to the rise

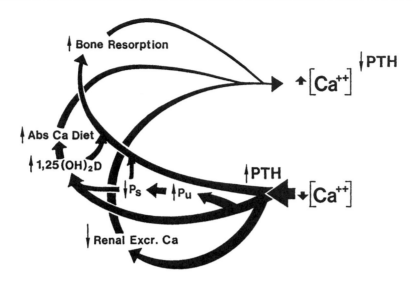

Fig. 2. Schematic depiction of the 3-arm control loop regulating extracellular fluid (ECF) [Ca^{2+}], showing specifically the response to a drop in [Ca^{2+}]. (P$_s$ is serum inorganic phosphorus concentration and P$_u$ is urinary phosphorus clearance.) (Adapted from Arnaud *[4]*. Copyright Robert P. Heaney, 1981. Used with permission.)

in serum calcium concentration, but even before that, in response to gut hormones signaling the digestive activity that will lead to absorption. This burst of CT slows or halts osteoclastic resorption, thus stopping bony release of calcium. Later, when absorption falls, CT levels fall also, and osteoclastic resorption resumes.

By contrast, CT has little significance in adults because calcium absorption is less efficient in adults to begin with, and the ECF is vastly larger. As a result, transient absorptive calcemia from a high calcium diet raises the ECF [Ca^{2+}] by only a few percentage points (approx 1% for each 100 mg calcium ingested at typical intakes). For this reason CT deficiency is not recognized as causing disease or dysfunction in adults consuming typical diets.

4. ENDOGENOUS FECAL CALCIUM LOSS

Calcium is contained in all of the digestive secretions, as well as in the mucosal cells themselves (which turn over approximately every 5 d). Together, these sources account for entry of endogenous calcium into the gut amounting to approx 0.05 mmol (2 mg)/kg/d, or in a typical middle-aged woman, approx 3.5 mmol (140 mg)/d *(5)*. Both because absorption efficiency for calcium is low (discussed later), and because some of the digestive juice calcium enters the lumen downstream of the sites of most active absorption, most of this endogenous calcium ends up in the feces and is generally designated "endogenous fecal calcium" (EFCa). The quantity entering the gut is not regulated to an appreciable extent by the hormones otherwise controlling the calcium economy. The principal factors known to influence that entry are phosphorus intake and mucosal mass *(6)*. Because most of the endogenous calcium entering the gut does so above the ileum, it is subject to absorption as if it were food calcium. Hence, EFCa is inversely related to absorption efficiency and directly to calcium intake. It constitutes one of the unregulated drains on the calcium economy to which the control system must react. EFCa is measurable only by isotopic tracer methods (*see* Chapter 9), and hence cannot be assessed clinically. Nevertheless, when it is measured, it is found to account for a somewhat greater share of the variability in total body calcium balance than does actual oral calcium intake.

5. URINARY LOSS

Calcium losses in the urine are dependent on filtered load, except during infancy and adolescence. During these periods of rapid growth, at calcium intakes typically ingested, most of the absorbed calcium is diverted to bone growth and little spills into the urine.

Machinery for calcium transport, most extensively studied in intestinal epithelial cells, is also present in the nephrons of the kidney, but it is not known to what extent it is functional there (*see* Chapter 11 for details). The process is calcium load dependent, stimulated by PTH and $1,25(OH)_2D$, and has a microvillar myosin I-calmodulin complex that could serve as a calcium transporter *(7)*. Active transport occurs in the distal convoluted tubule against a concentration gradient. Renal calcium clearance is increased when PTH concentration in blood is low, thereby protecting against hypercalcemia when bone resorption is high for reasons other than homeostasis. Tubular reabsorption is determined to some extent by sodium chloride excretion. For every 100 mmol of sodium chloride excreted, approx 0.5–1.5 mmol of calcium is pulled out with it in the urine *(2,3)*.

Urine calcium rises with absorbed calcium intake, but the relationship is loose and depends strongly on the circulating level of PTH at the time. This alimentary rise is partly due to the small increase in blood calcium following absorption of ingested calcium, with a corresponding increase in the filtered load of calcium. Available data from healthy adults indicates that urinary calcium rises on dietary intake with a slope of approx +0.045, meaning that, for every 400 mg (10 mmol) rise in intake, urine calcium rises by approx 18 mg (0.45 mmol). But there is much variability around this average figure and the range of normal is accordingly very broad. Table 1 sets forth observed ranges in healthy estrogen-replete and estrogen-deprived adult women, both as absolute values and as weight-adjusted values *(8)*. The latter can be applied to men because the difference in urine calcium between the sexes is due principally to the generally greater body weight of men.

6. CUTANEOUS LOSS

Calcium is contained in all cells, and for organs such as the intestinal mucosa, which turns over approximately every 5 d, loss to the body of the component cells means loss of their calcium as well. The same is true with epidermis and skin appendages (hair and nails), all of which contain some calcium. This shedding thereby produces a steady calcium drain on the system. It is the sum total of these cell-related cutaneous calcium losses which is represented in Fig. 1 by the rough estimate of 60 mg (1.5 mmol)/d. Sweat losses have not been extensively studied, but such data as are available indicate that heavy physical exercise in a hot environment, leading to extensive sweating, can increase sweat losses to levels as high as 200–400 mg (5–10 mmol)/d. In one study of athletes, these losses were sufficient to produce a measurable decrease in bone mineral density (BMD; i.e., a detectable reduction of the nutrient calcium reserve) across a playing season, despite the relatively high dietary calcium intakes typical of varsity athletes *(1)*. A controlled trial of calcium supplementation in the same athletes showed that supplemental

Table 1
Distribution of 24-h Urinary Calcium Values in Normal
Middle-Aged Women

Estrogen-replete Percentile	mmol(mg)/d	mmol(mg)/kg/d
97.5	6.3 (252)	0.104 (4.15)
95.0	5.4 (215)	0.093 (3.72)
90.0	4.9 (197)	0.081 (3.23)
50.0	2.9 (116)	0.046 (1.86)
10.0	1.5 (62)	0.024 (0.99)
5.0	1.3 (53)	0.021 (0.83)
2.5	1.1 (44)	0.017 (0.67)
Estrogen-deprived Percentile	mmol(mg)/d	mmol(mg)/kg/d
97.5	7.6 (303)	0.126 (5.05)
95.0	6.6 (264)	0.107 (4.27)
90.0	5.6 (225)	0.091 (3.66)
50.0	3.3 (134)	0.054 (2.15)
10.0	2.0 (81)	0.028 (1.12)
5.0	1.4 (55)	0.020 (0.80)
2.5	0.9 (38)	0.014 (0.56)

Reproduced from ref. 8

calcium, above that which could be provided by diet, was able to prevent this seasonal, exercise-related bone loss. This instance probably represents an extreme situation, but it illustrates nicely the function of bone as the body's calcium nutrient reserve, and also a point, to be discussed further below, that, given relatively inefficient dietary extraction of calcium, there are limits to how much calcium the organism can get from food to offset unregulated losses.

7. INTESTINAL ABSORPTION

The pathways for calcium absorption and its regulation are discussed in Chapter 11. The relationship between calcium intake and absorption fraction is shown in Fig. 3. At lower calcium intakes, the active component contributes importantly to absorbed calcium. As calcium intakes increase, the active component becomes saturated and vitamin D-mediated synthesis of calbindin drops. Thus an increasing proportion of absorption is accounted for by passive diffusion. The figure illustrates that, across most of the intake range, the adaptive component is rather small. This partly explains the inefficiency of human ability to compensate for a fall in calcium intake.

Another key feature of Fig. 3 is the fact that absorption is substantially incomplete (fractional absorption averaging less than 0.30 at intakes in the range of recommended values). Moreover, net absorption fraction is lower still, averaging in the range of 0.10–0.15. The difference is due to the counter-movement of calcium into the gut in the form of mucosal cells and digestive secretions (see Subheading 4.). Figure 4 presents a worked

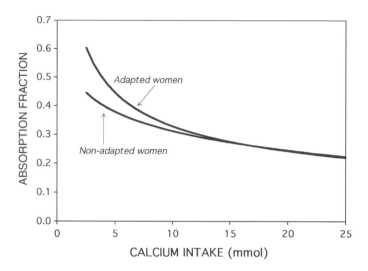

Fig. 3. Relationship between calcium intake and absorption fraction in women studied on their usual calcium intakes (adapted) and in women tested with no prior exposure to the test load (nonadapted). (Copyright Robert P. Heaney, 1999. Used with permission.)

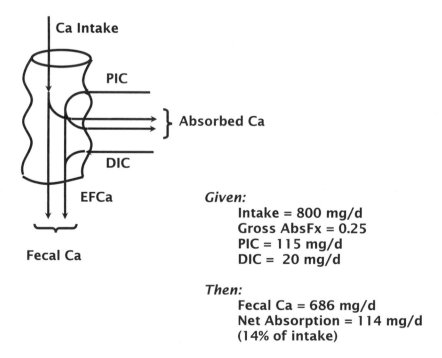

Given:
    Intake = 800 mg/d
    Gross AbsFx = 0.25
    PIC = 115 mg/d
    DIC = 20 mg/d

Then:
    Fecal Ca = 686 mg/d
    Net Absorption = 114 mg/d
    (14% of intake)

Fig. 4. Schematic depiction of the bidirectional movements of calcium into and out of the intestinal lumen. PIC, proximal intestinal calcium, i.e., calcium entering the gut effectively proximal to the principal absorption sites; and DIC, distal intestinal calcium, i.e., that calcium entering the gut distal to the principal absorption sites. (Copyright Robert P. Heaney, 2004. Used with permission.)

example in which a 25% gross extraction figure translates to 14% net absorption. The relative inefficiency of absorption of calcium is probably a reflection of the abundance of calcium in the foods available to the high primates and, presumably, to human hunter-gatherers. However, at the same time it is important to note that unabsorbed food calcium is not just wasted. As is described in Part VI of this book, luminal calcium binds with, and hence renders innocuous, potentially harmful byproducts of digestion.

Various host factors affect calcium absorption efficiency. Vitamin D status, intestinal transit time, mucosal mass, and stage of life are the best established. In infancy, absorption is dominated by paracellular diffusion. (For that reason, the vitamin D status of the mother has little effect on calcium absorption in young breast-fed infants.) Both active and passive calcium transport are increased during pregnancy and lactation. Calbindin and plasma $1,25(OH)_2D$ and PTH levels increase during pregnancy. From midlife on, absorption efficiency declines by approx 0.2 absorption percentage points per year, with an additional 2% decrease at menopause *(9)*.

It has long been recognized that calcium absorptive efficiency increases as the size of the ingested load falls. This relationship has two components: an effect of load itself and variation in vitamin D-mediated active absorption. Within individuals, absorptive efficiency generally varies approximately inversely with the logarithm of intake, but the *absolute* quantity of calcium absorbed increases nonlinearly with intake *(10,11)*. However, only 20% of the variation in calcium absorption can be accounted for by differences in intake. Individuals seem to have preset absorptive efficiencies, some high, others low.

The canonical inverse relationship between intake and absorption fraction has often been uncritically assumed to mean that the body can adapt perfectly well to reduced intake. However, extensive studies in which absorption has been measured by isotopic tracer methods show very clearly that, although fractional absorption does rise (Fig. 3), the increase is far short of what would be needed to maintain a constant mass transfer rate across the intestinal mucosa. Figure 5 illustrates this point with one such set of data. The regression line through the data in Fig. 5 is for a simple linear model, and more detailed investigations of the low intake end of the curve indicate that the rise is initially steeper, reflecting the active transport response to low intake discussed above. The slope of the line across the full range of intakes in Fig. 5 is +0.158, meaning that 15.8% of ingested calcium is absorbed, overall. If analysis is confined to intakes at the high end of the range, the slope drops to approx +0.12. This means that the body absorbs approx 12% of any additional amount of calcium that may be ingested. This value is the approximate midpoint of the range for net absorption noted above. At all intakes, the distribution of absorption values is broad, as the spread of the data in Fig. 5 demonstrates.

The relationship of absorption fraction to load size, and typical absorption values for a variety of sources, are illustrated in Fig. 6. First the figure summarizes the data from three groups of sources: milk calcium (the principal dietary source of calcium in the industrialized nations), calcium carbonate (the principal calcium salt used in calcium supplements), and finally calcium oxalate. What the figure clearly shows in this regard is that, altogether apart from the intrinsic absorbability of the calcium source, absorption varies linearly and inversely with the logarithm of the load size. Furthermore, because all of the studies summarized in Fig. 6 were acute studies, in which the subjects were not given an opportunity to habituate themselves to a particular calcium source or level of calcium intake, the relationships to load depicted are purely physical: there is no physi-

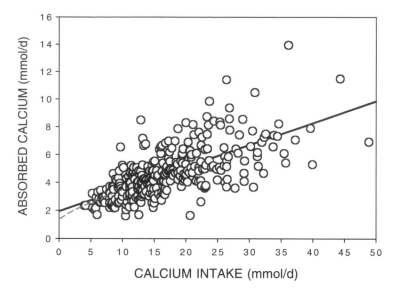

Fig. 5. Absorbed calcium plotted as a function of intake in 332 studies in middle-aged healthy women studied on their usual calcium intakes. (Copyright Robert P. Heaney, 2001. Used with permission.)

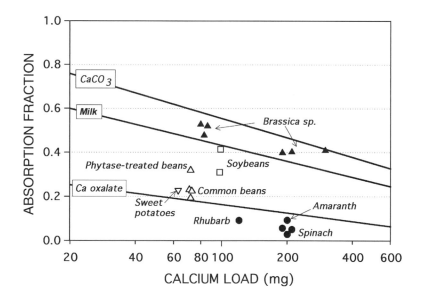

Fig. 6. Regression lines fitted to fractional absorption values at various load sizes for three families of calcium sources. Topmost is the line for plain calcium carbonate. Next is the line for milk calcium. The lowest is the line for calcium oxalate and the high oxalate vegetables (e.g., spinach and rhubarb). For all three groups there is an inverse linear relationship with the logarithm of load size (i.e., at low load sizes, a larger fraction of the load is absorbed than at high loads). Mean fractional absorption values for various other food sources are plotted for their respective intake loads. (Copyright Robert P. Heaney, 2001. Used with permission.)

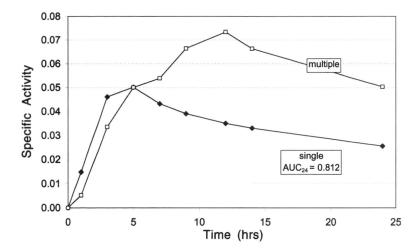

Fig. 7. Time course through 24 h for the mean specific activity values for two calcium dosing regimens. In the first (labeled "single"), 1000 mg Ca (25 mmol) was ingested as a single bolus at breakfast, and in the second (labeled "multiple"), the same total load was ingested in 17 equally spaced doses of 59 mg (1.5 mmol) each, ingested at 0.5-h intervals. (Copyright Robert P. Heaney, 2000. Used with permission.)

ological adjustment component, that is, no compensating alteration of $1,25(OH)_2D$-mediated active absorption.

There are several practical consequences of this load relationship. One is that dividing calcium intake into multiple doses over the course of a day results in much more efficient absorption than ingesting the same total quantity in a single dose. This point is illustrated in an experiment shown in Fig. 7, in which healthy individuals were given the same tracer-labeled calcium load (25 mmol), either as a single bolus at breakfast, or as 17 individual doses of 1.47 mmol at 30-min intervals, starting with the same breakfast and continuing for the next 8 h *(12)*. Figure 7 shows graphically, and pharmacokinetic calculation reveals explicitly, that the area under the curve (AUC) for the divided dose regimen was substantially higher than that for the single dose regimen. (At 24 h, AUC was approx 50% higher for the divided dose regimen, and for AUC^∞, the difference was nearly twofold.) A related consequence deals with the interpretation of published studies in which calcium supplements were used. Even if the aggregate daily doses were the same in two studies, when the dosing regimens are different, the effective *delivered* dose will be predictably different.

It is worth noting in passing that the primitive human diet, which would have been relatively calcium-rich in most of its constituents, would more closely have approximated the continuous dosing regimen. Hence, not only would the primitive calcium intake have been higher than we currently experience, but its pattern of ingestion would have likely delivered calcium into the body more efficiently than modern humans generally manage.

8. BONE CALCIUM TURNOVER

As the numbers in Fig. 1 indicate, the turnover of bone calcium, in the process of bone modeling and remodeling, accounts for roughly half of the total turnover of the ECF calcium in a typical healthy adult. (The proportion would be substantially higher during growth.) A single cubic centimeter of bone contains approx 400 mg (~10 mmol) calcium, equivalent to approx 40% of the total calcium in the entire ECF of an adult. Essentially all of that bone calcium is locked away in intimate association with the collagen fibers of the bone matrix, and for the most part it can be released into the blood only by physically tearing down a unit of bone through osteoclastic resorption. Similarly, calcium deposition in bone occurs as a result of another cellular activity, the osteoblastic deposition of collagen matrix, and its subsequent alteration to create crystal nuclei suitable for aggregating calcium and phosphate as hydroxyapatite.

Both processes are cell-mediated. However, with mineral deposition, the timing of the mineral entry lags behind the cell's deposition and activation of the matrix. Because hormonal control mechanisms, whether endocrine or paracrine, act only through functioning cells, it follows that mineral deposition in bone is much less *acutely* controllable than is mineral removal. Previously nucleated bone matrix creates a mineral drain, or debt, which is paid by extracting mineral from blood flowing past the new bone-forming site, and stopping osteoblastic bone formation will not stop mineralization of the last several days' accumulation of deposited matrix. By contrast, both PTH and calcitonin can act very promptly on osteoclastic resorption.

Hence, in the scheme of Fig. 1, it is the resorptive component of bone turnover which is the one most responsive to alterations of calcium movement into and out of the body. This is shown very nicely in the study by Wastney et al. *(13)* in adolescent girls, in which, across different calcium intakes, bone formation remained constant, whereas bone resorption varied inversely with calcium intake.

In the foregoing, we have emphasized transfers into and out of bone through bone remodeling. Quantitatively, this route seems by far the more important. However, there are competent bone biologists who believe physical–chemical dissolution plays an important role *(14)*. The most likely candidate for such an effect may involve the calcium carbonate of bone. Although bone mineral is commonly assumed to be hydroxyapatite, the fact is that bone contains a substantial amount of carbonate, which varies in magnitude from species to species and from one metabolic state to another. Presumably, the counter ion for the carbonate is calcium. Importantly, the carbonate content of bone appears to be substantially more labile than its phosphate content, being depleted quite rapidly under conditions of acidosis, and rising rapidly when the internal environment is alkalotic. This lability means that the carbonate is located mainly on bone surfaces, both anatomic and crystal. Calcium carbonate is more soluble than hydroxyapatite at prevailing pH and pCO_2 and may well be releasable without structural remodeling as a result of hypothesized lining cell activity. The anatomic surfaces of bone are so large that limited, *one-time* transfers of this sort could occur without leaving recognizable morphologic evidence. Thus, under conditions of acidosis, a limited amount of calcium may be available by dissolution. In brief, although calcium carbonate precipitation/dissolution may help buffer short-term oscillations in ECF [Ca^{2+}], it does not have the capacity required for effective, long-term ECF [Ca^{2+}] homeostasis.

9. QUANTITATIVE OPERATION OF THE SYSTEM

Although the operation of the calcium regulatory system, or any feedback loop for that matter, must first be sketched out *qualitatively* (as in Fig. 2), in the final analysis it is the *quantitative* operation of the system that will determine what ultimately happens (e.g., to the size of the calcium reserve, i.e., the mass of the skeleton). This *quantitative* working of the system for adjusting inputs and losses in response to dietary and other perturbations is often ignored. For example, it is commonly, if erroneously, assumed that, because intestinal calcium absorption efficiency varies inversely with intake, the body can fully compensate for declines in intake or increases in excretory loss. But quantitative analysis of the system (as well as data such as those assembled in Fig. 5) shows the fallacy of that assumption (discussed later). In the face of reduced intake, ECF [Ca^{2+}] tends to fall, and the prior rate of absorption of food calcium no longer suffices. The result is an increase in PTH secretion, which produces the three end-organ effects of Fig. 2, that is, more bone resorption, improved renal conservation, and increased calcium absorption efficiency. In brief, all three control loops are called upon to offset a shortfall originating in just one of them. The net effect with respect to total bone mass depends both on the relationship between the responsiveness of the three effector organs and on their capacity to provide the needed calcium *(15)*. *Sensitivity* of the effectors is genetically and hormonally determined, whereas *capacity* to respond is largely determined by unregulated factors outside the control loop, such as the calcium content of the diet and factors that influence obligatory loss.

If for some reason the response of one or the other of these effectors is blunted, PTH secretion must rise further, forcing more response from the other two effectors. Conversely, if one effector (such as bone) is highly responsive to PTH, the hormone level rises less because the needed calcium is readily supplied from the nearly limitless skeletal reserves. As a result, when the bone is more than usually responsive, less improvement in external calcium utilization ensues. Similarly, if the gut is unresponsive or the diet is so low in calcium that its capacity to yield the needed amount is exceeded, then PTH secretion rises further and bone is driven to meet the needs of the ECF [Ca^{2+}]. The three key insights here are: (1) it is ECF [Ca^{2+}] that is being regulated, not bone mass; (2) the dose–response curves for the three effector systems are independent of one another; and (3) PTH secretion is determined by the aggregate calcium output of all three end-organs, not by one or the other of them.

Examples of different patterns of effector responsiveness abound. Thus, American Blacks (and probably African Blacks as well) have a bony resorptive apparatus relatively resistant to PTH *(24–26)*. (*See* Chapter 7 for the impact of this difference on requirements.) As a result, they develop and maintain a somewhat higher bone mass than do Caucasians and Orientals, despite an often lower calcium intake. As predicted from the foregoing, African-Americans exhibit higher PTH and calcitriol levels, but lower levels of bone remodeling *(19)*. In brief, they utilize and conserve diet calcium more efficiently than Caucasians. Somewhat the opposite situation occurs in most women at normal menopause. Because estrogen acts to decrease bony responsiveness to PTH, estrogen loss at menopause increases the skeletal response to PTH. This is a part of the explanation for the increase in recommended calcium intake after menopause *(20,21)*. Obese individuals also increase their bone mass as they gain weight *(22)*, and they lose less bone at menopause *(23)*. Like blacks, they have high circulating PTH levels and (presumably) a relatively resistant bone remodeling apparatus.

10. AGE-RELATED CHANGES IN OPERATION OF THE CONTROL SYSTEM

Important changes occur both in the quantitative settings of the system with age and in the unregulated inputs. An example of the latter is the fall in calcium intake among women in the United States from early adolescence to the end of life. In National Health and Nutrition Examination Survey (NHANES)-II, median calcium intake was 793 mg (~20 mmol) in early adolescence, 550 mg (~14 mmol) in the 20s, and 474 mg (~12 mmol) at menopause (24). At the same time, absorption efficiency also falls with age. (Note: A part of this absorptive decline is due to estrogen deficiency, which both decreases renal 1α-hydroxylation of 25(OH)D and appears to have a small effect on the intestinal mucosa. A further part may be the result of a decrease in mucosal mass which, in animals, varies with food intake. Peripubertal girls absorb calcium with approx 45% greater efficiency for the same intake than do perimenopausal women (25). As already noted, after age 40 yr, absorption efficiency drops by approx 0.2 absorption percentage points per year, with an added 2.0 percentage point drop across menopause (9). In concrete terms, if a 40-yr-old woman absorbed a standard load at an efficiency of 30%, the same woman, at age 65 yr and deprived of estrogen, would absorb at an efficiency of 22.8%, or almost a 25% worsening in absorptive performance.

To complicate the situation further, renal calcium clearance rises at menopause (26), as shown in the differences between the estrogen-replete and estrogen-deprived values for urine calcium in Table 1. This effect is seen most clearly with low calcium intakes, when urinary calcium can be as much as 36% higher than premenopause (8). Vitamin D status deteriorates with age as well (27,28); this decline is a function of reduced solar exposure and falls in both cutaneous vitamin D synthetic efficiency and in milk consumption. In Europe, where solar vitamin D synthesis is low for reasons of latitude and climate, and milk is generally not fortified, serum 25(OH)D concentration drops from over 100 nmol/L (40 ng/mL) in young adults to under 40 nmol/L (16 ng/mL) in individuals over age 70 yr.

Not surprisingly, serum PTH rises with age as a consequence of this aggregate of age-related changes. Twenty-four-hour integrated PTH is 70% higher in healthy 65-yr-old US women consuming diets containing 800 mg Ca per day than in third-decade women on the same diets (29). That this difference is due to insufficient absorptive input is shown by the fact that the difference can be completely obliterated by increasing calcium intake (29).

11. TWO EXAMPLES OF SYSTEM OPERATION

As stressed in the foregoing, it is a *quantity* of calcium that is being optimized (i.e., ECF [Ca^{2+}]); this is accomplished by the algebraic sum of various quantitative inputs and outputs. Two examples will serve to illustrate further the importance of attending to quantities. One examines in more detail the contrast in calcium handling at menarche and menopause just described, and the second describes the response of the system at any given age to a fixed increase in obligatory loss.

11.1. Menarche and Menopause

True trabecular bone density increases by approx 15% across menarche (30), and approximately the same quantum of bone is lost across menopause (31). Curiously, administration of estrogen to women more than 3 yr postmenopausal has generally failed

Table 2
Net Calcium Absorption at Menarche and Menopause

	Menarche	Menopause
Ca intake[a]	793 mg/d	474 mg/d
	(19.8 mmol/d)	(11.8 mmol/d)
Ca absorption efficiency[b]	35.2%	30.5%
Endogenous fecal Ca[c]	67 mg/d	102 mg/d
	(1.7 mmol/d)	(2.5 mmol/d)
Net Ca absorption	212 mg/d	42 mg/d
	(53 mmol/d)	(10.5 mmol/d)

[a]National Health and Nutrition Examination Survey (NHANES)-II median values (24).
[b]Heaney et al. (9); O'Brien et al. (25).
[c]Heaney et al. (5).

to reproduce the pubertal increase in BMD, and in recent years it has been customary to say that, apart from whatever remodeling transient estrogen/hormone replacement therapy (ERT/HRT) may produce in postmenopausal women (32), the principal effect of ERT/HRT on bone is stabilization of bone mass, rather than restoration of what had been lost. But the quantitative aspects of the age-related changes in the calcium economy, summarized in the foregoing, were not attended to as this conclusion was drawn.

Table 2 assembles published data for median calcium intake and mean data for absorption efficiency and EFCa loss, and shows very clearly how quantitative changes occurring in the 40 yr from menarche to menopause account for the rather different performance of the two age groups. In brief (and despite an intake less than recommended), a peripubertal girl is able to achieve net absorption of over 200 mg (5 mmol) calcium from the median diet of her age cohort, whereas an early menopausal woman extracts less than one-fifth as much from hers. The drop in intake amounts to approx 40%, but the fall in net absorption is 80%. As Table 2 shows, this is the resultant of lower intake, lower absorption efficiency, and higher digestive juice calcium losses. Given the level of total body obligatory losses at midlife, this absorbed quantity is simply not sufficient to support an estrogen-stimulated increase in BMD. As would be predicted from this understanding, higher calcium intakes in postmenopausal women permit estrogen to produce bony increases closer to those seen at puberty (33).

11.2. Response to Augmented Losses

As already noted, it is commonly (and uncritically) considered that the absorptive apparatus is able to compensate either for a change in intake or a change in excretory loss. However, quantitative considerations make it clear that this depends entirely on the level of calcium in the diet. Thus, an individual increasing his/her salt intake by an amount equivalent to a single daily serving of a fast-food, fried chicken meal experiences an increase in urinary calcium of approx 1 mmol (40 mg)/d. Without compensating adjustments in input to the ECF, $[Ca^{2+}]$ would drop. PTH, of course, would rise, and with it, synthesis of $1,25(OH)_2D$, resulting ultimately in better extraction of calcium from the diet.

Published data allow rough estimation that a calcium drain of this magnitude produces an increase in $1,25(OH)_2D$ concentration of approx 6–7 pmol/L (34), and dose–response measurements for $1,25(OH)_2D$ indicate that this stimulus would increase calcium absorption efficiency by approx 2–3 absorption percentage points *(35)*. A 2–3% increase in extraction from a 50-mmol (2000-mg) diet yields 1–1.5 mmol (40–60 mg) of extra calcium, more than enough to offset the increased urinary loss, whereas from a 5-mmol (200-mg) diet, the same absorptive increase yields less than 0.1 mmol (4 mg). (Note: This is partly because extraction efficiency is already relatively high on low intakes, and partly because there is less calcium still unabsorbed on which the mucosa can work to extract additional calcium.) Thus, on a high-calcium diet, the body easily compensates for varying drains: both bone and ECF $[Ca^{2+}]$ are protected. But on a low-calcium diet, although the ECF $[Ca^{2+}]$ is protected, the bone is not. Why does serum $1,25(OH)_2D$ not rise more on a low-calcium diet? Simply because the 1α-hydroxylation step is responding to PTH. Bone calcium meets much (or most) of the ECF need, so $1,25(OH)_2D$ production is less than maximal. PTH secretion, as we have noted several times, is regulated by ECF $[Ca^{2+}]$, not by bone mass.

In brief, as the body adjusts to varying demands, the portion of the demand met by bone will be determined both by factors influencing bony responsiveness and by the level of diet calcium, the principal component of the system that is not regulated. However, it must also be stressed that, although an adequate calcium intake is a necessary condition for bone building and for adaptation to varying calcium demands, it is not by itself sufficient. Calcium alone will not stop estrogen-deficiency bone loss nor disuse bone loss (because neither is caused by calcium deficiency). However, recovery from immobilization or restoration of bone lost because of hormone deficiency will not be possible without an adequate supply of the raw materials needed to build bone substance.

12. CONCLUSIONS

The calcium economy consists of the traffic of calcium ions into and out of the blood, of the forces that alter that traffic, and of the control systems that regulate it. Central to the operation of the system is PTH, which stimulates calcium removal from bone, improves calcium absorption from food, and regulates loss of calcium through the kidneys. These three effects are independent of one another and their relative responsiveness to PTH differs between ethnic groups and at different life stages within individuals. Unregulated stresses to the system consist mainly of variable cutaneous losses (e.g., sweat), digestive juice losses, and obligatory urinary losses caused by interaction with other nutrients (e.g., sodium chloride). Ability to maintain constancy of both ECF $[Ca^{2+}]$ and the size of the skeletal reserve, that is, bone mass, depends on calcium intake. At intakes above the currently recommended values, both ECF $[Ca^{2+}]$ and bone are preserved. At lower intakes, bone mass may be sacrificed to sustain ECF $[Ca^{2+}]$.

REFERENCES

1. Klesges RC, Ward KD, Shelton ML, et al. Changes in bone mineral content in male athletes. JAMA 1996;276:226–230.
2. Itoh R, Suyama Y. Sodium excretion in relation to calcium and hydroxyproline excretion in a healthy Japanese population. Am J Clin Nutr 1996;63:735–740.
3. Nordin BEC, Need AG, Morris HA, Horowitz M. The nature and significance of the relationship between urinary sodium and urinary calcium in women. J Nutr 1993;123:1615–1622.

4. Arnaud CD. Calcium homeostasis: regulatory elements and their integration. Fed Proc 1978;37:2557–2560.

5. Heaney RP. Recker RR. Determinants of endogenous fecal calcium in healthy women. J Bone Miner Res 1994;9:1621–1627.

6. Davies KM, Rafferty K, Heaney RP. Determinants of endogenous calcium entry into the gut. Am J Clin Nutr 2004;80:919–923.

7. Coluccio LM. Identification of the microvillar 110-kDa calmodulin complex (myosin-1) in kidney. Eur J Cell Biol 1991;56:286–294.

8. Heaney RP, Recker RR, Ryan RA. Urinary calcium in perimenopausal women: normative values. Osteoporos Int 1999;9:13–18.

9. Heaney RP, Recker RR, Stegman MR, Moy AJ. Calcium absorption in women: relationships to calcium intake, estrogen status, and age. J Bone Miner Res 1989;4:469–475.

10. Heaney RP, Weaver CM, Fitzsimmons ML. The influence of calcium load on absorption fraction. J Bone Miner Res 1990;11(5):1135–1138.

11. Heaney RP, Saville PD, Recker RR. Calcium absorption as a function of calcium intake. J Lab Clin Med 1975;85:881–890.

12. Heaney RP, Berner B, Louie-Helm J. Dosing regimen for calcium supplementation. J Bone Miner Res 2000;15(11):2291.

13. Wastney ME, Martin BR, Peacock M, et al. Changes in calcium kinetics in adolescent girls induced by high calcium intake. J Clin Endocrinol Metab 2000;85:4470–4475.

14. Parfitt AM. Misconceptions (3): calcium leaves bone only by resorption and enters only by formation. Bone 2003;33:259–263.

15. Heaney RP. A unified concept of osteoporosis. Am J Med 1965;39:877–880.

16. Bell NH, Greene A, Epstein S, Oexmann MJ, Shaw S, Shary J. Evidence for alteration of the vitamin D-endocrine system in blacks. J Clin Invest 1985;76:470–473.

17. Aloia JF, Mikhail M, Pagan CD, Arunachalam A, Yeh JK, Flaster E. Biochemical and hormonal variables in black and white women matched for age and weight. J Lab Clin Med 1998;132:383–389.

18. Cosman F, Shen V, Morgan D, et al. Biochemical responses of bone metabolism to 1,25-dihydroxyvitamin D administration in black and white women. Osteoporos Int 2000;11:271–277.

19. Heaney RP. Ethnicity, bone status, and the calcium requirement. Nutr Res 2002;22 (1–2):153–178.

20. NIH Consensus Conference: Optimal Calcium Intake. J Am Med Assoc 1994;272:1942–1948.

21. Dietary Reference Intakes for Calcium, Magnesium, Phosphorus, Vitamin D, and Fluoride. Food and Nutrition Board, Institute of Medicine. National Academy Press, Washington, DC: 1997

22. Matkovic V, Jelic T, Wardlaw GM, et al. Timing of peak bone mass in Caucasian females and its implication for the prevention of osteoporosis. J Clin Invest 1994;93:799–808.

23. Ribot C, Tremollieres F, Pouilles JM, Bonneu M, Germain F, Louvet JP. Obesity and postmenopausal bone loss: the influence of obesity on vertebral density and bone turnover in postmenopausal women. Bone 1988;8:327–331.

24. Carroll MD, Abraham S, Dresser CM. Dietary intake source data: United States, 1976–80, Vital and Health Statistics. Series 11-No. 231. DHHS Pub. No. (PHS) 83-1681. National Center for Health Statistics, Public Health Service. Washington. U.S. Government Printing Office, 1983.

25. O'Brien KO, Abrams SA, Liang LK, Ellis KJ, Gagel RF. Increased efficiency of calcium absorption during short periods of inadequate calcium intake in girls. Am J Clin Nutr 1996;63:579–583.

26. Nordin BEC, Need AG, Morris HA, Horowitz M. Biochemical variables in pre- and postmenopausal women: reconciling the calcium and estrogen hypotheses. Osteoporos Int 1999;9:351–357.

27. McKenna MJ, Freaney R, Meade A, Muldowney FP. Hypovitaminosis D and elevated serum alkaline phosphatase in elderly Irish people. Am J Clin Nutr 1985;41:101–109.

28. Francis RM, Peacock M, Storer JH, Davies AEJ, Brown WB, Nordin BEC. Calcium malaborption in the elderly: the effect of treatment with oral 25-hydroxyvitamin D_3. European J Clin Invest 1983;13, 391–396.

29. McKane WR, Khosla S, Egan KS, Robins SP, Burritt MF, Riggs BL. Role of calcium intake in modulating age-related increases in parathyroid function and bone resorption. J Clin Endocrinol Metab 1996;81:1699–1703.

30. Gilsanz V, Gibbens DT, Roe TF, et al. Vertebral bone density in children: effect of puberty. Radiology 1988;166:847–850.
31. Genant HK, Cann CF, Ettinger B, et al. Quantitative computed tomography for spinal mineral assessment. In: Christiansen, C. et al., eds. Osteoporosis. Glostrup Hospital, Department of Chemistry, Copenhagen, Denmark: 1984; pp.65–72.
32. Heaney RP. The bone remodeling transient: implications for the interpretation of clinical studies of bone mass change. J Bone Miner Res 1994;9:1515–1523.
33. Nieves JW, Komar L, Cosman F, Lindsay R. Calcium potentiates the effect of estrogen and calcitonin on bone mass: review and analysis. Am J Clin Nutr 1998;67:18–24.
34. Dawson-Hughes B, Stem DT, Shipp CC, Rasmussen HM. Effect of lowering dietary calcium intake on fractional whole body calcium retention. J Clin Endocrinol Metab 1988;67:62–68.
35. Heaney RP, Barger-Lux MJ, Dowell MS, Chen TC, Holick MF. Calcium absorptive effects of vitamin D and its major metabolites. J Clin Endocrinol Metab 1997;82:4111–4116.

11 Molecular Regulation of Calcium Metabolism

James C. Fleet

KEY POINTS

- Molecular events in the intestine, kidney, and bone control calcium metabolism and influence bone health.
- Parathyroid hormone and 1,25 dihydroxyvitamin D_3 are the primary hormonal regulators of calcium metabolism.
- Other hormones (e.g., estrogen, growth hormone, prolactin) have specialized roles in the control of calcium metabolism during certain phases of life (i.e., growth, pregnancy and lactation, menopause).
- Cell surface and nuclear receptors are necessary for the molecular actions of hormones on intestine, kidney, and bone.

1. INTRODUCTION: THE CENTRAL ROLE OF INTESTINE–KIDNEY–BONE FOR THE CONTROL OF CALCIUM METABOLISM

In the other chapters in this book, it is apparent that bone is the tissue that is affected during periods of inadequate dietary calcium intake, as a result of changes in physiology or defects in calcium homeostasis. Based on this, one might reasonably—but incorrectly—believe that calcium homeostasis is regulated to maintain bone integrity. As Fig. 1 illustrates, and as Chapter 10 developed in some detail, bone, intestine, and kidney make up a three-tissue axis whose activities are coordinated to maintain serum calcium within a narrow range (8.9–10.2 mg/dL). In this model, calcium absorption from the intestine is a "disturbing" signal that elevates serum calcium after a meal while bone turnover (i.e., the balance between bone formation and resorption) and renal calcium excretion are "controlling" signals that respond to fluxes in serum calcium. The importance of this coordinated regulation can be seen in the table accompanying Fig. 1. This table is based on research by Bronner and Aubert who studied the influence of dietary calcium on calcium homeostasis in growing rats (1). Using calcium kinetics, their studies showed that when calcium intake is inadequate (a lack of Ca input into serum Ca), the body compensates by increasing calcium mobilization from the bone (resorption) as well

From: *Calcium in Human Health*
Edited by: C. M. Weaver and R. P. Heaney © Humana Press Inc., Totowa, NJ

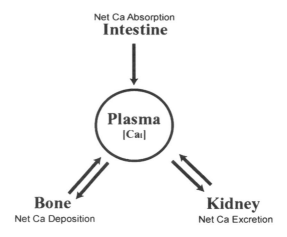

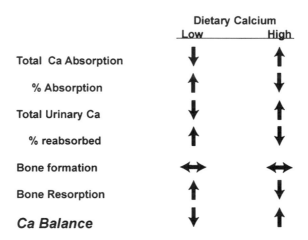

Fig. 1. Coordinate regulation of a three-tissue axis controls whole-body calcium metabolism. This is reflected in the response of calcium absorption, urinary calcium excretion, and bone formation/resorption to changes in the habitual dietary calcium intake. (The table is based on data in growing rats from Bronner and Aubert *[1]*.)

as the efficiency of both calcium reabsorption from the renal filtrate and calcium absorption from the diet. Similar types of compensatory adaptation would also occur if renal calcium output was too high (e.g., as a result of high dietary salt intake), leading to a drain on serum Ca that promotes compensation at the intestine and bone, or if bone resorption were elevated (e.g., owing to the loss of estrogen), leading to elevated serum Ca that would suppress the activities of the intestine and bone.

In Chapter 10, the integrated functioning of this tri-axial system is examined from a physiological perspective. In this chapter, the hormonal changes that lead to alterations in the way the bone, intestine, and kidney handle calcium and the molecular mechanisms of action of these hormones on these critical target tissues that control calcium homeostasis are discussed.

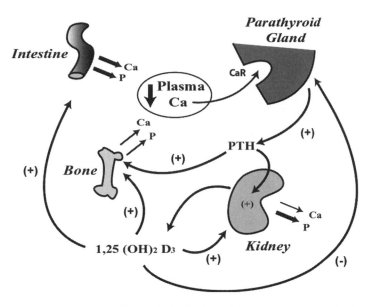

Fig. 2. Hormonal responses controlling whole-body calcium homeostasis during habitual low dietary calcium intake. CaR, calcium-sensing receptor; PTH, parathyroid hormone; 1,25(OH)$_2$D$_3$, 1,25(OH)$_2$ vitamin D.

2. VITAMIN D AND PARATHYROID HORMONE AS REGULATORS OF CALCIUM HOMEOSTASIS

Classical studies like the one using calcium deprivation, shown in Fig. 1, have identified the vitamin D metabolite, 1,25 dihydroxyvitamin D (1,25[OH]$_2$D$_3$) and parathyroid hormone (PTH) as the major hormonal regulators of calcium homeostasis. The response of these two hormones to a low calcium diet is shown in Fig. 2. Here, low serum calcium is sensed at the level of the parathyroid gland through a calcium-sensing receptor (CaSR; *see* Chapter 3). The CaSR relays a signal that leads to the increased production and release of PTH into the circulation. Once released, PTH has several important functions. First, it promotes bone resorption by stimulating osteoclastic activity. Second, it stimulates renal calcium reabsorption in the proximal renal tubule and also suppresses renal phosphate reabsorption (*see* Chapter 10, Fig. 2). Finally, PTH is a strong stimulator of the renal enzyme, 25 hydroxyvitamin D (25[OH]D)-1α hydroxylase, that catalyzes the conversion of 25(OH)D to 1,25(OH)$_2$D$_3$, the hormonally active form of vitamin D.g stimulates bone resorption, renal calcium reabsorption in the distal convoluted tubule, and active calcium absorption in the proximal small intestine. Collectively, the actions of 1,25(OH)$_2$D$_3$ and PTH serve to increase serum calcium at the expense of bone.

2.1. Vitamin D Metabolism

Figure 3 is a summary of vitamin D metabolism leading to the active production of 1,25(OH)$_2$D$_3$. Vitamin D has been termed the "sunshine vitamin" because it can be produced from 7-dehydrocholesterol when skin is exposed to ultraviolet (UV)-B light. In the presence of adequate sunlight exposure there is no dietary requirement for vitamin

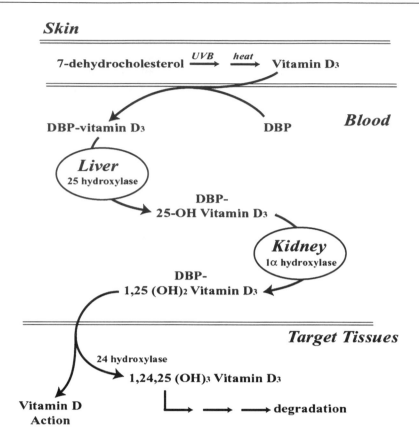

Fig. 3. A summary of vitamin D metabolism. DBP, vitamin D binding protein

D. However, it should be noted that there will be a dietary requirement for vitamin D when the skin production of vitamin D is inadequate, for example in people with highly pigmented skin, in those who cover their skin (i.e., with strong sunblocks or for religious reasons), in homebound elderly, and in areas where wintertime UV-B irradiation is inadequate (e.g., the Northern part of the United States) *(2)*.

Vitamin D and vitamin D metabolites are transported in the circulation by the vitamin D binding protein (DBP) *(3)*. It is not clear how vitamin D is transported from the serum into tissues. During renal filtration, vitamin D metabolite–DBP complexes are actively reabsorbed by the membrane receptor megalin; this system may also be important for other tissues as well *(4)*. Once delivered to the liver, vitamin D is hydroxylated by the 25-hydroxylase to form 25(OH)D. This is a very stable form of the vitamin D (biological-half-life of ~2 wk) and thus it is used as the functional measure of vitamin D status. The conversion of vitamin D to 25(OH)D appears to be driven primarily by the level of the substrate and is inhibited by the product, 25(OH)D *(5)*. In contrast, the production of the hormonally active form of vitamin D, $1,25(OH)_2D_3$, is highly regulated *(6)*. Classically, the production of $1,25(OH)_2D_3$ has been thought to be exclusively within the kidney. PTH stimulates and $1,25(OH)_2D_3$ suppresses renal $1,25(OH)_2D_3$ production. Finally, the $1,25(OH)_2D_3$ released into the serum acts on various target tissues—classically, intestine, bone, and kidney. The mechanisms used by $1,25(OH)_2D_3$ to modulate the biology of cells will be described later. The vitamin D signaling system is attenuated within each target tissue though the actions of another important enzyme, the 24-hydroxylase (7). This enzyme is induced by $1,25(OH)_2D_3$ and its role is to hydroxylate the hormone to form the short-lived metabolite $1,24,25(OH)_3D$. This metabolite is a substrate for other enzymes that lead to the degradation and inactivation of $1,25(OH)_2D_3$. 24-Hydroxylase can also act upon $25(OH)D$ to make the metabolite $24,25(OH)_2D$. Evidence suggests that this metabolite is important for activation of resting zone chondrocytes in the growth plate (8) and perhaps in the repair of bone fractures (9).

2.1.1. EXTRARENAL PRODUCTION OF $1,25(OH)_2D_3$

Although the classic model of vitamin D action is described as an endocrine system relying solely upon the renal production of $1,25(OH)_2D_3$ (as in Fig. 2), several clinical observations have caused researchers to expand this model. Several groups have shown that serum levels of $25(OH)D$ are inversely correlated with serum PTH levels (10,11) and positively correlated with intestinal calcium absorption (12–15). In several of these studies, serum $1,25(OH)_2D_3$ levels did not associate with PTH or calcium absorption, suggesting that renal conversion of $25(OH)D$ to the active form is not accounting for the change in biological function associated with high serum $25(OH)D$ levels, and that tissues other than kidney have the capacity to produce $1,25(OH)_2D_3$. Research in anephric patients (16,17), in cells from nonclassical target tissues like the prostate (18,19), and from immunohistochemical analysis of a variety of other tissues (20) have now confirmed this extrarenal capacity to produce $1,25(OH)_2D_3$. Recent evidence suggests that whereas the extrarenal expression of 1α hydroxylase is suppressed by $1,25(OH)_2D_3$, it is not regulated by the classical modulator of the renal 1α hydroxylase, PTH. This suggests that the functions of vitamin D could be controlled by $1,25(OH)_2D_3$ at two levels: as an endocrine system that is sensitive to PTH and is critical in times of inadequate dietary calcium intake, and as an autocrine or paracrine system that is sensitive to vitamin D status. In this model, the autocrine/paracrine function would reduce the need for the endocrine system, a scenario that is supported by data from rats showing that high serum $25(OH)D$ is associated with reduced serum $1,25(OH)_2D_3$ levels (21). Although these ideas are still being developed and tested by researchers, a model describing the two tiered system is presented in Fig. 4.

2.2. Vitamin D Action

2.2.1. VITAMIN D RECEPTOR-MEDIATED GENE TRANSCRIPTION

Within the cells of vitamin D target tissues is a receptor for $1,25(OH)_2D_3$. This receptor is a member of the steroid hormone receptor superfamily of ligand-activated transcription factors (22). Two lines of evidence demonstrate that this vitamin D receptor (VDR) is crucial for calcium economy. First, the molecular cause for the human genetic disease type II rickets is mutations with the coding region of the VDR gene (23). Second, the deletion of the VDR gene in mice leads to a phenotype identical to human type II rickets (e.g., alopecia, low bone mass, hypocalcemia, hyperparathyroidism) (24,25). Interestingly, the phenotype of rickets can be reversed in VDR-null mice by normalizing serum calcium through the use of diets with very high calcium intake. This demonstrates that one of the most important roles for $1,25(OH)_2D_3$ signaling through the VDR is the control of intestinal calcium absorption (26,27).

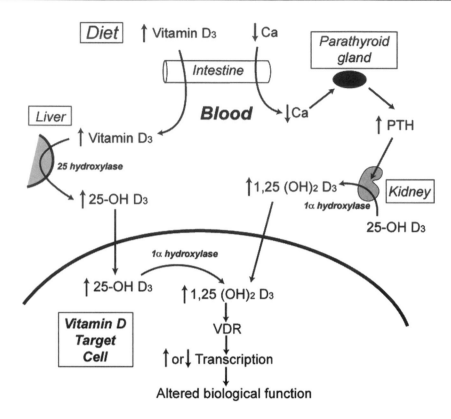

Fig. 4. Local and endocrine production of $1,25(OH)_2$ vitamin D may contribute to the physiological effects of vitamin D on calcium homeostasis. PTH, parathyroid hormone; $25(OH)D_3$, 25 hydroxyvitamin D3; $1,25(OH)_2D_3$, 1,25 dihydroxyvitamin D_3; VDR, vitamin D receptor.

The VDR can be found in both the cytoplasm and nucleus of vitamin D target cells. Binding of $1,25(OH)_2D_3$ to the VDR promotes association of VDR with the retinoid X receptor (RXR). This heterodimerization is required for migration of the RXR–VDR–ligand complex from the cytoplasm to the nucleus *(28–31)*. Once in the nucleus, the $1,25(OH)_2D_3$–VDR–RXR complex regulates gene transcription by interacting with specific vitamin D response elements (VDRE) in the promoters of vitamin D-responsive genes *(22)*. The steps leading to vitamin D-mediated gene transcription are summarized in Fig. 5.

Access to VDREs in their chromosomal context may be limited; Paredes et al. *(32)* used an ex vivo assay to show that although VDR–RXR binding to the osteocalcin VDRE in histone-free DNA was strong, this binding was minimal when the VDRE was in DNA assembled with histones into an artificial nucleosome. In vivo, release of chromosomal structure requires phosphorylation of histone H3, acetylation of histones H3 and H4, and phosphorylation events mediated by the SWI/SNF complex ATPases *(33–35)*. To overcome the constraints imposed by higher order chromatin structure, the VDR–RXR dimer recruits a complex with histone acetyl transferase (HAT) activity (e.g., CBP/p300, SRC1 *[36,37]*) as well as SWI/SNF complexes (e.g,. the BAF57 subunit of SWI/SNF directly interacts with SRC1 and steroid hormone receptors *[38]*). After chromosomal unwind-

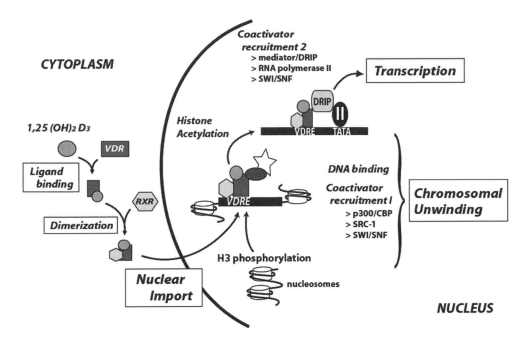

Fig. 5. A summary of the vitamin D receptor (VDR)-mediated molecular regulation of gene expression by 1,25(OH)$_2$ vitamin D$_3$ (1,25(OH)$_2$D$_3$). RXR, retinoid X receptor; VDRE, vitamin D response element; DRIP, vitamin D receptor-interacting protein; SRC-1, steroid receptor coactivator 1; p300/CBP, transcriptional coactivators with histone acetyl transferase activity; SWI/SNF, ATP-dependent chromatin remodeling factors; II, RNA polymerase II; TATA or "TATA box," binding site for RNA polymerase II.

ing, the VDR–RXR dimer recruits the 16 protein mediator complex (a.k.a. DRIP) and utilizes it to recruit and activate the basal transcription unit containing RNA polymerase II *(39)*.

2.2.2. Calcium Transport Across Intestinal and Renal Epithelial Cells: Regulation by 1,25(OH)$_2$D$_3$

The movement of calcium across the intestinal and renal epithelium has many similarities *(see also* Chapter 3). First, calcium movement can occur both between cells (paracellular) and through cells (transcellular). The paracellular movement is thought to be exclusively diffusional and nonregulated but sensitive to ion and electrical gradients as well as bulk fluid flow. Thus, a set percentage of any calcium present on the luminal side of the intestine or renal tubule will leak across the barrier (e.g., 16%/h in rat duodenum). This can become quantitatively important in the intestine when dietary intake is high. 1,25(OH)$_2$D$_3$ regulates only the transcellular movement of calcium in the proximal part of the human intestine *(40,41)*, and its impact on the kidney is less clear.

The mechanisms by which calcium crosses the intestinal and renal epithelial cell are currently under debate. However, the bulk of experimental data is consistent with the facilitated diffusion model *(40)*. This model, and the proteins mediating transport in both proximal small intestine intestine and distal convoluted tubule of the kidney, is shown in Fig. 6. The first step of transcellular transport is entry of free calcium into the cell through a calcium channel. Two related channels mediate this process in intestine and kidney:

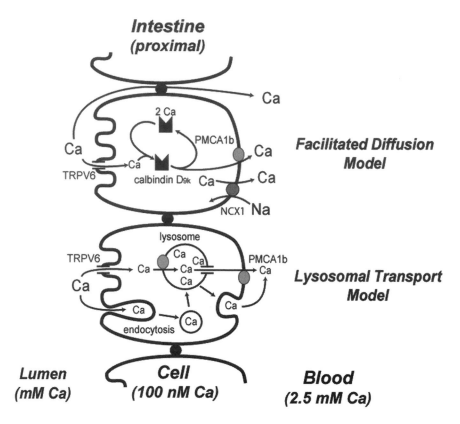

Fig. 6. Two models for transcellular calcium transport across the intestinal epithelial cell. TRPV6, transient receptor potential channel, vanilloid subfamily member 6; PMCA1b, plasma membrane calcium ATPase 1b; NCX1, sodium-calcium exchanger 1.

transient receptor potential channel, vanilloid subfamily member 6 (TRPV6) in the duodenum (a.k.a. CaT1 or ECaC2) and both TRPV6 and TRPV5 (a.k.a. CaT2 or ECaC1) in the kidney *(42)*. These channels are members of the vanilloid family of channels. The mRNA level for TRPV6 in the intestine, and to a lesser extent, TRPV6 and TRPV5 mRNA levels in the kidney, are regulated by $1,25(OH)_2D_3$ *(43)*. In the intestine, the induction of TRPV6 mRNA precedes the induction of active calcium absorption, suggesting that the two events are temporally linked. Both TRPV5 and TRPV6 are very effective at permitting calcium movement through membranes, but their activity is rapidly suppressed when intracellular calcium levels increase *(44)*. Calbindin D_{9k} (in intestine) and calbindin D28k are intracellular calcium binding proteins that may serve as intracellular buffers to prevent increases in cytosolic $[Ca^{2+}]$ that would shut down TRPV6 and TRPV5. Calbindin D_{9k} can bind two calcium ions per mole of protein, whereas calbindin D_{28k} can bind 4 moles of calcium per mole of protein. In their capacity as intracellular buffers, the calbindins also limit increases in intracellular calcium that could activate cellular signaling; this would be crucial to limit inadvertent signaling following calcium-rich meals *(45)*.

Based on a mathematical model by Bronner et al. *(40)*, the intracellular diffusion of calcium across the enterocyte is the rate-limiting step for intracellular calcium absorption. Experiments suggest that the calbindins may also promote intracellular diffusion of calcium across the cell *(46)*, and this is where the facilitated diffusion model gets its name. In animal experiments, the level of calbindin D_{9k} in the intestine has been shown to correlate closely with the efficiency of intestinal calcium absorption, as well as serum or plasma $1,25(OH)_2D_3$ levels *(40,43,47)*. These and other data suggest that calbindin D_{9k} protein and mRNA levels are inducible by $1,25(OH)_2D_3$; the lack of a functional vitamin D response element in the calbindin D_{9k} gene, as well as experimental data *(48)*, suggest that this regulation is primarily a posttranscriptional response. In the kidney of mice, calbindin D28k expression can be upregulated by diet-induced changes in serum $1,25(OH)_2D_3$ and by $1,25(OH)_2D_3$ injection *(43)*. However, this induction is small (two-fold under extreme conditions), and although the lack of VDR leads to a significant reduction in intestinal calbindin D_{9k}, no such decline is observed for calbindin D_{28k} in the kidney *(26)*. These data are consistent with evidence from cultured mouse distal tubule cells that showed that $1,25(OH)_2D_3$ did not alter calcium reabsorption *(49)*.

Although the facilitated diffusion model depends on the calbindins, more recent data reveal that high levels of calbindin D_{9k} in the intestine are not a guarantee that calcium absorption will be elevated *(43,50,51)*. This further supports the idea that there is a critical interplay between other parts of the transcellular calcium transport apparatus and the calbindins. The final step in the transcellular calcium transport is the active extrusion of calcium by the action of plasma membrane calcium ATPases (PMCA) or a sodium–calcium exchanger. Although both the activity and amount of the PMCAs are regulated by $1,25(OH)_2D_3$ *(52)*, this step appears to be the least sensitive to the hormone. Like TRPV6, the maximal activity of the PMCA isoforms in the intestine may require the presence of calbindin D_{9k}. Walters *(53)* demonstrated that binding of calbindin D_{9k} to PMCA stimulates the pump activity.

Other models have also been proposed to explain transcellular calcium movement in the intestine. This includes the lysosomal transport model where calcium is sequestered into lysomes and transcellular transport occurs by extrusion of calcium from the cell by exocitosis *(54)*. Another model is transcaltachia, the rapid transcellular movement of calcium in response to $1,25(OH)_2D_3$ treatment *(55)*. The transcaltachia model has been demonstrated only in chick intestine and suffers conceptually from the need to have controlled fluxes in $1,25(OH)_2D_3$ occurring simultaneous to consumption of calcium-rich meals.

2.2.3. RAPID ACTIONS OF $1,25(OH)_2D_3$

While research on VDR-mediated gene transcription continues to be fruitful, there is now compelling evidence for the existence of nongenomic $1,25(OH)_2D_3$-inducible signal transduction pathways within various cell types *(56,57)*. Figure 7 summarizes the kinase and second messenger pathways that have been shown to be activated through rapid $1,25(OH)_2 D_3$-mediated signaling. For example, in rat colonocytes *(58,59)* and in proliferating cultures of the intestinal cell line Caco-2 *(60,61)*, $1,25(OH)_2D_3$ rapidly (within seconds and minutes) activates phospholipase C (PLC), increases phosphoinositide turnover, generates the second messengers inositol 1,3,4-triphosphate (IP_3) and 1,2-diacylglycerol (DAG), activates protein kinase C (PKC) isoforms *(62)*, and activates the c-Jun-N-terminal kinase (JNK) and ERK family of MAP kinases *(63)*. The effect of $1,25(OH)_2D_3$ treatment on kinase activation may depend on adequate vitamin D status; rapid $1,25(OH)_2D_3$-induced changes in phosphoinositide turnover, PKC translocation,

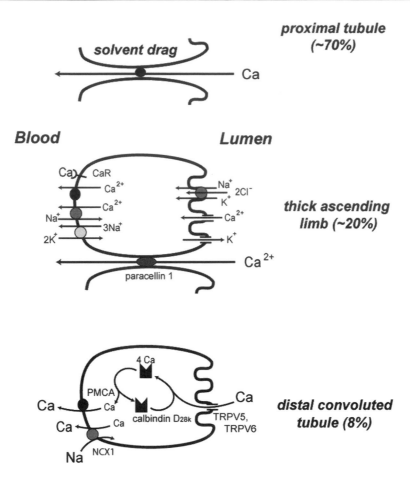

Fig. 7. Different modes of calcium reabsorption are used for renal calcium reabsorption in the proximal, middle, and distal segments of the nephron. TRPV6, transient receptor potential channel, vanilloid subfamily member 6; TRPV5, transient receptor potential channel, vanilloid subfamily member 5; PMCA, plasma membrane calcium ATPase; NCX1, sodium-calcium exchanger 1.

and changes in intracellular calcium do not occur in colonocytes from vitamin D-deficient, hypocalcemic rats *(64)*.

The rapid activation of kinases is a signaling system that has been traditionally used to explain the mechanism of action of peptide hormones and growth factors; however, it is now being recognized as important for the action of steroid hormones as well *(65)*. There is considerable controversy regarding the mechanism used by $1,25(OH)_2D_3$ to transduce a signal across the membrane of cells and activate kinase pathways. One line of evidence suggests that there may be a unique membrane receptor for $1,25(OH)_2D_3$. This protein, termed the membrane-associated rapid response steroid-binding protein (MARRS) *(66)*, binds $1,25(OH)_2D_3$ with high affinity, is distinct from the classical VDR, and is found on the membrane of a number of cells that respond to $1,25(OH)_2D_3$ treatment by activating kinase pathways and stimulating calcium fluxes. However, in addition to the MARRS protein, several recent papers have indicated that the classical VDR may be involved in at least some of the rapid $1,25(OH)_2D_3$ signaling pathways. For example,

Buitrago et al. *(67,68)* have demonstrated that the classical VDR is associated with src kinase and is also a target of src kinase activity in myocytes. In addition, Bettoun et al. found that in the Caco-2 intestinal cell line, the VDR is part of a ternary complex with proteins known to control movement of cells through the G1-S transition in cell cycle, i.e., the protein phosphatase PP1c and the p70 S6 kinase *(69)*. Finally, Erben et al. *(70)* found that 1,25(OH)2 D-mediated activation of calcium fluxes is blocked in osteoblasts from mice expressing a VDR that lacks the DNA binding domain. Although this observation conflicts with data generated by Wali et al. *(71)* in VDR-null mice, coupled with the other data from cell systems, it suggests that VDR may participate in at least some rapid signaling pathways.

Although the recent observations on rapid $1,25(OH)_2D_3$ signaling are interesting, the central importance of VDR-mediated signaling in calcium homeostasis appears to leave little room for an independent effect of these pathways. To date, two distinct areas support a unique biological role for the rapid activation of kinase pathways by $1,25(OH)_2D_3$. The first area is the modulation of growth zone chondrocyte biology *(72–74)*. Treatment of growth zone chondrocytes with $1,25(OH)_2D_3$ activates phospholipase A2 and causes an increase in membrane fluidity, activates PLC leading to the activation of PKC and release of intracellular calcium, and indirectly activates protein kinase A through production of prostaglandin E_2. These changes are important for activation of growth factors (i.e., latent transforming growth factor [TGF]-β in matrix), proteoglycan degradation, and matrix mineralization.

Another emerging area suggests that rapid, membrane-initiated actions of $1,25(OH)_2D_3$ can modulate adipocyte biology by controlling intracellular calcium levels. Shi et al. *(75)* showed that $1,25(OH)_2D_3$ stimulates lipogenesis and lipid loading of human adipocytes by causing a dose–responsive increase in intracellular calcium levels, increasing adipocyte fatty acid synthase expression/activity and glycerol-3-phosphate dehydrogenase activity, and inhibiting isoproterenol-stimulated lipolysis. These effects were mimicked by an analog with minimal ability to regulate the VDR-mediated transcriptional effects of $1,25(OH)_2D_3$ and they were completely prevented by 1β,25 dihydroxyvitamin D_3, a specific antagonist of the membrane-initiated actions of $1,25(OH)_2D_3$. Suppression of this pathway has been used as a mechanistic foundation to explain a controversial new observation that high dietary calcium intake can limit weight gain or promote weight loss in humans *(76,77)*.

2.2.3.1. POTENTIAL INTERACTIONS BETWEEN THE RAPID AND VDR PATHWAYS

Several studies support the hypothesis that signal transduction pathways are important regulators of VDR-mediated gene expression (Fig. 8). For example, suppression of PKC activity with staurosporine or H7 inhibited $1,25(OH)_2D_3$-regulated 25-hydroxyvitamin D 24-hydroxylase (CYP24) gene expression in proliferating, small intestine crypt-like, rat intestinal epithelial cell (IEC)-6 cells *(78)*, and activation of PKC with phorbol esters enhanced $1,25(OH)_2D_3$- regulated CYP24 gene transcription in IEC-6 and IEC-18 cells *(79)*. Similar findings have been observed for $1,25(OH)_2D_3$-mediated osteocalcin gene expression in the osteoblast-like reactive oxygen species (ROS) 17/2.8 cell *(80)*, CYP24 gene induction in COS-1 cells *(81)*, c-myc activation in proliferating skeletal muscle *(82)*, and CYP3A4 gene regulation in proliferating Caco-2 cells *(83)*. Specific cross-talk between rapid, membrane-initiated vitamin D actions and VDR-mediated genomic ac-

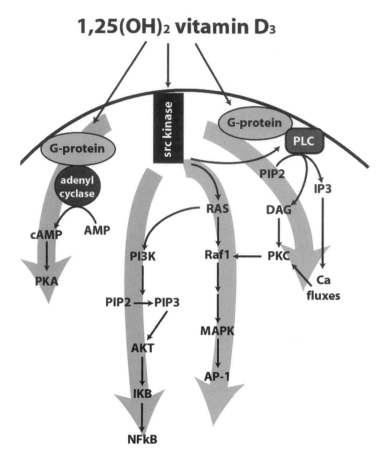

Fig. 8. 1,25(OH)$_2$ vitamin D$_3$ can rapidly activate a variety of signal transduction pathways. PKA, protein kinase A; PI3K, phosphatidylinositol 3 kinase; PIP2, phosphatidylinositol-4,5, bisphosphate; PIP3, phosphatidylinositol-3,4,5 trisphosphate; PLC, phospholipase C; IP3, inositol triphosphate; DAG, diacylglycerol; PKC, protein kinase C; AKT, protein kinase B; IκB, inhibitor of NFκB; NFκB, nuclear factor κB; MAPK, mitogen-activated kinase; AP-1, activator protein-1.

tions are also supported by the observation that an antagonist of the nongenomic pathway, 1β,25(OH)2 D, blocks 1α, 25(OH)$_2$D-mediated osteocalcin gene transcription in osteoblasts *(84)*. The mechanism for this interaction between 1,25(OH)$_2$D$_3$-induced kinase pathways and VDR-mediated gene transcription is unclear, but it likely results from the modulation of protein–protein interactions that are responsible for recruitment of coactivators necessary for disruption of higher order chromatin structure and transcriptional activation *(see* Fig. 3) *(81,85)*.

2.3. PTH (Kidney and Bone)

2.3.1. CONTROL OF PTH PRODUCTION AND RELEASE

As shown in Fig. 2, two factors have a strong influence on the production and release of PTH from the parathyroid gland: serum ionized calcium and 1,25(OH)$_2$D$_3$. Changes in serum calcium can alter three aspects of PTH biology in the parathyroid gland: intra-

cellular degradation, gene expression, and hormone secretion (86). In response to hypocalcemia, PTH secretion can increase within seconds, suppression of intracellular PTH
degradation leads to an increase in the amount of intact PTH available for secretion within
30 min, and both transcriptional regulation of the PTH gene and stabilization of the PTH
mRNA lead to increased PTH synthesis within hours.

Serum calcium and phosphorus have opposing effects on PTH mRNA levels. While
high serum phosphate levels increase PTH mRNA levels, high serum calcium levels
suppress PTH mRNA levels. These ions influence PTH mRNA stability through the
binding (hyperphosphatemia) and release (hypercalcemia) of proteins to the 3'
untranslated region of the PTH mRNA (87). Although the ability of high serum phosphate
levels to increase PTH levels suggests that high dietary phosphate may promote bone loss
by increasing PTH-mediated bone resorption, a short-term study by Whybro et al. (88)
found that a diet with 2000 mg of elemental phosphate did not increase a urinary marker
of bone resorption in young men.

Changes in serum calcium levels are sensed by the calcium-sensing receptor (CaR)
(89). The CaR is dimeric glycoprotein that belongs to the superfamily of G protein-
coupled receptors. It resides on the cell surface of many cell types, including the chief
cells of the parathyroid gland and the cells along the kidney tubules involved in mineral
ion homeostasis. Upon binding of Ca to the CaR, several intracellular signaling pathways
are activated—e.g., PLC-mediated activation of PKC signaling, PLD- and PLA2-medi-
ated generation of arachadonic acid for regulation of cyclooxygenase and lipoygenase
pathways, and activation of all three MAP kinase pathways (ERK, JNK, and p38). Unfortunately, it is not yet clear which of these intracellular signaling pathways are critical for
the control of PTH secretion or other aspects of parathyroid function.

As described earlier in the subsections on vitamin D, PTH secretion leads to an activation of the renal 1α hydroxylase and increases the production of $1,25(OH)_2D_3$. Whereas
this hormone influences bone, intestine, and kidney to improve calcium homeostasis, it
is also a potent signal for the suppression of PTH gene expression (90). Like vitamin D-
mediated gene activation, suppression of PTH mediated gene expression requires the
binding of the $1,25(OH)_2D_3$–VDR–RXR complex to two vitamin D response elements
in the promoter of the PTH gene (91). It is likely that these interactions recruit co-
repressors with histone deacetylase (HDAC) activity, which keeps the PTH gene in a
transcriptionally repressed state.

2.3.2. MOLECULAR ACTIONS OF PTH

PTH is known to influence mineral ion homeostasis by activating a membrane receptor, the PTH/PTH related protein (PTHrp) receptor (92). Figure 9 demonstrates schematically the signaling pathways utilized upon the activation of the PTH/PTHrp receptor in
osteoblasts. By utilizing both stimulatory (e.g., G_q and $G_{s\alpha}$) and inhibitory ($G_{i/o}$) G
proteins, PTH can activate either a protein kinase C/MAP kinase pathway or a protein
kinase A signaling pathway. Mahon et al. (93) have demonstrated that the PTH/PTHrp
receptor interacts with Na^+/H^+ exchanger regulatory factors (NHERF) 1 and 2. Upon
stimulation of cells with PTH, NHERF2 is responsible for the inhibition of adenyl cyclase
(and the protein kinase A pathway), whereas in kidney cells, NHERF1 is responsible for
the inhibition of phosphate uptake leading to increased phosphate excretion (93).

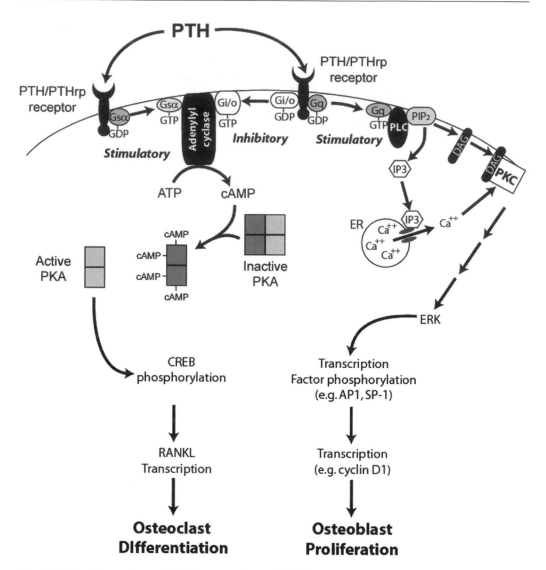

Fig. 9. Molecular actions of PTH in osteoblasts. PTH/PTHrp, parathyroid hormone/parathyroid hormone related peptide; PKA, protein kinase A; PLC, phospholipase C; IP3, inositol triphosphate; DAG, diacylglycerol; PKC, protein kinase C; ERK, extracellular signal-regulated kinase; CREB, cAMP response element binding protein; RANKL, ligand for the receptor for activation of nuclear factor κB; AP-1, activator protein-1.

2.3.2.1. STIMULATION OF RENAL CALCIUM REABSORPTION BY PTH

Figure 7 demonstrates that the bulk of calcium reabsorption in the kidney occurs in the proximal tubule as a result of solvent drag. However, PTH is known to activate both cellular and paracellular pathways of calcium reabsorption in the thick ascending limb of Henle *(94)*. In addition, PTH activates the fine-tuning mechanisms controlling calcium reabsorption in the distal convoluted tubule. PTH-activated calcium uptake in the distal tubule depends on the activation of both PKC and PKA *(49)*, and may require voltage-gated calcium channel family members. Antisense oligonucleotides against the calcium channel β accessory subunit ($\beta3$) inhibited PTH-mediated increases in intracellular calcium (95). Although TRPV5 and TRPV6 are co-localized with the other proteins thought to mediate active renal calcium reabsorption in the distal tubule (96), it is not yet clear whether PTH stimulates the production of these proteins or activates them. In VDR receptor-null mice with elevated PTH levels, both TRPV5 and TRPV6 mRNA levels are significantly elevated 50–100% in the kidney, suggesting the existence of a moderate PTH-mediated induction (26).

2.3.2.2. ACTIVATION OF RENAL $1,25(OH)_2D_3$ PRODUCTION

The impact of PTH on the intestine is mediated through its ability to stimulate the renal 1α hydroxylase gene expression and suppress 24-hydroxylase (CYP24) mRNA levels, leading to an increase in the renal production of $1,25(OH)_2D_3$ (97,98). The impact of PTH on CYP24 mRNA levels is due to a reduction in the half-life of the message while PTH activates 1α hydroxylase through a cAMP-dependent mechanism that leads to the activation of the cyclic AMP response element binding protein (CREB) transcription factor (*see* Fig. 9 for PTH signaling pathways).

2.3.2.3. INFLUENCE OF PTH ON BONE CELLS

It is an accepted principle of bone biology that the activities of osteoblasts and osteoclasts are coupled. The importance of coupling is clear when one considers the paradox that while $1,25(OH)_2D_3$ and PTH are classically thought to promote bone resorption, their receptors are found on osteoblasts but not osteoclasts. Cell cultures studies show that the formation of active osteoclasts requires direct cell-to-cell contact of osteoclast progenitors with osteoblasts (99). This osteoblast-induced differentiation of osteoclasts is mediated through the RANK–RANKL system (*see* Fig. 10) (100). RANK is a receptor for the activation of the nuclear factor (NF)κB signaling system and it resides on the cell surface of osteoclast progenitors. While RANK activation is one of several critical steps that stimulate the differentiation of cells from the monocyte/macrophage lineage into osteoclasts, it is the step that is sensitive to stimulation by PTH as well as other mediators like $1,25(OH)_2D_3$, cytokines (e.g., interleukin [IL]-11), and prostaglandin E (PGE)$_2$. Upon stimulation of osteoblasts with PTH, the cells increase their production of the ligand for RANK (RANKL), a cell-associated protein (101). Thus, close association of stimulated osteoblasts and osteoclast progenitors permits the binding of RANKL to RANK and the activation of the differentiation program. In addition to RANKL, PTH can also suppress the production of osteoprotegerin (OPG). OPG is a secreted protein produced by osteoblasts that binds to RANK, blocks RANKL binding to RANK, and prevents RANKL-mediated activation of osteoclast differentiation. Finally, PTH can stimulate the secretion of macrophage colony-stimulating factor (MCSF), another factor that promotes osteoclast differentiation (102). Collectively, it is the PTH-induced shift in the ratio of RANKL to OPG, coupled with the induced synthesis of MCSF, which promotes osteoclast differentiation and ultimately increased bone resorption.

The fact that PTH signals through the osteoblast may account for the paradoxical observation that although continuous PTH treatment promotes bone loss, intermittent administration of the hormone stimulates bone formation (103). As shown in Fig. 9, PTH can activate both the PKA signaling pathway that leads to the production of RANKL as

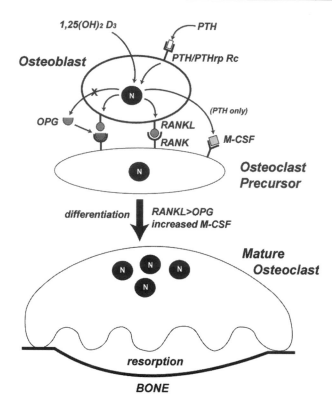

Fig. 10. Stimulation of osteoclast differentiation by 1,25(OH)$_2$ vitamin D$_3$ (1,25[OH]$_2$D$_3$) and parathyroid hormone (PTH)-mediated activation of the RANK–RANKL system. PTH/PTHrp Rc, PTH/PTHrp receptor; OPG, osteoprotegerin; RANK, receptor for activation of nuclear factor κB; RANKL, ligand for RANK; M-CSF, macrophage-colony stimulating factor; N, nucleus.

well as a PKC signaling pathway that activates transcription factors like AP-1 and SP-1, leading to the stimulation of osteoblast proliferation. Thus, continuous high level PTH (as seen during calcium deprivation) increases osteoclast number, but intermittent PTH administration increases the number of osteoblasts but not osteoclasts. This is the basis for the osteotrophic activity of intermittent PTH (or PTH fragment) use in treatment of osteoporosis. In addition to the effects on osteoblast proliferation, the increase in osteoblast number is also due to a suppression of apoptosis resulting from PKA-mediated phosphorylation and inactivation of the pro-apoptotic protein Bad and the CREB-mediated transcription of the anti-apoptotic proteins Bcl-2 and Runx *(104)*.

3. ESTROGEN

The loss of estrogen due to the menopause leads to increased bone turnover and bone loss *(105)*. This clearly demonstrates the importance of estrogen to bone health. Estrogen is thought to affect bone by its direct actions on bone cells as well as indirect actions on calcium homeostasis *(106)*. Estrogen's effect on bone may be mediated by changes induced in the expression of multiple regulatory factors. For example, estrogen increases the production and release of osteoprotegerin from osteoblasts *(107)*, suppresses the membrane form of MCSF in human bone marrow cultures *(108)*, and suppresses the production of cytokines by osteoblasts, monocytes, and T-cells that normally promote osteoclastogenesis (e.g., IL-1, tumor necrosis factor [TNF]-α, IL-6, and PGE_2). The impact of mechanical strain on bone may also depend on estrogen action *(106)*; thus, loss of estrogen results in loss of mechanotransduction and accelerated bone loss. Although estrogens presumably regulate bone biology by transcriptional activation of genes mediated through estrogen receptor α *(109)*, some of the bone protective actions of estrogen may be due to nongenomic actions of the hormone. Kousteni et al. *(110)* reported that an estrogen analog increased bone formation and strength in ovariectomized mice without stimulating transcription of estrogen regulated genes in bone and without causing uterine growth.

Estrogen is thought to impact calcium homeostasis through the intestine and kidney in several ways. First, during the early phase of menopause characterized by a rapid drop in estrogen levels, the increase in calcium release from the bone will increase serum calcium levels, suppress PTH levels and reduce the renal production of $1,25(OH)_2D_3$. By lowering PTH and $1,25(OH)_2D_3$ levels, estrogen indirectly reduces the efficiency of intestinal calcium absorption and renal calcium excretion, leading to increased urinary calcium loss at the expense of bone. Later, after the system has adapted to the loss of estrogen and bone loss has slowed, the loss of calcium absorption efficiency due to estrogen deficiency, coupled to enhanced renal calcium loss, will eventually lead to hypocalcemia and increased parathyroid activity *(111)*. At this stage, the loss of intestinal absorption efficiency may be due to disruption of vitamin D signaling. Gennari et al. *(112)* found that oophorectomy reduced basal and $1,25(OH)_2D_3$ induced intestinal calcium absorption in young women but that this could be reversed by estrogen repletion. Several groups have suggested that this is due to the reduction in VDR levels that results from estrogen deficiency *(113–115)*, although this hypothesis is not universally accepted *(116)*. Estrogen may also have vitamin D-independent effects on calcium absorption and excretion as well. Van Able et al. *(117)* found that whereas ovariectomy did not significantly reduce TRPV5 levels in the kidney of mice, estradiol injections elevated the level of this message twofold. Similarly, van Cromphaut et al. *(27)* found that intestine TRPV6 mRNA levels fell 55% in estrogen receptor α-null mice and that pharmacological treatment with estradiol increased duodenal TRPV6 mRNA levels four- to eightfold in both normal and VDR receptor-null mice, indicating the regulation is vitamin D-independent.

4. OTHER HORMONES

A number of other hormones are proposed to be important for the control of calcium metabolism. Most of these hormones have been studied primarily in the context of their effects on bone cells. In this light, any signaling molecule that can influence serum calcium indirectly through the accretion or loss of calcium from bone will theoretically modulate the PTH–vitamin D axis and regulate intestinal calcium absorption and renal calcium excretion. The following paragraphs provide a brief review of several hormones or physiological states that are known to influence calcium homeostasis.

4.1. Calcitonin

The discussion on PTH and vitamin D metabolites focused on compensatory changes that occur originating from a drop in serum calcium levels. In contrast, calcitonin is a peptide hormone produced from the thyroidal C-cells that inhibits osteoclastic activity by binding to a cell surface receptor on osteoclasts *(118)*. Secretion of calcitonin is regulated by binding of serum calcium to the calcium sensing receptor on C-cells. High serum calcium levels lead to CaR-mediated cellular depolarization, activation of voltage-dependent calcium channels, and calcitonin secretion. When bone turnover is very high, calcitonin-mediated suppression of osteoclast activity can lead to hypocalcemia and the stimulation of intestinal calcium absorption and renal calcium reabsorption through the PTH–vitamin D axis outlined in Fig. 2.

4.2. Growth Hormone

During childhood and adolescence, growth hormone and its physiological mediator, insulin-like growth factor (IGF)-1, have a major role in linear bone growth and accrual of bone mass. In children, serum IGF-1 levels are positively correlated with femur size *(119)*, and growth hormone deficiency is commonly associated with reduced bone density in children *(120)* and adults *(121)*. IGF-1 increases bone formation by increasing proliferation in osteoblast precursors, increasing the activity of mature osteoblasts, and suppressing osteoblast apoptosis *(122,123)*. In addition, growth hormone can also promote intestinal calcium absorption. Data from some studies suggest that this is indirectly due to the activation of the renal 1α hydroxylase and elevation of serum $1,25(OH)_2D_3$ levels *(124)*. However, we have shown that growth hormone treatment significantly increases intestinal calcium absorption and duodenal calbindin D_{9k} levels in aged rats without significantly increasing serum $1,25(OH)_2D_3$ levels *(47)*. Similarly, although calcium absorption is reduced by 70% in mice lacking the VDR, there is evidence for vitamin D-independent, growth-related regulation of intestinal calcium absorption in these mice *(26)*. The vitamin D-independent mechanism by which the growth hormone–IGF-1 axis may regulate intestinal calcium absorption is not clear at this time.

4.3. Hormones of Pregnancy and Lactation

During pregnancy and lactation, the three-tissue axis described in Figs. 1 and 2 becomes a four-tissue axis (Fig. 11). In addition, the normal coordination among the activities of the intestine, kidney, and bone are disrupted. This suggests that there are additional factors that regulate calcium homeostasis beyond simply vitamin D and PTH.

Not surprisingly, fetal skeletal development is a significant drain on maternal calcium metabolism; approx 80% of the 33 g of calcium that is deposited in the fetus is accumulated during the third trimester of pregnancy. As a result, serum $1,25(OH)_2D_3$ levels and intestinal calcium absorption are both elevated in an attempt to compensate for increased bone turnover in the mother (Fig. 11B) *(125)*. Several things are interesting about this period. First, the increase in serum $1,25(OH)_2D_3$ is due in part to extrarenal production by the placenta *(126)*, and this could explain why serum PTH levels, the normal physiological stimulus for renal production of $1,25(OH)_2D_3$, are not elevated. Second, although serum $1,25(OH)_2D_3$ levels are elevated, renal calcium loss is high. The high rate of calcium loss simply could be a reflection of high calcium absorption and a higher filtered calcium load, or it may be because PTH is a stronger regulator of renal calcium reabsorption and PTH levels are not elevated. Third, bone loss does not occur during pregnancy despite the considerable loss of calcium to the fetus and elevated serum $1,25(OH)_2D_3$ levels. This may be caused by the elevated calcitonin level observed during pregnancy *(127)* and calcitonin-mediated suppression of osteoclast activity. Finally, in

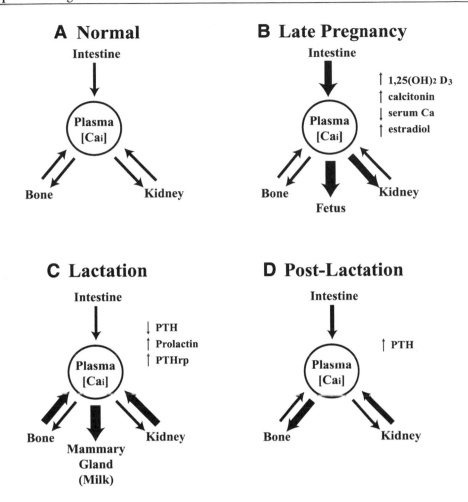

A Normal

Intestine

Plasma [Ca$_i$]

Bone   Kidney

B Late Pregnancy

Intestine

↑ 1,25(OH)$_2$ D$_3$
↑ calcitonin
↓ serum Ca
↑ estradiol

Plasma [Ca$_i$]

Bone   Kidney

Fetus

C Lactation

Intestine

↓ PTH
↑ Prolactin
↑ PTHrp

Plasma [Ca$_i$]

Bone   Kidney

Mammary Gland (Milk)

D Post-Lactation

Intestine

↑ PTH

Plasma [Ca$_i$]

Bone   Kidney

Fig. 11. Alterations in calcium homeostasis at the three-tissue axis of intestine, kidney, and bone during pregnancy, lactation, and postweaning in humans.

rats, the pregnancy-induced elevation in intestinal calcium absorption appears before fetal skeletal mineralization, changes in serum-ionized calcium, or changes in serum 1,25(OH)$_2$D$_3$ levels *(128)*. This suggests that there are vitamin D-independent factors controlling intestinal calcium absorption in pregnant rats. This is consistent with the data on TRPV6 gene expression in the intestine of mice; pregnancy increased TRPV6 mRNA levels more than 10-fold in both pregnant wild-type and VDR receptor-null mice *(27)*.

The lactation and postlactation periods are particularly interesting physiological states with regard to bone biology. During lactation, maternal bone loss can reach 7%, yet this loss is completely recovered once nursing is halted and there is no increased risk of osteoporosis associated with this process *(129)*. Figure 11C shows that during lactation, milk production puts a considerable drain on maternal bone and that this is compensated for by renal calcium conservation but not by elevated intestinal calcium absorption in humans *(125,130)*. Serum calcium levels are elevated, and serum PTH levels are lower than in nonlactating women *(131)*. In contrast to humans, lactating rats have both elevated serum $1,25(OH)_2D_3$ levels and a twofold higher level of calcium absorption *(132)*. However, whereas vitamin D deprivation can prevent the increase in serum $1,25(OH)_2D_3$ levels during lactation, calcium absorption is still high in vitamin D-deprived, lactating rats indicating the effect is vitamin D-independent *(132)*. Studies in rats have demonstrated that prolactin can directly stimulate transcellular calcium transport in the duodenum *(133)*. The mechanism for this regulation is unclear but includes the upregulation of duodenal calbindin D_{9k} and TRPV6 mRNA levels *(27)*. Finally, Fig. 11D shows the compensation that occurs in calcium homeostasis immediately following lactation and which permits the complete recovery of bone mass. Unfortunately, this recovery period has been only marginally studied and the mechanisms explaining this rapid recovery remain to be determined.

5. GENETIC CONTROL OF CALCIUM HOMEOSTASIS

Although the mechanisms controlling calcium homeostasis described above are well studied, it is clear that the individual variation in any given process controlling calcium metabolism is high. Family and twin studies examining the heritability of various components of calcium homeostasis strongly suggest a role for genetics in the control of bone mineral density, bone architecture, serum calcium, 24-h urinary calcium, and calcium absorption *(134–136)*. Many genetic studies of calcium metabolism have searched for the mutated genes that are responsible for the rare, heritable diseases affecting bone—e.g., vitamin D-resistant rickets (VDR), pseudovitamin D deficiency rickets (1α hydroxylase), osteogenesis imperfecta (collagen type Iα1). These mutations do not account for the variation in bone density seen in the general population. In an attempt to identify the genetic contributors to the variability in bone density that exists within the general population, other studies have searched for quantitative trait loci (QTL) in twins, in families with high or low bone density, or in mice that have large differences in their bone phenotypes *(136)*. These traditional approaches have identified a large number of chromosomal regions that influence bone phenotypes but only a few specific genes—e.g. the low-density lipoprotein (LDL) receptor-related protein 5 (LRP5) gene that accounts for very high bone mass observed in a specific kindred *(137)*.

Finally, researchers have conducted a large number of association studies to assess the role of common polymorphisms (single-base changes or nucleotide repeats) within candidate genes (e.g., those with known roles in normal calcium and bone metabolism) on bone mineral density and calcium homeostasis *(136)*. Although the mutations in the genes accounting for changes in bone density in heritable genetic diseases or in restricted subpopulations with high or low bone mass occur within the coding region of genes (leading to premature termination or deletion/replacement of critical amino acids) or in the regulatory regions of gene promoters, most common polymorphisms occur in noncoding, nonregulatory regions and do not have an obvious impact on the function or level of the protein encoded by the gene. Without a clear functional consequence to the polymorphism, one must be cautious about overinterpreting a positive association to mean that there is an alteration in the activity of a specific pathway. For example, although polymorphisms in the 3' untranslated region of the VDR gene have been associated with low bone density in some human studies (e.g., the B allele of the Bsm-I restriction fragment length polymorphism *[138]*), there is no strong evidence that demonstrates that these polymorphisms alter VDR level or signaling. As a result, the polymorphism in the VDR gene could be in linkage disequilibrium with a functional mutation in another gene that has a role in calcium or bone metabolism (i.e., the VDR gene polymorphism is a marker for the mutation in another gene). This could explain why many gene polymorphisms associate with bone density in one racial or ethnic group (where linkage may exist) but not in another (where linkage does not exist).

In contrast, a polymorphism in an Sp-1 binding site with the collagen type Iα1 gene promoter is associated with lower bone mass *(139)* and does so by reducing the binding of Sp-1 to the promoter and reducing collagen type Iα1 production *(140)*. Although the role of genetic variability in calcium and bone metabolism is likely to be crucial to our long-term understanding of individual responses to lifestyle and pharmacological treatments to improve bone health, at this time there are no genetic markers that can be utilized for this purpose. In the future, it is likely that researchers will find that the combined effects of polymorphisms in many genes with highly distinct functions are responsible for the individual variability we see in complex traits like intestinal calcium absorption, urinary calcium excretion, and bone density.

6. CONCLUSIONS

Whole-body calcium metabolism is controlled by the coordinated actions of a three-tissue axis of intestine, bone, and kidney. As such, to fully understand the control of whole-body calcium metabolism, one must understand the mechanisms controlling intestinal calcium absorption, renal calcium excretion, and bone turnover. These processes are controlled by a number of hormones—e.g., vitamin D metabolites, PTH, estrogens, calcitonin, growth hormone/IGF-1, and prolactin. This chapter reviewed the molecular actions of these hormones in the control of calcium absorption and excretion as well as bone biology.

REFERENCES

1. Bronner F, Aubert JP. Bone metabolism and regulation of the blood calcium level in rats. Am J Physiol 1963;209:887–889.
2. Holick MF. Vitamin D: a millenium perspective. J Cell Biochem 2003;88(2):296–307.
3. White P, Cooke N. The multifunctional properties and characteristics of vitamin D-binding protein. Trends Endocrinol Metab 2000;11(8):320–327.
4. Leheste JR, Melsen F, Wellner M, et al. Hypocalcemia and osteopathy in mice with kidney-specific megalin gene defect. FASEB J 2003;17(2):247–249.
5. Trang HM, Cole DE, Rubin LA, Pierratos A, Siu S, Vieth R. Evidence that vitamin D3 increases serum 25-hydroxyvitamin D more efficiently than does vitamin D2. Am J Clin Nutr 1998;68(4):854–858.
6. Hewison M, Zehnder D, Bland R, Stewart PM. 1alpha-Hydroxylase and the action of vitamin D. J Mol Endocrinol 2000;25(2):141–148.
7. Omdahl JL, Morris HA, May BK. Hydroxylase enzymes of the vitamin D pathway: expression, function, and regulation. Annu Rev Nutr 2002;22:139–166.
8. Boyan BD, Sylvia VL, Dean DD, Schwartz Z. 24,25-(OH)(2)D(3) regulates cartilage and bone via autocrine and endocrine mechanisms. Steroids 2001;66(3–5):363–374.
9. Norman AW, Okamura WH, Bishop JE, Henry HL. Update on biological actions of 1alpha,25(OH)2-vitamin D3 (rapid effects) and 24R,25(OH)2-vitamin D3. Mol Cell Endocrinol 2002;197(1–2):1–13.
10. Thomas MK, Lloyd-Jones DM, Thadhani RI, et al. Hypovitaminosis D in medical inpatients. N Engl J Med 1998;338(12):777–783.

11. Chapuy MC, Preziosi P, Maamer M, et al. Prevalence of vitamin D insufficiency in an adult normal population. Osteoporos Int 1997;7(5):439–443.

12. Heaney RP, Dowell MS, Hale CA, Bendich A. Calcium absorption varies within the reference range for serum 25-hydroxyvitamin D. J Am Coll Nutr 2003;22(2):142–146.

13. Barger-Lux MJ, Heaney RP, Lanspa SJ, Healy JC, DeLuca HF. An investigation of sources of variation in calcium absorption efficiency. J Clin Endocrinol Metab 1995;80(2):406–411.

14. Heaney RP, Barger-Lux.M.J., Dowell MS, Chen TC, Holick MF. Calcium absorptive effects of vitamin D and its major metabolites. J Clin Endocrinol Metab 1997;82:4111–4116.

15. Devine A, Wilson SG, Dick IM, Prince RL. Effects of vitamin D metabolites on intestinal calcium absorption and bone turnover in elderly women. Am J Clin Nutr 2002;75(2):283–288.

16. Dusso A, Lopez-Hilker S, Rapp N, Slatopolsky E. Extra-renal production of calcitriol in chronic renal failure. Kidney Int 1988;34(3):368–375.

17. Jongen MJ, Van der vijgh WJ, Lips P, Netelenbos JC. Measurement of vitamin D metabolites in anephric subjects. Nephron 1984;36(4):230–234.

18. Whitlatch LW, Young MV, Schwartz GG, et al. 25-Hydroxyvitamin D-1alpha-hydroxylase activity is diminished in human prostate cancer cells and is enhanced by gene transfer. J Steroid Biochem Mol Biol 2002;81(2):135–140.

19. Lou YR, Laaksi I, Syvala H, et al. 25-Hydroxyvitamin D3 is an active hormone in human primary prostatic stromal cells. FASEB J 2004;18(2):332–334.

20. Zehnder D, Bland R, Williams MC, et al. Extrarenal expression of 25-hydroxyvitamin d(3)-1 alpha-hydroxylase. J Clin Endocrinol Metab 2001;86(2):888–894.

21. Vieth R, Milojevic S, Peltekova V. Improved cholecalciferol nutrition in rats is noncalcemic, suppresses parathyroid hormone and increases responsiveness to 1, 25-dihydroxycholecalciferol. J Nutr 2000;130(3):578–584.

22. Haussler MR, Whitfield GK, Haussler CA, Hsieh et al. The nuclear vitamin D receptor: biological and molecular regulatory properties revealed. J Bone Miner Res 1998;13(3):325–349.

23. Malloy PJ, Feldman D. Hereditary 1,25-dihydroxyvitamin D-resistant rickets. Endocr Dev 2003;6:175–199.

24. Yoshizawa T, Handa Y, Uematsu Y, et al. Mice lacking the vitamin D receptor exhibit impaired bone formation, uterine hypoplasia and growth retardation after weaning. Nat Genet 1997;16:391–396.

25. Li YC, Pirro AE, Amling M, et al. Targeted ablation of the vitamin D receptor: An animal model of vitamin D-dependent rickets type II with alopecia. Proc Natl Acad Sci USA 1997;94:9831–9835.

26. Song Y, Kato S, Fleet JC. Vitamin D receptor (VDR) knockout mice reveal VDR-independent regulation of intestinal calcium absorption and ECaC2 and calbindin D(9k) mRNA. J Nutr 2003;133(2):374–380.

27. Bouillon R, Van Cromphaut S, Carmeliet G. Intestinal calcium absorption: Molecular vitamin D mediated mechanisms. J Cell Biochem 2003;88(2):332–339.

28. Barsony J, Pike JW, DeLuca HF, Marx SJ. Immunocytology with microwave-fixed fibroblasts shows 1 alpha,25-dihydroxyvitamin D3-dependent rapid and estrogen-dependent slow reorganization of vitamin D receptors. J Cell Biol 1990;111(6 Pt 1):2385–2395.

29. Prufer K, Barsony J. Retinoid X receptor dominates the nuclear import and export of the unliganded vitamin D receptor. Mol Endocrinol 2002;16(8):1738–1751.

30. Barsony J, Renyi I, McKoy W. Subcellular distribution of normal and mutant vitamin D receptors in living cells. J Biol Chem 1997;272:5774–5782.

31. Prufer K, Racz A, Lin GC, Barsony J. Dimerization with retinoid X receptors promotes nuclear localization and subnuclear targeting of vitamin D receptors. J Biol Chem 2000;275(52):41114–41123.

32. Paredes R, Gutierrez J, Gutierrez S, et al. Interaction of the 1alpha,25-dihydroxyvitamin D3 receptor at the distal promoter region of the bone-specific osteocalcin gene requires nucleosomal remodelling. Biochem J 2002;363(Pt 3):667–676.

33. Berger SL. Histone modifications in transcriptional regulation. Curr Opin Genet Dev 2002;12(2):142–148.

34. Dilworth FJ, Chambon P. Nuclear receptors coordinate the activities of chromatin remodeling complexes and coactivators to facilitate initiation of transcription. Oncogene 2001;20(24):3047–3054.

35. Rachez C, Freedman LP. Mediator complexes and transcription. Current Opinion in Cell Biology 2001;13:274–280.

36. Freedman LP. Increasing the complexity of coactivation in nuclear receptor signaling. Cell 1999;97:5–8.

37. Chen H, Lin RJ, Xie W, Wilpitz D, Evans RM. Regulation of hormone-induced histone hyperacetylation and gene activation via acetylation of an acetylase. Cell 1999;98(5):675–686.
38. Belandia B, Orford RL, Hurst HC, Parker MG. Targeting of SWI/SNF chromatin remodelling complexes to estrogen-responsive genes. EMBO J 2002;21(15):4094–4103.
39. Rachez C, Lemon BD, Suldan Z, et al. Ligand-dependent transcription activation by nuclear receptors requires the DRIP complex. Nature 1999;398:824–828.
40. Bronner F, Pansu D, Stein WD. An analysis of intestinal calcium transport across the rat intestine. Am J Physiol 1986;250(5 Pt 1):G561–G569.
41. Giuliano AR, Wood RJ. Vitamin D-regulated calcium transport in Caco-2 cells: unique in vitro model. Am J Physiol 1991;260(2 Pt 1):G207–G212.
42. Peng JB, Brown EM, Hediger MA. Apical entry channels in calcium-transporting epithelia. News Physiol Sci 2003;18:158–163.
43. Song Y, Peng X, Porta A, et al. Calcium transporter 1 and epithelial calcium channel messenger ribonucleic acid are differentially regulated by 1,25 dihydroxyvitamin D3 in the intestine and kidney of mice. Endocrinology 2003;144(9):3885–3894.
44. Hoenderop JG, Vennekens R, Muller D, et al. Function and expression of the epithelial Ca(2+) channel family: comparison of mammalian ECaC1 and 2. J Physiol 2001;537(Pt 3):747–761.
45. Christakos S, Gabrielides C, Rhoten WB. Vitamin D-dependent calcium binding proteins: Chemistry distribution, functional considerations, and molecular biology. Endocrine Rev 1989;10:3–26.
46. Feher JJ, Fullmer CS, Wasserman RH. Role of facilitated diffusion of calcium by calbindin in intestinal calcium absorption. Am J Physiol 1992;262(2):C517–C526.
47. Fleet JC, Bruns ME, Hock JM, Wood RJ. Growth hormone and parathyroid hormone stimulate intestinal calcium absorption in aged female rats. Endocrinology 1994,134.1755–1760.
48. Dupret JM, Brun P, Perret C, Lomri N, Thomasset M, Cuisinier-Gleizes P. Transcriptional and post-transcriptional regulation of vitamin D-dependent calcium-binding protein gene expression in the rat duodenum by 1,25-dihydroxycholecalciferol. J Biol Chem 1987;262(34):16,553–16,557.
49. Friedman PA, Gesek FA. Cellular calcium transport in renal epithelia: measurement, mechanisms, and regulation. Physiol Rev 1995;75(3):429–471.
50. Wang YZ, Li H, Bruns ME, et al. Effect of 1,25,28-trihydroxyvitamin D2 and 1,24,25-trihydroxyvitamin D3 on intestinal calbindin-D_{9k} mRNA and protein: Is there a correlation with intestinal calcium transport? J Bone Min Res 1993;8:1483–1490.
51. Fleet JC, Eksir F, Hance KW, Wood RJ. Vitamin D-inducible calcium transport and gene expression in three Caco-2 cell lines. Am J Physiol Gastrointest Liver Physiol 2002;283(3):G618–G625.
52. Pannabecker TL, Chandler JS, Wasserman RH. Vitamin D-dependent transcriptional regulation of the intestinal plasma membrane calcium pump. Biochem Biohphys Res Commun 1995;213:499–505.
53. Walters JRF. Calbindin-D_{9k} stimulates the calcium pump in rat enterocyte basolateral membranes. Am J Physiol 1989;256:G124–G128.
54. Nemere I. Vesicular calcium transport in chick intestine. J Nutr 1992;122(3 Suppl):657–661.
55. Zhou LX, Nemere I, Norman AW. A parathyroid-related peptide induces transcaltachia (the rapid, hormonal stimulation of intestinal Ca2+ transport). Biochem Biophys Res Commun 1992;186:69–73.
56. Nemere I, Farach-Carson MC. Membrane receptors for steroid hormones: a case for specific cell surface binding sites for vitamin D metabolites and estrogens. Biochem Biophys Res Comm 1998;248:443–449.
57. Sitrin MD, Bissonnette M, Bolt MJ, et al. Rapid effects of 1,25(OH)2 vitamin D3 on signal transduction systems in colonic cells. Steroids 1999;64(1–2):137–142.
58. Khare S, Bolt MJ, Wali RK, et al. 1,25 dihydroxyvitamin D3 stimulates phospholipase C-gamma in rat colonocytes: role of c-Src in PLC-gamma activation. J Clin Invest 1997;99(8):1831–1841.
59. Wali RK, Baum CL, Sitrin MD, Brasitus TA. 1,25(OH)2 vitamin D3 stimulates membrane phosphoinositide turnover, activates protein kinase C, and increases cytosolic calcium in rat colonic epithelium. J Clin Invest 1990;85(4):1296–1303.
60. Tien X-Y, Katnik C, Qasawa BM, Sitrin MD, Nelson DJ, Brasitus TA. Characterization of the 1,25 dihydroxycholecalcferol-stimulated calcium influx pathway in Caco-2 cells. J Membrane Biol 1993;136:159–168.

61. Wali RK, Bolt MJ, Tien XY, Brasitus TA, Sitrin MD. Differential effect of 1,25-dihydroxycholecalciferol on phosphoinositide turnover in the antipodal plasma membranes of colonic epithelial cells. Biochem Biophys Res Commun 1992;187(2):1128–1134.

62. Khare S, Bissonnette M, Scaglione-Sewell B, Wali RK, Sitrin MD, Brasitus TA. 1,25-dihydroxyvitamin D3 and TPA activate phospholipase D in Caco-2 cells: role of PKC-alpha. Am J Physiol 1999;276(4 Pt 1):G993–G1004.

63. Chen A, Davis BH, Bissonnette M, Scaglione-Sewell B, Brasitus TA. 1,25-Dihydroxyvitamin D(3) stimulates activator protein-1-dependent caco-2 cell differentiation. J Biol Chem 1999;274(50):35,505–35,513.

64. Wali RK, Baum CL, Sitrin MD, Bolt MJG, Dudeja PK, Brasitus TA. Effect of vitamin-D status on the rapid actions of 1,25-dihydroxycholecalciferol in rat colonic membranes. Am J Physiol 1992;262(6): G945–G953.

65. Harvey BJ, Alzamora R, Healy V, Renard C, Doolan CM. Rapid responses to steroid hormones: from frog skin to human colon. A homage to Hans Ussing. Biochim Biophys Acta 2002;1566(1–2):116–128.

66. Farach-Carson MC, Nemere I. Membrane receptors for vitamin D steroid hormones: potential new drug targets. Curr Drug Targets 2003;4(1):67–76.

67. Buitrago C, Vazquez G, de Boland AR, Boland RL. Activation of Src kinase in skeletal muscle cells by 1, 1,25-(OH(2))- vitamin D(3) correlates with tyrosine phosphorylation of the vitamin D receptor (VDR) and VDR-Src interaction. J Cell Biochem 2000;79(2):274–281.

68. Buitrago C, Vazquez G, de Boland AR, Boland R. The vitamin D receptor mediates rapid changes in muscle protein tyrosine phosphorylation induced by 1,25(OH)(2)D(3). Biochem Biophys Res Commun 2001;289(5):1150–1156.

69. Bettoun DJ, Burris TP, Houck KA, Buck DW, Stayrook KR, Khalifa B et al. Retinoid X Receptor is a Non-Silent Major Contributor to Vitamin D Receptor-Mediated Transcriptional Activation. Mol Endocrinol 2003.

70. Erben RG, Soegiarto DW, Weber K, Zeitz U, Lieberherr M, Gniadecki R et al. Deletion of deoxyribonucleic acid binding domain of the vitamin D receptor abrogates genomic and nongenomic functions of vitamin D. Molecular Endocrinology 2002;16(7):1524–1537.

71. Wali RK, Kong J, Sitrin MD, Bissonnette M, Li YC. Vitamin D receptor is not required for the rapid actions of 1,25-dihydroxyvitamin D3 to increase intracellular calcium and activate protein kinase C in mouse osteoblasts. J Cell Biochem 2003;88(4):794–801.

72. Boyan BD, Dean DD, Sylvia VL, Schwartz Z. Steroid hormone action in musculoskeletal cells involves membrane receptor and nuclear receptor mechanisms. Connect Tissue Res 2003;44 Suppl 1:130–135.

73. Boyan BD, Sylvia VL, Dean DD, t al. 1,25-(OH)2D3 modulates growth plate chondrocytes via membrane receptor- mediated protein kinase C by a mechanism that involves changes in phospholipid metabolism and the action of arachidonic acid and PGE2. Steroids 1999;64(1–2):129–136.

74. Boyan BD, Dean DD, Sylvia VL, Schwartz Z. Nongenomic regulation of extracellular matrix events by vitamin D metabolites. J Cell Biochem 1994;56:331–339.

75. Shi H, Norman AW, Okamura WH, Sen A, Zemel MB. 1alpha,25-Dihydroxyvitamin D3 modulates human adipocyte metabolism via nongenomic action. FASEB J 2001;15(14):2751–2753.

76. Loos RJ, Rankinen T, Leon AS, et al. Calcium intake is associated with adiposity in Black and White men and White women of the HERITAGE Family Study. J Nutr 2004;134(7):1772–1778.

77. Zemel MB. Role of calcium and dairy products in energy partitioning and weight management. Am J Clin Nutr 2004;79(5):907S–912S.

78. Koyama H, Inaba M, Nishizawa Y, Ohno S, Morii H. Protein kinase C is involved in 24-hydroxylase gene expression induced by $1,25(OH)_2D_3$ in rat intestinal epithelial cells. J Cell Biochem 1994;55:230–240.

79. Armbrecht HJ, Boltz MA, Hodam TL, Kumar VB. Differential responsiveness of intestinal epithelial cells to 1,25- dihydroxyvitamin D3—role of protein kinase C. J Endocrinol 2001;169(1):145–151.

80. Desai RK, van Wijnen AJ, Stein JL, Stein GL, Lian JB. Control of 1,25-dihydroxyvitamin D3 receptor-mediated enhancement of osteoclacin gene transcription: effects of perturbing phosphorylation pathwasy by okadaic acid and staurosporine. Endocrinology 1995;136:5685–5693.

81. Dwivedi PP, Hii CS, Ferrante A, et al. Role of MAP kinases in the 1,25-dihydroxyvitamin D3-induced transactivation of the rat cytochrome P450C24 (CYP24) promoter. Specific functions for ERK1/ERK2 and ERK5. J Biol Chem 2002;277(33):29,643–29,653.

82. Buitrago C, Boland R, de Boland AR. The tyrosine kinase c-Src is required for 1,25(OH)2-vitamin D3 signalling to the nucleus in muscle cells. Biochim Biophys Acta 2001;1541(3):179–187.

83. Hara H, Yasunami Y, Adachi T. Alteration of cellular phosphorylation state affects vitamin D receptor-mediated CYP3A4 mRNA induction in Caco-2 cells. Biochem Biophys Res Commun 2002;296(1):182–188.

84. Baran DT, Sorensen AM, Shalhoub V, Owen T, Stein G, Lian J. The rapid nongenomic actions of 1 alpha,25-dihydroxyvitamin D3 modulate the hormone-induced increments in osteocalcin gene transcription in osteoblast-like cells. J Cell Biochem 1992;50(2):124–129.

85. Barletta F, Freedman LP, Christakos S. Enhancement of VDR-mediated transcription by phosphorylation: correlation with increased interaction between the VDR and DRIP205, a subunit of the VDR-interacting protein coactivator complex. Mol Endocrinol 2002;16(2):301–314.

86. Juppner H, Gadella T, Brown E, Kronenberg H, Potts J. Parathyroid hormone and parathyroid hormone-related peptide in the regulation of calcium homeostasis and bone development. In: DeGroot L, Jameson J, eds. Endocrinology. W.B. Saunders Company, Philadelphia, PA: 2000; pp. 969–998.

87. Silver J, Yalcindag C, Sela-Brown A, Kilav R, Naveh-Many T. Regulation of the parathyroid hormone gene by vitamin D, calcium and phosphate. Kidney Int Suppl 1999;73:S2–S7.

88. Whybro A, Jagger H, Barker M, Eastell R. Phosphate supplementation in young men: lack of effect on calcium homeostasis and bone turnover. Eur J Clin Nutr 1998;52(1):29–33.

89. Hebert SC, Brown EM, Harris HW. Role of the Ca(2+)-sensing receptor in divalent mineral ion homeostasis. J Exp Biol 1997;200 (Pt 2):295–302.

90. Nishishita T, Okazaki T, Ishikawa T, et al. A negative vitamin D response DNA element in the human parathyroid hormone-related peptide gene binds to vitamin D receptor along with Ku antigen to mediate negative gene regulation by vitamin D. J Biol Chem 1998;273(18):10,901–10,907.

91. Russell J, Ashok S, Koszewski NJ. Vitamin D receptor interactions with the rat parathyroid hormone gene: synergistic effects between two negative vitamin D response elements. J Bone Miner Res 1999;14(11):1828-1837.

92. Gardella TJ, Juppner H. Molecular properties of the PTH/PTHrP receptor. Trends Endocrinol Metab 2001;12(5):210–217.

93. Mahon MJ, Cole JA, Lederer ED, Segre GV. Na+/H+ exchanger-regulatory factor 1 mediates inhibition of phosphate transport by parathyroid hormone and second messengers by acting at multiple sites in opossum kidney cells. Mol Endocrinol 2003;17(11):2355–2364.

94. Lau K, Bourdeau JE. Parathyroid hormone action in calcium transport in the distal nephron. Curr Opin Nephrol Hypertens 1995;4(1):55–63.

95. Barry EL, Gesek FA, Yu AS, Lytton J, Friedman PA. Distinct calcium channel isoforms mediate parathyroid hormone and chlorothiazide-stimulated calcium entry in transporting epithelial cells. J Membr Biol 1998;161(1):55–64.

96. Peng JB, Chen XZ, Berger UV, Vassilev PM, Brown EM, Hediger MA. A rat kidney-specific calcium transporter in the distal nephron. J Biol Chem 2000;275(36):28,186–28,194.

97. Zierold C, Mings JA, DeLuca HF. Regulation of 25-hydroxyvitamin D3-24-hydroxylase mRNA by 1,25-dihydroxyvitamin D3 and parathyroid hormone. J Cell Biochem 2003;88(2):234–237.

98. Armbrecht HJ, Boltz MA, Hodam TL. PTH increases renal 25(OH)D3-1alpha -hydroxylase (CYP1alpha) mRNA but not renal 1,25(OH)2D$_3$ production in adult rats. Am J Physiol Renal Physiol 2003;284(5): F1032–F1036.

99. Jimi E, Nakamura I, Amano H, et al. Osteoclast function is activated by osteoblastic cells through a mechamism involving cell-to-cell contact. Endocrinology 1996;137:2187–2190.

100. Boyle WJ, Simonet WS, Lacey DL. Osteoclast differentiation and activation. Nature 2003;423(6937): 337–342.

101. Fu Q, Jilka RL, Manolagas SC, O'Brien CA. Parathyroid hormone stimulates receptor activator of NFkappa B ligand and inhibits osteoprotegerin expression via protein kinase A activation of cAMP-response element-binding protein. J Biol Chem 2002;277(50):48,868–48,875.

102. Rubin J, Fan D, Wade A, et al. Transcriptional regulation of the expression of macrophage colony stimulating factor. Mol Cell Endocrinol 2000;160(1–2):193–202.

103. Hock JM, Gera I. Effects of continuous and intermittent administration and inhibition of resorption on the anabolic response of bone to parathyroid hormone. J Bone Miner Res 1992;7(1):65–72.

104. Bellido T, Ali AA, Plotkin LI, et al. Proteasomal degradation of Runx2 shortens parathyroid hormone-induced anti-apoptotic signaling in osteoblasts. A putative explanation for why intermittent administration is needed for bone anabolism. J Biol Chem 2003;278(50):50,259–50,272.
105. Heaney RP, Recker RR, Saville PD. Menopausal changes in bone remodeling. J Lab Clin Med 1978;92(6):964–970.
106. Riggs BL, Khosla S, Melton LJ, III. Sex steroids and the construction and conservation of the adult skeleton. Endocr Rev 2002;23(3):279–302.
107. Hofbauer LC, Khosla S, Dunstan CR, Lacey DL, Spelsberg TC, Riggs BL. Estrogen stimulates gene expression and protein production of osteoprotegerin in human osteoblastic cells. Endocrinology 1999;140(9):4367–4370.
108. Sarma U, Edwards M, Motoyoshi K, Flanagan AM. Inhibition of bone resorption by 17beta-estradiol in human bone marrow cultures. J Cell Physiol 1998;175(1):99–108.
109. McCauley LK, Tozum TF, Rosol TJ. Estrogen receptors in skeletal metabolism: lessons from genetically modified models of receptor function. Crit Rev Eukaryot Gene Expr 2002;12(2):89–100.
110. Kousteni S, Chen JR, Bellido T, et al. Reversal of bone loss in mice by nongenotropic signaling of sex steroids. Science 2002;298(5594):843–846.
111. Riggs BL, Khosla S, Melton LJ. A unitary model for involutional osteoporosis: estrogen deficiency causes both type I and type II osteoporosis in postmenopausal women and contributes to bone loss in aging men. J Bone Min Res 1998;13:763–773.
112. Gennari C, Agnusdei D, Nardi P, Civitelli R. Estrogen preserves a normal intestinal responsiveness to 1,25- dihydroxyvitamin D3 in oophorectomized women. J Clin Endocrinol Metab 1990;71(5):1288–1293.
113. Chen C, Noland KA, Kalu DN. Modulation of intestinal vitamin D receptor by ovariectomy, estrogen and growth hormone. Mech Ageing and Develop 1997;99:109–122.
114. Arjmandi BH, Holis BW, Kalu DN. In vivo effect of 17 β-estradiol on intestinal calcium absorption in rats. Bone and Mineral 1994;26:181–189.
115. Liel Y, Shany S, Smirnoff P, Schwartz B. Estrogen increases 1,25-dihydroxyvitamin D receptors expression and bioresponse in the rat duodenal mucosa. Endocrinology 1999;140(1):280–285.
116. Colin EM, van den Bemd GJ, Van Aken M, et al. Evidence for involvement of 17beta-estradiol in intestinal calcium absorption independent of 1,25-dihydroxyvitamin D3 level in the Rat. J Bone Miner Res 1999;14(1):57–64.
117. Van Abel M, Hoenderop JG, van der Kemp AW, van Leeuwen JP, Bindels RJ. Regulation of the epithelial Ca2+ channels in small intestine as studied by quantitative mRNA detection. Am J Physiol Gastrointest Liver Physiol 2003.
118. Inzerillo AM, Zaidi M, Huang CL. Calcitonin: the other thyroid hormone. Thyroid 2002;12(9):791–798.
119. Mora S, Pitukcheewanont P, Nelson JC, Gilsanz V. Serum levels of insulin-like growth factor I and the density, volume, and cross-sectional area of cortical bone in children. J Clin Endocrinol Metab 1999;84(8):2780–2783.
120. Boot AM, Engels MA, Boerma GJ, Krenning EP, De Muinck Keizer-Schrama SM. Changes in bone mineral density, body composition, and lipid metabolism during growth hormone (GH) treatment in children with GH deficiency. J Clin Endocrinol Metab 1997;82(8):2423–2428.
121. Rudman D, Feller AG, Nagrajm H.S., et al. Effects of human growth hormone in men over 60 years old. N Engl J Med 1990;323:1–6.
122. Hock JM, Gera I, Fonseca J, Raisz LG. Human parathyroid hormone-(1-34) increases bone mass in ovariectomized and orchidectomized rats. Endocrinology 1988;122(6):2899–2904.
123. Hill PA, Tumber A, Meikle MC. Multiple extracellular signals promote osteoblast survival and apoptosis. Endocrinology 1997;138(9):3849–3858.
124. Zoidis E, Gosteli-Peter M, Ghirlanda-Keller C, Meinel L, Zapf J, Schmid C. IGF-I and GH stimulate Phex mRNA expression in lungs and bones and 1,25-dihydroxyvitamin D(3) production in hypophysectomized rats. Eur J Endocrinol 2002;146(1):97–105.
125. Ritchie LD, Fung EB, Halloran BP, et al. A longitudinal study of calcium homeostasis during human pregnancy and lactation and after resumption of menses. Am J Clin Nutr 1998;67(4):693–701.
126. Breslau NA, Zerwekh JE. Relationship of estrogen and pregnancy to calcium homeostasis in pseudohypoparathyroidism. J Clin Endocrinol Metab 1986;62(1):45–51.

127. Whitehead M, Lane G, Young O, et al. Interrelations of calcium-regulating hormones during normal pregnancy. Br Med J (Clin Res Ed) 1981;283(6283):10–12.
128. Quan-Sheng D, Miller SC. Calciotrophic hormone levels and calcium absorption during pregnancy in rats. Am J Physiol 1989;257(1 Pt 1):E118–E123.
129. Kalkwarf HJ, Specker BL. Bone mineral changes during pregnancy and lactation. Endocrine 2002;17(1):49–53.
130. Kalkwarf HJ, Specker BL, Heubi JE, Vieira NE, Yergey AL. Intestinal calcium absorption of women during lactation and after weaning. Am J Clin Nutr 1996;63(4):526–531.
131. Kalkwarf HJ, Specker BL, Ho M. Effects of calcium supplementation on calcium homeostasis and bone turnover in lactating women. J Clin Endocrinol Metab 1999;84(2):464–470.
132. Boass A, Toverud SU, Pike JW, Haussler MR. Calcium metabolism during lactation: enhanced intestinal calcium absorption in vitamin D-deprived, hypocalcemic rats. Endocrinology 1981;109(3):900–907.
133. Charoenphandhu N, Limlomwongse L, Krishnamra N. Prolactin directly stimulates transcellular active calcium transport in the duodenum of female rats. Can J Physiol Pharmacol 2001;79(5):430–438.
134. Wood RJ, Fleet JC. The genetics of osteoporosis: vitamin D receptor polymorphisms. Annu Rev Nutr 1998;18:233–258.
135. Hunter DJ, Lange M, Snieder H, et al. Genetic contribution to renal function and electrolyte balance: a twin study. Clin Sci (Lond) 2002;103(3):259–265.
136. Liu YZ, Liu YJ, Recker RR, Deng HW. Molecular studies of identification of genes for osteoporosis: the 2002 update. J Endocrinol 2003;177(2):147–196.
137. Little RD, Carulli JP, Del Mastro RG, et al. A mutation in the LDL receptor-related protein 5 gene results in the autosomal dominant high-bone-mass trait. Am J Hum Genet 2002;70(1):11–19.
138. Morrison NA, Qi JC, Tokita A, et al. Prediction of bone density from vitamin D receptor alleles. Nature 1994;367(6460):284–287.
139. Grant SF, Reic DM, Blake G, Herd F, Fogelman I, Ralston SH. Reduced bone density and osteoporosis associated with a polymorphic Sp1 binding site in the collagen type I alpha 1 gene. Nat Genet 1996;14:203–205.
140. Mann V, Hobson EE, Li B, et al. A COL1A1 Sp1 binding site polymorphism predisposes to osteoporotic fracture by affecting bone density and quality. J Clin Invest 2001;107(7):899–907.

12 Influence of Total Diet on Calcium Homeostasis

Zamzam K. (Fariba) Roughead

KEY POINTS

- Recent data from controlled feeding studies have demonstrated that, despite common belief, common sources of protein do not adversely affect calcium homeostasis.
- The effects of dietary salt on calcium homeostasis may be modulated by accompanying factors in the diet, such as calcium and potassium.
- The beneficial effects of fruits and vegetables on bone health is thought to be related to either their contribution to acid–base balance or the essential nutrients that they provide, such as magnesium, potassium, vitamin C, and so on.
- Most of the emphasis on the influence of diet on bone health has been on the acid–base (renal) effects. However, dietary factors such as iron, copper, and zinc also have systemic and endocrine influences important for bone health.
- Carefully controlled feeding studies are needed to unravel the complexity of the interaction of nutrients in whole foods and to give evidence-based advice to the public.

1. INTRODUCTION

Changes in dietary practices offer a sensible, food-based, low-cost approach for modification of risk factors and prevention of osteoporosis. However, defining the effects of diet on bone health has not been a simple task becauseof the following reasons:

1. *Bone is complex.* Bone is a composite material with both organic and inorganic components. By weight, bone is 70% mineral and 5–8% water, and the rest is organic material. The inorganic phase of bone is approx 95% calcium hydroxyapatite arranged in plate-like crystals; the organic phase is primarily proteins with approx 98% type I collagen, plus a variety of noncollagenous proteins including important regulatory proteins, cytokines, and growth factors *(1)*.

   This specialized, vital, metabolically active, connective tissue provides not only structural framework, protection for vital organs, locomotion, and hematopoesis, but also serves as a buffering reservoir and aids the kidneys and lungs in the tight regulation of the body's hydrogen ion concentration. This latter metabolic function of bone has received considerable attention in the area of nutrition research and bone health.

From: *Calcium in Human Health*
Edited by: C. M. Weaver and R. P. Heaney © Humana Press Inc., Totowa, NJ

2. *Food is complex.* In addition to energy, food provides a host of essential nutrients and bioactive nonnutrients with multifaceted metabolic functions and interactions. These components can affect calcium homeostasis not only through a direct effect on acid–base balance, but also through systemic or cellular processes. Previously, the bulk of studies investigating the effects of diet on bone metabolism have focused primarily on the influence of single nutrients on calcium homeostasis. The strength of this reductionistic approach is that it affords a focused investigation of both the specific role and the mechanism of action of a given nutrient; however, this approach does not address the various interactions between nutrients and nonnutrients that result when we consume whole foods in a mixed diet.

3. *The body is complex and adaptable.* The response of the body to dietary stimuli spans the entire range from localized cellular responses such as changes in osteoblast and/or osteoclast activity and paracrine/autocrine signals, to systemic, whole-body responses such as changes in renal acid–base excretion, and endocrine (hormonal/growth factor) changes. The recent observations that renal acid excretion adapts over time in response to dietary changes point to the often understated quality of the human body—its innate capability to adapt to a given stimulus over time.

2. DIETARY PROTEIN

Investigations of the effects of diet on bone health and prevention of osteoporosis have primarily centered on the regulation of acid–base balance and the need to "neutralize" the acid load produced by common Western diets. Dietary practices that lead to chronic production of acid ash residue, such as diets high in animal protein, are hypothesized to tap into the alkali reservoir in bone, cause gradual dissolution of bone mineral *(2,3)*, and are considered a risk for excessive urinary calcium loss and thus osteoporosis *(4–6)*. This concern is based primarily on evidence from studies using *purified* proteins, in which a clear hypercalciuric effect has been established *(7–10)*. Until recently, the results of the few controlled feeding studies testing the effects of *common* sources of protein (such as meat) on calcium retention were inconclusive *(11–15)*. Methodological approaches such as equalization of the phosphorus content of the experimental diets, use of inherently insensitive balance methodology, short duration of controlled diets, and few test subjects contributed to the lack of clarity on this issue *(11–15)*. Recent evidence, from a controlled feeding study of several weeks' duration and using sensitive radiotracer methodology, has demonstrated that high protein intake (as meat) does not adversely affect calcium retention *(16)*. Additionally, data from prospective trials *(17,18)* have indicated a potential positive role for high protein intake in bone metabolism. Key findings from intervention and observational studies are highlighted as follows.

2.1. Feeding Studies

The earliest feeding study examining the effects of dietary protein on urinary calcium reported that a high dietary intake of meat increased urinary calcium loss *(19)*. It is thought that the sulfates in protein increase calcium excretion by reducing the reabsorption of calcium in the kidneys and eventually cause loss of calcium from bone (Fig. 1). This hypercalciuric effect of sulfates has been demonstrated in studies using purified proteins *(10)* as well as those using common sources of protein when phosphorus intakes were held constant *(12)*. In the latter study, which compared three sources of dietary

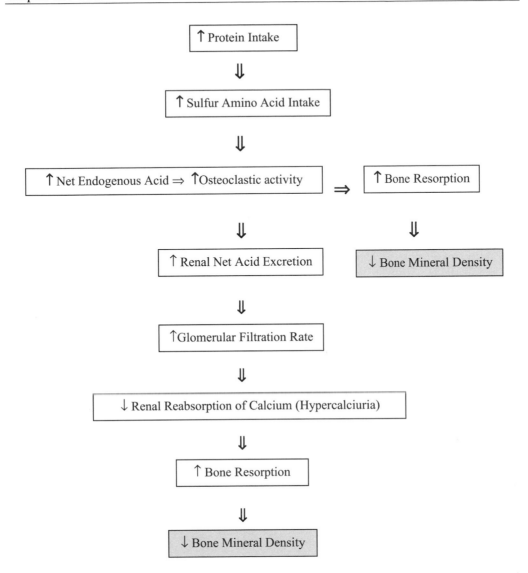

Fig. 1. The proposed mechanism for the negative effect of dietary protein on calcium homeostasis and bone health.

protein (vegetables, vegetables plus egg protein, and animal proteins), with equalized phosphorus content, it was found that the animal protein-rich diet was associated with the highest sulfate content and resulted in the highest excretion of urinary acids and calcium. Dietary phosphorus in meat, on the other hand, is thought to counteract this calciuric effect of sulfates and reduce the urinary excretion of calcium *(20)*. Previous studies *(11,13,21)* have demonstrated that when increased protein is added as common foods, particularly meat, *without manipulation of the phosphorus content*, hypercalciuria is not observed. It has also been suggested that the favorable effects of phosphorus from meat on urinary calcium loss maybe offset by increased fecal calcium losses, resulting in a negative calcium *balance (22)*. However, in two recent controlled feeding studies,

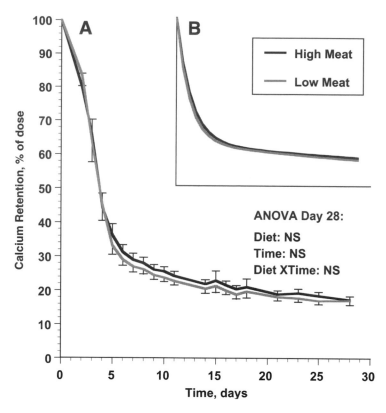

Fig. 2. Whole-body retention of a calcium radiotracer (^{47}Ca) administered to healthy postmeno-pausal women at the midpoints of controlled high and low meat diets consumed for 8 wk each in a crossover design. **(A)** The whole-body calcium retention, as % of dose (means ± SEM, $n = 15$) over time. Calcium retention was not different between the high and low meat diets at all weekly time points tested. **(B)** The two component exponential models ($y = 74.5\ e^{-0.0188t} + 25.7\ e^{-0.0006t}$ for high meat and $y = 74.0\ e^{-0.0211t} + 26.0\ e^{-0.0008t}$ for low meat, where t is expressed in hours). (Reprinted from ref. *16*, with permission.)

addition of meat to the diet did not decrease whole-body calcium retention as measured by sensitive radiotracer methodology *(23,24)*. In the first study *(16)*, healthy postmeno-pausal women ($N = 15$) ate diets with similar calcium content (~ 600 mg), but either low or high in meat (12 vs 20% of energy as protein or 0.9 vs 1.6 g protein/kg body weight) for 8 wk each, in a randomized crossover design. The women were allowed to equilibrate on each diet for 4 wk and subsequently, calcium retention was measured by extrinsically labeling the entire menu with ^{47}Ca, followed by whole-body scintillation counting for several weeks. Calcium retention was not different during the high and low meat intake dietary periods (day 28, mean ± pooled SD: 17.1 vs 15.6%, ± 0.6%, respectively; $p = 0.09$; Fig. 2A and B represent the observed and modeled data, respectively). Although renal acid excretion (defined as sum of urinary titratable acidity plus ammonium) was approx 45% higher during week 3 of the high meat intake period, urinary calcium excretion was not different between the two diets. This difference in renal acid excretion abated to only 18% by week 8 of the study, indicating adaptation in renal acid excretion over time *(16)*.

In a study of similar design, calcium retention was similar from diets in which 25 g of soy protein was substituted for an equivalent amount of meat protein (25), despite a consistently lower renal acid excretion (approx 15–20%) with soy consumption. These collective findings from these two studies indicate that changes in urinary acidity within the range that may result from common, practical dietary practices do not reach a "threshold" which triggers an increase in glomerular filtration rate and/or use of body calcium as a buffering agent. Remer and Manz have suggested that a net acid excretion of more than 120 mEq/d is required for the depletion of plasma bicarbonate and use of alkali from the skeleton (26). Furthermore, protein is shown to increase the renal capacity by increasing the endogenous supply of ammonia (27). Ammonium is released upon deamination of glutamine to glutamic acid in renal tubules and is converted to ammonium ion in the tubular lumen by accepting a hydrogen ion. Under controlled conditions, ammonium excretion accounted for at least 50% of the total acid excretion and was approx 15% higher when subjects consumed high meat versus low protein diets without altering urinary calcium loss (16).

In addition to influence of quantity of dietary protein in the diet, the effects of protein source (animal vs plant) has been the subject of much scientific debate. Although many of commonly consumed plant proteins, such as wheat and rice, have similar or even higher sulfur amino acid content as meats (28), the counteracting alkali in plants are thought to reduce the dietary acid load (29) (Table 1). Therefore, the net effect of any protein source on calcium balance is determined by many co-existing factors in the protein source as well as the rest of the diet and thus is difficult to predict. As mentioned above, incorporation of plant protein (as soy protein) in place of animal protein (as meat) for several weeks, in a mixed diet with typical calcium intakes of approx 700 mg/d, did not improve calcium retention and did not affect biomarkers of bone turnover (25). However, several studies have suggested a bone sparing effect for high-isoflavone soy protein compared to milk proteins in peri- and postmenopausal women (30–32). Studies in ovariectomized rats have also indicated protection from estrogen deficiency bone loss in animals fed intact soy protein vs casein (33–35). Although the results of the human studies cited previously (30–32) must be interpreted with full recognition of their short duration and small sample size, the favorable effects of soy protein supplementation on bone are intriguing and imply improved calcium retention as compared to isolated milk proteins. This difference may be related to the higher calciuric effect of isolated milk-based proteins vs soy protein (32). Again, because of the use of isolated milk proteins instead of milk as a whole food, these results must be interpreted with caution. Alternatively, the putative beneficial effect of soy protein may depend on higher combined doses of both soy protein (40 g/d) and supplemental calcium (650–1400 mg/d) used (30–32).

2.2. Synergistic Interaction of Dietary Protein With Calcium

The results of two recent studies (36,37) suggest that calcium intake may modulate the effect of protein on the skeleton and that, at high intakes, dietary calcium and protein may synergistically interact to favorably affect bone mass. Meyer et al. (36) noted no association between protein intake and risk of hip fracture in most women, but among those with very low calcium intakes (400 mg/d), a higher protein intake was associated with an increased risk of hip fracture. In a recent calcium and vitamin D supplementation trial of the elderly, higher protein intake was significantly associated with a favorable 3-yr

Table 1
Sulfur Amino Acid Content of Select Common Foods[a]

Food item	mEq/serving	mEq/100 g edible portion	mEq/100 g protein
Almonds, dry-roasted	2.1	7.5	33.8
Peanuts, dry-roasted	2.5	8.9	37.7
Tofu, regular	4.0	3.2	40.0
Tofu, firm	5.3	6.3	40.0
Soy protein isolate	9.2	32.5	40.2
Corn, yellow, cooked	2.3	1.4	41.3
Potato, baked	1.5	1.0	41.9
Walnuts	1.9	6.6	43.4
Cheddar cheese	3.1	10.8	43.4
Soy milk, fluid	3.2	1.3	47.8
Milk, whole	3.9	1.6	48.9
Milk, 1%	3.9	1.6	48.9
Milk, 2%	4.0	1.6	49.2
Milk, skim	4.1	1.7	49.4
Beef, cooked	13.4	15.8	52.9
Pork, cooked	14.1	16.6	56.6
Tuna, water-packed	22.6	14.6	57.4
Millet, cooked	3.6	2.0	58.3
Chicken, roasted	14.3	16.9	58.3
Wheat (whole) flour	9.7	8.1	59.0
Barley, pearled, cooked	2.2	1.4	62.1
Oatmeal, cooked	3.9	1.7	64.2
White rice, cooked	1.8	1.8	65.2
Egg, poached	5.0	10.0	80.3

[a]Total sulfur amino acid (cysteine+ methionine) and total protein content are from the USDA Nutrient Database, Standard Reference, Release 14 (2001).

change in total body bone mineral density in the supplemented group, but not in the placebo group (37) (Fig. 3). Also, at the lower calcium intakes of approx 800 mg/d, a 20% higher protein intake was associated with a 23% (25 mg/d) lower absorbed calcium (using single stable isotope method), whereas at the higher calcium intake, absorbed calcium was greater overall and did not change significantly with increasing protein intake (37). The results of these studies (36,37) suggest that higher protein intake, when combined with moderately low intake of calcium, has an antagonistic effect on the calcium economy. However, under controlled feeding conditions, many investigators have found little or no effect of dietary protein on calcium absorption or excretion (13,15) even when calcium intake is low (16,25).

2.3. Low Protein Intake

The effects of low protein intake on calcium absorption have also been tested. Some studies have suggested that low protein intakes decrease calcium absorption. Women in National Health and Nutrition Examination Survey (NHANES) III survey (N = 1822) with lower protein intake (calcium intake below or above 800 mg/d) had significantly

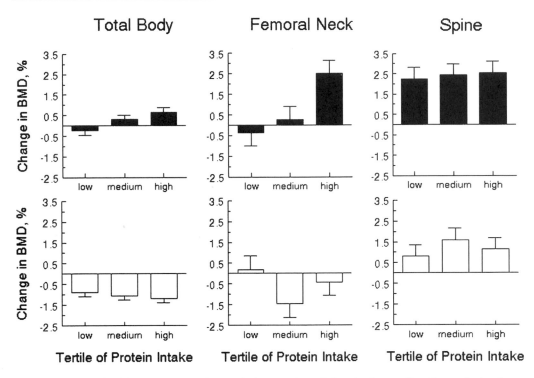

Fig. 3. Mean (± SEM) percentage change in bone mineral density by tertile of protein intake as a percentage of total energy intake (adjusted for sex, age, weight, total energy intake, and dietary calcium intake) in 342 men and women treated with calcium citrate malate and vitamin D (black bars) or placebo (white bars) for 3 yr. For the total body, there was a significant interaction of treatment group X protein tertile (p + 0.044); in the supplemented group, the high tertile differed from the low tertile (p + 0.042; adjusted for multiple comparisons). For the femoral neck, the interaction term was not significant, but the pattern of change in bone mineral density (BMD) in the supplemented group was similar to that for the total body: the high tertile differed from the low (p = 0.011) and middle (p = 0.042) tertiles. (Reprinted from ref. *37*, with permission.)

reduced femoral neck bone mineral density (BMD) *(38)* (Fig. 4). The authors concluded that diminished calcium absorption and secondary hyperparathyroidism at low levels of dietary protein intake cause a reduction in BMD. In women with mean calcium intakes of 800 g/d, lowering protein intake from 158 to 52 g/d lowered calcium absorption (using dual stable isotopes) within 4 d *(39)*. Because of the very short duration of this study, it is not clear if calcium absorption would improve as an adaptive response over time. Other mechanisms for the adverse effect of low protein status on bone health may be that adequate protein is needed to supply the amino acids needed for the maintenance of the organic matrix of bone which is approx 50% protein by volume *(40)*. A low protein intake may also compromise bone health through a reduction in serum insulin-like growth factor (IGF)-1 *(41)* or increasing propensity for falls *(42)*, and thus fractures.

2.4. Observational Studies

Epidemiologic studies have not been helpful in clarifying the effect of protein consumption on bone health. Although several studies have identified an association be-

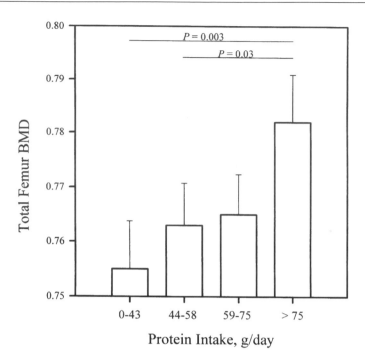

Fig. 4. Relationship between dietary protein intake and total femur BMD (expressed as mean g/cm^2 ± SEM) in non-Hispanic white women older than 50 (NHANES-III). Number individuals for each of the levels of protein intake are 0–43 g, $n = 480$; 44–58 g $n = 471$; 59–75 g, $n = 446$; >75 g, $n = 425$. (Printed with permission from ref. *38*.)

tween dietary protein intake and bone mineral density *(43)*, rates of bone loss *(6,44)*, and fracture incidence *(6,44,45)*, there is no clear consensus on what this effect may be. In the Framingham study, subjects with lower total and animal protein intakes had higher rates of bone loss from the femoral neck and spine than did subjects consuming more protein *(44)*. In contrast, a high intake ratio of animal to plant protein was associated with greater bone loss for the femoral neck and a greater risk of hip fracture in women over the age of 65 *(6)*. Higher total and animal protein intakes were also associated with an increased risk of forearm fracture in younger postmenopausal women *(45)*. However, in an earlier study of Seventh Day Adventists, no significant differences or trends were found between early or current dietary protein and bone mineral content (BMC) *(46)*. Munger et al. *(17)* reported that higher total (and animal) protein intake was associated with a reduced incidence of hip fracture in postmenopausal women. Similarly, a positive association between low-protein status, as indicated by serum albumin and the incidence of hip fractures *(47)*, has been observed.

Abelow described a positive association between hip fractures and animal protein intake in 16 industrialized countries *(48)*, later Frassetto et al. *(49)* described a similar positive association between animal protein with hip fractures incidence in women over age 50 in 33 countries *(49)*. Approximately 70% of variation in hip fracture incidence was accounted for by the vegetable to animal protein ratio. However, the findings may be confounded by many co-variables, such as race, exercise, key dietary variables (e.g., potassium, sodium, calcium), as well as cultural differences.

3. SODIUM

Sodium is consumed in a variety of forms such as a sodium chloride (salt), sodium bicarbonate, and common food additives such as monosodium glutamate, sodium phosphate, sodium carbonate, and sodium benzoate. Of these, sodium chloride is by far the major form of sodium consumed. Based on several intervention studies, there is general consensus that excessive dietary sodium intake as NaCl induces hypercalciuria *(50–55)*. This hypercalciuric effect is attributed to a shared renal reabsorption pathway with calcium in the proximal tubule and ascending loop of Henle *(56)*. Furthermore, an increase in urinary excretion of sodium has been shown to be accompanied with an increase in urinary calcium loss *(53)*. Both salt-loading studies and reports of free-living populations find that urinary calcium excretion increases approximately 1 mmol (40 mg) for each 100 mmol (2300 mg) increase in dietary sodium in normal adults. Renal calcium stone-formers with hypercalciuria appear to have greater proportional increases in urinary calcium (approx 2 mmol) per 100 mmol increase in salt intake. Thus, reduction of dietary NaCl may be a useful strategy to decrease the risk of forming calcium-containing kidney stones *(57)*. In an observational study of women, linear regression analysis indicated that for each 1-g increment increase in sodium intake, 26.3 mg calcium was lost daily in the urine *(56)*. Thus, in adult women, 1 g of extra sodium would result in an additional rate of bone loss of 1%/yr if bone is the source of the urinary calcium. Moreover, urinary calcium loss does not appear to be corrected by a compensatory increase in calcium absorption or reduced endogenous fecal secretion, despite one report that high sodium diet resulted in increased 1,25 dihydroxyvitamin D (1,25[OH]$_2$D) levels *(51)*. The relationship between urinary sodium and urinary calcium excretion remained significant in multivariate analysis after controlling for sex, age, body weight, and protein, calcium, and phosphorus intakes in 20- to 79-yr-old women *(58)*. In one longitudinal study (Rancho Bernardo cohort), no association between sodium intake, as assessed by 24-h recall, and BMD was observed *(59)*; however, urinary sodium excretion was not measured in this study. In another longitudinal study of postmenopausal women, a negative correlation between urinary sodium excretion and bone mineral density of the hip was detected, suggesting that bone loss could have been prevented by either a daily dietary calcium increase of 891 mg calcium or by halving the daily sodium excretion of 2110 mg/d *(60)*. It is not clear how much of the calciuric effect of table salt is due to the co-existing chloride anion. For example, addition of bicarbonate or citrate forms of sodium did not increase urinary calcium excretion *(61)*. Moreover, addition of potassium citrate to constant diets increased net calcium retention in postmenopausal women *(62)*. These findings indicate that the net effect of dietary minerals (such as sodium) is modulated by the accompanying anions.

4. FRUITS AND VEGETABLES

Cross-sectional studies have indicated a positive association between nutrients found in fruits and vegetables (potassium, magnesium, vitamin C, and fiber) and bone mass in premenopausal women *(63)* and in children *(64)*. In the Framingham Heart Study, greater intakes of potassium, magnesium, and fruit and vegetables were each associated with less decline in BMD in hip of men. Although similar associations were not found in women, results support the hypothesis that alkaline-producing dietary components, specifically, potassium, magnesium, and fruit and vegetables, may contribute to maintenance of BMD *(18,65)*. Vegetables have been shown to be rich in bicarbonate and organic anions which also produce bicarbonate when metabolized *(29,66,67)* and neutralize sulfuric acid generated by consumption of high-protein foods *(68)*. Potassium bicarbonate in particular has been shown to decrease urinary calcium excretion, improve calcium balance, decrease bone resorption, and increase the rate of bone formation *(69)*. Epidemiological studies also have shown a positive relationship between potassium intake and BMD in children *(70)*, and in pre- and perimenopausal women *(71,72)*. A higher potassium intake was also associated with slower decline in BMD of femoral neck in a 4-yr longitudinal study of the Framingham cohort *(65)*.

The net effect of a diet may also depend on the relative abundance of these key nutrients in the diet. In a recent cross-sectional study, diets with a lower dietary protein to potassium ratio, as assessed from food frequency questionnaires, were associated with greater femoral, lumbar, and forearm BMD *(72)*. These findings suggest that the critical determinant of hip fracture risk in relation to the acid–base effects of diet is the net load of acid in the diet, when the intake of both acid and base precursors is considered. The authors concluded that a moderation of animal food consumption and an increased ratio of vegetable/animal food consumption may confer a protective effect *(49)*.

Ascorbic acid, another key nutrient present in fruits and vegetables, is a required cofactor in the hydroxylations of lysine and proline necessary for collagen formation *(73)*. In women from the Postmenopausal Estrogen/Progestin Interventions Trial, a positive association of vitamin C with BMD was observed in postmenopausal women with dietary calcium intakes of at least 500 mg *(73)*. In a cross-sectional study, there was no evidence that vitamin C from the diet was associated with BMD, although long term use of vitamin C supplements was associated with a higher BMD in the early postmenopausal years and among never-users of estrogen *(74)*. In a recent 3-yr longitudinal study of elderly White men and women, no effect of fruit and vegetable intake on bone loss was detected; however, in women, low intake of vitamin C was associated with greater bone loss *(75)*.

A higher intake of magnesium is associated with lower bone resorption. Low magnesium intakes have been associated with low vertebral BMD in postmenopausal women *(44)*. Although the mechanism is unknown, it is likely that magnesium plays a role as an alkaline cation and a buffering agent in the kidneys *(26)*. Also, the effect of magnesium may occur at the cellular level as a deficiency of magnesium is speculated to impair the ATPase activity and thus transport of potassium ions into the skeletal interstitial space in exchange for hydrogen ion *(76)* This movement could result in a decrease in pH and enhanced bone resorption *(77)*. In animals, magnesium deficiency impairs bone growth and strength *(78)* and has been shown to increase bone resorption through inflammatory cytokines such as substance P and tumor necrosis factor *(79)*. In clinical trials, magnesium supplementation has also been shown to improve trabecular bone density *(80)*. In a recent observational study, after adjusting for several covariates, magnesium intake accounted for about 12% of variability in biomarkers of bone resorption in perimenopausal women *(76)*.

5. ENDOCRINE AND SYSTEMIC EFFECTS OF DIET

Although the majority of the debate over the effects of diet on bone health has focused on the acid vs alkali load, diet may also have other endocrine and systemic effects that have not been as extensively studied. One such response is the already mentioned acute secondary hyperparathyroidism observed with low protein intakes *(81)*. Experimental and clinical studies suggest that protein intake affects both the production and action of growth factors, particularly the IGF-1 axis, and thus dietary proteins are involved in the control of bone anabolism *(82)*. Both the hepatic production and the total level of IGF-1 are under the influence of dietary proteins, and protein restriction has been shown to reduce plasma IGF-1 in humans *(83)*, inducing a resistance of target organs to the action of growth hormone *(82)*. In a controlled, 1-yr intervention study, 20 g of supplemental dietary protein/d improved hip BMD (and serum IGF-1) in elderly patients with recent hip fracture *(84)*. IGF-1 is essential for longitudinal bone growth, as it stimulates proliferation and differentiation of bone cells *(85)*. It is well established that a decreased serum concentration of IGF-1 is strongly associated with decreased bone strength in animals *(86)* and an increase in risk of osteoporotic fractures in humans *(87)*. In addition to growth hormone, the principal hormonal regulator of circulating IGF-1 *(88)*, and dietary protein, the intake of other nutrients can also profoundly affect serum IGF-1 *(89,90)*. For example, dietary zinc has a strong influence on serum IGF-1 concentration in humans *(91–94)* and animals *(95,96)*. Matsui and co-workers have shown that the anabolic effects of IGF-1 in osteoblastic-like cells are mediated and enhanced by zinc *(97)*. Zinc is also a known constituent of about 300 enzymes, including those essential for bone metabolism such as bone alkaline phosphatase *(98)*.

Copper deficiency has been shown to result in reduced bone strength in rats *(14,15)* and osteoporotic lesions in other animals *(16)*. In humans, skeletal disorders such as osteopenia have been noted in Menke's syndrome, a genetic copper deficiency disease *(17)*. Short term supplementation trials with copper have indicated both no effect *(99,100)* and favorable changes in biomarkers of bone health in healthy adults *(101)*. The effect of copper on skeletal health occur directly at the tissue level as copper is a cofactor for lysyl oxidase (EC 1.4.3.13), one of the principal enzymes involved in collagen crosslinking *(13)*. Roughead and Lukaski have demonstrated reduced bone strength and serum IGF-1 in growing female rats fed copper deficient diets, which suggest that the effect of copper on the skeleton may also be mediated systemic and endocrine factors *(86)*.

Iron, a commonly deficient trace element in American diets, may have an important impact upon bone health, and this effect may be exacerbated by a calcium-restricted diet *(102)*. In a small observational study of postmenopausal women, iron was a positive predictor of BMD in the femoral neck, and iron, zinc, and magnesium intake were positively correlated with forearm BMC in premenopausal women by multiple regression analysis. Iron and magnesium were significant predictors of forearm BMC in premenopausal and postmenopausal women, respectively, by multiple regression analysis *(103)*.

6. NONNUTRITIVE FACTORS IN FOOD

In addition to nutrients already mentioned, nonnutrient components in food may also affect calcium homeostasis. For examples, recent evidence from animal studies suggest that inulin, a soluble, nondigestible polyfructan present in a number of vegetables and plants, and also used in dairy and cheese industries, may enhance calcium absorption *(104,105)* and improve BMD *(106)*. The mechanisms by which inulin and other nondigestible oligosaccharides exert their putative beneficial effects are not known. These compounds resist intestinal digestion and undergo fermentation in the large intestine where they form volatile short-chain fatty acids (SCFA) that increase colon acidity *(107)*. The solubility and bioavailability of trace minerals *(108,109)* and calcium *(108)* are thought to be increased by this increase in acidity. Furthermore, both the low pH and SCFA are thought to induce hypertrophy of the mucosal cells, leading to increased surface area and enhanced calcium absorption. It is also possible that the paracellular calcium diffusion is enhanced in the ileum leading to increased permeability of the tight junctions in the presence of nondigestible fibers. An increase in the ceco–colorectal calbindin –D9K protein expression in the presence of inulin has also been reported *(110)*. In addition to increasing calcium retention, nondigestible oligosaccharides have also been shown to reduce bone resorption in ovariectomized rats *(111)*.

Human studies examining the effects of oligofructose on calcium absorption have been contradictory. Three human studies have shown a beneficial effect on calcium absorption *(105,112,113)* whereas two recent human studies have shown no effect on calcium absorption *(114,115)*. Because of the potential for health promotion by inulin and oligofructose *(116)*, an increased use in various types of foods such as confectionery, fruit preparations, milk desserts, yogurt and fresh cheese, baked goods, chocolate, ice cream, and sauces can be expected. Thus, a clear definition of the effects of these additives on health including mineral bioavailability is of great interest.

7. CONCLUSIONS AND FUTURE DIRECTIONS

In recent years, our understanding of the effects of various components in food has increased dramatically. However, the challenges of defining the intricate interrelationships between food constituents and their effect on the body including bone metabolism remain. The recent findings from observational studies describing the effects of dietary patterns on bone health *(65,72,117)* can serve as hypothesis-generating platforms for future controlled trials. Only under carefully controlled conditions in which the composition of the diets is well-defined and intakes are tightly controlled can we begin to unravel the complexity of the interaction of whole foods and to give evidence-based advice to the public. Even then, we are reminded that, "As we analyze a thing into its parts and properties, we tend to magnify these, to exaggerate their apparent independence and to hide from ourselves the essential integrity and individuality for the composite whole. We may study them apart but it is a concession to our weakness and the narrow outlook of our minds" *(118)*.

REFERENCES

1. Lee CA, Einhorn TA. The bone organ system, form and function. In: Marcus R, Feldman D, Kelsey J, eds. Osteoporosis, 2nd ed. Academic, San Diego: 2001; pp. 3–20.
2. Goto K. Mineral metabolism in experimental acidosis. J Biol Chemistry 1918;36:355–376.
3. Wachman A, Bernstein DS. Diet and osteoporosis. Lancet 1968;1:958–959.
4. Hegsted DM. Fractures, calcium, and the modern diet. Am J Clin Nutr 2001;74(5):571–573.
5. Bunker VW. The role of nutrition in osteoporosis. Br J Biomed Sci 1994;51(3):228–240.
6. Sellmeyer DE, Stone KL, Sebastian A, Cummings SR. A high ratio of dietary animal to vegetable protein increases the rate of bone loss and the risk of fracture in postmenopausal women. Am J Clin Nutr 2001;73(1):118–122.
7. Walker RM, Linkswiler HM. Calcium retention in the adult human male as affected by protein intake. J Nutr 1972;102(10):1297–1302.

8. Johnson NE, Alcantara EN, Linkswiler H. Effect of level of protein intake on urinary and fecal calcium and calcium retention of young adult males. J Nutr 1970;100(12):1425–1430.

9. Allen LH, Oddoye EA, Margen S. Protein-induced hypercalciuria: a longer term study. Am J Clin Nutr 1979;32:741–749.

10. Schuette SA, Zemel MB, Linkswiler HM. Studies on the mechanism of protein-induced hypercalciuria in older men and women. J Nutr 1980;110:305–315.

11. Pannemans DL, Schaafsma G, Westerterp KR. Calcium excretion, apparent calcium absorption and calcium balance in young and elderly subjects: influence of protein intake. Br J Nutr 1997;77(5):721–729.

12. Breslau NA, Brinkley L, Hill KD, Pak CY. Relationship of animal protein-rich diet to kidney stone formation and calcium metabolism. J Clin Endocrinol Metab 1988;66(1):140–146.

13. Spencer H, Kramer L, Osis D, Norris C. Effect of a high protein (meat) intake on calcium metabolism in man. Am J Clin Nutr 1978;31:2167–2180.

14. Spencer H, Kramer L, DeBartolo M, Norris C, Osis D. Further studies of the effect of a high protein diet as meat on calcium metabolism. Am J Clin Nutr 1983;37(6):924–929.

15. Heaney RP, Recker RR. Effects of nitrogen, phosphorus, and caffeine on calcium balance in women. J Lab Clin Med 1982;99(1):46–55.

16. Roughead ZK, Johnson LK, Lykken GI, Hunt JR. Controlled high meat diets do not affect calcium retention or indices of bone status in healthy postmenopausal women. J Nutr 2003;133(4):1020–1026.

17. Munger RG, Cerhan JR, Chiu BC. Prospective study of dietary protein intake and risk of hip fracture in postmenopausal women. Am J Clin Nutr 1999;69(1):147–152.

18. Tucker KL, Hannan MT, Kiel DP. The acid-base hypothesis: diet and bone in the Framingham Osteoporosis Study. Eur J Nutr 2001;40(5):231–237.

19. Sherman HC. Calcium requirement of maintenance in man. J Biol Chem 1920;44:21.

20. Spencer H, Kramer L, Osis D, Norris C. Effect of phosphorus on the absorption of calcium and on the calcium balance in man. J Nutr 1978;108:447–457.

21. Spencer H, Kramer L, Osis D. Do protein and phosphorus cause calcium loss? J Nutr 1988;118:657–660.

22. Heaney RP. Protein intake and the calcium economy. J Am Dietet Assoc 1993;93(11):1259–1260.

23. Roughead Z, Hunt J. Controlled high meat diets do not adversely affect calcium retention or indicators of bone metabolism in postmenopausal women. J Trace Elem Exp Med 2001;14:329–330.

24. Roughead ZK. Substituting soy protein for meat protein did not affect calcium retention in a controlled feeding study of healthy postmenopausal women (Abstract). J Bone Mineral Res 2002;17:S266.

25. Roughead ZK, Hunt JR, Johnson LK, Badger TM, Lykken GI. Controlled substitution of soy protein for meat protein: effects on calcium retention, bone and cardiovascular health indices in postmenopausal women. J Clin Endocrinol Metab 2005;90:181–189.

26. Remer T, Dimitriou T, Manz F. Dietary potential renal acid load and renal net acid excretion in healthy, free-living children and adolescents. Am J Clin Nutr 2003;77(5):1255–1260.

27. Remer T. Influence of nutrition on acid-base balance—metabolic aspects. Eur J Nutr 2001;40(5):214–20.

28. Massey LK. Dietary animal and plant protein and human bone health: a whole foods approach. J Nutr 2003;133(3):862S–865S.

29. Remer T. Influence of diet on acid-base balance. Semin Dial 2000;13(4):221–226.

30. Potter SM, Baum JA, Teng H, Stillman RJ, Shay NF, Erdman JW, Jr. Soy protein and isoflavones: their effects on blood lipids and bone density in postmenopausal women. Am J Clin Nutr 1998;68(6 Suppl):1375S–1379S.

31. Alekel DL, Germain AS, Peterson CT, Hanson KB, Stewart JW, Toda T. Isoflavone-rich soy protein isolate attenuates bone loss in the lumbar spine of perimenopausal women [see comments]. Am J Clin Nutr 2000;72(3):844–852.

32. Arjmandi BH, Khalil DA, Smith BJ, et al. Soy protein has a greater effect on bone in postmenopausal women not on hormone replacement therapy, as evidenced by reducing bone resorption and urinary calcium excretion. J Clin Endocrinol Metab 2003;88(3):1048–1054.

33. Arjmandi BH, Alekel L, Hollis BW, et al. Dietary soybean protein prevents bone loss in an ovariectomized rat model of osteoporosis. J Nutr 1996;126(1):161–167.

34. Arjmandi BH, Getlinger MJ, Goyal NV, et al. Role of soy protein with normal or reduced isoflavone content in reversing bone loss induced by ovarian hormone deficiency in rats. Am J Clin Nutr 1998;68(6 Suppl):1358S–13563S.

35. Arjmandi BH, Birnbaum R, Goyal NV, et al. Bone-sparing effect of soy protein in ovarian hormone-deficient rats is related to its isoflavone content. Am J Clin Nutr 1998;68(6 Suppl):1364S–1368S.
36. Meyer HE, Pedersen JI, Loken EB, Tverdal A. Dietary factors and the incidence of hip fracture in middle-aged Norwegians. A prospective study. Am J Epidemiol 1997;145(2):117–123.
37. Dawson-Hughes B, Harris SS. Calcium intake influences the association of protein intake with rates of bone loss in elderly men and women. Am J Clin Nutr 2002;75(4):773–779.
38. Kerstetter JE, Looker AC, Insogna KL. Low dietary protein and low bone density. Calcif Tissue Int 2000;66(4):313.
39. Kerstetter JE, O'Brien KO, Insogna KL. Dietary protein affects intestinal calcium absorption. Am J Clin Nutr 1998;68(4):859–865.
40. Heaney RP. Protein and calcium: antagonists or synergists? Am J Clin Nutr 2002;75(4):609–610.
41. Bonjour JP, Rizzoli R. Inadequate protein intake and osteoporosis:Possible involvement of the IGF system. In: Burckhardt P, Heaney RP, eds. Nutritional aspects of osteoporosis. Rome: Ares-Serono Symposia Publications; 1995:399–406.
42. Eastell R, Lambert H. Strategies for skeletal health in the elderly. Proc Nutr Soc 2002;61(2):173–180.
43. Cooper C, Atkinson EJ, Hensrud DD, et al. Dietary protein intake and bone mass in women. Calcif Tissue Int 1996;58(5):320–325.
44. Hannan MT, Tucker KL, Dawson-Hughes B, Cupples LA, Felson DT, Kiel DP. Effect of dietary protein on bone loss in elderly men and women: the Framingham Osteoporosis Study. J Bone Miner Res 2000;15(12):2504–2512.
45. Feskanich D, Willett WC, Stampfer MJ, Colditz GA. Protein consumption and bone fractures in women. Am J Epidemiol 1996;143(5):472–479.
46. Hunt IF, Murphy NJ, Henderson C, et al. Bone mineral content in postmenopausal women: comparison of omnivores and vegetarians. Am J Clin Nutr 1989;50:517–523.
47. Huang Z, Himes JH, McGovern PG. Nutrition and subsequent hip fracture risk among a national cohort of white women. Am J Epidemiol 1996;144(2):124–134.
48. Abelow BJ, Holford TR, Insogna KL. Cross-cultural association between dietary animal protein and hip fracture: A hypothesis. Calcif Tissue Int 1992;50:14–18.
49. Frassetto LA, Todd KM, Morris RC, Jr., Sebastian A. Worldwide incidence of hip fracture in elderly women: relation to consumption of animal and vegetable foods. J Gerontol A Biol Sci Med Sci 2000;55(10):M585–M592.
50. Castenmiller JJ, Mensink RP, van der Heijden L, et al. The effect of dietary sodium on urinary calcium and potassium excretion in normotensive men with different calcium intakes. Am J Clin Nutr 1985;41(1):52–60.
51. Breslau NA, McGuire JL, Zerwekh JE, Pak CY. The role of dietary sodium on renal excretion and intestinal absorption of calcium and on vitamin D metabolism. J Clin Endocrinol Metab 1982;55(2):369–373.
52. McCarron DA, Rankin LI, Bennett WM, Krutzik S, McClung MR, Luft FC. Urinary calcium excretion at extremes of sodium intake in normal man. Am J Nephrol 1981;1(2):84–90.
53. Nordin BE, Need AG, Morris HA, Horowitz M. The nature and significance of the relationship between urinary sodium and urinary calcium in women. J Nutr 1993;123(9):1615–1622.
54. Zarkadas M, Gougeon-Reyburn R, Marliss EB, Block E, Alton-Mackey M. Sodium chloride supplementation and urinary calcium excretion in postmenopausal women. Am J Clin Nutr 1989;50(5):1088–1094.
55. McParland BE, Goulding A, Campbell AJ. Dietary salt affects biochemical markers of resorption and formation of bone in elderly women. BMJ 1989;299(6703):834–835.
56. Shortt C, Madden A, Flynn A, Morrissey PA. Influence of dietary sodium intake on urinary calcium excretion in selected Irish individuals. Eur J Clin Nutr 1988;42(7):595–603.
57. Massey LK, Whiting SJ. Dietary salt, urinary calcium, and bone loss. J Bone Miner Res 1996;11(6):731–736.
58. Itoh R, Suyama Y. Sodium excretion in relation to calcium and hydroxyproline excretion in a healthy Japanese population. Am J Clin Nutr 1996;63(5):735–740.
59. Greendale GA, Barrett-Connor E, Edelstein S, Ingles S, Haile R. Dietary sodium and bone mineral density: results of a 16-year follow-up study. J Am Geriatr Soc 1994;42(10):1050–1055.

60. Devine A, Criddle RA, Dick IM, Kerr DA, Prince RL. A longitudinal study of the effect of sodium and calcium intakes on regional bone density in postmenopausal women. Am J Clin Nutr 1995;62(4):740–745.

61. Lemann J, Jr., Gray RW, Pleuss JA. Potassium bicarbonate, but not sodium bicarbonate, reduces urinary calcium excretion and improves calcium balance in healthy men. Kidney Int 1989;35(2):688–695.

62. Sebastian A, Harris ST, Ottaway JH, Todd KM, Morris RC, Jr. Improved mineral balance and skeletal metabolism in postmenopausal women treated with potassium bicarbonate. N Engl J Med 1994;330(25): 1776–1781.

63. New SA, Bolton-Smith C, Grubb DA, Reid DM. Nutritional influences on bone mineral density: a cross-sectional study in premenopausal women. Am J Clin Nutr 1997;65(6):1831–1839.

64. Tylavsky FA, Holliday K, Danish R, Womack C, Norwood J, Carbone L. Fruit and vegetable intakes are an independent predictor of bone size in early pubertal children. Am J Clin Nutr 2004;79(2):311–317.

65. Tucker KL, Hannan MT, Chen H, Cupples LA, Wilson PW, Kiel DP. Potassium, magnesium, and fruit and vegetable intakes are associated with greater bone mineral density in elderly men and women. Am J Clin Nutr 1999;69(4):727–736.

66. Remer T, Manz F. Estimation of the renal net acid excretion by adults consuming diets containing variable amounts of protein. Am J Clin Nutr 1994;59:1356–1361.

67. Remer T, Manz F. Potential renal acid load of foods and its influence on urine pH. J Am Diet Assoc 1995;95:791–797.

68. Institute of Medicine FaNB. Dietary Reference Intakes for Water, Potassium, Choloride and Sulfate. National Academy Science, Washington, DC: 2004.

69. Lemann J, Jr. Relationship between urinary calcium and net acid excretion as determined by dietary protein and potassium: a review. Nephron 1999;81 Suppl 1:18–25.

70. Jones G, Riley MD, Whiting S. Association between urinary potassium, urinary sodium, current diet, and bone density in prepubertal children. Am J Clin Nutr 2001;73(4):839–844.

71. Macdonald HM, New SA, Golden MH, Campbell MK, Reid DM. Nutritional associations with bone loss during the menopausal transition: evidence of a beneficial effect of calcium, alcohol, and fruit and vegetable nutrients and of a detrimental effect of fatty acids. Am J Clin Nutr 2004;79(1):155–165.

72. New SA, MacDonald HM, Campbell MK, et al. Lower estimates of net endogenous non-carbonic acid production are positively associated with indexes of bone health in premenopausal and perimenopausal women. Am J Clin Nutr 2004;79(1):131–138.

73. Hall SL, Greendale GA. The relation of dietary vitamin C intake to bone mineral density: results from the PEPI study. Calcif Tissue Int 1998;63(3):183–189.

74. Leveille SG, LaCroix AZ, Koepsell TD, Beresford SA, Van Belle G, Buchner DM. Dietary vitamin C and bone mineral density in postmenopausal women in Washington State, USA. J Epidemiol Community Health 1997;51(5):479–485.

75. Kaptoge S, Welch A, McTaggart A, et al. Effects of dietary nutrients and food groups on bone loss from the proximal femur in men and women in the 7th and 8th decades of age. Osteoporos Int 2003;14(5):418–428.

76. New SA, Robins SP, Campbell MK, et al. Dietary influences on bone mass and bone metabolism: further evidence of a positive link between fruit and vegetable consumption and bone health? Am J Clin Nutr 2000;71(1):142–151.

77. Bushinsky DA. Acid-base imbalance and the skeleton. Eur J Nutr 2001;40(5):238–244.

78. Kenney MA, McCoy H, Williams L. Effects of magnesium deficiency on strength, mass, and composition of rat femur. Calcif Tissue Int 1994;54(1):44–49.

79. Rude RK, Gruber HE, Norton HJ, Wei LY, Frausto A, Mills BG. Bone loss induced by dietary magnesium reduction to 10% of the nutrient requirement in rats is associated with increased release of substance P and tumor necrosis factor-alpha. J Nutr 2004;134(1):79–85.

80. Stendig-Lindberg G, Tepper R, Leichter I. Trabecular bone density in a two year controlled trial of peroral magnesium in osteoporosis. Magnes Res 1993;6(2):155–163.

81. Kerstetter JE, Svastisalee CM, Caseria DM, Mitnick ME, Insogna KL. A threshold for low-protein-diet-induced elevations in parathyroid hormone. Am J Clin Nutr 2000;72(1):168–173.

82. Rizzoli R, Ammann P, Chevalley T, Bonjour JP. Protein intake and bone disorders in the elderly. Joint Bone Spine 2001;68(5):383–392.

83. Ammann P, Bourrin S, Bonjour JP, Meyer JM, Rizzoli R. Protein undernutrition-induced bone loss is associated with decreased IGF-I levels and estrogen deficiency. J Bone Miner Res 2000;15(4):683–690.

84. Schurch MA, Rizzoli R, Slosman D, Vadas L, Vergnaud P, Bonjour JP. Protein supplements increase serum insulin-like growth factor-I levels and attenuate proximal femur bone loss in patients with recent hip fracture. A randomized, double-blind, placebo-controlled trial. Ann Intern Med 1998;128(10):801–809.

85. Canalis. Insulin-like growth factors and osteoporosis. Bone 1997;21:215–216.

86. Roughead ZK, Lukaski HC. Inadequate Copper Intake Reduces Serum Insulin-Like Growth Factor-I and Bone Strength in Growing Rats Fed Graded Amounts of Copper and Zinc. J Nutr 2003;133(2):442–448.

87. Gamero P, Sornay-Rendu E, Delmas PD. Low serum IGF-1 and occurrence of osteoporotic fractures in postmenopausal women. Lancet 2000;355(9207):898–899.

88. Chenu C, Valentin-Opran A, Chavassieux P, Saez S, Meunier PJ, Delmas PD. Insulin like growth factor I hormonal regulation by growth hormone and by 1,25(OH)2D3 and activity on human osteoblast-like cells in short-term cultures. Bone 1990;11(2):81–86.

89. Rosen CJ. IGF-I and osteoporosis. Clin Lab Med 2000;20(3):591–602.

90. Roughead Z, Lukaski H. Inadequate copper intake reduces serum insulin-like growth factor-1 (IGF-1) and bone Strength in growing rats (abstract). J Bone Mineral Res 2002;17:S240.

91. Devine A, Rosen C, Mohan S, Baylink D, Prince RL. Effects of zinc and other nutritional factors on insulin-like growth factor I and insulin-like growth factor binding proteins in postmenopausal women. Am J Clin Nutr 1998;68(1):200–206.

92. Ninh NX, Thissen JP, Collette L, Gerard G, Khoi HH, Ketelslegers JM. Zinc supplementation increases growth and circulating insulin-like growth factor I (IGF-I) in growth-retarded Vietnamese children. Am J Clin Nutr 1996;63(4):514–519.

93. Nishiyama S, Kiwaki K, Miyazaki Y, Hasuda T. Zinc and IGF-I concentrations in pregnant women with anemia before and after supplementation with iron and/or zinc. J Am Coll Nutr 1999;18(3):261–267.

94. Estivariz CF, Ziegler TR. Nutrition and the insulin-like growth factor system. Endocrine 1997;7(1):65–71.

95. Cha MC, Rojhani A. Failure of IGF-I infusion to promote growth in Zn deficient hypophysectomized rats. J Trace Elem Med Biol 1998;12(3):141–147.

96. Ninh NX, Thissen JP, Maiter D, Adam E, Mulumba N, Ketelslegers JM. Reduced liver insulin-like growth factor-I gene expression in young zinc-deprived rats is associated with a decrease in liver growth hormone (GH) receptors and serum GH-binding protein. J Endocrinol 1995;144(3):449–456.

97. Matsui T, Yamaguchi M. Zinc modulation of insulin-like growth factor's effect in osteoblastic MC3T3-E1 cells. Peptides 1995;16(6):1063–1068.

98. Vallee BL, Falchuk KH. The biochemical basis of zinc physiology. Physiol Rev 1993;73(1):79–118.

99. Cashman KD, Baker A, Ginty F, et al. No effect of copper supplementation on biochemical markers of bone metabolism in healthy young adult females despite apparently improved copper status. Eur J Clin Nutr 2001;55(7):525–531.

100. Baker A, Turley E, Bonham MP, et al. No effect of copper supplementation on biochemical markers of bone metabolism in healthy adults. Br J Nutr 1999;82(4):283–290.

101. Baker A, Harvey L, Majask-Newman G, Fairweather-Tait S, Flynn A, Cashman K. Effect of dietary copper intakes on biochemical markers of bone metabolism in healthy adult males. Eur J Clin Nutr 1999;53(5):408–412.

102. Medeiros DM, Plattner A, Jennings D, Stoecker B. Bone morphology, strength and density are compromised in iron-deficient rats and exacerbated by calcium restriction. J Nutr 2002;132(10):3135–3141.

103. Angus RM, Sambrook PN, Pocock NA, Eisman JA. Dietary intake and bone mineral density. Bone Miner 1988;4(3):265–277.

104. Younes H, Coudray C, Bellanger J, Demigne C, Rayssiguier Y, Remesy C. Effects of two fermentable carbohydrates (inulin and resistant starch) and their combination on calcium and magnesium balance in rats. Br J Nutr 2001;86(4):479–485.

105. Griffin IJ, Davila PM, Abrams SA. Non-digestible oligosaccharides and calcium absorption in girls with adequate calcium intakes. Br J Nutr 2002;87 Suppl 2:S187–S191.

106. Roberfroid MB, Cumps J, Devogelaer JP. Dietary chicory inulin increases whole-body bone mineral density in growing male rats. J Nutr 2002;132(12):3599–3602.

107. Van Loo J, Cummings J, Delzenne N, et al. Functional food properties of non-digestible oligosaccharides: a consensus report from the ENDO project (DGXII AIRII-CT94-1095). Br J Nutr 1999;81(2): 121–132.
108. Greger JL. Nondigestible carbohydrates and mineral bioavailability. J Nutr 1999;129(7 Suppl):1434S–1435S.
109. Morais MB, Feste A, Miller RG, Lifschitz CH. Effect of resistant and digestible starch on intestinal absorption of calcium, iron, and zinc in infant pigs. Pediatr Res 1996;39(5):872–876.
110. Ohta A, Motohashi Y, Sakai K, Hirayama M, Adachi T, Sakuma K. Dietary fructooligosaccharides increase calcium absorption and levels of mucosal calbindin-D9k in the large intestine of gastrectomized rats. Scand J Gastroenterol 1998;33(10):1062–1068.
111. Zafar TA, Weaver CM, Zhao Y, Martin BR, Wastney ME. Nondigestible oligosaccharides increase calcium absorption and suppress bone resorption in ovariectomized rats. J Nutr 2004;134(2):399–402.
112. Coudray C, Bellanger J, Castiglia-Delavaud C, Remesy C, Vermorel M, Rayssignuier Y. Effect of soluble or partly soluble dietary fibres supplementation on absorption and balance of calcium, magnesium, iron and zinc in healthy young men. Eur J Clin Nutr 1997;51(6):375–380.
113. van den Heuvel EG, Muys T, van Dokkum W, Schaafsma G. Oligofructose stimulates calcium absorption in adolescents. Am J Clin Nutr 1999;69(3):544–548.
114. van den Heuvel EG, Schaafsma G, Muys T, van Dokkum W. Nondigestible oligosaccharides do not interfere with calcium and nonheme-iron absorption in young, healthy men. Am J Clin Nutr 1998;67(3):445–451.
115. Tahiri M, Tressol JC, Arnaud J, et al. Effect of short-chain fructooligosaccharides on intestinal calcium absorption and calcium status in postmenopausal women: a stable-isotope study. Am J Clin Nutr 2003;77(2):449–457.
116. Kaur N, Gupta AK. Applications of inulin and oligofructose in health and nutrition. J Biosci 2002;27(7):703–714.
117. Tucker KL, Chen H, Hannan MT, et al. Bone mineral density and dietary patterns in older adults: the Framingham Osteoporosis Study. Am J Clin Nutr 2002;76(1):245–252.
118. Thompson DW. On Growth and Form. Cambridge University Press, London: 1942.

13 Influence of Lifestyle Choices on Calcium Homeostasis

Smoking, Alcohol, and Hormone Therapies

D. Lee Alekel and Oksana Matvienko

KEY POINTS

- Smoking and alcohol intake affect bone turnover and calcium homeostasis, particularly with heavier use.
- Duration of smoking and alcohol use appear to be important factors in determining their negative effects on bone.
- Provided smoking and alcohol ingestion have not caused permanent end-organ damage, deleterious effects on calcium homeostasis are apparently reversible.
- Hormone therapy in postmenopausal women exerts beneficial effects on bone and calcium homeostasis.

1. INTRODUCTION

Much of the research in the area of smoking, alcohol intake, and estrogen/progesterone hormone therapies (HTs) concentrates on bone mineral density (BMD) and osteoporotic risk rather than on calcium homeostasis *per se*. Heavy smoking and excessive alcohol intake are key risk factors for bone loss and osteoporotic fractures. However, the effect of light smoking on bone is not as clear, whereas very moderate alcohol intake has been shown to either increase BMD or not have adverse effects on bone. Nonetheless, smoking and alcohol intake affect bone turnover and calcium homeostasis, although this primarily has been observed with heavier use. Duration of smoking and alcohol use appear to be important factors in determining their negative effects on bone. Provided smoking and alcohol ingestion have not caused permanent end-organ damage (i.e., lung disease, cancer, cirrhosis, osteoporosis), deleterious effects on calcium homeostasis are apparently reversible. Coexistent lifestyle factors, such as heavy coffee drinking and physical inactivity, may also contribute synergistically to osteopenia in smokers and drinkers. Although estrogen deficiency plays a key role in osteoporosis and other menopause-related chronic diseases, HT is often accompanied by side effects and increases the risks of breast and uterine cancer. Because of adverse effects as revealed by results from the Women's Health Initiative (WHI; increased risk of breast cancer, coronary heart disease,

From: *Calcium in Human Health*
Edited by: C. M. Weaver and R. P. Heaney © Humana Press Inc., Totowa, NJ

stroke, and venous thromboembolism) and the fear of cancer, noncompliance is a major obstacle with HTs. The current thinking is that HT should not be used to prevent or treat osteoporosis, but may be indicated short-term to alleviate vasomotor symptoms. Still, HT in postmenopausal women exerts beneficial effects on bone and calcium homeostasis. This chapter reviews studies on the effects of smoking, alcohol, and HT on BMD, as well as those involving calcium homeostasis and its link to BMD in humans.

2. CIGARETTE SMOKING

2.1. Effect of Cigarette Smoking on Bone and Calcium Homeostasis: Proposed Mechanisms

Cigarette smoking is a frequently cited risk factor for osteoporosis (1) and has been implicated as such in several retrospective (2,3) and prospective (4–7) studies. The mechanism by which smoking exerts its debilitating effect on bone is unclear. The adverse effect of smoking could be attributable to the tendency of smokers to have poorer health and eating habits compared with nonsmokers. Some researchers have suggested that the effect of smoking on bone mass is influenced by the low body weight so common among smokers (8,9). It has also been speculated that smoking reduces the peak bone mass attained in early adulthood (4).

Perhaps the most convincing evidence is that smoking alters estrogen metabolism and hence may modify estrogen effects on bone mass. Smoking is associated with early natural menopause (10), greater risk of oligomenorrhea (11), and infertility (12). It is not, however, known whether this anti-estrogenic effect of smoking is due to a decrease in estrogen production or an increase in estrogen degradation. Evidence for a decrease in production is suggested by direct inhibition of human granulosa cell aromatase activity and the consequent reduction in androgen to estrogen conversion (13). Alternatively, there is evidence for an increase in deactivation of estrogens via enhanced 2-hydroxylation of estradiol (14).

More recently, evidence indicates that smoking accelerates bone loss by lowering intestinal calcium absorption (15,16). Studies in the elderly and postmenopausal women report a 1.7–13% difference in mean fractional calcium absorption between smokers and nonsmokers, after adjustment for various confounding factors (15,17). Need and colleagues proposed that the smoking-mediated impairment in calcium absorption might be caused by the suppression of the parathyroid hormone (PTH)–1,25 dihydroxyvitamin D $(1,25[OH]_2D)$–endocrine axis (16). Although there was no significant difference in calcium absorption between postmenopausal female smokers and nonsmokers who had similar serum $1,25(OH)_2D$ concentrations, they observed significantly lower concentrations of circulating PTH and $1,25(OH)_2D$ in smokers. Likewise, Brot et al. reported that serum concentrations of 25 hydroxyvitamin D (25[OH]D) and $1,25[OH]_2D$ were approx 10% lower, and PTH 20% lower in Danish perimenopausal female smokers than nonsmokers, with serum ionized calcium concentrations being similar in the two groups (18). In contrast, Rapuri et al. did not find significant differences in $1,25(OH)_2D$, intact PTH, serum calcium, or ionized calcium concentrations between elderly female smokers and nonsmokers (17). However, they reported a significant 12% decrease in circulating 25(OH)D in the smoking group.

2.2. Cigarette Smoking and Risk of Bone Fracture

The impact of cigarette smoking on bone, vitamin D status, and calcium homeostasis appears to be more pronounced in postmenopausal women and the elderly, particularly in heavy smokers (at least one pack per day) or long-term smokers (at least 2 yr), whereas it is less apparent in younger individuals *(4,19,20)*. Although studies that have examined the association between cigarette smoking and BMD differ somewhat in their reports of bone sites most susceptible to the deleterious effect of smoking, there is general agreement that smoking accelerates the rate of bone loss. A significant, smoking-mediated decrease in BMD has been noted at the total proximal femur *(7,17,20)*, femoral neck *(15,21)*, total body *(15,17)*, lumbar spine *(21)*, and the radius *(5)*. Some earlier studies, however, did not show that smoking had an independent effect on bone mass *(22,23)*. The magnitude of the difference in BMD between postmenopausal or elderly nonsmokers and heavy smokers depends on age and bone site, and ranges from 4 to 6% *(21,17)*. Pocock and colleagues *(24)* compared twin pairs discordant for tobacco use (subject age was not reported). They found that twins who were heavy smokers had a 2.4% lower BMD in the lumbar spine than their siblings who were light smokers. The researcher equated this smoking-related difference in lumbar BMD to approx 3 to 4 yr of normal postmenopausal bone loss. In their meta-analysis, Law and Hackshaw *(19)* estimated that postmenopausal female smokers lose an additional 0.2% of bone mass per year compared with nonsmokers. This loss of bone mass is associated with an increased relative risk of hip fracture in current smokers compared with nonsmokers that ranges from 17% at age 60 yr to 108% at age 90 yr. They also estimated that among postmenopausal women, smoking accounts for every eighth fracture.

2.3. Effect of Smoking Cessation on Fracture Risk

Evidence suggests that the adverse effect of smoking on bone is at least partially reversible when smoking is discontinued *(20,21)*. As the duration of smoking cessation increases, the risk of a bone fracture decreases and, after 14–15 yr, may approach the risk of never-smokers. The age-adjusted risk of hip fracture is increased 35% for current and 15% for past (quit within past 14 yr) elderly smokers compared with never-smokers, after correcting for body mass index and HT. Duration of smoking appears to be a stronger predictor of hip fracture risk than the number of cigarettes smoked, and may account for an incremental increase of 6% in fracture risk for every 5 yr of smoking *(20)*.

3. ALCOHOL INTAKE

3.1. Chronic Alcohol Abuse and Bone Disease

Osteoporosis is associated with alcohol abuse, as first proposed by Saville *(25)*. Alcoholics have reduced bone mass, which has been confirmed radiographically *(26,27)* by bone mineral measurements *(28)*, and histomorphometrically *(28–30)* in each study uncomplicated by osteomalacia or cirrhosis. In contrast, another study did not find that heavy alcohol intake, in the absence of liver disease, significantly affected bone mass in black men *(31)*. However, in white men, *duration* of alcohol intake had an independent negative effect on BMD. The authors concluded that prolonged heavy alcohol intake resulted in bone loss in white but not black men, likely illustrating racial differences in calcium homeostasis. Similarly, Laitinen and co-workers *(32)* reported that mean BMD at the lumbar spine and proximal femur sites was not different between noncirrhotic alcoholics ($n = 27$) and controls (($n = 100$). However, those alcoholics who had a longer history (>20 yr) of alcohol consumption had significantly lower BMD than those with a shorter history (<10 yr or 10–20 yr duration) of alcohol intake, particularly at the trochanter. Likewise, Laitinen and colleagues *(33)* studied 24- to 48-yr-old noncirrhotic alcoholic ($N = 19$) women, 16 of whom had regular menstrual cycles, hospitalized for withdrawal. Bone mineral content and BMD did not differ between patients and controls at any measurement site, whereas the alcoholics had depressed bone formation on admission compared with controls, as reflected by lower (48%) serum osteocalcin, a vitamin K-dependent protein synthesized by osteoblasts. After 2 wk of abstinence, osteocalcin completely normalized.

Nonetheless, in the presence of alcoholic liver disease, BMD may very well be lower as a result of reduced bone formation rate and turnover *(34)* owing to depressed osteoblastic activity *(35,36)*. Circulating osteocalcin is reduced with both chronic *(33,37)* and acute *(38,39)* alcohol ingestion, suggesting a direct toxic effect of alcohol on bone formation. Furthermore, the rate of skeletal fractures is higher among alcoholics than in the normal population *(40,41)*. The high prevalence of fractures among alcoholics also may be the result of the increased risk of falling superimposed on alcohol-associated osteopenia. Lifestyle factors that co-exist with alcohol ingestion, such as cigarette smoking, heavy coffee drinking, and physical inactivity, may also contribute to osteopenia.

3.2. Alcohol Abuse and Calcium Metabolism

Many factors may contribute to the development of alcohol-induced bone disease, and thus it is critical to understand how alcohol affects mineral metabolism. Certainly, nutritional deficiencies and altered mineral metabolism are common among alcoholics. Chronic alcohol intake is associated with low serum concentrations of vitamin D metabolites 25(OH)D *(30,33,42)*, 1,25(OH)$_2$D *(30,34,42)*, and 24,25(OH)$_2$D *(43)*. The low concentrations of 25(OH)D and 1,25(OH)$_2$D may be the result of the inhibition of hydroxylase activities in the liver *(42)* and kidney *(44)*, respectively, or perhaps owing to the degradation of vitamin D metabolites in the liver via induction of the cytochrome P450 system *(42)*. One would presume that low-circulating 1,25(OH)$_2$D results in impaired intestinal calcium absorption, hypocalcemia/hypocalciuria *(43)*, and elevated PTH concentrations *(30)*. However, 37% greater calcium absorption as measured by stable strontium has been demonstrated in noncirrhotic male alcoholics compared with controls *(32)*. An explanation for this surprising finding may be alcohol-induced injury to the intestinal mucosal cells, thereby allowing greater calcium absorption via the nonsaturable para- or intercellular route *(45)*. The effect of alcohol on nutrient absorption varies widely, depending on the nutrient, the amount of alcohol ingested, and the nutritional status of the host, rendering generalizations difficult. However, iron absorption appears to be increased via the paracellular route, contributing to the iron overload in chronic alcoholics *(46)*. Yet, the absorption of other nutrients that have been studied is likely to be decreased or unchanged *(47)*. Further discussion of the transcellular (active, saturable) vs paracellular (passive) calcium absorption is described elsewhere in this volume.

Acute alcohol ingestion induces acute hypocalcemia and hypermagnesemia, which in turn stimulates PTH, with subsequent hypercalciuria and hypermagnesuria *(38)*, but not necessarily with the expected change in serum calcium *(48)*. Chronic alcohol ingestion results in elevated *(49)*, normal *(33)*, or reduced *(34)* PTH concentrations, with discrepancies perhaps related to the duration and extent of drinking, as well as the age of the individuals examined. For example, Bikle and colleagues proposed that PTH may stimulate bone remodeling in younger alcoholics, but that with sustained abuse, bone loses its responsiveness to PTH, resorption is impaired, and serum calcium cannot be maintained *(50)*. Thus, PTH does not correct the alcohol-induced hypocalcemia, indicating that alcohol may impair the response of the parathyroid glands to hypocalcemia *(51,52)*. Laitinen and colleagues suggested that alcohol caused an influx of calcium into the intracellular space, particularly within the parathyroid gland, explaining the reduced PTH concentrations *(51)*. Some of these apparent discrepancies may also be due to which fragment of PTH was measured, because PTH is metabolized in the liver, which may be damaged. In contrast with PTH, calcitonin is more consistently elevated with chronic *(53)* and acute *(48)* alcohol ingestion, but this effect is not likely to be sustained over time. The main biological effect of calcitonin is to inhibit osteoclastic bone resorption 54*)*, producing hypocalcemia and hypophosphatemia when bone turnover is sufficiently high. Nonetheless, the exact physiologic role of calcitonin in calcium homeostasis in adult humans has not been clearly established *(55)*.

3.3. Abstinence From Alcohol and Reversal of Disturbances

Lindholm et al. examined men who were current alcohol abusers (drinkers) and compared results to men who had previously abused alcohol but abstained (abstainers) for at least 2 yr and compared with normal controls *(34)*. They found no differences in bone mineral content of the distal forearm or lumbar spine among these three groups, although a number of the drinkers and abstainers had subnormal values. Although the drinkers had lower serum PTH, 1,25(OH)$_2$D, and osteocalcin concentrations, the abstainers had results similar to those of controls. Similarly, Laitinen and coworkers reported that 2 wk of abstinence in men resulted in increased serum ionized calcium, urinary phosphate, serum osteocalcin, and procollagen I carboxyterminal propeptide (PICP; a marker of bone formation) *(32)*. Likewise, Laitinen et al. examined young and middle-aged women who abstained for 2 wk, with results indicating increased serum-ionized calcium, serum phosphate, urinary phosphate, serum osteocalcin, and PICP *(33)*. Serum concentrations of vitamin D metabolites (25[OH] and 1,25[OH]$_2$) did not normalize during abstention, but control values were higher in the women *(33)* than the men *(32)*. Thus, the effects of chronic alcohol abuse on calcium homeostasis appear to be reversible with abstinence, whereas the effect on bone may be dependent on the duration of alcohol abuse.

3.4. Moderate Alcohol Intake and Bone

An adverse effect of more moderate alcohol consumption on BMD has not been established. May et al. reported that moderate alcohol intake (one to two drinks per day) did not have a detrimental effect on BMD in older men *(56)*. In fact, femoral neck, trochanter, and Ward's triangle were higher ($p = 0.02$) in drinkers than nondrinkers when adjusted for age and body weight. When further adjusted for covariates (smoking, physical activity, caffeine), the only site that remained higher in drinkers was the trochanter. Likewise, elderly women who consumed alcohol had higher spine (10%), total body (4.5%), and mid-radius (6%) BMD than did nondrinkers *(17)*. The maximum effect was noted with moderate intakes (>28.6 to ≤57.2 g/wk), although this was also the group with the lowest percentage of smokers. Serum 25(OH)D tended to be lower (albeit not significantly) in alcohol consumers than in nondrinkers, and in those with an alcohol intake greater than 57.2 to 142.9 g or less per week. Serum PTH concentrations were significantly lower in drinkers (>28.6 to ≤57.2 g/wk) than nondrinkers, whereas serum $1,25(OH)_2D$ concentrations were not different between drinkers and nondrinkers and the amount of alcohol intake did not have an effect. This study also provided evidence that the bone effects were likely mediated by a decrease in bone remodeling, as indicated by a marked reduction in serum osteocalcin, urinary cross-linked *N*-telopeptides of type I collagen (NTx; a marker of bone resorption), and serum PTH concentrations. Similar evidence has been provided for middle-aged women, with moderate alcohol use associated with low serum osteocalcin concentrations *(57)*.

Felson et al. examined long-term alcohol intake in 1154 participants from the Framingham Study who received bone density assessments at the radius, proximal femur, and lumbar spine *(58)*. Women who drank at least 7 oz (207 mL/wk) of alcohol had higher lumbar spine, trochanter, and radius BMD than women in the lightest category (<1 oz or 29.6 mL/wk) of intake, after adjusting for age, weight, height, smoking, and estrogen exposure. Men who drank at least 14 oz (414 mL/wk) of alcohol tended to have higher BMD, but these differences were less than in the women and were not significant once adjustments were made for covariates. Likewise, in 7598 elderly ambulatory women from five centers in France, moderate drinking (11–29 g or one to three glasses of wine daily) was associated with higher trochanteric BMD, whereas heavy alcohol intake (30 g/d) was associated with lower total body BMD *(59)*. These results were unrelated to various lifestyle or sociodemographic factors. In premenopausal American and Indian/Pakistani Caucasian women, Alekel et al. *(60,61)* reported that usual but moderate (defined as no more than six alcoholic beverages, equivalent to 255 g alcohol, per week) alcohol intake was positively and consistently related to lumbar spine *(60)* and femoral *(61)* areal BMD. Gavaler and VanThiel have found that moderate alcohol intake in postmenopausal women significantly increased circulating estradiol, presumably due to the stimulating effect of alcohol on peripheral aromatization of androgens to estrogens and may also increase adrenal stimulation, thus offering a partial explanation of the reported beneficial effect on bone *(62)*.

To examine the acute effects of moderate social drinking on calcium homeostasis and bone metabolism, Laitinen and co-workers examined 10 healthy males *(63)*. Serum concentrations of intact PTH increased from the start to the end of the 3-wk drinking period and returned to baseline within 1 wk of subsequent abstention. Serum vitamin D metabolites and intestinal absorption of calcium remained unchanged. Serum osteocalcin concentrations decreased by 30% during the drinking period and then recovered by 25% following the abstinence period. Thus, moderate alcohol intake acutely affects serum PTH and osteocalcin, suggestive of increased osteoclastic bone resorption and decreased osteoblastic bone formation, in accord with the proposed toxic effect of alcohol on osteoblasts. However, moderate alcohol intake may not have negative effects on vitamin D or calcium metabolism.

3.5. Alcohol Intake and Fracture Risk

The evidence for a deleterious effect of moderate alcohol consumption on fracture risk in women appears puzzling, given the beneficial effect on BMD. Seeman and colleagues conducted a retrospective case–control study of risk factors for spinal osteoporosis in men and found a statistically elevated relative risk (RR) among smokers (RR = 2.3) and those who drank alcoholic beverages (RR = 2.4) (3). Hernandez-Avila and colleagues assessed the relationship between alcohol intake and risk of forearm and hip fractures using prospectively collected data on almost 85,000 women 34–59 yr of age (64). They found that alcohol was independently associated with increased risk of both hip and forearm fractures. Women consuming at least 25 g alcohol per day had a relative risk of 2.33 for hip fractures and a relative risk of 1.38 for forearm fractures compared with nondrinkers. Paganini-Hill and coworkers observed a positive trend in the risk of fractures with increasing number of shots of liquor per week after menopause (65). Women who drank no less than eight shots per week had a relative risk of 1.85 compared with women who never imbibed. In an analysis of the Framingham Study data relating alcohol intake to hip fractures, Felson and associates reported an increased risk as alcohol consumption rose (trend test, $p < 0.05$) (58). In contrast, Baron et al. reported that age-adjusted odds ratio for postmenopausal women who consumed alcohol was 0.80 (95% confidence interval [CI], 0.69–0.93), suggesting that moderate alcohol consumption modestly decreased risk for hip fracture (20). Certainly, heavy alcohol intake (65) and alcoholism (66) are associated with increased risk, whereas the case for moderate alcohol intake is not as clear. Collectively, these findings indicate how complex the relationships are among lifestyle factors, calcium homeostasis, and bone metabolism.

4. HORMONE THERAPIES

4.1. Estrogen Deficiency

Fuller Albright first recognized the association between osteoporosis and estrogen deficiency in 1941 (67). It is widely accepted that estrogen deficiency plays a central role in the pathogenesis of osteoporosis and that estrogen therapy is effective in preventing menopausal bone loss and reducing fracture risk (68). The menopause is the transition from the reproductive to the nonreproductive stage of a woman's life, characterized clinically by permanent cessation of menstruation. The decline in ovarian activity may begin as early as 35–40 yr of age, long before menopause in most women. However, there is conflicting evidence as to when bone loss starts and whether premenopausal bone loss occurs. Most studies, however, have demonstrated that during and after menopause there is an accelerated rate of bone loss in the spine, with rates of between 1 and 6% (69–72) during natural menopause and as high as 10% after oophorectomy (73). A longitudinal study indicated annual rates of loss from the proximal radius in excess of 1% in the majority of postmenopausal women (74). The femoral neck shows annual rates of loss similar to those observed for the radius (75,76). Thus, the majority of evidence not only supports increased rates of bone loss during and after menopause, but that the highest rates occur in trabecular bone. This bone loss may continue for the next decade, accounting for 20–30% loss in cancellous (trabecular) bone and 5–10% loss in cortical bone (77). The median age at menopause in most industrialized societies occurs around 50 yr (78). Because the average life expectancy of women is approx 75 yr, most women will be postmenopausal for one-third of their lifetime (79).

4.2. Estrogen Therapy, Estrogen/Progestin Therapy, Bone, and Fracture Risk

Estrogen plays a critical role in bone health as evidenced by an accelerated loss in bone mass during the perimenopausal years. Estrogen alone or in combination with progestin prevents bone loss at the hip and spine *(80)* and reduces hip fracture rates *(81)*. The mechanism of estrogen to reduce bone loss is unclear, but locally active growth factors and cytokines modulate its effects on osteoblasts and osteoclasts *(82)*. Although estrogen deficiency plays a key role in osteoporosis and other menopause-related chronic diseases, HT increases the risks of breast *(83)* and uterine *(84)* cancer and is often accompanied by side effects *(85)*. Indeed, HT or estrogen therapy alleviates vasomotor symptoms *(86)*, exerts some cardioprotective effects *(87)*, and prevents bone loss *(88)*. Yet, because of adverse effects as revealed by results from the WHI *(89)* and the fear of cancer, noncompliance is a major obstacle with traditional HTs *(90)*. Indeed, the global index of benefits and risks of HT in the WHI revealed a net harm (hazards ratio 1.15, 95% CI 1.03–1.28) and women taking HT had an increased risk of breast cancer (26%), coronary heart disease (29%), stroke (41%), and venous thromboembolism (double). However, women taking HT had a 33, 29, 35, and 24% decline in hip, forearm, vertebral, and total fracture rate, respectively *(91*; Fig. 1), and 37% decline in colorectal cancer rate. Nonetheless, many of the women in the WHI had stopped the study medication during the trial (42% in the HT group, 38% in the placebo group), illustrating problems with compliance. Previous surveys indicate that two-thirds of women discontinue treatment within 5 yr of initiation as a result of undesirable side effects *(92)*. The current thinking is that HT should not be used to prevent or treat osteoporosis, but may be indicated short-term to alleviate vasomotor symptoms. Nevertheless, HT in postmenopausal women clearly exerts beneficial effects on bone and calcium homeostasis. Furthermore, the data from a meta-analysis are convincing that supplemental calcium potentiates the positive effect of estrogen on bone mass at the lumbar spine, femoral neck, and forearm *(93*; Fig. 2). This report indicated that the benefit was for calcium intakes of approx 1200 mg/d, with a synergistic relation between high calcium intake and estrogen treatment. Calcium is not only thought to decrease bone resorption, but it is likely that an additional calcium supply may allow an increase in the deposition of mineral in newly formed and perhaps previously formed bone. However, research indicates that estrogen treatment provided at the onset of menopause, continued for less than 10 yr, but then discontinued, has little if any effect on fracture incidence by age 70 yr *(81)*. Hence, when HT is discontinued, bone loss ensues and is similar to what occurs immediately after menopause *(94)*.

4.3. Menopause, Hormone Therapy, and Calcium Homeostasis

Studies by Heaney and co-workers confirmed that ovarian failure was associated with a 20% increase in bone resorption and a 15% increase in bone formation, leading to a net loss of bone *(95)*. Calcium balance averaged –0.020 g/d in 207 studies with premenopausal women, whereas this balance was significantly more negative *(p* < 0.02) at –0.043 g/d in 41 studies with postmenopausal (untreated) women. These alterations in skeletal metabolism are accompanied by an increased urinary loss of calcium and decline in intestinal calcium absorption *(96)*. The rise in urinary calcium with menopause is caused by a decline in tubular reabsorption of calcium, rather than a rise in filtered load *(97)*. These authors concluded that estrogens likely promote tubular reabsorption of calcium

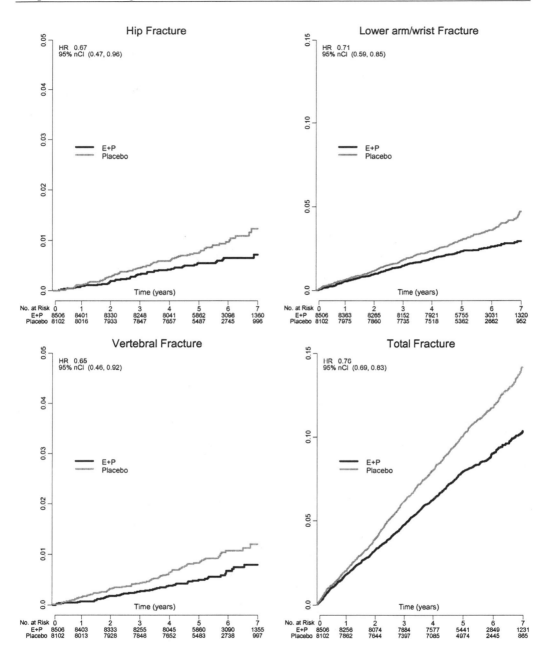

Fig. 1. Kaplan-Meier estimates of cumulative hazards for fracture.
HR indicates hazard ratio; nCI indicates nominal confidence interval; dark line indicates placebo arm; light line indicates hormone therapy arm. (Adapted from ref. *91*, with permission.)

and that this renal calcium leak contributes to subsequent bone resorption with estrogen lack. Consequently, premenopausal and treated postmenopausal women have an apparent calcium requirement of 0.990 g/d, whereas untreated postmenopausal women require approx 1.504 g/d *(96)*. These changes in calcium metabolism are accompanied by alterations in the biochemical markers of bone turnover: serum osteocalcin, serum tartrate-

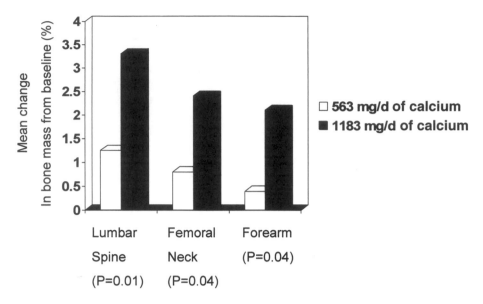

Fig. 2. Mean (+ SEM) annual percentage change in bone mass at the lumbar spine, femoral neck, and forearm in postmenopausal women treated with estrogen alone (white bars; total average calcium intake: 563 mg/d) compared with women treated with estrogen and calcium (black bars; total average calcium intake: 1183 mg/d). (Adapted from ref. *93*, with permission of the *American Journal of Clinical Nutrition.*)

resistant acid phosphatase, serum alkaline phosphatase, urinary NTx, urinary hydroxyproline, and urinary pyridinoline and deoxypyridinoline (collagen crosslinks) *(98,99)*.

Aloia and co-workers have shown that HT within 6 mo to 6 yr after menopause decreases serum calcium, osteocalcin, and urinary hydroxyproline, and increases concentrations of calcitonin, PTH, and 1,25(OH)$_2$D, indicating a reduction in bone remodeling *(100)*. In addition, whether daily continuous or sequential estrogen/progestin therapy was taken by postmenopausal women, indices of bone turnover (osteocalcin, alkaline phosphatase, urinary calcium, urinary hydroxyproline) declined, whereas PTH rose, from baseline through 1 yr of treatment *(101)*. Women with the highest bone resorption rates achieved the greatest increment in BMD in response to therapy. Marshall et al. found more marked lowering effects of ethinyl oestradiol on plasma total and ionized calcium and phosphate and urinary calcium excretion in postmenopausal compared with perimenopausal women *(102)*. Another study examined the effects of oral estriol and conjugated estrogen in early postmenopausal women and found that the former was not as effective in lowering serum alkaline phosphatase or urinary hydroxyproline, but had similar effects on serum osteocalcin and urinary calcium excretion *(103)*. However, both treatments exerted lumbar bone-preserving effects after 24 mo of treatment.

4.4. Calcitonin and Calcium Homeostasis

The effect of calcitonin on calcium homeostasis has not been well studied and the role of calcitonin in adult mineral and bone homeostasis is not well understood. Nonetheless, calcitonin is a bone active, US Food and Drug Administration-approved, antiresorptive agent to treat but not prevent osteoporosis *(104)*. One report indicated that calcitonin therapy regulated circulating magnesium, copper, and zinc and these minerals were more useful for evaluating response to treatment in women with postmenopausal osteoporosis *(105)*. Thus, calcitonin may be involved with minerals other than calcium in decreasing bone resorption. A single dose of nasal calcitonin has been shown to decrease bone resorption by 15% as evidenced by biochemical markers of bone turnover *(106)*, whereas the anabolic action of calcitonin has not been clearly demonstrated. Calcitonin reduces the risk of vertebral fractures up to 40%, but does not affect nonvertebral (i.e., hip) BMD or fractures *(107)*. Long-term efficacy appears to be reduced with calcitonin and thus its use is limited. However, advantages of calcitonin are that it is bone-specific, may be used as an alternative to estrogen, and may be used in men. Calcitonin is typically administered intranasally, obviating the problems of parenteral administration, and has analgesic benefits *(108)*. Interestingly, calcitonin therapy for 6 mo decreased serum interleukin (IL)-10 and IL-6r, but increased serum IL-2, IL-8, and tumor necrosis factor (TNF)-α, illustrating that calcitonin may influence bone through the action of cytokines and that cytokines may be affected in different directions *(109)*.

4.5. Potential Mechanisms for Bone Resorption and Perturbation of Calcium Homeostasis With Menopause and Hormone Therapy

Estrogen deficiency is associated with increased cytokine production. For this reason, there are numerous studies of the relative contribution of cytokines to bone loss, the potential cell sources of cytokines in the bone microenvironment, and the mechanism of action of various cytokines. The inflammatory cytokines (IL-6, IL-1, and TNF-α in particular) are thought to be involved in stimulating bone resorption. IL-1 was one of the first to be identified and most potent bone-resorbing cytokines *(110,111)*, causing osteoclast formation, differentiation, and activation *(112,113)*. The effects of IL-1 are enhanced by two orders of magnitude when IL-6 is present in the medium *(114)*. Under estradiol-deficient conditions (i.e., menopause), IL-6 plays a role as a local regulator of bone turnover *(115)*. TNF is necessary for stimulating osteoclastogenesis and also stimulates osteoblasts such that their bone-formative action is hindered. TNF suppresses recruitment of osteoblasts from progenitor cells, inhibits the expression of matrix protein genes, and stimulates expression of genes that amplify osteoclastogenesis. Thus, TNF assails bone at many levels *(116)*. As indicated previously, many postmenopausal women experience hypercalciuria and it may very well be that cytokines play a role in this process *(117)*. The action of HT to reduce bone resorption may be mediated by inhibiting cytokines *(118)*. Further research is needed to understand the connections between HT, cytokines, and calcium homeostasis in postmenopausal women.

Another area that should be investigated is that of perturbations in acid–base balance with menopause because one metabolic consequence is a rise in the venous bicarbonate concentration *(97,119)*, which is reversed by HT *(119,120)*. Orr-Walker and colleagues examined the changes in acid–base metabolism in normal postmenopausal women starting on HT regimens *(121)*. Groups receiving either medroxyprogesterone acetate alone or combined with estrogen exhibited a decrease in arterialized venous blood bicarbonate and P_{CO2}, whereas those receiving estrogen only or placebo did not change. Accompanying changes in blood pH were noted only in those who received combined therapy. With respect to calcium metabolism, only the combined therapy group showed consistent changes, with reductions in urinary calcium excretion and serum phosphate. Bone turnover indexes (i.e., bone-specific alkaline phosphatase, hydroxyproline, osteocalcin, deoxypyridinoline) decreased in both the estrogen only and combined groups, with more consistent and larger changes in the combined therapy group. Thus, the changes in acid–base balance correlated with the suppression of bone resorption, suggesting that acid–base balance may contribute to the effect of HT on bone and calcium balance.

5. CONCLUSIONS

Both heavy smoking and excessive alcohol intake are risk factors for bone loss and osteoporotic fractures. Yet, very moderate alcohol intake has been shown to either not have adverse effects on bone or increase BMD, whereas the effect of light smoking on bone is not clear. Smoking and alcohol intake, particularly with heavier use, affect bone turnover and calcium homeostatis. The deleterious effects on bone seem to be related to the duration of smoking and alcohol use, although coexistent lifestyle factors may also contribute to osteopenia in smokers and drinkers. Hormone therapy in postmenopausal women exerts beneficial effects on bone and calcium homeostasis, but is no longer recommended to prevent or treat osteoporosis because of the increased risk of breast cancer, coronary heart disease, stroke, and venous thromboembolism.

REFERENCES

1. Kelsey JL. Risk factors for osteoporosis and associated fractures. Public Health Rep 1989;104(Suppl): 14–20.
2. Aloia JF, Cohn SH, Vaswani A, Yeh JK, Yuen K, Ellis K. Risk factors for postmenopausal osteoporosis. Am J Med 1985;78:95–100.
3. Seeman E, Melton LJ 3rd, O'Fallon WM, Riggs BL. Risk factors for spinal osteoporosis in men. Am J Med 1983;75:977–983.
4. Slemenda CW, Hui SL, Longcope C, Johnston CC. Cigarette smoking, obesity, and bone mass. J Bone Miner Res 1989;4:737–741.
5. Krall EA, Dawson-Hughes B. Smoking and bone loss among postmenopausal women. J Bone Miner Res 1991;6:331–337.
6. Mazess RB, Barden HS. Bone density in premenopausal women: Effects of age, dietary intake, physical activity, smoking, and birth-control pills. Am J Clin Nutr 1991;53:132–142.
7. Hollenbach KA, Barrett-Connor E, Edelstein SL, Holbrook T. Cigarette smoking and bone mineral density in older men and women. Am J Public Health 1993;83:1265–1270.
8. Garvey AJ, Bosse R, Seltzer CC. Smoking, weight change, and age: A longitudinal analysis. Arch Environ Health 1974;28:327–329.
9. Jensen GF. Osteoporosis of the slender smoker revisited by epidemiologic approach. Eur J Clin Invest 1986;16:239–242.
10. Kaufman DW, Slone D, Rosenberg L, Meittinen OS, Shapiro S. Cigarette smoking and age at natural menopause. Am J Public Health 1980;70:420–422.
11. Hartz AJ, Kelber S, Borkowf H, Wild R, Gillis BL, Rimm AA. The association of smoking with clinical indicators of altered sex steroids—a study of 50,145 women. Public Health Rep 1987;102:254–259.
12. Tokuhata G. Smoking in relation to infertility and fetal loss. Arch Environ Health 1968;17:353–359.
13. Barbieri RL, McShane RM, Ryan KJ. Constituents of cigarette smoke inhibit human granulosa cell aromatase. Fertil Steril 1986;46:232–236.
14. Michnovicz JJ, Hershcopf RJ, Naganuma H, Bradlow HL, Fishman J. Increased 2-hydroxylation of estradiol as a possible mechanism for the anti-estrogenic effect of cigarette smoking. N Engl J Med 1986;315:1305–1309.
15. Krall EA, Dawson-Hughes B. Smoking increases bone loss and decreases intestinal calcium absorption. J Bone Miner Res 1999;14:215–220.

16. Need AG, Kemp A, Giles N, Morris HA, Horowitz M, Nordin BE. Relationships between intestinal calcium absorption, serum vitamin D metabolites, and smoking in postmenopausal women. Osteopors Int 2002;13:83–88.
17. Rapuri P, Gallagher JC, Balhorn KE, Ryschon KL. Alcohol intake and bone metabolism in elderly women. Am J Clin Nutr 2000;72:1206–1213.
18. Brot C, Rye Jørgensen N, Helmer Sørensen O. The influence of smoking on vitamin D status and calcium metabolism. Eur J Clin Nutr 1999;53:920–926.
19. Law MR, Hackshaw AK. A meta-analysis of cigarette smoking, bone mineral density and risk of hip fracture: Recognition of a major effect. Br Med J 1997;315:841–846.
20. Baron J, Farahmand BY, Weiderpass E, et al. Cigarette smoking, alcohol consumption, and risk of hip fracture in women. Arch Intern Med 2001;161:983–988.
21. Nguyen TV, Kelly PJ, Sambrook PN, Gilbert C, Pocock NA, Eisman JA. Lifestyle factors and bone density in the elderly: Implications for osteoporosis prevention. J Bone Miner Res 1994;9:1339–1346.
22. McDermott MT, Witte MC. Bone mineral content in smokers. So Med J 1988;81:477–480.
23. Daniel M, Martin AD, Drinkwater DT. Cigarette smoking, steroid hormones, and bone mineral density of young women. Calcif Tissue Int 1992;50:300–305.
24. Pocock NA, Eisman JA, Kelly PJ, Sambrook PN, Yeates MG. Effects of tobacco use on axial and appendicular bone mineral density. Bone 1989;10:329–331.
25. Saville PD. Changes in bone mass with age and alcoholism. J Bone Joint Surg 1965;47:492–299.
26. Dalen N, Lamke B. Bone mineral losses in alcoholics. Acta Orthop Scand 1976;47:469–471.
27. Spencer H, Rubio N, Rubio E, Indreika M, Seitam A. Chronic alcoholism. Frequently overlooked cause of osteoporosis in men. Am J Med 1986;80:393–397.
28. Crilly RG, Anderson C, Hogan D, Delaquerriere-Richardson L. Bone histomorphometry, bone mass, and related parameters in alcoholic males. Calcif Tissue Int 1988;43:269–276.
29. Verbanck M, Verbanck J, Brauman J, Mullier JP. Bone histology and 25-OH vitamin D plasma levels in alcoholics without cirrhosis. Calcif Tissue Res 1977;22(Suppl):538–541.
30. Lalor BC, France MW, Powell D, Adams PH, Counihan TB. Bone and mineral metabolism and chronic alcohol abuse. Q J Med 1986;59:497–511.
31. Odvina CV, Safi I, Wojtowicz CH, et al. Effect of heavy alcohol intake in the absence of liver disease on bone mass in black and white men. J Clin Endocrinol Metab 1995;80:2499–2503.
32. Laitinen K, Lamberg-Allardt C, Tunninen R, Harkonen M, Välimäki M. Bone mineral density and abstention-induced changes in bone and mineral metabolism in noncirrhotic male alcoholics. Am J Med 1992;93:642–650.
33. Laitinen K, Kärkkäinen M, Lalla M, et al. Is alcohol an osteoporosis-inducing agent for young and middle-aged women? Metabolism 1993;42:875–881.
34. Lindholm J, Steiniche T, Rasmussen E, et al. Bone disorder in men with chronic alcoholism: A reversible disease? J Clin Endocrinol Metab 1991;73:118–124.
35. Bikle DD, Genant HK, Cann C, Recker RR, Halloran BP, Strewler GJ. Bone disease in alcohol abuse. Ann Intern Med 1985;103:42–48.
36. Diamond T, Stiel D, Lunzer M, Wilkinson M, Posen S. Ethanol reduces bone formation and may cause osteoporosis. Am J Med 1989;86:282–288.
37. Labib M, Abdel-Kader M, Ranganath L, Teale D, Marks V. Bone disease in chronic alcoholism: The value of plasma osteocalcin measurement. Alcohol Alcohol 1989;24:141–144.
38. Laitinen K, Lamberg-Allardt C, Tunninen R, et al. Transient hypoparathyroidism during acute alcohol intoxication. N Engl J Med 1991;324:721–727.
39. Rico H, Cabranes JA, Cabello J, Gomez-Castresana F, Hernandez ER. Low serum osteocalcin in acute alcohol intoxication: A direct toxic effect of alcohol on osteoblasts. Bone Miner 1987;2:221–225.
40. Israel Y, Orrego H, Holt S, MacDonald DW, Meema HE. Identification of alcohol abuse: Thoracic fractures on routine X-rays as indicators of alcoholism. Alcoholism 1980;4:420–422.
41. Johnson RD, Davidson S, Saunders JB, Williams R. Fractures on chest radiography as indicators of alcoholism in patients with liver disease. Br Med J 1984;288:365–366.
42. Bjørneboe GE, Bjorneboe A, Johnsen J, et al. Calcium status and calcium-regulating hormones in alcoholics. Alcohol Clin Exp Res 1988;12:229–232.

43. Laitinen K, Välimäki M, Lamberg-Allardt C, Kivisaari et al. Deranged vitamin D metabolism but normal bone mineral density in Finnish noncirrhotic male alcoholics. Alcoholism 1990;14:551–556.
44. Gascon-Barré M. Influence of chronic ethanol consumption on the metabolism and action of vitamin D. J Am Coll Nutr 1985;4:565–574.
45. Persson J, Berg NO, Sjolund K, Stenling R, Magnusson PH. Morphologix changes in the small intestine after chronic alcohol consumption. Scand J Gastroenterol 1990;25:173–184.
46. Duane P, Raja KB, Simpson RJ, Peters TJ. Intestinal iron absorption in chronic alcoholics. Alcohol Alcohol 1992;27:539–544.
47. Bode C, Bode JC. Effect of alcohol consumption on the gut. Best Pract Res Clin Gastroenterol. 2003;17:575–592.
48. Williams GA, Bowser EN, Hargis GK, et al. Effect of ethanol on parathyroid hormone and calcitonin secretion in man. Proc Soc Exp Biol Med 1978;159:187–191.
49. Feitelberg S, Epstein S, Ismail F, D'Amanda C. Deranged bone mineral metabolism in chronic alcoholism. Metabolism 1987;36:322–326.
50. Bikle DD, Stesin A, Halloran BP, Steinbach L, Recker R. Alcohol-induced bone disease: Relationship to age and parathyroid hormone levels. Alcohol Clin Exp Res 1993;17:690–695.
51. Laitinen K, Tahtela R, Luomanmaki K, Välimäki M. Mechanisms of hypocalcemia and markers of bone turnover in alcohol-intoxicated drinkers. Bone Miner 1994;24:171–179.
52. Thomas S, Movsowitz C, Epstein S, Jowell P, Ismail F. The response of circulating parameters of bone mineral metabolism to ethanol- and EDTA-induced hypocalcemia in the rat. Bone Miner 1990;8:1–6.
53. Jorge-Hernandez JA, Gonzalez-Reimers CE, Torres-Ramirez A, et al. Bone changes in alcoholic liver cirrhosis: A histomorphometrical analysis of 52 cases. Dig Dis Sci 1988;33:1089–1095.
54. Inzerillo AM, Zaidi M, Huang CL. Calcitonin: the other thyroid hormone. Thyroid 2002;12:791–798.
55. Deftos LJ. Calcitonin. In: Favus MJ, ed. American Society for Bone and Mineral Research's Primer on the Metabolic Bone Diseases and Disorders of Mineral Metabolism, 5th ed. American Society for Bone and Mineral Research, Washington, DC: 2003; pp. 137–141.
56. May H, Murphy S, Khaw K-T. Alcohol consumption and bone mineral density in older men. Gerontology 1992;41:152–158.
57. Leino A, Impivaara O, Jarvisalo J, Helenius H. Factors related to risk of osteoporosis in 50-year-old women. Calcif Tissue Int 1991;49 (Suppl):S76–S77.
58. Felson DT, Zhang Y, Hannan MT, Kannel WB, Kiel DP. Alcohol intake and bone mineral density in elderly men and women. The Framingham Study. Am J Epidemiol 1995;142:485–492.
59. Ganry O, Baudoin C, Fardellone P. Effect of alcohol intake on bone mineral density in elderly women. The EPIDOS Study. Am J Epidemiol 2000;151:773–780.
60. Alekel DL, Peterson CT, Werner RK, Mortillaro E, Ahmed N, Kukreja SC. Frame size, ethnicity, lifestyle, and biologic contributors to areal and volumetric lumbar spine bone mineral density in Indian/ Pakistani and American Caucasian premenopausal women. J Clin Densit 2002;5:175–186.
61. Alekel DL, Mortillaro E, Hussain EA, et al. Lifestyle and biologic contributors to proximal femur bone mineral density and hip axis length in two distinct ethnic groups of premenopausal women. Osteoporos Int 1999;9:327–338.
62. Gavaler JS, VanThiel DH. The association between moderate alcoholic beverage consumption and serum estradiol and testosterone levels in normal postmenopausal women: relationship to the literature. Alcohol Clin Exp Res 1992;16:87–92.
63. Laitinen K, Lamberg-Allardt C, Tunninen R, Karonen SL, Ylikahri R, Välimäki M. Effects of 3 weeks' moderate alcohol intake on bone and mineral metabolism in normal men. Bone Miner 1991;13:139–151.
64. Hernandez-Avila M, Colditz GA, Stampfer MJ, Rosner B, Speizer FE, Willett WC. Caffeine, moderate alcohol intake, and risk of fractures of the hip and forearm in middle-aged women. Am J Clin Nutr 1991;54:157–163.
65. Paganini-Hill A, Ross RK, Gerkins VR, Henderson BE, Arthur M, Mack TM. Menopausal estrogen therapy and hip fractures. Ann Intern Med 1981;95:28–31.
66. Laitinen K, Välimäki M. Alcohol and bone. Calcif Tissue Int 1991;49:S70–S73.
67. Albright F, Smith PH, Richardson AM. Postmenopausal osteoporosis. JAMA 1941;116:2465–2474.
68. Compston JE. HRT and osteoporosis. Br Med Bull 1992;48:309–344.
69. Riggs BL, Melton III LJ. Involutional osteoporosis. N Engl J Med 1986;314:1676–1686.

70. Aloia JF, Vaswani A, Ellis K, Yuen K, Cohn SH. A model for involutional bone loss. J Lab Clin Invest 1985;106:630–637.

71. Hui SL, Slemenda CW, Johnston CC, Appledorn CR. Effects of age and menopause on vertebral bone density. Bone Miner 1987;2:141–146.

72. Nilas L, Christiansen C. Rates of bone loss in normal women: Evidence of accelerated trabecular bone loss after the menopause. Eur J Clin Invest 1988;18:529–534.

73. Genant HK, Cann CE, Ettinger B, Gilbert SG. Quantitative computed tomography of vertebral spongiosa: a sensitive method for detecting early bone loss after oophorectomy. Ann Intern Med 1982;97:699–705.

74. Sowers MFR, Clark MK, Wallace RB, Jannausch ML, Lemke J. Prospective study of radial bone mineral density in a geographically defined population of postmenopausal Caucasian women. Calcif Tissue Int 1991;48:232–239.

75. Riggs BL, Wahner HW, Seeman E, et al. Changes in bone mineral density of the proximal femur and spine with age. Differences between the postmenopausal and senile osteoporosis syndromes. J Clin Invest 1982;70:716–723.

76. Pun KK, Wong FHW, Loh T. Rapid postmenopausal loss of total body and regional bone mass in normal southern Chinese females in Hong Kong. Osteoporosis Int 1991;1:87–94.

77. Riggs BL, Khosla S, Melton LJ III. A unitary model for involutional osteoporosis: Estrogen deficiency causes both type I and type II osteoporosis in postmenopausal women and contributes to bone loss in aging men. J Bone Miner Res 1998;13:763–773.

78. Ginsburg J. What determines age at menopause? Br Med J 1991;302:1288–1289.

79. Khaw K-T. The menopause and hormone replacement therapy. Postgrad Med J 1992;68:615–623.

80. Komulainen M, Kroger H, Tuppurainen MT, et al. Prevention of femoral and lumbar bone loss with hormone replacement therapy and vitamin D_3 in early postmenopausal women: a population-based 5-year randomized trial. J Clin Endocrinol Metab 1999; 84:546–552.

81. Cauley JA, Seeley DG, Ensrud K, Ettinger B, Black D, Cummings SR. Estrogen replacement therapy and fractures in older women. Study of Osteoporotic Fractures Research Group. Ann Intern Med 1995;122:9–16.

82. Manolagas SC, Jilka RL. Mechanisms of disease: bone marrow, cytokines, and bone remodeling: Emerging insights into the pathophysiology of osteoporosis. N Engl J Med 1995;332:305–311.

83. Collaborative Group on Hormonal Factors in Breast Cancer (CGHFBC). Breast cancer and hormone replacement therapy: Collaborative reanalysis of data from 51 epidemiological studies of 52,705 women with breast cancer and 108,411 without breast cancer. Lancet 1997;350:1047–1059.

84. Beresford SAA, Weiss NS, McKnight B. Risk of endometrial cancer in relation to use of oestrogen combined with cyclic progestagen therapy in postmenopausal women. Lancet 1997;349:458–461.

85. Scharbo-DeHaan M. Hormone replacement therapy. Nurse Pract 1996;21(12 Pt 2):1–13.

86. McNagny SE. Prescribing hormone replacement therapy for menopausal symptoms. Ann Intern Med 1999;131:605–616.

87. Bush TL. Preserving cardiovascular benefits of hormone replacement therapy. J Reprod Med 2000;45(Suppl 3):259–273.

88. Eastell R. Treatment of postmenopausal osteoporosis. N Engl J Med 1998;338:736–746.

89. Writing Group for the Women's Health Initiative Investigators. Risks and benefits of estrogen plus progestin in healthy postmenopausal women: principal results from the Women's Health Initiative randomized controlled trial. JAMA 2002;288:321–333.

90. Kessel B. Alternatives to estrogen for menopausal women. Proc Soc Exp Biol Med 1998;217:38–44.

91. Cauley JA, Robbins J, Chen Z, et al., Women's Health Initiative Investigators. Effects of estrogen plus progestin on risk of fracture and bone mineral density: the Women's Health Initiative randomized trial. JAMA. 2003;290:1729–1738.

92. Groeneveld FP, Bareman FP, Barentsen R, Dokter HJ, Drogendijk AC, Hoes AW. Duration of hormonal replacement therapy in general practice: a follow-up study. Maturitas 1998;29:125–131.

93. Nieves JW, Komar L, Cosman F, Lindsay R. Calcium potentiates the effect of estrogen and calcitonin on bone mass: review and analysis. Am J Clin Nutr 1998;67:18–24.

94. Schneider DL, Barrett-Connor EL, Morton DJ. Timing of postmenopausal estrogen for optimal bone mineral density. The Rancho Bernardo Study. JAMA 1997;277:543–547.

95. Heaney RP, Recker RR, Saville PD. Menopausal changes in bone remodeling. J Lab Clin Med 1978;92:964–970.

96. Heaney RP, Recker RR, Saville PD. Menopausal changes in calcium balance performance. J Lab Clin Med 1978;92:953–963.

97. Nordin BE, Need AG, Morris HA, Horowitz M, Robertson WG. Evidence for a renal calcium leak in postmenopausal women. J Clin Endocrinol Metab 1991;72:401–407.

98. Riis BJ. Biochemical markers of bone turnover in diagnosis and assessment of therapy. Am J Med 1991;91(Suppl5B):64S–68S.

99. Delmas PD. Biochemical markers of bone turnover: methodology and clinical use in osteoporosis. Am J Med 1991;91(5B):59S–63S.

100. Aloia JF, Vaswani A, Yeh JK, McGowan DM, Ross P. Biochemical short-term changes produced by hormonal replacement therapy. J Endocrinol Invest 1991;14:927–934.

101. El-Hajj Fuleihan G, Brown EM, Curtis K, et al. Effect of sequential and daily continuous hormone replacement therapy on indexes of mineral metabolism. Arch Intern Med 1992;152:1904–1909.

102. Marshall RW, Selby PL, Chilvers DC, Hodgkinson A. The effect of ethinyl oestradiol on calcium and bone metabolism in peri- and postmenopausal women. Horm Metab Res 1984;16:97–99.

103. Itoi H, Minakami H, Sato I. Comparison of the long-term effects of oral estriol with the effects of conjugated estrogen, 1-α-hydroxyvitamin D3 and calcium lactate on vertebral bone loss in early menopausal women. Maturitas 1997;28:11–17.

104. Overgaard K, Hansen MA, Jensen SB, Christiansen C. Effect of calcitonin given intranasally on bone mass and fracture rates in established osteoporosis: a dose response study. Br Med J 1992;305:556–561.

105. Gur A, Colpan L, Nas K, et al. The role of trace minerals in the pathogenesis of postmenopausal osteoporosis and a new effect of calcitonin. J Bone Miner Metab 2002;20:39–43.

106. Thamsborg G. Effect of nasal salmon calcitonin on calcium and bone metabolism. Dan Med Bull 1999;46:118–126.

107. Silverman SL. Calcitonin. Rheum Dis Clin North Am 2001;27:187–196.

108. Pontiroli AE, Pajetta E, Scaglia L, Rubinacci et al. Analgesic effect of intranasal and intramuscular salmon calcitonin in post-menopausal osteoporosis: a double-blind, double-placebo study. Aging Clin Exp Res 1994;6:459–463.

109. Gur A, Denli A, Cevik R, Nas K, Karakoc M, Sarac AJ. The effects of alendronate and calcitonin on cytokines in postmenopausal osteoporosis: a 6-month randomized and controlled study. Yonsei Med J 2003;44:99–109.

110. Gowen M, Meikle MC, Reynolds JJ. Stimulation of bone resorption in vitro by a non-prostanoid factor released by human monocytes in culture. Biochim Biophy Acta 1983;762:471–474.

111. Gowen M, Mundy GR. Actions of recombinant interleukin 1, interleukin 2, and interferon-γ on bone resorption in vitro. J Immunol 1986;136:2478–2482.

112. Pfeilschifter J, Chen U, Bird A, Mundy GR, Roodman GD. Interleukin-1 and tumor necrosis factor stimulate the formation of human osteoclast-like cells in vitro. J Bone Miner Res 1989;4:113–118.

113. Thomson BM, Saklatvala J, Chambers TJ. Osteoblasts mediate interleukin-1 stimulation of bone resorption by rat osteoclasts. J Exp Med 1986;164:104–112.

114. Black K, Mundy GR, Garrett IR. Interleukin-6 causes hypercalcemia in vivo and enhances the bone resorbing potency of interleukin-1 and tumor necrosis factors by two orders of magnitude in vitro. J Bone Miner Res 1990;5(Suppl 2):Abstract 787.

115. Girasole G, Jilka RL, Passeri G, et al. 17-β estradiol inhibits interleukin-6 production by bone marrow-derived stromal cells and osteoblasts in vitro: a potential mechanism for the antiosteoporotic effect of estrogens. J Clin Invest 1992;89:883–891.

116. Nanes MS. Tumor necrosis factor-alpha: Molecular and cellular mechanisms in skeletal pathology. Gene 2003;321:1–15.

117. Weisinger JR, Alonzo E, Bellorin-Font E, et al. Possible role of cytokines on the bone mineral loss in idiopathic hypercalciuria. Kidney Int 1996;49:244–250.

118. Rogers A, Eastell R. Effects of estrogen therapy of postmenopausal women on cytokines measured in peripheral blood. J Bone Miner Res 1998;13:1577–86.

119. Adami S, Gatti D, Bertoldo F, et al. The effects of menopause and estrogen replacement therapy on the renal handling of calcium. Osteoporos Int 1992;2:180–185.

120. McKane WR, Khosla S, Burritt MF, et al. Mechanism of renal calcium conservation with estrogen replacement therapy in women in early postmenopause—a clinical research center study. J Clin Endocrinol Metab 1995;80:3458–3464.

121. Orr-Walker BJ, Horne AM, Evans MC, et al. Hormone replacement therapy causes a respiratory alkalosis in normal postmenopausal women. J Clin Endocrinol Metab 1999;84:1997–2001.

14 Influence of Physical Activity on Calcium and Bone

Matthew Vukovich and Bonny Specker

KEY POINTS

- Both exercise intensity and duration impact calcium and bone metabolism.
- Exercise early in life leads to increased bone mass at sites that are loaded.
- Cortical bone density and bone size is dependent on interactions between hormonal changes as well as loads placed on the skeleton.
- Calcium intake may modify the bone response to loading. It is speculated that protein intake also may modify the bone response to loading, possibly by influencing insulin-like growth factor-1 concentrations.

1. INTRODUCTION

The degree of bone gain and loss over an individual's lifetime is thought to determine the risk of osteoporosis and fracture as an adult. Traditionally, two major factors thought to determine whether an individual is at increased risk for fracture are the peak bone mass achieved early in life, which is determined from the gain in bone during childhood, and the rate of loss later in life. For many years, research has focused on strategies or interventions for decreasing the rate of bone loss that occurs later in life.

Childhood fractures are increasingly recognized as a significant problem. The incidence of childhood distal forearm fractures was recently reported to have increased 32% among males and 56% among females in the years 1999–2001 compared with 1969–1971 *(1)*. Although the cause is unclear, this dramatic increase in forearm fractures may be due to the adverse bone effects of decreased activity levels or poor dietary intake during childhood.

Recently, the importance of bone size, rather than just bone mineral content (BMC) and bone mineral density (BMD), has been recognized as an important factor in determining bone strength. Although numerous cross-sectional and longitudinal studies have shown a relationship between BMD and physical activity levels *(2–5)*, recent pediatric activity trials indicate that physical activity also may increase bone size, thereby increasing bone strength. A clearer picture of how activity and diet influence bone is emerging with the ability to measure subtle changes in bone size through the development of software to perform, for example, hip structural analyses (HSA) using data obtained from

From: *Calcium in Human Health*
Edited by: C. M. Weaver and R. P. Heaney © Humana Press Inc., Totowa, NJ

dual energy X-ray absorptiometry (DXA) hip scans or by the use of peripheral quantitative computed tomography (pQCT) technology.

Physical activity is defined as any form of muscular activity that results in an increase in energy expenditure. Exercise is planned physical activity, with a goal of improving or maintaining fitness. When prescribing exercise programs, the frequency, intensity, and duration (time) principle is followed. These three criteria are used to ensure that a proper dose of exercise is performed to bring about a desired effect. To achieve the desired effect, the system must include overload, or a degree of stress to which the individual is unaccustomed. For example, for muscle to hypertrophy, the muscle must be overloaded by increasing the intensity, frequency, or duration of the strength training program. Mechanical loading of bone stimulates remodeling, and, as with muscle, for bone to adapt, physical activity must produce enough of a stress to overload the bone.

The purpose of this chapter is to (1) provide an overview on the effect of exercise on calcium homeostasis, growth, and bone; (2) describe the effects of mechanical loading on bone; (3) provide an overview of pediatric activity studies; and (4) discuss factors that may modify the bone response to loading.

2. EFFECT OF EXERCISE ON CALCIUM HOMEOSTASIS AND GROWTH FACTORS

2.1. Relationship Between Calcium Homeostasis and Exercise

The homeostatic mechanisms involved in calcium metabolism are discussed in Chapters 10 and 11. With regard to the effects of exercise on serum calcium and parathyroid hormone (PTH) concentrations, the data are somewhat equivocal, and said effects may depend on the intensity and duration of the exercise regimen and the training status of the individual. Increases in ionized calcium during exercise appear to be related directly to exercise-induced acidosis and therefore, exercise intensity (6,7). However, the increase in serum ionized calcium concentrations during and following prolonged endurance exercise does not result in a decrease in serum PTH concentrations, possibly because of the increase in catecholamines. Short-duration, high-intensity exercise increases ionized calcium with a concomitant decrease in serum PTH concentrations (8). Training status appears to affect the exercise-associated response of PTH (9,10). Salvesen and co-workers found that following 50 min of running, well-trained men experienced an increase in serum PTH concentration whereas fire-fighters, who were less trained, did not (10). Both groups of men experienced an increase in serum calcium (10). However, other studies report that resting PTH concentrations are actually lower in trained vs untrained individuals (9). It can be concluded from these studies, as well as others, that endurance exercise must last at least 30 min in order to elicit an increase in circulating PTH concentrations (8,11,12).

Studies involving the effect of resistance training on serum PTH concentrations are conflicting. Rong and co-workers reported an increase in serum PTH concentrations immediately following a period of strength training (13), whereas others report a decrease (14). Bell and co-workers studied a relatively small number of male weight-lifters compared with age-matched controls, and although they did not find statistically different PTH concentrations, they did speculate that subtle differences in PTH concentrations may have been of sufficient magnitude to produce the increases in serum 1,25 dihydroxyvitamin D (1,25-$(OH)_2$ D) and urinary cyclic AMP concentrations that were observed *(15)*. These differences in PTH response to exercise could be due to differences in the intensity and duration of the training periods, as well as acute vs long-term exercise effects on PTH.

2.2. Relationship Between Growth Factors and Exercise

Growth hormone (GH) and insulin-like growth factor (IGF)-1 have major influences on bone growth and mineralization and are reviewed in detail elsewhere *(16,17)*. Briefly, GH and IGF-1 have direct and indirect effects on osteoblasts and osteoclasts. Bone formation and resorption increase when GH is given to GH-deficient individuals, indicating an increase in bone modeling and/or remodeling *(18)*. GH and IGF-1 increase bone size and BMC, but not BMD *(19)*. Whereas the GH–IGF axis is likely responsible for the large increases in bone length and bone circumference during early puberty, increased concentrations of estrogen may decrease endosteal resorption and lead to increased cortical thickness in mid to late puberty. Estrogen also plays an important role in the closure of the growth plates *(20)*.

Duration and intensity of exercise have significant impacts on GH and IGF-1 secretion. Acute endurance exercise results in a significant increase in serum GH concentrations *(21,22)*, whereas acute resistance exercise results in a significant decrease in serum IGF-1 and IGF-binding protein (IGFBP)-3 concentrations *(23)*. Furthermore, skeletal muscle IGF-1 expression is downregulated at the mRNA level during the initial recovery phase following resistance exercise *(24)*, but increases to levels higher than pre-exercise values at 24 and 48 h after the exercise bout *(24,25)*. Treadmill running appears to produce similar results *(26)*. It is not known what happens to IGF-1 mRNA in bone cells after acute bouts of exercise.

Exercise training, both resistance and endurance, results in significant increases in serum IGF-1 concentrations, which have been observed in both young and older individuals *(27–29)*. The role that nutritional status plays in modifying this hormonal response to exercise is described below.

3. EFFECTS OF MECHANICAL LOADING ON BONE

3.1. Methodological Issues With Measuring Bone

Cross-sectional and longitudinal studies of factors influencing bone accretion or BMD changes during infancy and childhood have been reported *(30–34)*. It is often difficult to interpret the findings of BMD changes during childhood because most studies use DXA technology, which measures bone in two, rather than three, dimensions, and therefore cannot measure true volumetric density. A larger bone size may artificially inflate areal bone mineral density (aBMD) measurements as shown in Fig. 1. This is illustrated in studies that show that aBMD increases with age, but volumentric bone mineral density (vBMD) measured by computed tomography is relatively constant during childhood until the time of puberty, when there is a large increase between Tanner stages 2 and 3 *(35)*. Several mathematical methods have been proposed with which to adjust this two-dimensional aBMD to more closely reflect vBMD *(36,37)*; however, it is not evident that these adjustments are satisfactory. These methods include the calculation of bone mineral apparent density for the spine or femoral neck, dividing the BMC by the projected bone

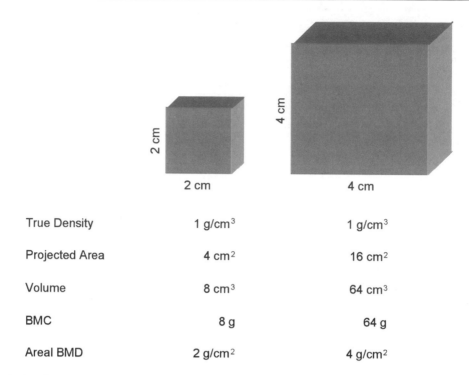

Fig. 1. Areal measurements of bone mineral density (BMD) are influenced by the size of the bone being measured. BMC, bone mineral content.

area to the power of 1.5 for spine *(38)* or 2.0 for the femoral neck *(39)*; application of formulas for the femoral neck measurements that assume a cylinder shape *(40)*; or inclusion of bone and body size parameters in a regression approach (size-adjusted bone mineral content [SA-BMC]) *(37)*. This limitation of DXA-derived bone measurements, as well as the possibility of subtle changes in bone conformation that are not detected using DXA, must be considered when reviewing results of activity trials, especially during growth.

3.2. Cortical Bone Changes During Growth

Garn and co-workers conducted many of the original studies on human cortical bone growth and estimated periosteal and endosteal circumferences in cortical bone (Fig. 2) with age, based on more than 25,000 hand radiographs that they collected throughout the life cycle *(41)*. Briefly, increases in periosteal growth resemble increases in axial growth, with a period of rapid growth early in infancy followed by a period of more moderate growth until the hormone-mediated growth spurt occurs. The hormone-mediated increase in periosteal diameter occurs earlier in females than in males, although the final size in males is greater. Resorption along the endosteal surface occurs from birth until the second decade in both sexes, whereas estrogen is thought to decrease resorption along the endosteal surface among females at the time of adolescence leading to a smaller

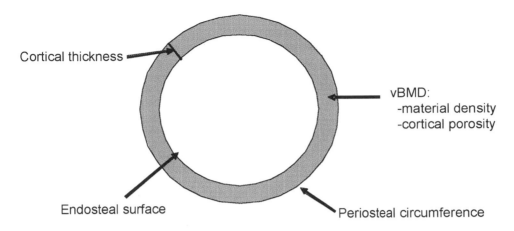

Fig. 2. Schematic of the cross-section of the shaft of a long bone, illustrating the periosteal and endosteal surfaces and the thickness of the cortical shell. The volumetric bone mineral density (vBMD) is a measure of the material density and the cortical porosity.

endocortical diameter. The changes that occur in the periosteal and endosteal circumferences during the pubertal growth spurt lead to a gradual increase in cortical thickness, which is generally greater in males than in females *(41)*. This growth in cortical bone and bone size is dependent on interactions between hormonal changes that are occurring, as well as the loads that are placed on the skeleton, and possibly substrate availability (i.e., calcium and phosphorus).

3.3. Animal Studies of Bone Loading

Animal studies show that skeletal loading can increase bone remodeling within a short time *(42,43)*. In general, these studies find that the responses to increased loading consist of an increase in periosteal circumference and cortical thickness, translating into increased bone strength *(43–45)*. Some investigators find that the loading effect on increasing periosteal expansion appears to be greater at distal vs proximal sites *(46,47)*.

The *amount* of load that is necessary to increase mineralization and change bone conformation appears to be small. In a study by Umemura et al., rats performing five jumps per day to a 40 cm platform for 8 wk had similar increases in tibial and femoral bone mineral as rats that jumped 100 times per day (42). The *frequency* of the load also appears to be important. Srinivasan et al. found insertion of a 10-s interval between low magnitude loads in an avian model lead to significantly greater periosteal bone formation compared with a similar number of loads occurring at 1/s *(48)*. They concluded that these data support the hypothesis that fluid flow near osteocytes underlies the mechanotrans-duction within bone, and that there must be sufficient time between loads for the viscous fluid flow to recover from inertial damping. The *type* of load may also affect bone conformational changes. Loading activities that result in high bending and torsional loads put greater strains on the bone's outer surface, and bone will respond through periosteal expansion. Compression loads place strains on the bone that are more uniform throughout the bone and may induce bone apposition on the endosteal surfaces.

4. OVERVIEW OF PEDIATRIC ACTIVITY STUDIES

4.1. Cross-Sectional and Longitudinal Studies of Childhood Activity and Adult Bone

Many cross-sectional studies have shown a role of early physical activity on BMD later in life. Kriska and co-workers reported in the 1980s that the radius BMD of postmenopausal women was more strongly correlated with recall of adolescent activity levels than activity levels during the postmenopausal years (49). Over the last decade, numerous studies have reported associations between adult BMD and early activity levels (2,50–55). Many of these studies involved women or men who participated in competitive sports around the time of puberty, whereas other studies find that recreational activities early in life also increase BMD. A case–control study conducted by Neives et al. found that recreational activities in adolescence and early adulthood afford greater protection against hip fracture than either teenage calcium intake or milk-drinking (56).

Joakimsen and co-workers summarized the available literature (17 studies) on hip fracture risk and activity levels (57). Overall, the results indicated that increased physical activity is protective against hip fracture and that this association was present for activity from childhood through adult life. These studies indicated that women who were physically active earlier in life have a higher BMD and decreased fracture risk compared with women who categorized themselves as less active. However, because activity levels appear to track throughout life, it is difficult to separate the effect of childhood and adult activity on BMD, or to determine at what age increased activity leads to beneficial bone effects. Another disadvantage to cross-sectional studies is the possible bias in recalling activity levels early in life.

The advantage of the longitudinal study design is the prospective collection of activity data. Some studies have made use of activity data collected longitudinally during childhood to determine whether adult BMD was associated with previous activity levels (4,5). Information on physical activity levels and dietary intake were obtained in the Cardiovascular Risk in Young Finns Study Group at three occassions over 11 yr in subjects 9 to 18 yr of age (4). Lumbar spine and femoral neck BMD were measured when these subjects were 20 to 29 yr of age and childhood physical activity was found to be a significant predictor of adult BMD. Similar results were obtained in the Amsterdam Growth and Health Study, which consisted of 182 males and females who were followed from 13 to 28 yr of age (5). Weight-bearing activity and calcium intakes were assessed during three periods: 13–17 yr, 13–21 yr, and 13–27 yr of age. Only weight-bearing activity, and not calcium intake, was significantly associated with lumbar spine BMD at age 27 yr, and this was true for activity in all three age groupings.

Although these older studies used primarily DXA technology to show an effect of childhood activity on adult BMD, recent studies using pQCT have shown that the effect of activity is primarily on bone size and cortical thickness, and not true vBMD (58). A study of female tennis and squash players found that the effect of bone loading on bone size, as measured by total cross-sectional area of the humerus, was greater if the women started playing racquet sports prior to or at the time of menarche (59). Although there was no difference in cortical vBMD by pQCT, the larger bone size and cortical wall thickness resulted in greater aBMD in the young vs old starters. These studies are important in understanding how physical activity and bone loading may influence bone strength.

Unfortunately, there are limitations of measuring the cortical vBMD of the small bones of children owing to a partial volume effect, which results in underestimation of cortical density when the cortex is too thin *(60)*.

4.2. Pediatric Trials of Physical Activity on Bone

Fourteen activity trials are summarized in Table 1. Sample sizes ranged from 38 to 178, and trials were of varying length, ranging from 3 to 12 mo. An assortment of bone sites was measured using various methods to adjust for bone size. DXA technology was used in the majority of studies, although HSA and pQCT technology were used in some in order to determine more subtle activity effects on bone size *(61–64)*.

Overall, there appears to be no consistent pattern in the effects measured by DXA (Table 2). Neither of the two studies conducted in boys found an effect of activity on bone size, whereas only one study in girls found a larger bone size in the exercise group, but only at the femoral neck. None of the studies conducted in pubertal children found an effect of activity on bone size, and only two of the three studies among prepubertal children reported a larger bone size among the exercise group at the femoral neck. Although one study did not report a bone size effect with exercise using DXA technology *(65)*, a further analysis of the same cohort using HSA found a greater increase in femoral neck cross-sectional area among pubertal girls randomized to jumping *(63)*. One study using pQCT reported a greater periosteal circumference at the 20% distal tibia among young prepubertal children and concluded that this supported the findings of animal studies showing an effect at more distal bone sites *(62)*. BMD and BMC results are conflicting, both for girls and boys, except at the leg where all studies that have reported this site find a greater BMC and BMD in the intervention vs control group.

It is likely that there are numerous factors that may be influencing the bone response to activity or bone loading. As described above the amount, frequency and type of load that is applied to the skeleton may influence its response to the load. In addition, there may be other factors that modify the relationship between bone and physical activity.

5. FACTORS THAT MAY MODIFY THE BONE RESPONSE TO LOADING

5.1. Body Mass Index

One study found that the bone benefit in prepubertal boys varied depending on the child's body mass index (BMI) *(66)*. In boys with a low or average BMI, an exercise intervention resulted in greater increases in hip and trochanter BMD and total body and spine BMC compared with controls, whereas no exercise effect was found among boys with a high BMI. The authors speculated that one reason for the lack of findings in the high BMI group was that the skeleton of the heavy boys may not respond to an exercise program, because it is under substantial adaptive stress because of greater body weight.

The idea that the loads the skeleton is accustomed to determines the bone response to exercise also would explain the findings of Van Langendonck and co-workers, who observed that the bone benefit from exercise was only significant when the analysis was limited to girls who had minimal weight-bearing activity during their leisure time *(67)*. In this situation, the girl's skeleton would not have been under adaptive stress prior to intervention, which may lead to a greater response to the intervention.

Table 1

Summary of Pediatric Activity Intervention Trials

Reference	Study design	Description of intervention	Bone measurement method	Bone sites measured	Significant findings	Comments
Morris et al. (70)	Longitudinal, nonrandomized trial with exercise group within specific schools (N = 4) 10 mo duration 73 premenarcheal girls aged 9–10 yr (71 completed)	N = 38 for I N = 33 for C I = high impact and strength exercises 30 min three times per week C = encouraged not to change activity patterns	DXA for BMC, BA, BMD, and BMAD (spine & neck)	Total body Hip (total, femoral neck) Lumbar spine	Greater increases in total body BMC & BMD; spine BMD, and BMAD; hip BMC and BMD, and femoral neck BMC and BA in I vs C Regional TB results: greater increases in leg, arm and pelvic BMD in I vs C	I group gained more lean mass in total body, trunk and leg than C and lost more TB fat mass Mean Ca intake approx 980 mg/d Mean attendance (midway) was 96%
Bradney et al. (64)	Controlled prospective study 8 mo duration 38/40 boys aged 8.4–11.8 yr from 2 schools (I vs C) completed study All prepubertal (Tanner & serum testosterone & E2)	N = 19 for I N = 19 for C 30 min weight bearing activity three times a week for 32 wk	DXA for BMC, aBMD and areal vBMD (femoral midshaft & L3 vertebrate) Estimates of periosteal & endocortical widths, cortical thickness, CSMI, section modulus, and strength index made from hip scan	Total body Hip Spine	Total body aBMD, leg aBMD from TB scan, and spine aBMD greater in I vs C Femoral midshaft: endocortical thickness and medullary area and volume less, while cortical thickness, cortical volume, BMC, aBMD, and areal vBMD greater in I vs C	Mean attendance was 96 Groups matched for age, standing height, sitting height, weight and baseline aBMD
Specker et al. (32)	RCT 12 mo duration 72 infants 69/72 infants completed 9 mo of intervention	N = 34 for I N = 35 for C I = bone loading activities for 15–20 min/d, five times	DXA for SA-BMC	Total body	Significant interaction between Ca intake and activity group No difference between ac-	Infants tolerated bone loading activities approx 65% of the time

	All infants enrolled prior to 6 mo of age, with interventions beginning at 6 mo	a week C = infants held for equivalent time		tivity groups in TB SA-BMC gain for high Ca intake; TB SA-BMC gain was lower in I vs C for low Ca intake infants had less SA-BMC gain	More compliant
Heinonen et al. (61)	Controlled trial 9 mo duration 139 girls both pre- and post-menarcheal (126 completed)	Premenarcheal: N = 25 for I N = 33 for C Postmenarcheal: N = 39 for I C = 29 for C I = 2 50-min step-aerobic sessions/wk C = usual activities	DXA for BMC pQCT midshaft of tibia for cortical BMD, cortical area, and polar section modulus (BSI) Spine Hip (total, femoral neck) Midshaft of tibia (pQCT)	Pre-menarcheal girls: gains in spine and femoral neck BMC greater in I vs C, no differences in midshaft tibia Postmenarcheal girls: no significant group differences	Mean Ca intake approx 1040 mg/d Compliance 70% and 65% in pre- and postmenarcheal groups
Witzke and Snow (84)	Nonrandomized trial 9 mo 56 girls aged 13–15 yr from 2 high schools (53 completed)	N = 25 for I N = 28 for C I = 30–45 min three times a week using weighted vests and plyometrics C = usual activities	DXA for BMC Total body Spine Hip (femoral neck, trochanter, & femoral midshaft)	No significant differences between groups in BMC change I group gained trochanter BMC, while C group did not (groups did not differ)	Controls matched by age and months past menarche Average of 22.7 mo past menarche
McKay et al. (85)	RCT with school as unit 8 mo duration 144 boys and girls aged 6.9–10.2 yr from 10 schools All boys T1; 66/74 girls T1, 8 girls T2	N = 63 for I N = 81 for C I = 10 tuck jumps three times a week + loading activities twice a week C = regular physical education classes	DXA for BMC, BA BMD Total body Lumbar spine Hip (total, femoral neck, trochanter)	Trochanter BMD greater in I vs C	Children in C schools had higher baseline activity levels & greater vertical jump than children in I schools Height gain was greater in C vs I Mean Ca intake = 988 mg/d

(continued)

Table 1 (Continued)

Reference	Study design	Description of intervention	Bone measurement method	Bone sites measured	Significant findings:	Comments
MacKelvie et al. (65)	RCT with school as unit 7 mo duration 383 boys and girls from 14 schools, 191 girls aged 8.7–11.7 yr included in this analysis (177 completed)	Prepubertal (T1): N = 44 for I N = 26 for C Early pubertal (T2 & T3): N = 43 for I C = 64 for C I = 10–12 min/d three times a week high-impact jumping C = stretching	DXA for BMC, aBMD, and areal vBMD (femoral neck)	Total body Lumbar spine Hip (total, femoral neck, trochanter)	Prepubertal: No differences between I and C Early Puberty: greater increases in spine BMC and aBMD and femoral neck BMC, and aBMD areal vBMD in I vs C	Compliance averaged approx 80%
MacKelvie et al. (66)	RCT with school as unit 7 mo duration 383 boys and girls from 14 schools, 133 boys aged 8.8–11.7 yr included in this analysis (121 completed) All T1 at baseline	N = 61 for I N = 60 for C I = 10–12 min/d three times a week high-impact jumping C = stretching	DXA for BMC, aBMD, & areal vBMD (femoral neck)	Total body Lumbar spine Hip (total, femoral neck, trochanter)	Greater increases in TB BMC and hip aBMD in I vs C	Compliance averaged approx 80% Approx 40% of boys advanced to T2 during study Boys with low/average BMI had greater change in LS BMC and trochanter BMD in I vs C No differences between I and C in any measure for high BMI boys
Fuchs et al. (69)	RCT with classroom as unit 7 mo duration 100 consenting boys and girls aged 5.9–9.8yr in 5 classrooms (89 completed) All were T1 at baseline and final visits	N = 45 for I (25 boys) N = 44 for C (26 boys) I = 20 min three times a week of 100 jumps off 61 cm box C = 20 min three times a week of stretching	DXA for BMC, BA, aBMD	Femoral neck Lumbar spine	Greater increases in femoral neck BMC, BA and spine BMC and aBMD in jumping vs stretching group	Mean Ca intake approx 1265 mg/d Overall attendance 86–100%
Petit et al. (63) (See also ref. 65)	RCT with school as unit 7 mo duration 383 boys and girls from 14	Prepubertal: N = 44 for I N = 26 for C	HSA from DXA hip scan including areal vBMD, CSA, subperiosteal	DXA HSA of neck, intertrochanter and femoral shaft	Prepubertal girls: no effect of activity on any bone measure	

	schools, 177 girls included in this analysis. Prepubertal (T1) and early pubertal (T2 & T3) girls. Mean age of both groups = 10 yr. Early pubertal: $N = 43$ for I, $N = 64$ for C, I = 10–12 min/d three times a week high-impact jumping, C = stretching	width, endosteal diameter, CWT, section modulus		Early pubertal girls: greater gains in FN and intertrochanter BMD; greater increases in CSA, CWT, and section modulus of the femoral neck	Baseline Ca intake = 940 mg/d
Specker et al. (62)	2×2 RCT with calcium and activity as main effects. 12 mo duration. 239 boys and girls 3–5 yr (178 completed with >50% attendance). Mean age = 4 yr. $N = 88$ for I, $N = 90$ for C, I = 30 min loading/d, 5d/wk (gross motor), C = arts and crafts activities (fine motor)	DXA for SA-BMC, BA pQCT % for PC, EC, cortical area, CWT	Total body pQCT of 20% tibia	Interaction between Ca and activity in change of leg SA-BMC, and cortical area and CWT at study completion. Interaction indicated a greater gain in leg SA-BMC and larger cortical area and CWT in Ca+gross motor group vs other groups	
Iuliano-Burns et al. (81)	2×2 RCT with calcium and activity as main effects. 8.5 mo duration. 73 girls aged 7–11 yr (66 completed). Mean age = 8.8y (T1 & T2). $N = 34$ for I, $N = 36$ for C, I = 20 min three times a week of high-impact activities, C = 20 min three times a week of low-impact activities	DXA for BMC	Total body and spine	Ca-by-exercise interaction detected at the femur. Main effect of exercise at tibia-fibula	Ca was fortified (434 mg/d) vs nonfortified foods. Baseline Ca approx 640 mg/d. Sample size not based on detecting interaction. Mean attendance was 93%
Van Langendonck et al. (67)	RCT. 9 mo duration. 21 prepubertal female monozygotic twins aged 8.7 yr. $N = 21$ for I, $N = 21$ for C, I = 10 min of high impact exercise three times a week	DXA for BMC, BA, & aBMD	Total body (total and right arm) Spine Hip (total, femoral neck)	No group differences except among 12 twin pairs who did not do high-impact leisure time activities.	Mean attendance approx 69%

(continued)

Table 1 (Continued)

Reference	Study design	Description of intervention	Bone measurement method	Bone sites measured	Significant findings:	Comments
					For these girls there was a greater hip BMC and aBMD in I vs C	
Stear et al. (82)	2 × 2 RCT with calcium and exercise as main effects 15.5 mo duration 144 females aged 16–18 yr (131 completed)	N = 75 for I N = 56 for C (N = 20 for >50% attendance) I = 45min exercise class 3 times/wk C = no intervention Results are for good attendance only	DXA for BMC, BA, and SA-BMC	Total body Spine Radius (total, distal & ultradistal) Hip (total, neck, trochanter, intertrochanter)	No effect if intent-to-treat analysis performed Based on good compliance (>50% attendance with exercises): no effect of loading on BMC or BA at any site. SA-BMC was greater with loading at the total hip and trochanter	Mean attendance was 36% Baseline Ca intake = 938 mg/d No Ca-by-activity interaction, although authors note that study was not sized to detect interaction
Johannsen et al. (83)	RCT 3 mo duration 55 boys & girls aged 3–5, 7–8, 11–12, & 15–18 yr (54 completed) 26 prepubertal (T1), 12 peripubertal T2&T3; 16 pubertal (T4&T5)	N = 26 for I N = 28 for C I = 25 jumps/d five times a week for 12 wk C = no intervention	DXA for SA-BMC & BA pQCT 4% tibia measures of total BMC, vBMD and bone area; 20% tibi a measures of periosteal & endosteal circumferences & cortical area	Total body (total & leg) Spine Hip (femoral neck) 4% and 20% distal tibia	Greater increases in total body and leg SA-BMC Pubertal status-by -activity interaction significant for spine SA-BMC and 4% tibia total BMC & BMD: changes greater with I vs C in pubertal, but less in peripubertal children.	Mean Ca intake = 1130 mg/d Change in leg BMC correlated with Ca intake in I group, but no correlation in C group Mean attendance was 76%

T, Tanner stage; N, number; I, intervention group; C, control group; DXA, dual energy x-ray absorptiometry; BMC, bone mineral content; BA, bone area; BMD, bone mineral density; BMAD, bone mineral apparent density; CSMI, cross-sectional moment of inertia; aBMD, areal bone mineral density; RCT, randomized clinical trial; SA-BMC, size-adjusted bone mineral content; pQCT, peripheral quantitative computed tomography; PC, periosteal circumference; EC, endosteal circumference; CSA, cross-sectional area; CWT, cortical wall thickness; E2, estradiol; TB, total body.

Table 2

Percent of Studies Finding a Positive Effect of Exercise Based on DXA Findings (number/number conducted)

	Bone Size				BMD or SA-BMC					BMC				
	TB	HIP	FN	LS	TB	HIP	FN	LS	LEG	TB	HIP	FN	LS	LEG
Boys	0	0	0	0	50% (1/2)	100% (1/1)	0% (0/1)	50% (1/2)	100% (1/1)	100% (1/1)	0% (0/1)	0% (0/1)	50% (1/2)	100% (1/1)
Girls	0% (0/3)	0% (0/3)	50% (1/2)	0% (0/3)	20% (1/5)	20% (3/5)	60% (1/4)	25% (2/4)	50% (1/1)	17% (1/6)	40% (2/5)	50% (3/6)	29% (2/7)	100% (1/1)
Gender not separated	0% (0/3)	0% (0/3)	33% (1/3)	0% (0/3)	0% (0/5)	100% (1/1)	0% (0/4)	25% (1/4)	100% (1/1)	67% (2/3)	0% (0/1)	50% (2/4)	75% (3/4)	100% (2/2)
TOTAL	0% 0/6	0% 0/6	40% 2/5	0% 0/6	17% 2/12	71% 5/7	11% 1/9	40% 4/10	100% 2/2	40% 4/10	29% 2/7	45% 5/11	46% 6/13	100% 4/4
Prepubertal	0% (0/4)	0% (0/2)	57% (2/3)	0% (0/4)	29% (2/7)	80% (4/5)	0% (0/6)	43% (3/7)	100% (2/2)	50% (3/6)	50% (2/4)	67% (4/6)	50% (4/8)	100% (3/3)
Pubertal	0% (0/2)	0% (0/1)	0% (0/2)	0% (0/2)	0% (0/3)	50% (1/2)	50% (1/2)	33% (1/3)	0	25% (1/4)	0% (0/3)	20% (1/5)	40% (2/5)	100% (1/1)

BMD, bone mineral density; BMC, bone mineral content; SA-BMC, size adjusted BMC; TB, total body; FN, femoral neck; LS, lumbar spine.

5.2. Pubertal or Hormonal Status

As described earlier, there appear to be different responses to bone loading activities among prepubertal and pubertal children, especially with regard to the effect on bone size. None of the studies conducted in pubertal children has found a benefit of bone loading activities on bone size. However, many of these studies did not measure distal sites, which are thought to be more likely to increase in periosteal circumference in response to bone-loading activities (46,47). The difficulty with assessing the influence of puberty on bone response to loading is that the definition of puberty varies from one study to the other. In some studies puberty is defined based on menarcheal status, whereas others considered Tanner stages 2 and 3 to be pubertal.

Some investigators have proposed that estrogen augments the bone response to loading (68). If estrogen modifies the bone response to loading, it may explain why some trials find beneficial bone effects in pubertal, but not prepubertal children (65). However, several trials report beneficial bone effects of activity in prepubertal children and not pubertal children (64,69,70), leading to the speculation that increased activity may enhance bone formation during the prepubertal years by acting synergistically with GH (71). During puberty, there appears to be decreased resorption along the endosteal surface as well as an increase in vBMD of cortical bone among girls (72). Cortical bone vBMD reflects not only the material density of cortical bone, but also cortical porosity. Jarvinen and co-workers recently proposed that estrogen packs bone into the cortex and that this increase in cortical vBMD and thickness actually leads to a bone that is less responsive to mechanical strain (73). This may explain why some of the activity trials among pubertal girls do not find a beneficial effect of activity on changes in bone size.

5.3. Energy and Protein Intake

The synthesis and secretion of IGF-1 is dependent on GH and the availability of adequate nutrient intake (74). The increase in IGF-1 concentrations may, therefore, signal target cells that adequate nutrients are available for growth and repair. Factors that influence IGF-1 concentrations or its binding proteins will be important modulators of biological activity. Research has found that the plasma concentrations of IGF-1 and the IGFBPs are largely affected by dietary energy and protein intake (75).

Energy intake appears to alter plasma IGF-1 concentrations as well as its physiological action. Isley and co-workers reported an approx 60% decrease in IGF-1 concentrations with 5 d of fasting (76). Refeeding returned serum IGF-1 concentrations toward baseline, but at 5 d, levels were still approx 30% below prefasting conditions. Energy balance during exercise training also has an effect on IGF-I levels. Nemet et al. reported a significant reduction in IGF-1 concentrations, and an increase in IGFBP-1, during 7 d of exercise training with a negative energy balance of 2000 kcal (77).

A reduction in protein consumption with or without adequate energy intake also results in a decrease in plasma IGF-1I concentrations. This decrease in circulating IGF-1 may be the result of a decrease in synthesis or release of IGF-1 by the liver or both. Furthermore, protein restriction also may increase receptor resistance to GH at the liver or to IGF-1 at target tissues. In the study by Isley et al. described above, the investigators compared the effect of low protein, isocaloric diets during refeeding on IGF-1 concentrations (76). They reported that dietary protein reduction (1.35 g/kg body weight/d vs 0.43 g/kg/d) during the refeeding phase resulted in a blunted IGF-1 response. At the end of the 5 d of refeeding IGF-1 concentrations in the low protein diet group were 25% below the higher protein diet group, and 52% lower than pre-fasting levels. The difference in the two groups' IGF-1 response to protein has resulted in subsequent studies focusing on the effects of protein under-nutrition on IGF-1 concentrations.

Harp et al. reported a reduction in IGF-1 mRNA and IGF-1 release in cultured hepatocytes when essential amino acids were eliminated from the culture medium *(78)*. Subsequent research in rats supported the work by Harp et al.—rats fed a casein-based diet had 50% and 2.5-fold higher plasma IGF-1 concentrations compared with rats fed a soy protein-based diet and a protein-free diet, respectively *(79)*.

Over-nutrition, as well as under-nutrition, appears to affect IGF-1 concentrations. Kraemer and co-workers found that positive energy balance increases IGF-1 concentrations *(80)*. They conducted a controlled study in which they provided either a protein/carbohydrate supplement or a placebo for 7 d and during the last 3 d of supplementation, the subjects participated in a resistance training program. The protein/carbohydrate supplement provided 600 kcals (50 g protein, 100 g carbohydrate, 0 g fat) per serving and subjects consumed this supplement three times per day in addition to their normal diet. Serum IGF-1 concentrations increased 25% by the third day of resistance training in subjects consuming the protein/carbohydrate supplement. There was no change in serum IGF-1 concentrations during the 3 d of resistance training in subjects who consumed the placebo.

Results from our lab indicate that protein intake during training also has a significant effect on circulating IGF-1 concentrations. Individuals were randomized to consume either an additional 84 g of protein (casein) per day or placebo while participating in a 6-mo strength and conditioning program. On average, the treatment group consumed 2.25 g/kg body weight vs 1.12 g/kg among the controls. Total caloric intake was identical in the two groups. We observed that protein supplementation resulted in a significant increase in serum IGF-1 concentrations over the 6-mo study, whereas the placebo group experienced a significant decrease.

In summary, both energy intake and protein consumption alter circulating IGF-1 concentrations. Dietary protein intake appears to have a greater affect on IGF-1 concentrations than energy intake alone. Protein supplementation increases circulating IGF-1 levels during short- and long-term resistance training. Whether prolonged protein supplementation in conjunction with exercise affects bone metabolism via IGF-1 has yet to be determined.

5.4. Calcium Intake

Calcium intake appears to modify the bone response to loading activities. One 2×2 trial that was sized to detect a calcium-by-activity interaction found significant effects in leg SA-BMC and cortical area and thickness at the 20% distal tibia site *(62)*. In this study there was a greater increase in leg SA-BMC and cortical area and thickness among children who were randomized to gross motor (i.e., bone-loading) activities vs fine motor activities if they received supplemental calcium, whereas there was no effect of exercise on leg SA-BMC if they received a placebo (Fig. 3). Although two additional trials of calcium supplementation and exercise have been reported *(81,82)*, neither were sized to detect a significant interaction and one had an average attendance at the exercise intervention of 36% *(82)*. One study found a similar calcium-by-activity interaction as Specker and co-workers with femur BMC measured from a DXA total body scan *(81)*.

A study conducted in infants actually found that those infants who were consuming low levels of calcium and were randomized to bone loading activities had less gain in total

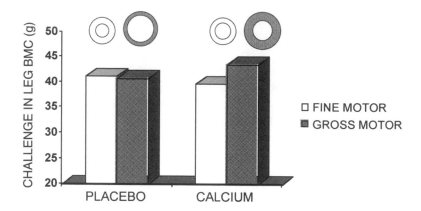

Fig 3. The change in leg bone mineral content (BMC) shows the interaction of activity-by-calcium intake. The cross-sectional images above the bars illustrates the pQCT findings of the cross-section of the tibia at study completion. (Adapted from ref. *86.*)

body BMC than those infants randomized to nonloading activities *(32)*. At higher calcium intakes, there was no difference between the intervention groups in total body bone accretion. Infants at this age (6–18 mo) are undergoing the most rapid gain in linear growth that they would experience throughout their lifetimes. The authors speculated that during this period of rapid growth, a low calcium intake may limit the bone gain and actually lead to a decrease in bone accretion with increased loading. Six-hour urinary calcium excretion tended to be lower, and PTH marginally higher, in the infants randomized to bone-loading activities vs controls and the higher PTH may have lead to increased urinary phosphate excretion thereby limiting the substrate available for mineralization (B. Specker, unpublished data).

The study by Johannsen and co-workers also found that the results of the exercise intervention varied by calcium intake *(83)*. They observed a relationship between change in leg BMC by calcium intake among those children in the intervention group who jumped daily, but no correlation among those children in the control group.

The results of these trials suggest that calcium intake may play a role in modifying the bone response to loading. However, the mechanism behind this effect is not clear. High calcium intakes are thought to decrease bone turnover, especially at the endosteal surface and may explain the greater cortical wall thickness observed in the study by Specker and co-workers *(62)*. However, this increase in cortical wall thickness theoretically should have made the bone less likely to expand at the periosteal surface, yet exercise resulted in similar periosteal circumferences whether they child was receiving supplemental calcium or not. Unfortunately, cortical vBMD could not be accurately determined owing to the small cortical wall thicknesses.

6. CONCLUSIONS

In conclusion, exercise has a significant impact on calcium metabolism, growth, and bone. However, the mechanisms by which exercise affects bone or the specific types of loading (amount vs frequency) that is best to improve bone health are not known. Exercise of different intensities and durations as well as different forms of exercise (strength vs endurance) have resulted in different responses in ionized calcium, PTH, and growth factors. Animal studies show that bone remodeling can be increased within a short time with minimal load. High bending and torsional loads lead to increases in periosteal expansion, whereas compression loads lead to bone apposition on endosteal surfaces. The lack of consistent findings among pediatric activity trials is likely to be due to the different types of loads, different technologies used to measure bone, and the possibility that the bone response to activity is dependent upon pubertal status, BMI and baseline activity levels, or the nutrient intakes of the children.

REFERENCES

1. Khosla S, Melton III LJ, Dekutoski MB, Achenbach SJ, Oberg AL, Riggs BL. Incidence of childhood distal forearm fractures over 30 years. JAMA 2003;290:1479–1485.
2. Haapasalo H, Kannus P, Sievanen H, et al. Effect of long-term unilateral activity on bone mineral density of female junior tennis players. J Bone Miner Res 1998;13:310–319.
3. Cassell C, Benedict M, Specker B. Bone mineral density in elite 7–9 year old female gymnasts and swimmers. Med Sci Sports Exerc 1996;28:1243–1246.
4. Valimaki MJ, Karkkainen M, Lamberg-Allardt C, et al. Exercise, smoking, and calcium intake during adolescence and early adulthood as determinants of peak bone mass. BMJ 1994;309:230–231.
5. Welten DC, Kemper HCG, Post GB, et al. Weight-bearing activity during youth is a more important factor for peak bone mass than calcium intake. J Bone Miner Res 1994;9:1089–1096.
6. Nielsen SP, Christiansen TF, Harting O, Trap-Jensen J. Increase in serum ionized calcium during exercise. Clin Sci Mol Med 1977;53:579–586.
7. Ljunghall S, Joborn H, Benson L, Fellstrom B, Wide LE, Akerstroem G. Effects of physical exercise on serum calcium and parathyroid hormone. Eur J Clin Invest 1984;14:469–473.
8. Rong H, Berg U, Torring O, Sundberg CJ, Granberg B, Bucht E. Effect of acute endurance and strength exercise on circulating calcium-regulating hormones and bone markers in young healthy males. Scan J Med Sci Sports 1997;7:152–159.
9. Brahm H, Strom H, Piehl-Aulin K, Mallmin H, Ljunghall S. Bone metabolism in endurance trained athletes: a comparison to population-based controls based on DXA, SXA, quantitative ultrasound, and biochemical markers. Calcif Tissue Int 1997;61:448–454.
10. Salvesen H, Joahnsson AG, Foxdal P, Wide LE, Piehl-Aulin K, Ljunghall S. Intact serum parathyroid hormone levels increase during running exercise in well-trained men. Calcif Tissue Int 1994;54:256–261.
11. Bouassida A, Zalleg D, AZaouali Ajine M, et al. Parathyroid hormone concentrations during and after two periods of high intensity exercise with and without an intervening recovery period. Eur J Appl Physiol 2003;88:339–344.
12. Franck H, Beuker F, Gurk S. The effect of physical activity on bone turnover in young adults. Exp Clin Endocrinol 1991;98:42–46.
13. Rong H, Berg U, Torring O, Sundberg CJ, Granberg B, Bucht E. Effect of acute endurance and strength exercise on circulating calcium-regulating hormones and bone markers in young healthy males. Scand J Med Sci Sports 1997;7:152–159.
14. Ashizawa N, Fujimura R, Tokuyama K, Suzuki M. A bout of resistance exercise increases urinary calcium independently of osteoclastic activation in men. J Appl Physiol 1997;83:1159–1163.
15. Bell NH, Godsen RN, Henry DP, Shary J, Epstein S. The effects of muscle-building exercise on vitamin D and mineral metabolism. J Bone Min Res 1988;3:369–373.
16. Mundy GR, Oyajobi B, Traianedes K, Dallas S, Chen D. Cytokines and bone remodeling. In: Marcus R, Feldman D, Kelsey J, eds. Osteoporosis. Vol. 1. Academic, San Diego: 2001; pp. 373–404.
17. Turner RT, Riggs BL, Spelsberg TC. Skeletal effects of estrogen: Update 1995. Endocrine Rev 1995;4:155–158.
18. Johannsson G, Bengtsson BA. Growth hormone and the acquisition of bone mass. Horm Res 1997;48: 72–77.
19. Libanati C, Baylink DJ, Lois-Wenzel E, Srinivasan N, Mohan S. Studies on the potential mediators of skeletal changes occurring during puberty in girls. J Clin Endocrinol Metab 1999;84:2807–2814.

20. Smith EP, Boyd J, Frank GR, et al. Estrogen resistance caused by a mutation in the estrogen-receptor gene in a man. N Engl J Med 1994;331:1056–1061.

21. Gotshalk LA, Loebel CC, Nindl BC, et al. Hormonal responses of multiset versus single-set heavy resistance exercise protocols. Can J Appl Physiol 1997;22:244–255.

22. Kanaley JA, Weltman JY, Veldhuis JD, Rogol AD, Hartman ML, Weltman A. Human growth hormone response to repeated bouts of aerobic exercise. J Appl Physiol 1997;83:1756–1761.

23. Kraemer WJ, Hakkinen K, Newton RU, et al. Effects of heavy-resistance training on hormonal response patterns in younger vs. older men. J Appl Physiol 1999;87:982–992.

24. Psilander N, Damsgaard R, Pilegaard H. Resistance exercise alters MRF and IGF-I mRNA content in human skeletal muscle. J Appl Physiol 2003;95:1038–1044.

25. Bamman MM, Shipp JR, Jiang J, et al. Mechanical load increases muscle IGF-I and androgen receptor mRNA concentrations in humans. Am J Physiol Endocrinol Metab 2001;280:E383–E390.

26. Anthony TG, Anthony JC, Lewitt MS, Donovan SM, Layman DK. Time course changes in IGFBP-1 after treadmill exercise and postexercise food intake in rats. Am J Physiol Endocrinol Metab 2001;280:E650–E656.

27. Borst SE, De Hoyos DV, Garzarella L, et al. Effects of resistance training on insulin-like growth factor-I and IGF binding proteins. Med Sci Sports Exerc 2001;33:648–653.

28. Koziris LP, Hickson RC, Chatterton Jr RT, et al. Serum levels of total and free IGF-I and GIFBP-3 are increased and maintained in long-term training. J Appl Physiol 1999;86:1436–1442.

29. Poehlman ET, Rosen CJ, Copeland KC. The influence of endurance training on insulin-like growth factor-1 in older individuals. Metabolism 1994;43:1401–1405.

30. Specker BL, Johannsen N, Binkley T, Finn K. Total body bone mineral content and tibial cortical bone measures in preschool children. J Bone Miner Res 2001;16:2298–2305.

31. Ellis KJ, Shypailo RJ, Hergenroeder A, Perez M, Abrams S. Total body calcium and bone mineral content: comparison of dual-energy x-ray absorptiometry with neutron activation analysis. J Bone Miner Res 1996;11:843–848.

32. Specker BL, Mulligan L, Ho ML. Longitudinal study of calcium intake, physical activity, and bone mineral content in infants 6–18 months of age. J Bone Miner Res 1999;14:569–576.

33. Molgaard C, Thomsen BL, Prentice A, Cole TJ, Michaelsen KF. Whole body bone mineral content in healthy children and adolescents. Arch Dis Child 1997;76:9–15.

34. Bailey DA. The Saskatchewan Pediatric Bone Mineral Accrual Study: bone mineral acquisition during the growing years. Intern J Sports Med 1997;18:S191–S194.

35. Gilsanz V, Roe TF, Mora S, Costin G, Goodman WG. Changes in vertebral bone density in black girls and white girls during childhood and puberty. N Engl J Med 1991;325:1597–1600.

36. Cowell CT, Lu PW, Lloyd-Jones SA, et al. Volumetric bone mineral density—a potential role in paediatrics. Acta Paediatr Suppl 1995;411:12–16.

37. Prentice A, Parsons T, Cole T. Uncritical use of bone mineral density in absorptiometry may lead to size related artifacts in the identification of bone mineral determinants. Am J Clin Nutr 1994;60:837–842.

38. Carter DR, Bouxsein ML, Marcus R. New approaches for interpreting projected bone densitometry data. J Bone Miner Res 1992;7:137–145.

39. Katzman DK, Bachrach LK, Carter DR, Marcus R. Clinical and anthropometric correlates with bone mineral acquisition in healthy adolescent girls. J Clin Endocrinol Metab 1991;73:1332–1339.

40. Sievanen H, Kannus P, Nieminen V, Heinonen A, Oja P, Vuori I. Estimation of various mechanical characteristics of human bones using dual energy x-ray absorptiometry: methodology and precision. Bone 1996;18:17s–27s.

41. Garn SM. The Earlier Gain and the Later Loss of Cortical Bone. Charles C. Thomas, Springfield, IL: 1970; p. 146.

42. Umemura Y, Ishiko T, Yamauchi T, Kurono M, Mashiko S. Five jumps per day increases bone mass and breaking force in rats. J Bone Miner Res 1997;12:1480–1485.

43. Jarvinen TLN, Kannus P, Sievanen H, Jolma P, Heinonen A, Jarvinen M. Randomized controlled study of effects of sudden impact loading on rat femur. J Bone Miner Res 1998;13:1475–1482.

44. Burr DB, Turner CH. Biomechanics of bone. In: Lian JB, Goldring SR, eds. Primer on the Metabolic Bone Diseases and Disorders of Mineral Metabolism American Society for Bone and Mineral Research. Washington, DC: 2003; pp. 58–64.

45. Robling AG, Duijvelaar KM, Geevers JV, Ohashi N, Turner CH. Modulation of appositional and longitudinal bone growth in the rat ulna by applied static and dynamic force. Bone 2001;29:105–113.
46. Mosley JR, March BM, Lynch J, Lanyon LE. Strain magnitude related changes in whole bone architecture in growing rats. Bone 1997;20:191–198.
47. Heinonen A, McKay HA, MacKelvie KJ, Whittall KP, Forster BB, Khan KM. High-impact exercise and tibial polar moment of inertia in pre-and early pubertal girls: A quantitative MRI study. J Bone Miner Res 2001;16:S482.
48. Srinivasan S, Weimer DA, Agans SC, Bain SD, Gross TS. Low-magnitude mechanical loading becomes osteogenic when rest is inserted between each load cycle. J Bone Miner Res 2002;17:1613–1620.
49. Kriska AM, Sandler RB, Dauley JA, LaPorte RE, Hom DL, Pambianco G. The assessment of historical physical activity and its relation to adult bone parameters. Am J Epidemiol 1988;127:1053–1063.
50. McCulloch RG, Bailey DA, Houston CS, Dodd BL. Effects of physical activity, dietary calcium intake and selected lifestyle factors on bone density in young women. Can Med Assoc J 1990;142:221–227.
51. Cooper C, Cawley M, Bhalla A, et al. Childhood growth, physical activity, and peak bone mass in women. J Bone Miner Res 1995;10:940–947.
52. Teegarden D, Proulx WR, Kern M, et al. Previous physical activity relates to bone mineral measures in young women. Med Sci Sports Exerc 1996;28:105–113.
53. Puntila E, Kroger H, Lakka T, Honkanen R, Tuppurainen M. Physical activity in adolescence and bone density in peri and postmenopausal women: A population based study. Bone 1997;21:363–367.
54. Kirchner EM, Lewis RD, O'Connor PJ. Effect of past gymnastics participation on adult bone mass. J Appl Physiol 1996;80:226–232.
55. Bass S, Pearce G, Bradney M, et al. Exercise before puberty may confer residual benefits in bone density in adulthood: Studies in active prepubertal and retired female gymnasts. J Bone Miner Res 1998;13:500–507.
56. Nieves JW, Grisso JA, Kelsey JL. A case-control study of hip fracture: Evaluation of selected dietary variables and teenage physical activity. Osteoporosis Int 1992;2:122–127.
57. Joakimsen RM, Magnus JH, Foonebo V. Physical activity and predisposition for hip fractures: A review. Osteoporos Int 1997;7:503–513.
58. Haapasalo H, Kontulainen S, Sievanen H, Kanus P, Jarvinen M, Vuori I. Exercise-induced bone gain is due to enlargement in bone size without a change in volumetric bone denstiy: a peripheral quantitative computed tomography study of the upper arms of male tennis players. Bone 2000;27:351–357.
59. Kontulainen S, Sievanen H, Kannus P, Pasanen M, Vuori I. Effect of long-term impact-loading on mass, size, and estimated strength of humerus and radius of female racquet-sports players: A peripheral quantitative computed tomography study between young and old starters and controls. J Bone Miner Res 2002;18:352–359.
60. Binkley TL, Specker BL. pQCT measurement of bone parameters in young children: validation of technique. J Clin Densit 2000;3:9–14.
61. Heinonen A, Sievaenen H, Kannus P, Oja P, Pasanen M, Vuori I. High-impact exercise and bones of growing girls: A 9-month controlled trial. Osteoporos Int 2001;11:1010–1017.
62. Specker B, Binkley T. Randomized trial of physical activity and calcium supplementation on bone mineral content in 3–5 year old children. J Bone Miner Res 2003;18:885–892.
63. Petit MA, McKay HA, MacKelvie KJ, Heinonen A, Khan KM, Beck TJ. A randomized school-based jumping intervention confers site and maturity-specific benefits on bone structural properties in girls: a hip structural analysis study. J Bone Miner Res 2002;17:363–372.
64. Bradney M, Pearce G, Naughton G, et al. Moderate exercise during growth in prepubertal boys: Changes in bone mass, size, volumetric density, and bone strength: A controlled prospective study. J Bone Miner Res 1998;13:1814–1821.
65. MacKelvie KJ, McKay HA, Khan KM, Crocker PRE. A school-based exercise intervention augments bone mineral accrual in early pubertal girls. J Pediatr 2001;139:501–508.
66. MacKelvie KJ, McKay HA, Petit MA, Moran O, Khan KM. Bone mineral response to a 7-month randomized controlled, school-based jumping intervention in 121 prepubertal boys: associations with ethnicity and body mass index. J Bone Miner Res 2002;17:834–844.
67. Van Langendonck L, Claessens AL, Vlietinck R, Derom C, Beunen G. Influence of weight-bearing exercises on bone acquisition in prepubertal monozygotic female twins: a randomized controlled prospective study. Calcif Tissue Int 2003;72:666–674.

68. Bassey EJ, Rothwell MC, Littlewood JJ, Pye DW. Pre- and postmenopausal women have different bone mineral density responses to the same high-impact exercise. J Bone Miner Res 1998;13:1805–1813.
69. Fuchs RK, Bauer JJ, Snow CM. Jumping improves hip and lumbar spine bone mass in prepubescent children: a randomized controlled trial. J Bone Miner Res 2001;16:148–156.
70. Morris FL, Naughton GA, Gibbs JL, Carlson JS, Wark JD. Prospective ten-month exercise intervention in premenarcheal girls: Positive effects on bone and lean mass. J Bone Miner Res 1997;12:1453–1462.
71. Bass SL. The prepubertal years: A uniquely opportune stage of growth when the skeleton is most responsive to exercise. Sports Med 2000;30:73–78.
72. Schoenau E, Neu CM, Rauch F, Manz F. Gender-specific pubertal changes in volumetric cortical bone mineral density at the proximal radius. Bone 2002;31:110–113.
73. Jarvinen TL, Kannus P, Sievanen H. Estrogen and bone—a reproductive and locomotive perspective. J Bone Miner Res 2003;18:1921–1931.
74. Clemmons DR, Underwood LE. Nutritional regulation of IGF-I and IGF binding proteins. Ann Rev Nutr 1991;11:393–412.
75. Takenaka A, Takahashi SI, Noguichi T. Effects of protein nutrition on insulin-like growth factor-1 (IGF-1) receptor in various tissues of rats. J Nutr Sci Vitaminol 1996;42:347–357.
76. Isley WL, Underwood LE, Clemmons DR. Dietary components that regulate serum somatomedin-C concentrations in humans. J Clin Invest 1983;71:175–182.
77. Nemet D, Connolly PH, Pontello-Pescatello AM, et al. Negative energy balance plays a major role in IGF-I response to exercise training. J Appl Physiol 2004;96:276–282.
78. Harp JB, Goldstein S, Phillips LS. Nutrition and Somatomedian XXIII. Molecular regulation of IGF-I by amino acid availability in cultured hepatocytes. Diabetes 1991;40:95–101.
79. Miura Y, Kato H, Noguchi T. Effect of dietary proteins on insulin-like growth factor I messenger ribonucleic acid content in the rat liver. Br J Nutr 1992;67:257–265.
80. Kraemer WJ, Volek JS, Bush JA, Putukian M, Sebastianelli WJ. Hormonal responses to consecutive days of heavy-resistance exercise with or without nutritional supplementation. J Appl Physiol 1998;85:1544–1555.
81. Iuliano-Burns S, Saxon L, MNaughton G, Gibbons K, Bass S. Regional specificity of exercise and calcium during skeletal growth in girls: A randomized controlled trial. J Bone Miner Res 2003;18:156–162.
82. Stear SJ, Prentice A, Jones SC, Cole TJ. Effect of a calcium and exercise intervention on the bone mineral status of 16–18 y old adolescent girls. Am J Clin Nutr 2003;77:985–992.
83. Johannsen N, Binkley T, Englert V, Niederauer G, Specker B. Bone response to jumping is site-specific in children: A randomized trial. Bone 2003;33:533–539.
84. Witzke KA, Snow CM. Effects of plyometric jump training on bone mass in adolescent girls. Med Sci Sports Exerc 2000;32:1051–1057.
85. McKay HA, Petit MA, Schutz RW, Prior JC, Barr SI, Khan KM. Augmented trochanteric bone mineral density after modified physical education classes: A randomized school-based exercise intervention study in prepubescent and early pubescent children. J Pediatr 2000;136:156–162.
86. Specker B. Nutritional influences on bone development from infancy through toddler years. J Nutr 2004;134:691S–695S.

15 The Case for a Calcium Appetite in Humans

Michael G. Tordoff

KEY POINTS

- Anthropological and clinical studies suggest humans increase calcium intake in response to calcium deficiency.
- Calcium appetite can be expressed as an increase in preference and consumption of (a) calcium, (b) compounds that taste like calcium, (c) compounds that promote calcium metabolism, or (d) compounds that have been associated with calcium consumption in the past.
- Such "sublimated" expression of calcium appetite might explain why humans consume so much salt and fat.

1. INTRODUCTION

Other chapters in this book discuss calcium requirements and sources, the physiological mechanisms of calcium homeostasis, and diseases that are caused or exacerbated by insufficient calcium consumption. There is often an implicit assumption made that if only people consumed as much calcium as they need—or as much as nutritionists tell them they need—homeostatic mechanisms could maintain calcium balance and the diseases would be ameliorated. But there has been very little attention paid to the question of *why* people consume less calcium than they need. This chapter examines this critical but neglected question.

There are at least two logical possibilities for why calcium intakes are insufficient to meet needs. First, it may be that people do not recognize their need for calcium. Second, they may recognize the need but either cannot find calcium or are not motivated enough to obtain it. It would be nice to evaluate these possibilities by referring to rigorous clinical studies of humans, but this is not possible; the requisite experiments have not been conducted. Instead, frequent use is made of the pertinent animal literature to illustrate mechanisms, and where possible suggestive evidence from studies of humans is pointed out.

From: *Calcium in Human Health*
Edited by: C. M. Weaver and R. P. Heaney © Humana Press Inc., Totowa, NJ

1.1. Nutritional Wisdom and Specific Appetites

The notion of "wisdom of the body" was introduced by Cannon *(1)* to summarize diverse observations showing that environmental perturbations produce physiological responses that maintain homeostasis. In the 1930s, Richter extended this idea by showing that homeostasis involved behavioral as well as physiological components (for reviews, *see* refs. *2–4*). A seminal observation was that rats thrive and grow normally if allowed to choose among several food ingredients (Richter usually used casein, sucrose, olive oil, NaCl, Na_2HPO_4, KCl, calcium lactate, baker's yeast, cod liver oil, and wheat germ oil *[3]*). Moreover, rats with an induced physiological need for a particular nutrient selectively increased consumption of the needed nutrient. The most cited examples are studies in which rats increased consumption of NaCl solution after adrenalectomy, which prevents sodium retention and thus increases the animal's sodium requirement *(3–5)*. Less well known are similar studies in which rats chose appropriate nutrients in response to vitamin B deficiency *(6–8)*, pregnancy and lactation *(3,9)*, and, most pertinent here, after parathyroidectomy *(10–14)*. During pregnancy and lactation, intake of several nutrient sources increased including calcium lactate. After parathyroidectomy, intake of calcium lactate increased dramatically whereas intakes of other nutrients were either unaltered or decreased. Although Richter did not have the equipment to show it, we now know that the loss of parathyroid hormone (PTH) produced by parathyroidectomy causes hypocalcemia, and this can be ameliorated by calcium consumption. Richter's rats with parathyroidectomy displayed "nutritional wisdom" with respect to their physiological requirement for calcium. They consumed what they needed.

Later findings added weight to the notion that rats with parathyroidectomy have a specific hunger for calcium. First, Richter demonstrated that the increased intake of calcium was reversed by treatments that would be expected to influence calcium homeostasis (e.g., reimplantation of the parathyroid glands, injection of parathyroid extract, injection of vitamin D). Indeed, in the era before radioimmunoassay, he suggested that calcium intake of rats with parathyroidectomy was a sensitive bioassay for PTH *(2)*. Second, Lewis *(15)* showed that rats with parathyroidectomy worked (i.e., pressed a lever) to obtain calcium, and that these animals worked harder after they were calcium-deprived for a few hours. Third, Emmers and Nocenti *(16)* demonstrated that the increase in calcium intake observed after parathyroidectomy was abolished by lesions of the "taste" region of the ventrobasal thalamus. This argues that rats that could not distinguish calcium by taste could not select it. Fourth, Leshem and colleagues demonstrated that adult rats after parathyroidectomy had greater increases in consumption of $CaCl_2$ than NaCl or $MgCl_2$ solutions in choice tests *(17)*, and that this specific $CaCl_2$ preference in response to parathyroidectomy developed at approx 6 d of age *(18)*. Taken together, these studies make a compelling case that calcium hunger is innate and specific in the rat.

A comprehensive review of dozens of additional studies in which calcium appetite has been studied after manipulations that perturb calcium metabolism was published recently *(19)* and so will not be reiterated here. In addition to parathyroidectomy, a variety of methods have been used to induce a calcium appetite (e.g., dietary calcium deficiency, acute hypocalcemia, pregnancy and lactation). Moreover, although most of this work has been conducted using rats or chickens, there is confirmatory evidence from diverse vertebrate species including the iguana *(20)*, rabbit *(21)*, pig *(22)*, great tit *(23)*, marmoset

Table 1
Manipulations That Influence Blood Calcium Levels and Calcium Intake in the Rat

Target	Manipulation	Plasma total calcium	Plasma ionized calcium	Calcium intake
Calcium	Low-calcium diet	↓	↓	↑
	High-calcium diet	↑	↑	↓
	Calcium infusions	↑	↑	↓
Parathyroid	Parathyroidectomy	↓↓	↓↓	↑↑
hormone (PTH)	PTH infusion	↑	↑	↓
Calcitonin	Thyroidectomy	0	0	0
	Calcitonin infusion (acute)	↓	↓	↑
	Calcitonin infusion (chronic)	0	0	0
Vitamin D	Vitamin D deficient diet	↓	↓	↑
	High doses of 1,25(OH)$_2$D	↑	↑	↓
Calcium binding				
to blood	Low-protein diet	↓	0	0
proteins	Estrogen (chickens)	0	↓	↑
Miscellaneous	Polyethylene glycol	0	↓↓	↑↑
	Furosemide	↓	↓	↑

↑↑, large increase; ↑, moderate increase; 0, no change; ↓, moderate decrease; ↓↓, large decrease. Note that calcium intake is always inversely related to blood ionized calcium concentrations. The results are compiled from the following sources: refs. *59,87,88,122,123,* and unpublished results. A more detailed survey can be found in ref. *19.*

(24), and gorilla *(25).* It does not seem extravagant, then, to generalize that all vertebrates, including humans, have the physiological substrate to support a calcium appetite.

1.2. Physiological Basis for Calcium Appetite

The physiological event that triggers calcium appetite has not been unequivocally characterized, but the preponderance of evidence supports a mechanism sensitive to blood ionized calcium concentrations *(19).* Calcium intake is increased by manipulations that decrease blood ionized calcium concentrations and decreased by manipulations that increase blood-ionized calcium concentrations (Table 1).

Both rats and human have extracellular calcium receptors in the parathyroid gland that respond to calcium deficiency by releasing parathyroid hormone *(26,27).* Work with the rat has found the same receptors in many brain regions including the subfornical organ *(28),* an area that has been implicated in the control of several ingestive behaviors including calcium appetite *(29).* Perhaps they provide the signal that informs the brain when calcium is needed.

The response to calcium deficiency involves behavioral activation and direction, and also a change in oral sensitivity to calcium in such a manner that the taste of calcium is more acceptable *(30,31).* It is intriguing in this regard that the calcium receptor shares moderate homology with bitter and sweet taste receptors *(32).* It is tempting to speculate that the extracellular calcium receptor acts to detect calcium on the tongue as well as in the blood.

1.3. Nutritional Wisdom in Humans

Contemporaneously with Richter's studies on nutritional wisdom in rats, Davis showed that human infants could select a nutritionally reasonable diet and thrive when allowed to choose among several foodstuffs for several months *(33,34)*. Moreover, Wilkins and Richter *(35)* described a child with adrenal hyperplasia (probably a 21-hydroxylase deficiency) who consumed salt by the handful. When the child was hospitalized his salt intake was restricted and he died. These results looked like examples of human nutritional wisdom in action.

Despite the promising start, the study of nutritional wisdom in humans has not progressed much. Davis' work has been criticized because (a) the foods made available to her subjects were chosen so as to avoid those that might be overwhelmingly preferred (i.e., there were no sweet foods), and (b) the same outcomes would probably have occurred if the children selected foods randomly (*see* ref. *36*). Moreover, despite Wilkins and Richter's *(35)* ill-fated but dramatic demonstration of the importance of salt ingestion, the majority of patients with Addison's and other salt-wasting diseases manifest no noticeable increase in salt intake *(37)*.

Problems have also arisen with the animal literature on nutritional wisdom. There are many examples of animals that select inappropriate diets (*see* refs. *38–41* for examples). Factors such as the food's palatability and availability, and the animal's past experience and social communication can often override physiological needs.

So, is nutritional wisdom a useful concept for understanding food choice? There is a rift between "animal" and "human" researchers in interpretation that appears to be based more on philosophy than data. Investigators studying animals tend to have backgrounds in physiology, where the biological basis of behavior is stressed. Moreover, studies in animals tend to involve long-term investigations with relatively few simple food choices available, tightly controlled environments (including social isolation), and little extraneous past experience to worry about. On the other hand, investigators studying humans tend to have backgrounds in psychology and other cognitive sciences. They rarely conduct long-term studies, provide much more complex foods for subjects to choose from, and have to contend with the diverse social, cultural, and past experiences of their subjects. Nutritional wisdom in humans is also held to a higher standard than nutritional wisdom in animals. It is usually enough that animals engage in compensatory behaviors so that they (a) don't die and (b) appear normal, but for humans we ask for optimal health into old age. The result is that nutritional wisdom continues to be the major theoretical underpinning of most research involving food selection by animals but it is usually dismissed as irrelevent for human food selection. A conciliatory interpretation is that humans still show nutritional wisdom, but that its influence is often overwhelmed or masked by other, nonregulatory factors influencing food choice (*see*, for example, ref. *39*). The implication is that calcium appetite and other examples of nutritional wisdom will be evident in humans only if the physiological perturbation is large, the influence of other factors is reduced, and/or large numbers of subjects are tested to allow statistical disentanglement of subtle components.

2. RECOGNIZING CALCIUM APPETITE

A major issue is how to recognize calcium appetite. What food choices can be used to infer that a calcium appetite is present? The researcher is confronted with a circular argument: If nutritional wisdom is at play and the subjects have access to calcium, then they will select appropriate calcium-containing foods and thus are never calcium-deficient. If they are never calcium-deficient, then calcium appetite will never be observed. This means that in an environment where calcium is easily available the evidence for calcium appetite will be, at best, subtle. In environments where calcium is unavailable, calcium appetite either cannot be expressed (because there is no calcium to ingest) or will be expressed obliquely, by the ingestion of compounds that indirectly influence calcium metabolism. In other words, calcium appetite is most likely to be expressed as consumption of substances that influence calcium metabolism rather than by consumption of calcium itself.

2.1. Recognizing Calcium

The human tongue is exquisitely sensitive to calcium. It can detect micromolar concentrations of calcium salts dissolved in water *(42)*. Indeed, detection thresholds are lower than those typically found in saliva or tap water. In general, the taste of calcium is not easy to describe although it clearly differs from the taste of other minerals *(43)*. Most people have tasted blackboard chalk or masonry lime, so have an idea of what "pure" sources of calcium taste like. Humans consider the primary taste qualities of calcium salts to be bitterness and sourness, but the contribution of each quality varies with the calcium salt tested and its concentration *(42,44)*. Low concentrations of some calcium salts are considered to be more pleasant than water *(45)*, whereas high concentrations of all calcium salts are rated as unpleasant *(42)*. This unpleasant taste is a serious barrier to the production of high-calcium foods and drinks.

All studies of human calcium psychophysics have involved nutritionally replete subjects. However, electrophysiological recordings of rat gustatory sensory nerves and gustatory brain nuclei suggest that the animal's physiological calcium status influences its perception of calcium. Thus, relative to replete controls, calcium-deficient rats are more sensitive to low concentrations of calcium and less sensitive to high ones *(31)*. Moreover, applying calcium to the tongue of calcium-deprived, relative to replete, rats produces greater activity in "sweet-best" neurons, which are associated with pleasant tastes *(30)*. These results suggest that calcium tastes better to the calcium-deficient than replete rat. There is no reason to suspect the same is not true of calcium-deficient humans (*see* ref. *19* for discussion of mechanisms underlying calcium taste transduction).

Despite the low threshold for calcium detection, it is an open question whether calcium is ever detected in human foods. For example, skim milk contains roughly 30 mmol/L calcium, but more than 90% is bound to proteins or phosphates and so probably cannot be tasted. Moreover, the taste of other ingredients most likely masks any free calcium. Not being able to taste calcium is obviously a problem for the recognition of calcium, but it does not necessarily prevent the identification of sources of calcium if appropriate cues are available (*see* Subheading 2.4.).

2.2. Calcium Taste Mimics

There may be compounds that mimic the taste of calcium sufficiently closely that confusion occurs. Two are strontium and lead. A similarity between the taste of calcium and strontium appears probable given that both elements belong to the same group of the periodic table. Moreover, several studies involving long-term choice tests suggest that animals respond to strontium as if it were calcium *(10,46,47)*. Confusion between the taste of lead and calcium has been suggested *(19)*, based on findings that rats consider these two salts to have similar taste profiles *(48)*, and that calcium-deficient rats avidly lick lead acetate solution in a brief-exposure test *(49)*.

Whether humans confuse the tastes of calcium, strontium, and lead has not been tested. However, this is not without practical importance. Based on data that calcium-deprived rats and monkeys consume lead acetate solution, it has been suggested that calcium deficiency is a cause of lead poisoning in children *(50,51)*.

2.3. Compounds That, When Ingested, Promote Calcium Homeostasis

The primary goal of calcium homeostasis is to protect blood-ionized calcium concentrations. This is most easily achieved by consuming calcium, but if calcium is not available, consumption of some other compounds can help, at least temporarily. One reason that calcium-deprived animals consume strontium and lead is that these can be incorporated into bone *(52)*, which allows the calcium they replace to increase blood calcium concentrations. Blood calcium can also be increased by compounds that enhance the absorption of calcium from the gastrointestinal tract. Increased calcium absorption can be achieved by consuming compounds that slow gastrointestinal transit, such as lactose and clay (discussed later), or increase the concentration of 1,25-dihydroxyvitamin D, such as lead *(53)* and cod liver oil (discussed later). The opposite is also true. Calcium-deficient rats avoid solutions containing phosphorus *(10,14,16,54)*, which is entirely appropriate because phosphorus counteracts calcium homeostasis at several levels.

An important example of a compound that promotes calcium homeostasis when ingested is NaCl. Rats fed a low-calcium diet voluntarily and progressively increase intake of hypertonic NaCl solutions from just a few milliliters a day to more than 200 mL/d (Fig. 1). If calcium is reintroduced to the diet or made available as a separate source, NaCl intake returns to baseline levels within 24 h *(55)*.

There has been considerable effort to discover the mechanism underlying this dramatic phenomenon *(55–64)*. It appears, however, that the mechanism is quite simple. Ingested sodium enters the blood stream where it interferes with the distribution of calcium. Normally, a substantial proportion of circulating calcium is bound to proteins but in the presence of elevated sodium levels, some of this bound calcium is released into the free (ionized) pool. Because it is ionized calcium that is the mediator of calcium appetite (*see* Table 1), the rat has effectively ameliorated its deficiency *(64)*. It therefore learns to ingest NaCl in order to gain relief from its malady (*see* Subheading 2.4). Unfortunately for the rat, this is only temporary, because the excess sodium is excreted, and even more unfortunately this also results in calcium loss because sodium and calcium excretion are linked *(61)*. Thus, the rat is caught in a vicious cycle in which it drinks sodium for a short-term and superficial gain in calcium status but this leads to a long-term loss in calcium reserves.

2.4. Flavors Associated With Calcium

The fact that calcium may not be tasted is not a problem for the expression of calcium appetite. This is because flavors presented together with calcium (e.g., the flavor of milk) become associated with its beneficial effects. This has been investigated extensively in poultry *(46,65)* and rats *(66–69)*. For example, poultry can recognize the calcium content of a food by its color *(46)*. Rats can acquire a preference for an arbitrary flavor of Kool

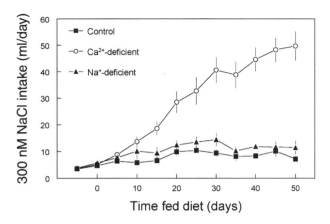

Fig. 1. Intake of NaCl solution by Fischer-344 rats fed nutritionally complete diet (Control), low-calcium diet (Ca^{2+}-deficient), or low-sodium diet (Na^+-deficient). Note the progressive increase in NaCl intake of the group of rats fed low-calcium diet. Water intakes for the three groups were similar (data not shown; *see* ref. *57* for methodological details). A similar phenomenon may exist in humans (*see* Subheading 3.5).

Aid (a fruit-flavored drink mix) when this is either mixed with $CaCl_2$ or always followed by an intragastric infusion of calcium *(68,69)*. The mechanism for the acquisition of these taste preferences appears to involve Pavlovian association, akin to the much-studied conditioned taste aversion. The learned preference for foods associated with calcium has not been demonstrated in humans, but once again, there is no reason to suspect that it does not occur.

2.5. The Specificity of Calcium Appetite

The previous three subsections describe reasons why animals that are calcium-deficient ingest noncalcium compounds. To some investigators, this appears counterintuitive because a hallmark of a specific appetite is that it is specific. The appetite for sodium—the "gold standard" for specific appetites—encompasses ingestion of just sodium and lithium compounds. How can the appetite for calcium be considered specific when it includes many compounds, including arbitrary flavors that happen to have been paired with calcium? The answer to this conundrum is that specificity applies when animals have an appropriate choice. When calcium is available, calcium-deficient rats select it. When given a choice between separate drinking tubes containing appropriate concentrations of $CaCl_2$ and $MgCl_2$, or between $CaCl_2$ and NaCl, intact rats drink roughly the same of each choice, but rats with parathyroidectomy drink more of the $CaCl_2$ solution *(17)*. Similarly, replete rats given a choice between 30 mM $CaCl_2$ and 30 mM $MgCl_2$ drink roughly the same of each solution, whereas rats fed a low-calcium diet drink more $CaCl_2$ than $MgCl_2$, and rats fed a low-magnesium diet drink more $MgCl_2$ than $CaCl_2$ *(70)*. Rats fed a low-calcium diet drink large volumes of hypertonic NaCl solutions if this is the only solution available (as well as water), but not if a calcium lactate solution is also available, and the high NaCl intakes dissipate within a few hours of providing a source of calcium *(55,56)*. These studies demonstrate that rats can choose specifically and appropriately to correct their deficit when calcium is available, but "make do" with alternatives if it is not.

3. THE EVIDENCE FOR A CALCIUM APPETITE IN HUMANS

The previous sections outline the mechanisms by which an appetite for calcium is expressed in animals. It is now time to consider whether humans use similar mechanisms. Ideally, the way to observe calcium appetite in humans would be to compare the food choices of large groups of calcium-deficient and replete individuals. One might expect that, relative to controls, the calcium-deficient subjects would choose more foods that contain calcium or increase calcium status. Of course, deliberately depriving humans of calcium is unethical and this experiment has not been done. Less perfect strategies must be entertained. The investigator must observe human populations that have calcium metabolism perturbed "naturally" or as a consequence of malnutrition or disease. Unfortunately, the evidence collected to date is not concerted and far from conclusive. It may be better to consider much of it as "promising hints" for guiding future studies than as proof.

3.1. Liking Cod Liver Oil

When calcium is scarce, it is important to make the most of what is available. Cod liver oil is a source of vitamin D, and vitamin D improves gastrointestinal absorption of calcium, so ingesting cod liver oil helps to maintain calcium homeostasis. Along these lines, it has been shown that calcium intake of rats is increased by vitamin D deficiency *(59,71)* and decreased by injections of vitamin D *(13)* or chronic infusions of high doses of 1,25-dihydroxyvitamin D.

Although vitamin D deficiency is now relatively rare in the United States, its physical manifestation as rickets was prevalent in big cities in the 1920s and 1930s. The most common "cure" was to give cod liver oil. Well-nourished children find the odor and taste of cod liver oil to be very unpleasant, making its administration a nasty experience for all involved. However, the dislike of cod liver oil is not universal. In the seminal study by Clara Davis of human food selection (*see* Subheading 1.3 and ref. *34*), one of the three orphan infants tested started the experiment with active rickets, which resolved over the 6 mo of the experiment. The results are meticulously documented: "Earl H. [chose] cod liver oil and a milk (S.M.A.) containing cod liver oil served on his tray during the first months of the experiment and ... he took voluntarily 47 $^1/_2$ drachms (178 cc) of the pure cod liver oil and 21 $^1/_3$ drachms (80 cc) of cod liver oil incorporated in S.M.A., a total of 68 $^5/_8$ drachms (258 cc) in 101 d. About the time the blood calcium and phosphorus reached normal and the roentgenogram showed the rickets had healed, he ceased to take any pure cod liver oil."

Following up on Davis' lead, Richter *(3)* found that cod liver oil was accepted almost universally by 5-yr-olds (who were probably from inner-city Baltimore), but that this acceptance decreased with age. He also reported that "some children ... had an almost insatiable appetite for cod liver oil. When allowed to satisfy their craving they took as much as 16 tablespoonfuls in one day, and continued to take high amounts for 5–10 days. After that they took only small amounts, and finally stated that they no longer liked it. Rats kept on diets deficient in vitamins A or D responded in much the same way when offered cod liver oil" (ref. *3*, pp. 96–97).

Thus, both rats and children consume cod liver oil when it does them good, but refuse it when it does not. There are other explanations for the results, but the most obvious one is that cod liver oil consumption is self-medication directed by the need for calcium.

3.2. Consuming Clay

The ingestion of dirt (geophagy) has been described for diverse species from parrots *(72)* to primates *(73)* and is particularly prevalent among ungulates *(74,75)*. However, little attention has been paid to the significance of this behavior in humans. The preparation of tortillas in many parts of Central America involves soaking them in lime. Similarly, the Quechua Indians from the high Peruvian Andes supplement their diet by eating a powdered rock porridge (*cal*), and chewing ashed stalks (*llipta*) along with coca *(76)*. These culinary procedures may help alleviate calcium deficiency, but they are probably not the only purpose. Soaking tortillas increases their calcium content but also makes dough that is more easily rolled out. The Quechua may chew lime because it increases the availability of active alkaloids from coca.

A more convincing argument for clay consumption as a behavioral response to calcium deficiency has been made based on pregnant women from many African (and some African-American *[77,78]*) societies *(79–82)*. Pregnant women report they have a "strong desire" for clay and indicate that consumption provides them with feelings of well-being *(78)*. They consume it in small amounts throughout the day rather than as a single meal. Hunter *(81)* reported that societies showing geophagy in southern Africa frequently lived in areas with low soil calcium content but chose to consume clays high in calcium, particularly those formed by colonies of termites, which accumulate calcium carbonate. Clay from termite mounds is traded throughout western and southern sub-Saharan Africa in much the same manner as is salt *(75,83)*. Indeed, one source suggests that "In East Africa the search for edible earths rich in calcium was frequently a cause of tribal raids and the evidence points to these products being instinctively consumed to make good the lack of lime in the customary diet" *(84)*.

An elegant survey of the relationship between dairy farming and clay consumption by African societies has been published by Wiley and Katz *(82)*. They compared 15 societies that farmed cows for milk ("dairying") with 45 that did not ("nondairying"). As Fig. 2 shows, there were significant differences between the milk drinkers and nondrinkers in the frequency distribution of clay consumption, with the practice being much more common in nondairying societies than dairying ones.

The simplest interpretation of the inverse relationship between dairying and geophagy is that societies that do not drink milk compensate for the lack of calcium by consuming clay. Of course, it is also possible to consider the advent of dairy farming as a manifestation of human calcium appetite.

It is unfortunate that calcium intakes of most of the African societies surveyed have not been measured. Values for some of them range from 200 to 2030 mg/d calcium (*see* ref. *82*). However, the utility of intake measurements is questionable because such figures do not account for the differences in availability of calcium from different sources. The plant diets of nondairying societies are high in fiber, phytates, and oxalates, which all reduce calcium absorption. They thus increase the effective difference between dairying and non-dairying societies *(82)*. Another problem is that not all the clay consumed is high in calcium (*see* ref. *82* and Table 15.4 therein). However, even calcium-free clays are beneficial because clay slows gastrointestinal transit and probably binds to, and thus effectively deactivates, phytates and oxalates. This allows more complete absorption of calcium from other components of the diet.

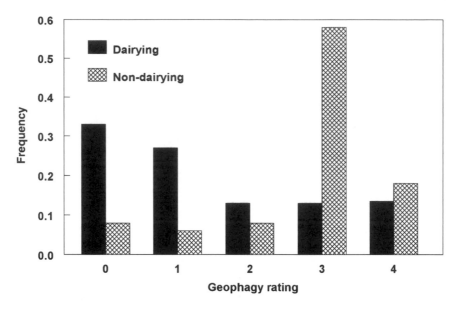

Fig. 2. Distribution of geophagy (clay consumption) by 60 African societies split into those that raise cows for milk (dairying) and those that do not (nondairying). Geophagy rating scale: 0, absent; 1, rare; 2, occasional; 3, common; 4, virtually universal. The impact of dairying to reduce geophagy is probably underestimated because several dairying tribes limit or prohibit women from consuming dairy products. (Data extracted from ref. *82.*)

This is not to say that the *only* function of geophagy is to provide calcium. Clays often contain magnesium and iron. They also have other benefits. Clay sequesters toxic plant compounds in the gastrointestinal tract, thereby detoxifying them. Some of these compounds may be teratogenic to the embryo. Moreover, geophagy can prevent pregnancy-related vomiting and diarrhea and so it is an appropriate response to gastrointestinal discomfort or malaise. Indeed, geophagy has been used as a proxy measure of illness in the rat (e.g., ref. *85*). Finally, perhaps by virtue of reducing feelings of malaise, geophagy can markedly increase the total energy intake of pregnant women *(86)*. Both the increased energy intake and reduced vomiting are likely to increase effective calcium intake.

3.3. Calcium in the Clinic: Choosing Chalky Cheese

Animal studies suggest that chelation and other treatments that produce hypocalcemia also induce a calcium appetite *(87,88)*. Recently, Leshem and colleagues *(89)* have investigated the effects on calcium preferences and calcium intensity ratings of chronic hemodialysis treatments that incidentally reduced plasma calcium concentrations. Ten patients and 10 age-matched controls were asked to choose their most and least favorite of three cream cheeses that were prepared with different amounts of calcium. Figure 3 shows the results: most of the controls reported the "best" cheese to be the one with the lowest calcium concentration and the "worst" cheese to be the one with the highest calcium concentration. In contrast, several of the patients reported the "best" cheese to have moderate or high concentrations of calcium and the "worst" cheese to have the lowest calcium concentration. Consistent with these rankings, patients described the cheese with the highest calcium concentration as significantly tastier than did controls. Despite the difference in cheese preference, there were no differences between patients

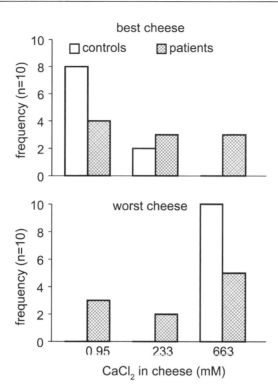

Fig. 3. Cheese choice of 10 controls and 10 patients undergoing hemodialysis. Three cheeses differing in calcium concentration were tested. Top panel, number of subjects who considered each cheese as the "best" one. Bottom panel, number of subjects who considered each cheese as the "worst" one. (Reproduced with permission from ref. *89*, with permission.)

and controls in ratings of taste intensity of the cheeses, in ratings of the intensity of five concentrations of $CaCl_2$ or sucrose in solution, in the ranking of the pleasantness of these solution concentrations, or in ratings of whether the solutions would be acceptable "in a health drink."

This study is open to criticism on several grounds: There were only a few subjects tested, there were no physiological data to corroborate that calcium metabolism was perturbed at the time patients were tested, and there were inadequate controls to characterize the specificity of the physiological deficit or the calcium preference. Nevertheless, this is an encouraging first attempt at concerted psychophysical testing for changes in calcium appetite in a clinical population.

Other clinical populations with disturbances of calcium metabolism have not been studied in detail. Richter stated that "children with parathyroid deficiency have been reported to show a craving for chalk, plaster, and other substances with a high calcium content" (ref. *3*, p. 98). Unfortunately, however, no evidence for this is presented. There is one study showing that patients with pseudohypoparathyroidism have reduced sensitivity to selected odors and sour and bitter tastes *(90)*. Perhaps these changes are owing to an underlying altered sensitivity to calcium, but this was not tested directly, and there were equivocal effects on sensitivity to sweetness and saltiness, which makes interpretation difficult.

Table 2
Intake of Energy and Nutrients by Women During Breast-Feeding Either
a Single Child or Twins

Intake	Single	Twin	Increase (%)
Energy, kcal	1859 ± 364	2386 ± 705	28%
Protein, g	84 ± 27	103 ± 31	23%
Ca, mg	996 ± 455	1790 ± 671	80%
P, mg	1430 ± 521	1797 ± 553	26%
Mg, mg	222 ± 82	247 ± 94	11%

Data extracted from ref. 98. Values are average daily intakes based on 19 mothers of singletons and 15 mothers of twins, collected during the first 6 wk of lactation. Similar results were found up to 26 wk lactation. Note that mothers of twins ate 80% more calcium but only approx 25% more of other food ingredients than did mothers of singletons, suggesting that the extra demands of breast-feeding twins causes a specific increase in calcium intake.

3.4. Calcium Intake During Pregnancy and Lactation

Several studies show that calcium intakes are higher in lactating than nonlactating women, and that calcium intakes increase as the children become older (and suckle more milk [91–97]). Women nursing twins consume significantly more calcium than do women with only one child to nurse (98). Intriguingly, the ratio of calcium intake to energy intake is higher in mothers of twins than singletons (Table 2), suggesting that there may be preferential intake of calcium during lactation. Of course, it is unclear whether this is due to changes in diet selection to favor calcium-containing products or the result of nutritional counseling directed specifically at increasing calcium intake.

3.5. Sodium Intake as a Response to Calcium Deficiency

The previous examples of calcium appetite in humans have involved special populations with poor nutritional status, clinically induced hypocalcemia, or a demand for calcium enhanced by lactation. The question thus arises of whether calcium appetite has relevance for the majority of the well-nourished, healthy US population and other Westernized societies.

As discussed under Subheading 2.3., there is considerable evidence that rats progressively increase NaCl intake when fed a low-calcium diet. Data showing that ingested sodium liberates calcium from plasma proteins led to the proposal that an appropriate response to calcium deficiency is to consume sodium because this temporarily alleviates calcium deficiency (64). Consuming sodium would reduce the appetite for calcium until the additional sodium was excreted. Under these circumstances, salty foods would become preferred during calcium deficiency even though saltiness does not signal calcium (see Subheading 2.3.).

There are indirect but persuasive data to support this hypothesis. Populations with a high demand for calcium have elevated NaCl preferences (e.g., pregnant and lactating women [99], children [100–102]). Moreover, subjects with low calcium intakes prefer significantly higher concentrations of NaCl in tomato juice and other salted foods than do subjects with high calcium intakes (61,103).

3.6. Fat Intake as a Response to Calcium Deficiency

The previous examples of calcium appetites have some basis in human research. A highly speculative further possibility is that low calcium intakes lead people to consume more fat. There are two reasons to believe this, both based on animal studies. First, calcium-deficient rats avoid sweet things, including sweet carbohydrates *(104)*. This switches preferences away from carbohydrates and thus towards fat. Second, as discussed previously, studies with rats and poultry show that arbitrary flavors can become associated with the beneficial postingestive effects of calcium consumption *(46,68,69)*. It is therefore quite possible that human infants associate the fatty texture of breast milk with the benefits of calcium consumption. When later in life they require calcium, they may seek out this fatty texture. It seems reasonable to assume this would include dairy products as well as other fatty foods. Excess fat consumption is a cause of obesity *(105)*. Several investigators have reported inverse correlations between calcium intakes and body weight in epidemiological studies *(106–112)* and there are also reports of reductions in body weight during clinical trials involving calcium supplementation *(108,109,113)*. It has been hypothesized that the lipogenic action of high circulating concentrations of 1,25-dihydroxyvitamin D is responsible for the obesity *(109,114)*, but this does not appear to be supported by recent animal research *(115,116)*. Perhaps, instead, the mechanism involves a misguided attempt to find calcium in the many foods with a fatty texture.

4. IF HUMANS HAVE A CALCIUM APPETITE, THEN WHY DON'T THEY CONSUME AS MUCH CALCIUM AS THEY NEED?

Based on the existence of a demonstrated calcium appetite in other mammals, there is good reason to believe that humans have the physiological and anatomical substrate for a calcium appetite. For the remainder of this chapter, it is assumed that humans have a calcium appetite and the question "What is wrong?" is addressed. Why don't people consume as much calcium as they need?

Of course, there is no answer to this question at present. As mentioned in the introduction, there are two logical possibilities. One is that there is an internal problem: humans may not recognize they need calcium; that is, they are never sufficiently deficient to activate calcium appetite. The other is an external one: that is, humans may be motivated to seek calcium but either cannot find it or make inappropriate choices for other reasons. Each of these possibilities is addressed separately.

4.1. Are Humans Ever Calcium-Deficient Enough for Calcium Appetite To Be Activated?

Identifying the internal stimulus controlling calcium appetite is crucial for understanding the problem of why humans do not eat enough calcium to prevent chronic diseases. The animal data suggest the stimulus triggering calcium appetite is related to hypocalcemia (*see* Subheading 1.2.). It is quite possible that abnormal depletion of bone stores (i.e., ultimately, osteoporosis) or even elevated intracellular calcium concentrations (i.e., ultimately, hypertension) can occur without detectable hypocalcemia, and thus without activating calcium appetite. It is difficult to see how calcium appetite could have evolved as an adaptive strategy to prevent chronic diseases, because these usually strike after the reproductive years, when death or disability has little influence on gene transmission.

Living to be old enough to have brittle bones is a new development in human evolution. Calcium appetite might prevent death from calcium deprivation, but modern diets must also provide optimal health and a long life. Maybe calcium appetite serves to help us survive only until we reproduce and wean our children.

Assuming that an anatomical substrate for calcium appetite is present, when, if ever, is it used? There are three possible answers to this question: Never, sometimes, or always. The "never" answer implies that humans differ from other animals, and that the examples of cod liver oil, clay, cheese, calcium, and salt intake listed in Subheading 3 are epiphenomena caused by other factors accompanying calcium deficiency. One reason for believing that humans never need a calcium appetite is that they are relatively large and slow-growing. Nearly all work on the mechanisms underlying calcium appetite has been conducted using small, rapidly growing or egg-laying animals. It is difficult to demonstrate a calcium appetite in other large mammals, such as cows and pigs *(22,117,118; see also* discussion in ref. *19)*. Large animals have large bones and thus large calcium reserves. It may be that with large calcium reserves, large animals rarely if ever need to resort to behavior to maintain calcium status. The counter-argument to this is that large animals also live longer and so they have longer to accumulate a calcium imbalance if faced with marginal dietary deficiency. By analogy, large animals have large fat (energy) stores that can protect them during long periods of starvation, but this does not mean they are immune to the hunger for energy. It may be that investigators simply need to be more patient to see calcium appetite in large animals.

The possibility that humans "sometimes" activate a calcium appetite implies that there may be certain populations with a high demand for calcium but this is not important for most well-nourished people. Exactly which populations have high enough demand is unclear, but the examples listed under Subheading 3 suggest that such populations include marginally malnourished children, pregnant women from African societies without dairy products, hypocalcemic dialysis patients, and lactating women in the United States. The "sometimes" answer is consistent with the notion that physiological counterregulation occurs in response to smaller perturbations of homeostasis than does behavioral counterregulation. The argument goes that, in the face of a modest calcium deficiency, it is more efficient to absorb a little more calcium from the gut or reabsorb more from bone than to activate calcium-seeking behavior. Behavior is required only to stave off frank depletion. Although this makes teleological sense, there is little evidence to support it. Indeed, for some homeostatic systems it is clearly incorrect (e.g., the natriuretic thresholds for thirst and antidiuretic hormone secretion are identical *[119]*; many animals avoid the sun rather than sweat; many humans eat rather than deplete fat stores).

The possibility that calcium appetite is "always" active implies that small changes in physiological calcium status are reflected by rapid changes in behavior. This might be akin to the allesthesia demonstrated for sweetness *(120)*. Just as recent consumption of sugar reduces the preference for sweet tastes, recent consumption of calcium may reduce the preference for the taste of calcium. This is consistent with the changes in the electrophysiological activity of gustatory afferent nerves in response to oral calcium observed in rats *(30,31)*. A simple, but untested, hypothesis is that when calcium has not been consumed for awhile, salivary calcium concentrations drop and this reduces the detection threshold for oral calcium and increases calcium preference. Such minute-to-minute changes in sensitivity to calcium might explain some of the intra-subject variability observed in psychophysical tests *(42)*.

4.2. Can Humans Find Calcium in a World of Many Food Choices?

In order to satisfy an internally detected need for calcium, humans must be able to detect calcium (or a marker for calcium) in the environment. There is no doubt that we can do this (42), but the real question is can we recognize calcium for what it is worth? Can we distinguish calcium incorporated into the diet from other nutrients and food-stuffs? Rats and poultry have no problems finding calcium when given several cups of food, some with it and some without it. The most complex study found that rats ingested sufficient calcium to grow normally when allowed to choose from among eight separate nutrient sources (16). However, this is a far cry from the complex diet of humans, or at least those humans living in the United States. The average US supermarket stocks more than 30,000 items (121).

It is important to remember that the search is for foods that ameliorate low calcium status, but these foods do not have to contain calcium itself. Almost as satisfactory are foods that favorably influence calcium metabolism and foods that have done so in the past. This could include a very large range of compounds. Discussed previously were compounds such as cod liver oil, clay, and NaCl, which enhance gastrointestinal absorption of calcium, slow gastrointestinal transit (allowing more calcium to be absorbed), or increase circulating ionized calcium concentrations by interfering with the binding of calcium to blood proteins. There are probably several other calcium-metabolism-"favoring" foods. There are also foods that have been associated with calcium in the past, even though they are not necessarily still associated with calcium. Finally, foods that taste similar to foods that beneficially influence calcium metabolism may be sought because of taste generalization.

Of course, many of the flavor cues for calcium in the diet are masked by other flavors. It is also likely that subtle physiological signals for calcium will be overridden by many factors including the motivation to consume palatable foods, advertising, and cultural constraints. Understanding the interactions underlying food choice is a formidable task, but nevertheless a vital one, if we are to understand how calcium appetite is expressed outside the laboratory.

5. CONCLUSIONS

A calcium appetite has been demonstrated in many animals, and there is therefore good reason to believe that the anatomical and physiological substrate for the appetite also exists in humans. There are several intriguing observations suggesting humans that require calcium seek out, ingest, and prefer foods that either contain calcium or promote calcium status. However, the case for a calcium appetite is by no means proven. In general, the idea of nutritional wisdom in humans has received little support. Relative to laboratory animals, humans have stronger social and cultural constraints as well as a much larger choice of foods. In such a complex world, it is unclear when or how a calcium appetite would be observed. One possibility is that it would be seen only under conditions of extreme calcium demand, such as during malnutrition, lactation, or disease. Another is that it would be seen all the time but it would be subtly expressed. Calcium appetite can be observed most obviously as an increase in preference and consumption of calcium, but it may also produce an increase in preference and consumption of compounds that taste like calcium, compounds that promote calcium metabolism, or compounds that have been associated with calcium consumption in the past. Such "sublimated" expression of calcium appetite might explain both why evidence for a human calcium appetite has not been recognized, and also why humans consume so much salt and fat.

ACKNOWLEDGMENTS

The author's studies on calcium appetite in rodents are supported by National Institutes of Health (NIH) grant DK-46791. Thanks to Drs. Sue Coldwell, Stuart McCaughey, and Qinmin Zhang for many years of help with these studies. Special thanks to Dr. Danielle Reed for her insightful comments on earlier versions of the manuscript.

REFERENCES

1. Cannon W. The wisdom of the body. Norton, New York: 1939.
2. Richter CP (ed.). The self-selection of diets. Essays in biology (In honor of Herbert M Evans). University of California Press, Berkeley, CA: 1943; pp. 500–505.
3. Richter CP. Total self-regulatory functions in animals and human beings. Harvey Lectures 1942–1943; Series 38:63–103.
4. Richter CP. Salt appetite of mammals: its dependence on instinct and metabolism. In: Cie Me, ed. L'instinct dans le comportement des animaux et de l'homme. Librares de l'Academie de Medécine, Paris, France: 1956; pp. 577–629.
5. Richter CP, Eckert JF. Mineral metabolism of adrenalectomized rats studied by the appetite method. Endocrinol 1938;22:214–224.
6. Richter C, Hawkes C. The dependence of the carbohydrate, fat, and protein appetite of rats on the various components of the vitamin B complex. Am J Physiol 1941;131:639–649.
7. Richter C, Barelare B. Further observations on the carbohydrate, fat, and protein appetite of vitamin B deficient rats. Am J Physiol 1939;127:199–210.
8. Richter C, Holt L, Barelare B, Hawkes C. Changes in fat, carbohydrate, and protein appetite in vitamin B deficiency. Am J Physiol 1938;124:596–602.
9. Barelare B, Richter CP. Increased sodium chloride appetite in pregnant rats. Am J Physiol 1938;121:185–188.
10. Richter CP, Eckert JF. Mineral appetite of parathyroidectomized rats. Am J Med Sci 1932;9:9–16.
11. Richter CP, Eckert JF. Increased calcium appetite of parathyroidectomized rats. Endocrinol 1937;21:50–54.
12. Eckert J. Further observations on the calcium appetite of parathyroidectomized rats. Am J Physiol 1938;123:59.
13. Richter CP, Birmingham JR. Calcium appetite of parathyroidectomized rats used to bioassay substances which affect blood calcium. Endocrinol 1941;29:655–666.
14. Richter CP, Helfrick S. Decreased phosphorus appetite of parathyroidectomized rats. Endocrinol 1943;33:349–352.
15. Lewis M. Behavior resulting from calcium deprivation in parathyroidectomized rats. J Comp Physiol Psychol 1964;57:348–352.
16. Emmers R, Nocenti MR. Role of thalamic gustatory nucleus in diet selection by normal and parathyroidectomized rats. Proc Soc Exp Biol Med 1967;125:1264–1270.
17. Leshem M, Del Canho S, Schulkin J. Calcium hunger in the parathyroidectomized rat is specific. Physiol Behav 1999;67:555–559.
18. Leshem M, del Canho S, Schulkin J. Ontogeny of calcium preference in the parathyroidectomized rat. Dev Psychobiol 1999;34:293–301.
19. Tordoff MG. Calcium: taste, intake and appetite. Physiol Rev 2001;81
20. Oftedal O, Chen T, Schulkin J. Preliminary observations on the relationship of calcium ingestion to vitamin D status in the green iguana (*Iguana iguana*). Zoo Biol 1997;16:201–207.
21. Denton DA, Nelson JF. Effects of pregnancy and lactation on the mineral appetites of wild rabbits [*Oryctolagus cuniculus (L.)*]. Endocrinol 1971;88:31–40.
22. Pickard DW, Hedley WG, Skilbeck S. Calcium appetite in growing pigs. Proc Nutr Soc 1977;36:87A.
23. Graveland J, Berends AE. Timing of the calcium intake and effect of calcium deficiency on behaviour and egg laying in captive great tits, *Parus major*. Physiol Zool 1997;70:74–84.

24. Power ML, Tardif SD, Layne DG, Schulkin J. Ingestion of calcium solutions by common marmosets (*Callithrix jacchus*). Am J Primatol 1999;47:255–261.

25. Magliocca F, Gautier-Horn A. Mineral content as a basis for food selection by Western Lowland Gorillas in a forest clearing. Am J Primatol 2002;57:67–77.

26. Brown EM, MacLeod RJ. Extracellular calcium sensing and extracellular calcium signaling. Physiol Rev 2001;81:239–297.

27. Hofer AM, Brown EM. Extracellular calcium sensing and signalling. Nature Reviews: Molecular Cell Biology 2003;4:530–538.

28. Rogers K, Dunn C, Hebert S, Brown E. Localization of calcium receptor mRNA in the adult rat central nervous system by in situ hybridization. Brain Res 1997;744:47–56.

29. McCaughey SA., Fitts DA, and Tordoff MG. Lesions of the subfornical organ decrease the calcium appetite of calcium-deprived rats. Physiol Behav 2003;79:605–12.

30. McCaughey SA, Tordoff MG. Calcium deprivation alters gustatory-evoked activity in the rat nucleus of the solitary tract. Am J Physiol Regul Integr Comp Physiol 2001;281:R971–978.

31. Inoue M, Tordoff MG. Calcium deficiency alters chorda tympani nerve responses to oral calcium chloride. Physiol Behav 1998;63:297–303.

32. Nelson G, Hoon MA, Chandrashekar J, Zhang Y, Ryba NJ, Zuker CS. Mammalian sweet taste receptors. Cell 2001;106:381–390.

33. Davis CM. Results of self-selection of diets by young children. Canadian Medical Association Journal 1939;41:257–261.

34. Davis CM. Self-selection of diet by newly weaned infants. American Journal of Diseases of Children 1928;36:651–679.

35. Wilkins L, Richter CP. A great craving for salt in a child with corticoadrenal insufficiency. JAMA 1940;114:866–868.

36. Story M, Brown JE. Do young children instinctively know what to eat? The studies of Clara Davis revisited. N Engl J Med 1987;316:103–106.

37. Beauchamp GK, Bertino M, Engelman K. Human salt appetite. In: Friedman MI, Tordoff MG, Kare MR, eds. Chemical senses: appetite and nutrition. Marcel Dekker, New York: 1991; pp. 85–107.

38. Galef BG, Jr. A contrarian view of the wisdom of the body as it relates to dietary self-selection. Psych Rev 1991;98:218–223.

39. Tordoff MG. Obesity by choice: The powerful effect of nutrient availability on nutrient intake. Am J Physiol Regul Integr Comp Physiol 2002;282:R1536–R1539.

40. Reed DR, Friedman MI, Tordoff MG. Experience with a macronutrient source influences subsequent macronutrient selection. Appetite 1992;18:223–232.

41. Richter C, Rogers P, Hall C. Failure of salt replacement therapy in adrenalectomized recently captured wild Norway rats. Endocrinol 1950;46:233–242.

42. Tordoff MG. Some basic psychophysics of calcium salts. Chem Senses 1996;21:417–424.

43. Schiffman SS, Erickson RP. A psychophysical model for gustatory quality. Physiol Behav 1971;7:617–633.

44. Hettinger T, Frank M, Myers W. Are the tastes of Polycose and monosodium glutamate unique? Chem Senses 1996;21:341–347.

45. Zoeteman BCJ, de Grunt FE, Köster EP, Smit KGJ, Punter PH. Taste assessment of individual salts in water. Methodology and preliminary findings by a selected national panel. Chem Senses Flavour 1978;3:127–139.

46. Hughes BO, Wood-Gush DGM. A specific appetite for calcium in domestic chicken. Anim Behav 1971;19:490–499.

47. Coldwell SE, Tordoff MG. Acceptance of minerals and other compounds by calcium-deprived rats: 24-h tests. Am J Physiol 1996;271:R1–R10.

48. Morrison GR. Behavioral response patterns to salt stimuli in the rat. Can J Psychol 1967;21:141–152.

49. Coldwell SE, Tordoff MG. Immediate acceptance of minerals and HCl by calcium-deprived rats: brief exposure tests. Am J Physiol 1996;271:R11–R17.

50. Snowdon CT, Sanderson BA. Lead pica produced in rats. Science 1974;183:92–94.

51. Snowdon CT. A nutritional basis for lead pica. Physiol Behav 1977;18:885–893.

52. Lederer LG, Bing FC. Effect of calcium and phosphorus on retention of lead by growing organism. JAMA 1940;114:2457–2461.

53. Fulmer CS. Lead-calcium interactions: involvement of 1,25-dihydroxyvitamin D. Environ Res 1997;72:45–55.
54. Wilens SL, Waller RK. Voluntary intake of calcium and phosphorus in partially nephrectomized and parathyroidectomized rats. Endocrinol 1941;28:828–834.
55. Tordoff MG, Ulrich PM, Schulkin J. Calcium deprivation increases salt intake. Am J Physiol 1990;259:R411–R419.
56. Tordoff MG. Influence of dietary calcium on sodium and calcium intake of spontaneously hypertensive rats. Am J Physiol 1992;262:R370–R381.
57. Tordoff MG. Calcium deprivation increases NaCl intake of Fischer-344 rats. Physiol Behav 1991;49:113–115.
58. Tordoff MG. Salt intake of rats fed diets deficient in calcium, iron, magnesium, phosphorus, potassium, or all minerals. Appetite 1992;18:29–41.
59. Tordoff MG, Hughes RL, Pilchak DM. Independence of salt intake from the hormones regulating calcium homeostasis. Am J Physiol 1993;264:R500–R512.
60. Tordoff MG, Pilchak DM, Hughes RL. Independence of salt intake induced by calcium deprivation from the renin-angiotensin-aldosterone system. Am J Physiol 1993;264:R492–R499.
61. Tordoff MG. The importance of calcium in the control of salt intake. Neurosci Biobeh Rev 1996;20:89–99.
62. Tordoff MG. Adrenalectomy decreases NaCl intake of rats fed low-calcium diets. Am J Physiol 1996;270:R11–R21.
63. Tordoff MG, Okiyama A. Daily rhythm of NaCl intake in rats fed low-Ca^{2+} diet: relation to plasma and urinary minerals and hormones. Am J Physiol 1996;270:R505–R517.
64. Tordoff MG. NaCl ingestion ameliorates plasma indexes of calcium deficiency. Am J Physiol 1997;273:R423–R432.
65. Hughes BO, Wood-Gush DGM. Hypothetical mechanisms underlying calcium appetite in fowls. Rev Comp Animal 1972;6:95–106.
66. Scott EM, Verney EL, Morissey PD. Self selection of diet. XI. Appetites for calcium, magnesium and potassium. J Nutr 1950;41:187–202.
67. Rodgers WL. Specificity of specific hungers. J Comp Physiol Psychol 1967;64:49–58.
68. Coldwell SE, Tordoff MG. Latent learning about calcium and sodium. Am J Physiol 1993;265:R1480–R1484.
69. Tordoff MG. Intragastric calcium infusions support flavor preference learning by calcium-deprived rats. Physiol Behav 2002;76:521–529.
70. McCaughey SA, Tordoff MG. Magnesium appetite in the rat. Appetite 2002;38:29–38.
71. Brommage R, DeLuca HF. Self-selection of a high calcium diet by vitamin D-deficient lactating rats increases food consumption and milk production. J Nutr 1984;114:1377–1385.
72. Diamond JM. Dirty eating for healthy living. Nature 1999;400:120–121.
73. Krishnaman R, Mahaney WC. Geophagy among primates: adaptive significance and ecological consequences. Anim Behav 1999;59:899–915.
74. Jones RL, Harrison HC. Mineral licks, geophagy, and biogeochemistry of North American ungulates. Iowa State University Press, Ames, IA: 1985.
75. Denton D. The hunger for salt: An anthropological, physiological and medical analysis. Springer-Verlag, Berlin: 1984.
76. Baker PT, Mazess RB. Calcium: unusual sources in the Highland Peruvian diet. Science 1963;142:1466–1467.
77. Hunt JN. Geophagy in Africa and in the United States: a culture-nutrition hypothesis. Geographical Review 1973;63:170–195.
78. Lagercrantz S. Geophagical customs in Africa and among the Negroes in America. Studia Ethnographica Upsaliensia 1958;17:24–81.
79. Vermeer DE. Geophagy among the Tiv of Nigeria. Annals of the Association of American Geographers 1966;56:197–204.
80. Vermeer DE. Geophagy among the Ewe of Ghana. Ethnology 1971;10:56–72.
81. Hunter JM. Marcroterme geophagy and pregnancy clays in Southern Africa. Journal of Cultural Geography 1993;14:69–92.

82. Wiley AS, Katz SH. Geophagy in pregnancy: a test of a hypothesis. Curr Anthropol 1998;39:532–545.

83. Kurlansky M. Salt: a world history: Penguin, New York: 2003.

84. Drummond JC. Lane medical lectures: biochemical studies of nutritional problems. Stanford University Press, Stanford, CA: 1934; p. 106.

85. McCaffrey RJ. Appropriateness of kaolin consumption as an index of motion sickness in the rat. Physiol Behav 1985;35:151–156.

86. Edwards CH, Mitchell JB, Jones L, Mason L, Trigg L. Effect of clay and cornstarch intake on women and their infants. J Am Dietetic Assoc 1964;44:109–115.

87. Lobaugh B, Joshua IG, Mueller WJ. Regulation of calcium appetite in broiler chickens. J Nutr 1981;111:298–306.

88. Tordoff MG. Polyethylene glycol-induced calcium appetite. Am J Physiol 1997;273:R587–R596.

89. Leshem M, Rudoy J, Schulkin J. Calcium taste preference and sensitivity in humans: II. hemodialysis patients. Physiol Behav 2003;78:409–414.

90. Henkin RI. Impairment of olfaction and of the tastes of sour and bitter in pseudohypoparathyroidism. J Clin Endocr 1968;28:624–628.

91. Kalkwarf HJ, Specker BL, Bianchi DC, Ranz J, Ho M. The effect of calcium supplementation on bone density during lactation and after weaning. N Engl J Med 1997;337:523–528.

92. Laskey MA, Prentice A, Hanratty LA, et al.. Bone changes after 3 mo of lactation: influence of calcium intake, breast-milk output, and vitamin D-receptor genotype. Am J Clin Nutr 1998;67:685–692.

93. Kolthoff N, Eiken P, Kristensen B, Nielsen SP. Bone mineral changes during pregnancy and lactation: a longitudinal cohort study. Clin Sci (Colch) 1998;94:405–412.

94. Sowers M, Corton G, Shapiro B, et al. Changes in bone density with lactation. JAMA 1993;269:3130–3135.

95. Affinito P, Tommaselli GA, di Carlo C, Guida F, Nappi C. Changes in bone mineral density and calcium metabolism in breastfeeding women: a one year follow-up study. J Clin Endocrinol Metab 1996;81:2314–2318.

96. Lopez JM, Gonzalez G, Reyes V, Campino C, Diaz S. Bone turnover and density in healthy women during breastfeeding and after weaning. Osteoporos Int 1996;6:153–159.

97. Krebs NF, Reidinger CJ, Robertson AD, Brenner M. Bone mineral density changes during lactation: maternal, dietary, and biochemical correlates. Am J Clin Nutr 1997;65:1738–1746.

98. Greer FR, Lane J, Ho M. Elevated serum parathyroid hormone, calcitonin, and 1,25-dihydroxyvitamin D in lactating women nursing twins. Am J Clin Nutr 1984;40:562–568.

99. Rodin J, Radke-Sharpe N. Changes in appetitive variables as a function of pregnancy. In: Friedman MI, Tordoff MG, Kare MR, eds. Chemical senses: appetite and nutrition. Marcel Dekker, New York: 1991; pp. 325–340.

100. Beauchamp GK, Cowart BJ. Preference for extremely high levels of salt among young children. Develop Psychobiol 1990;26:539–545.

101. Cowart BJ, Beauchamp GK. Factors affecting acceptance of salt by human infants and children. In: Kare MR, Brand JG, eds. Interaction of the chemical senses with nutrition. Academic, New York: 1986; 25–40.

102. Desor JA, Greene LS, Maller O. Preferences for sweet and salty in 9- to 15-year-old and adult humans. Science 1975;190:686–687.

103. Chan MM-Y, Garey JG, Levine B, McRae JE, Terpenning I. Moderate dietary salt reduction and salt taste perception of normotensive individuals with family history of hypertension. Nutr Res 1985;5:1309–1319.

104. Tordoff MG, Rabusa SH. Calcium-deprived rats avoid sweet compounds. J Nutr 1998;128:1232–1238.

105. Reed DR, Bachmanov AA, Beauchamp GK, Tordoff MG, Price RA. Heritable variation in food preferences and their contribution to obesity. Behav Genet 1997;27:373–387.

106. Lin YC, Lyle RM, McCabe LD, McCabe GP, Weaver CM, Teegarden D. Dairy calcium is related to changes in body composition during a two-year exercise intervention in young women. J Am Coll Nutr 2000;19:754–760.

107. Carruth BR, Skinner JD. The role of dietary calcium and other nutrients in moderating body fat in preschool children. Int J Obes Relat Metab Disord 2001;25:559–566.

108. Davies KM, Heaney RP, Recker RR, et al. Calcium intake and body weight. J Clin Endocrinol Metab 2000;85:4635–4638.

109. Zemel MB, Shi H, Greer B, Dirienzo D, Zemel PC. Regulation of adiposity by dietary calcium. FASEB J 2000;14:1132–1138.
110. McCarron DA, Morris CD, Henry HJ, Stanton JL. Blood pressure and nutrient intake in the United States. Science 1984;224:1392–1398.
111. Lovejoy JC, Champagne CM, Smith SR, de Jonge L, Xie H. Ethnic differences in dietary intakes, physical activity, and energy expenditure in middle-aged, premenopausal women: the Healthy Transitions Study. Am J Clin Nutr 2001;74:90–95.
112. Heaney RP. Normalizing calcium intake: projected population effects for body weight. J Nutr 2003;133:268S–270S.
113. Pereira MA, Jacobs DR, Jr., Van Horn L, Slattery ML, Kartashov AI, Ludwig DS. Dairy consumption, obesity, and the insulin resistance syndrome in young adults: the CARDIA Study. JAMA 2002;287:2081–2089.
114. Zemel MB. Mechanisms of dairy modulation of adiposity. Jounal of Nutrition 2003;133:252S–256S.
115. Papakonstantinou E, Flatt WP, Huth PJ, Harris RB. High dietary calcium reduces body fat content, digestibility of fat, and serum vitamin D in rats. Obesity Research 2003;11:387–394.
116. Zhang Q, Tordoff MG. Effect of dietary calcium on body weight of lean and obese mice and rats. Am J Physiol 2004;286:R669–R667.
117. Coppock CE, Everett RW, Merrill WG. Effect of ration on free choice consumption of calcium-phosphorus supplements by dairy cattle. J Dairy Sci 1972;55:245–256.
118. Coppock CE, Everett RW, Belyea RL. Effect of low calcium or low phosphorus diets on free choice consumption of dicalcium phosphate by lactating dairy cows. J Dairy Sci 1976;59:571–580.
119. Thompson CJ, Bland J, Burd J, Baylis PH. The osmotic thresholds for thirst and vasopressin release are similar in healthy man. Clin Sci (Lond) 1986;71:651–656.
120. Cabanac M. The physiological role of pleasure. Science 1971;173:1103–1107.
121. The Food Marketing Institute. Facts and figures: Supermarket facts: Industry overview 2001 [Online]. www.fmi.org/facts_figs/superfact.htm.
122. Tordoff M, Hughes R, Pilchak D. Calcium intake by the rat: Influence of parathyroid hormone, calcitonin, and 1,25-dihydroxyvitamin D. Am J Physiol 1998;274:R214–R231.
123. Okiyama A, Torii K, Tordoff MG. Increased NaCl preference of rats fed low-protein diet. Am J Physiol 1996;270:R1189–R1196.

V CALCIUM THROUGH DEVELOPMENT

16 Infancy and Childhood

Steven A. Abrams and Keli M. Hawthorne

KEY POINTS

- Human milk is an excellent source of calcium for full-term infants.
- Premature infants, especially those weighing less than 1500 g at birth, require additional calcium and phosphorus for adequate bone mineralization.
- In older children, calcium deficiency is uncommon but can be a factor in the development of nutritional rickets.

1. INTRODUCTION

When considering patterns of lifetime calcium intake, most attention has been paid to ensuring adequate intakes during puberty and thereafter. This is rational because the greatest total amount of calcium is accreted to the skeleton during puberty, and optimizing peak bone mass and osteoporosis prevention are crucial in enhancing the bone health of a large portion of the population. From a pediatric perspective, however, infancy and early childhood can be a time at which calcium issues are also important, primarily to ensure that overt deficiency and rickets do not occur, but also to develop good dietary habits for later adolescence and adulthood. In this chapter, we will consider three time periods in infancy and early childhood and what is known regarding calcium nutrition during these periods. These three are (1) early life in premature infants, (2) the first 6 mo of life in full-term infants, and (3) 6 mo to 8 yr of age. Each of these poses unique challenges to our understanding of calcium needs. Although there is not a sudden change in needs at the boundaries between these life periods, they nevertheless are useful when considering calcium requirements.

2. PREMATURE INFANTS

Premature infants are defined as those delivered at less than 37 wk gestation. They may or may not be of low birth weight (<2500 g), although most infants less than 35 wk gestation will also be less than 2500 g at birth. In general, severe mineral deficiencies are most commonly identified in babies who are of very low birth weight (VLBW), that is, less than 1500 g, regardless of gestational age. Inadequate mineral intake in VLBW infants places them at risk for low bone mass, often called "osteopenia of prematurity." In this condition, the bone mineral content (BMC) of a premature infant is significantly

From: *Calcium in Human Health*
Edited by: C. M. Weaver and R. P. Heaney © Humana Press Inc., Totowa, NJ

decreased relative to the expected level of mineralization for a fetus or infant of comparable size or gestational age. It may occur in as many as one-half of infants less than 1000 g birth weight who are fed either unfortified human milk or formulas that are designed for full-term rather than preterm infants (1,2). Most cases of osteopenia in VLBW infants are related to a deficiency in the two primary bone minerals, calcium and phosphorus. Vitamin D deficiency is an extremely uncommon clinical problem in VLBW infants. Phosphorus deficiency may be a problem equal to or greater than calcium deficiency. The frequency of osteopenia is increased in VLBW infants who require long-term parenteral nutrition, who are severely fluid restricted (as a result of chronic cardiorespiratory problems), or who require medications—especially loop diuretics—that may affect mineral metabolism (3,4).

Calcium and phosphorus are rapidly accreted during the third trimester of gestation. A premature infant born at 24–26 wk gestation, despite having completed 60% of his/her gestational time, will weigh only approx 800 g (~25% of the weight of a full-term infant) and have a whole-body calcium of 6–7 g (~20% of that of a full-term infant). During the peak time of calcium accumulation, from approx 30 to 36 wk of gestation, the fetus will accrete 100–120 mg/kg/d of calcium or approx 250–300 mg/d (5,6). This rate, with regard to body weight, is unmatched at any other time in life. The 300 mg/d added to the skeleton *in utero* is much greater than in infancy and early childhood, and is comparable with the maximum amount accreted during the peak of the pubertal growth spurt. In other words, the 2-kg, third-trimester fetus must accumulate daily approximately as much calcium as a pubertal adolescent. This is a remarkable rate, and is achieved via rates of bone formation that are comparable with that of adults with extremely low rates of bone resorption (7). Phosphorus accretion follows the same pattern as calcium, with net phosphorus accretion being approx 50–60 mg/kg/d during the third trimester of pregnancy (5).

This need for a large amount of calcium and phosphorus cannot readily be met by human milk (8). Human milk contains approx 220 mg calcium per liter and 140 mg phosphorus per liter. These concentrations are not altered significantly in the milk of mothers who deliver prematurely (9,10). Fortifying human milk with additional nutrients can minimize mineral deficiencies and the risk of osteopenia (11). Although no data exist from which to conclude exactly which infants should receive fortified human milk, the general consensus is that infants weighing less than 1500 g at birth would benefit from the fortification (12,13).

Various methods of human milk fortification have been developed. The most commonly used approaches in the United States are (1) multinutrient packaged powdered fortifiers, (2) special high-mineral liquid formulas that are mixed with human milk, and (3) alternating feedings of human milk and specialized high mineral-containing formulas. In other countries, these approaches are used, but it is also common to add minerals individually to human milk rather than use commercial products (14). Currently, several commercial fortifiers of human milk for premature infants are marketed to increase calories, protein, calcium, phosphorus, sodium, vitamins, and other minerals. Those available in the United States are shown in Table 1.

Growth measures and nutrient retention are key factors to consider when evaluating a method of human milk fortification. Premature infants are typically provided with adequate nutrients when they are fed 150–160 mL/kg/d of human milk fortified with one of the commercial fortificants shown in Table 1 (15). Infants consuming fortified human

Table 1
Comparison of Breast Milk and Commercially Available Human Milk Fortifiers When Fed at 150 mL/kg/d

Nutrient	Term human milk	Human milk plus Enfamil® Human milk fortifier (HMF)[a]	Human milk plus Similac® HMF[b]	Human Milk plus Similac Natural Care (25:75 ratio)[b]
Mixture	N/A	4 pkts HMF: 100 mL human milk	4 pkts HMF: 100 mL human milk	25 mL human milk:75 mL formula
Volume	150 mL/kg	150 mL/kg	150 mL/kg	150 mL/kg
Energy	102 kcal/kg	120 kcal/kg	124 kcal/kg	117 kcal/kg
Protein	1.57 g/kg	3.14 kg/kg	2.94 g/kg	2.87 g/kg
Calcium	42 mg/kg	172 mg/kg	230 mg/kg	202 mg/kg
Phosphorus	21 mg/kg	94 mg/kg	130 mg/kg	111 mg/kg
Magnesium	5.2 mg/kg	6.5 mg/kg	15.7 mg/kg	12.3 mg/kg
Calcium:Phos	2.0	1.8	1.8	1.8

[a]Mead Johnson Nutritionals, Evansville, IN.
[b]Ross Products Division of Abbott Laboratories, Columbus, OH.

271

Table 2
Typical Calcium Absorption and Retention in Premature Infants Receiving Different Calcium Sources[a]

	Calcium intake (mg/kg/d)	Percent retained (%)	Total retained (mg/kg/d)	Reference
In utero	N/A	N/A	100-120	21
Human milk	40	60	24	22
Fortified human milk	160	50–60	80–95	11,12,15
Parenteral nutrition	80	approx 95	75	5,12
Preterm formula	200–220	40–50	Up to 110	7,11

[a]Intakes assume typical full volume feeding and usual rates of urinary mineral excretion.

milk show improved gains in weight, length, and head circumference (16–18). Adequate retention of key nutrients has also been achieved with fortified human milk.

Not all studies have shown a benefit to adding minerals to human milk given to premature infants. In one randomized, blinded intervention study, researchers found that mineral supplementation either with phosphorus alone or with a multinutrient fortifier did not significantly improve bone mineralization in premature infants (19). However, the authors speculate that the high volume of intake achieved (200 mL/kg/d) in this study could account for the lack of effect of the supplementation on bone mineral content. Poor bioavailability of the added minerals and the use of phosphorus without adequate calcium could also have decreased the effectiveness of the approach in that study. It is clear that, regardless of bioavailability, there is limited ability even of high volume to meet the mineral requirement of premature infants. Calculations (see Table 2) show that using available bioavailability data, human milk can only provide about one-fourth of the needed calcium for VLBW infants. Even if 80% of the calcium were to be retained (a nonphysiological amount), the total would only reach about one-third of the requirement.

There are several important points to be considered regarding Table 1. First, it is not necessarily the case that the in utero rates of calcium and phosphorus accretion must be met for VLBW infants to grow well and avoid osteopenia. VLBW infants usually do not grow as rapidly after birth as they do in utero. However, once full enteral nutrition is established, growth rates often increase rapidly to in utero levels, and it is likely that skeletal growth is optimized by matching the in utero rates of mineral accretion.

The second is that although infants receiving full-volume feeding of enteral and even parenteral nutrition have a relatively small gap between their calcium retention and in utero rates, this gap can easily become much larger in the presence of fluid restriction, such as is widely used for infants with bronchopulmonary dysplasia. In response to this, approaches have recently been developed to "super-fortify" human milk and even preterm formula by either concentrating the formula or by adding high mineral-containing formula to human milk that is already fortified at usual levels with commercial human milk fortifiers. Neither of these approaches is practical for nonenterally fed babies (e.g.. those with short guts) and for infants with feeding intolerance. Such babies may be at very high risk of mineral deficiency and clinical rickets.

The final point is that not all human milk fortifiers or preterm formulas have comparable mineral bioavailability or content. Some products may have low mineral bioavailability and may not lead to the same clinical benefit. A recent European study found that human milk fortification did not meet mineral needs of infants born weighing less than1000 g (23). However, this fortifier has considerably less total calcium and phosphorus compared with fortifiers available in the United States, and may also have lower mineral bioavailability because of poor solubility of the mineral sources (24).

There has been concern regarding the safety of human milk fortification. A recent report from Finland evaluated the frequency of and risk for necrotizing enterocolitis (NEC) in preterm infants and found that fortified human milk feedings were an overall risk factor for all cases of NEC, but not for severe cases of NEC (Bell grades II–III) (25). Only the severe cases usually have major impact on the ultimate outcomes of infants. This was not a blinded, controlled trial, and there was a large weight difference ($p < 0.001$) between patients with severe NEC and controls (926 vs 1440 g, respectively). Infants with birth weights less than1000 g were more likely to receive fortified human milk as a result of their low birth weights in an effort to help them achieve their growth potentials. In addition, the frequency of dexamethasone use, well established as a risk factor for intestinal perforation (26–28), was significantly increased ($p < 0.001$) in the group of infants with NEC compared with controls (42 vs 5%, respectively). In another study, investigators (29) evaluated developmental outcomes in a randomized trial and found that premature infants who consumed fortified human milk had a slightly but not significantly higher incidence of NEC ($p - 0.12$) compared with control infants consuming preterm formula.

In contrast, other investigations have reported a protective effect of human milk, even if fortified, over preterm formula. Infection was less frequently observed in human milk-fed infants compared to formula-fed infants (26 vs 49%, respectively) (30). In a large prospective trial, investigators reported a lower incidence of NEC among human-milk fed premature infants compared to exclusively formula-fed infants (31). A prospective, double-blind, placebo-controlled trial (32) evaluated the growth and nutritional status of preterm infants receiving different types of fortifier added to their mother's milk. Investigators found no statistically significant differences in the incidence of NEC, and concluded that premature infants tolerate both of the powdered fortifiers very well. Researchers also report an 84% reduction in the incidence of NEC after implementing a specific feeding protocol in their nursery (33). Although the authors did not address human milk fortification specifically in their report, they did note that there was a 60% reduction in the risk of NEC among human milk-fed infants.

In one large-scale study (34) on growth, nutritional status, and feeding tolerance of premature infants, investigators compared outcomes of infants consuming fortified human milk vs preterm formula. The group fed fortified human milk had a lower incidence ($p < 0.01$) of NEC and sepsis than the formula-fed group. One possible reason for this increase in protection in the human milk-fed group is the high immunoglobulin A content of human milk. In addition, infants fed human milk may experience more frequent skin-to-skin interactions with the mother, which is valuable in increasing maternal milk output. This contact may lead to increased stimulation of maternal antibodies in breast milk against nosocomial pathogens in the hospital's nursery.

Taken together, we strongly believe that the currently available data support the safety and efficacy of human milk fortification for all human milk-fed VLBW infants. Fortified human milk makes the numerous health, nutritional, immunological, and developmental benefits (35) of human milk available to the smallest of infants while improving their growth rates and protecting their bones from significant risk of underdevelopment.

With current neonatal practices, the majority of VLBW infants born at more than 24 wk gestation will be discharged home. Those born weighing less than 1000 g are frequently discharged requiring fluid restriction and loop diuretics well after hospitalization. To meet the needs of this population, as well as larger preterm infants in which faster "catch-up mineralization" may be desired, several infant formulas have been developed that are specifically designed for use at home after hospital discharge. These formulas, often called "transitional" or "enriched" formulas, generally contain an amount of calcium and phosphorus midway between that of routine term-infant formulas and those designed for in-hospital feeding of premature infants. Several recent studies have evaluated these formulas and found improved growth and catch-up mineralization in infants to whom they were fed, compared with infants fed routine term-infant formulas. The benefit appears to be present for up to 8 mo of use of these formulas (36–38). The benefits may be greater in male than female infants (39,40). However, there are few data on which to base a decision as to which babies should receive these transitional formulas and how long they should be continued. We generally recommend that they be used in infants weighing less than 1500 g who are formula-fed, and that they be continued until at least 6 mo corrected gestational age. Use for infants between 1500–2000 g birth weight is reasonable, although less critical. For healthy infants weighing more than 2000 g at birth, routine infant formula will usually suffice.

A special situation to consider is the VLBW infant (especially <1000 g birth weight) whose mother intends to breastfeed exclusively after hospital discharge. Although most VLBW infants will do very well at home under this circumstance, it is prudent to assess these infants for evidence of mineral deficiency at some point, perhaps 4–8 wk after discharge (by measuring serum phosphorus and alkaline phosphatase). Such infants need careful postdischarge monitoring for laboratory evidence of inadequate bone mineral status. Supplemental minerals can be given by adding a small number of daily feedings of a transitional formula, using a bottle or specialized infant feeding device. If the mother is giving the infant breast milk via a bottle, powdered transitional formula can be added to the milk prior to feeding; although use of this approach postdischarge has not been evaluated in a controlled trial. In circumstances in which supplemental formula is not feasible (i.e., severe cow milk protein allergy) or desired, direct mineral supplementation of both calcium and phosphorus (and possibly zinc) may be advisable with careful follow-up of growth and bone mineralization.

3. FULL-TERM INFANTS LESS THAN 6 MO OF AGE

The challenge of determining the role of calcium absorption in bone health begins with infants. In this case, two potentially conflicting guidelines come into consideration. The first is the global consensus that human milk is the optimal nutritional source as a single food source in the first 6 mo of life and as the primary milk source throughout the first year of life (35). For calcium, this means that dietary requirements are based primarily on the intake from their mother's milk *(20,41)*, because relatively little calcium is derived from most solid infant foods.

In potential conflict with this, however, is the guideline that increasing calcium absorption and bone mineralization is beneficial in childhood. In this case, the demonstration that infant formulas have led to slightly greater bone mineralization in both the whole body and some skeletal regions than that obtained by human milk-fed babies. However, this increased BMC may not persist even during later infancy *(20,41)*.

There is a consensus also that calcium is well absorbed from human milk, with values for net calcium retention of about 50–60% of intake *(21,22)*. Calcium absorption values from infant formulas are highly variable as a result of the various carbohydrate, protein, and mineral sources of these formulas. Although it is generally stated that calcium bioavailability of formulas is lower than that of human milk, this may not always be the case. Early findings may have been related to the greater concentration of calcium in infant formulas than in human milk *(20,21)*. (*See also* Chapter 10 for a discussion of the effect of calcium load size on absorption.) In general, however, values of 30–40% absorption are typical for cow's milk-based infant formulas or whole cow's milk *(13)*.

Since the Infant Formula Act of 1980 in the United States, numerous expert committees have recommended higher concentrations of calcium in formulas than in human milk *(13,20,42)*. Calcium bioavailability comparisons at identical calcium concentration in human milk and formula have not been performed. However, several studies *(43,44)* have shown fractional calcium absorption vaules from infant formulas to be very similar to those for human milk.

These data indicate that it is possible for formula-fed infants to accumulate more calcium and bone mass during the first 6 mo of life than human milk-fed infants. It remains unknown, however, whether that is a worthwhile goal. There are no data to support any long-term benefit, in terms of either increased peak bone mass or the prevention of osteoporosis, of high calcium absorption or bone mass in early infancy *(45)*. Animal data further support the idea that increases in calcium intake in early childhood do not have beneficial effects on long-term bone mass *(46)*. Ultimately, long-term research must be done before it is appropriate to advocate or target a higher calcium retention or bone mass accretion in artificially fed infants relative to the human milk-fed standard. There are no data regarding the long-term consequences of different calcium intake levels or feeding sources provided to full-term infants. In a group of healthy, breast-fed, 5- to 7-mo-old infants, we calculated net calcium retention of approx 70 mg/d, and concluded that calcium from human milk is well absorbed by infants after the introduction of solid foods *(47)*.

Studies evaluating the BMC of full-term infants during the first year of life have generally found a slightly greater value for those fed infant formulas than in those fed human milk *(42)*. However, it is uncertain if this difference is maintained later in childhood. At present, there is no reason to recommend that high levels of calcium be given to infants less than 6 mo of age.

4. CHILDREN 6 MO TO 8 YR OF AGE

For several decades, the existence of a specific calcium deficiency—rickets—has been recognized, based on both case reports *(48,49)* and strong epidemiological data, especially from South Africa *(50)*. Recently, however, a series of studies conducted in Nigeria has provided compelling evidence for this entity. In these studies, it has been shown that despite an incidence of rickets of about 10% in Nigeria, vitamin D deficiency was very uncommon *(51)*. The 25 hydroxyvitamin D concentrations are similar in Nigerian children with and without rickets *(52,53)*. Finally, it was recently shown in Nigeria that the clinical response to vitamin D supplementation in children with rickets was lower than the response to calcium or to a combination of calcium and vitamin D *(54)*. The minimum calcium intake needed to prevent calcium-deficiency rickets has not been precisely identified. Egyptian children 1–2 yr of age who had mean calcium intakes of 290 mg/d with adequate vitamin D status did not develop rickets *(55)*. Among black South Africans, biochemical abnormalities associated with rickets occurred in 7- to 12-yr-old children with calcium intakes of 125 mg/d, but not those with 337 mg/d. None of the children with rickets or controls were vitamin D-deficient (50). In Nigerian children, calcium intakes averaging 200 mg/d were found in rachitic children *(51,52,56)*. These results suggest that calcium intakes below 300 mg/d in infants and small children may pose a high risk of rickets, especially among children who might have marginal or low vitamin D status.

Few data are available regarding calcium requirements in children prior to puberty. We recently found an increase in net calcium absorption when the intake of calcium in 3- to 5-yr-old children was increased from 500 to 1200 mg/d *(57)*. The benefit was relatively modest, however, and intermediate intake levels, as might more readily be achieved in preschool children, were not evaluated in this study. The potential benefit to ultimate peak bone mass of increasing calcium intake in this age group has been studied in groups of prepubertal children. In one controlled calcium supplementation trial, an increase in bone mass was found when calcium supplements were given to children as young as 6 yr of age *(58)*. However, relatively few children this young were studied, and the duration of effect of this supplementation and its impact on peak bone mass are uncertain. Further studies are needed to evaluate different levels of calcium intake in this age group.

High levels of calcium intake may negatively affect the absorption of other minerals such as iron and zinc. These minerals may be marginal in toddlers and preschool children, especially in developing countries. Therefore, more data regarding the risks and benefits of high calcium intake are needed in children and adolescents. It is likely, however, that adaptation to high calcium intakes occurs such that iron status and iron absorption are not harmed over a long period of time *(57,59)*. It is reasonable to conclude that greater consumption of calcium-rich foods and beverages can safely be encouraged in small children.

Recently, investigators reported the results of a follow-up study conducted more than 3 yr after the original controlled calcium supplementation trial was completed in prepubertal girls *(60)*. The initial study randomly assigned 149 girls (mean age, 7.9 yr) to calcium-enriched foods (average increase in calcium intake, 850 mg/d) or placebo for 48 k. BMCt and areal bone mineral density (aBMD)at six skeletal sites were measured by dual-energy X-ray absorptiometry (DXA) at the beginning and end of the study in 144 subjects, and mean changes at each site were calculated. In the supplemented group, a positive effect on aBMD was observed, along with an increased mean gain in BMC and bone size, with a trend for greater progression in standing height. When the girls ($N = 116$)

were re-examined 3.5 yr after the initial intervention concluded (with pubertal maturation and spontaneous calcium intake taken into consideration), the increase in bone mineral mass and skeletal longitudinal growth was maintained at a highly significant level in the calcium-supplemented group compared with the placebo group (179 mg/cm^2 vs 151 mg/cm^2, respectively). Thus, according to this study, the beneficial effects of calcium supplementation can persist for at least several years after discontinuation. The authors noted that they used a calcium phosphate extract from milk and that a qualitative difference in bone response according to the calcium salt used might account for the different result obtained in this trial, compared with other studies (60).

5. CONCLUSION

Calcium is an important nutrient for infants and children of all ages. Calcium deficiencies can lead to osteopenia of prematurity and rickets. Comparisons of formula-fed infants with human milk-fed infants show that infant formulas contain calcium adequate to produce appropriate net retention, although human milk remains the ideal nutrition source for infants. For hospitalized premature infants receiving breast milk, additional fortification using commercially available fortifiers provides extra calories, protein, vitamins, and minerals, and leads to improved growth parameters and nutrient retention. Young children with inadequate intake of calcium, although sufficient in vitamin D, may be at risk for rickets. Finally, although few studies have addressed calcium requirements in prepubertal children, the potential benefits of adequate calcium upon entering the peak bone mass phase underscore the importance of further research with this age group.

ACKNOWLEDGMENT/DISCLAIMER

This work is a publication of the US Department of Agriculture (USDA)/Agricultural Research Service (ARS) Children's Nutrition Research Center, Department of Pediatrics, Baylor College of Medicine and Texas Children's Hospital, Houston, TX. This project has been funded in part with federal funds from the USDA/ARS under Cooperative Agreement number 58-6250-6-001. Contents of this publication do not necessarily reflect the views or policies of the USDA, nor does mention of trade names, commercial products, or organizations imply endorsement by the US government.

REFERENCES

1. Abrams SA. Using stable isotopes to assess mineral absorption and utilization by children. Am J Clin Nutr 1999;70:955–964.
2. Heaney RP. Factors influencing the measurement of bioavailability, taking calcium as a model. J Nutr 2001;131:1344S–1348S.
3. Caksen H, Ozturk A, Kurtoglu S, Tuncel M. Reports of osteopenia/rickets of prematurity are on the increase because of improved survival rates of low birthweight infants. J Emerg Med 2002;23:305–306.
4. Toomey F, Hoag R, Batton D, Vain N. Rickets associated with cholestatis and parenteral nutrition in premature infants. Radiology 1982;142:85–88.
5. Salle BL, Senterre J, Putet G. Calcium, phosphorus, magnesium, and vitamin D requirements in premature infants. Nutrition of the low birthweight infant. Nestle Nutrition Workshop Series 1992, Vol. 32:125–135.
6. Abrams SA. Enteral feeding of the preterm infant: an update of recent findings. Bailliere's Clin Paediatr 1997;5:305–316.

7. Abrams SA, Schanler RJ, Yergey AL, Vieira NE, Bronner F. Compartmental analysis of calcium metabolism in very low birth weight infants. Pediatr Res 1994;36:424–428.
8. Atkinson SA, Radde IC, Anderson GH. Macromineral balances in premature infants fed their own mothers' milk or formula. J Pediatr 1983;102:99–106.
9. Butte NF, Garza C, Johnson CA, Smith EO, Nichols BL. Longitudinal changes in milk composition of mothers delivering preterm and term infants. Early Hum Dev 1986;9:153–164.
10. Koo WWK, Sherman R, Succop P, et al. Sequential bone mineral content in small preterm infants with and without fractures and rickets. J Bone Miner Res 1988;3:193–197.
11. Schanler RJ, Abrams SA, Garza C. Bioavailability of calcium and phosphorus in human milk fortifiers and formula for very low birth weight infants. J Pediatr 1988;113:95–100.
12. Schanler RJ. Human milk fortification for premature infants. Am J Clin Nutr 1996;64:249–250.
13. Life Sciences Research Office (LSRO) report. Assessment of nutrient requirements for infant formulas. J Nutr 1998;128:2059S–2293S.
14. Trotter A, Pohlandt F. Calcium and phosphorus retention in extremely preterm infants supplemented individually. Acta Paediatr 2002;91:680–683.
15. Schanler RJ. The use of human milk for premature infants. Pediatr Clin North Am 2001;48:207–219.
16. Porcelli P, Schanler R, Greer F, et al. Growth in human milk-fed very low birth weight infants receiving a new human milk fortifier. Ann Nutr Metab 2000;44:2–10.
17. Kashyap S, Forsyth M, Zucker C, Ramakrishnan R, Dell RB, Heird WC. Effects of varying protein and energy intakes on growth and metabolic response in low birth weight infants. J Pediatr 1986;108:955–963.
18. Charles P. Calcium absorption and calcium bioavailability. J Intern Med 1992;231:161#-168.
19. Faerk J, Petersen S, Peitersen B, Fleischer Michaelsen K. Diet and bone mineral content at term in premature infants. Pediatr Res 2000;47:148–156.
20. Institute of Medicine Food and Nutrition Board's Standing Committee on the Scientific Evaluation of Dietary Intervals: Calcium. Dietary Reference Intervals for Calcium, Phosphorus, Magnesium, Vitamin D and Fluoride. National Academy Press, Washington, DC: 1997; pp. 71–146.
21. Fomon SJ, Nelson SE. Calcium, phosphorus, magnesium, and sulfur. In: Fomon SJ. Nutrition of normal infants. Mosby-Year Book, St. Louis: 1993; 192–218.
22. Abrams SA, Wen J, Stuff JE. Absorption of calcium, zinc and iron from breast milk by 5- to 7-month-old infants. Pediatr Res 1997;41:384–390.
23. Loui A, Raab A, Obladen M, Bratter P. Calcium, phosphorus and magnesium balance: FM 85 fortification of human milk does not meet mineral needs of extremely low birthweight infants. Euro J Clin Nutr 2002;56:228–235.
24. DeCurtis M, Candusso M, Pieltain C, Rigo J. Effect of fortification on the osmolality of human milk. Arch Dis Child Fetal Neonatol Ed 1999;81:F141–F143.
25. Hallstrom M, Koivisto AM, Janas M, Tammela O. Frequency of and risk factors for necrotizing enterocolitis in infants born before 33 weeks of gestation. Acta Paediatr 2003;92:111–113.
26. De Laet MH, Dassonville M, Johanasson A, et al.. Small-bowel perforation in very low birth weight neonates treated with high-dose dexamethasone. Eur J Pediatr Surg 2000;10:323–327.
27. Gordon P, Rutledge J, Sawin R, Thomas S, Woodrum D. Early postnatal dexamethasone increases the risk of focal small bowel perforation in extremely low birth weight infants. J Perinatol 1999;19:573–577.
28. Stark AR, Carlo WA, Tyson JE, et al. Adverse effects of early dexamethasone in extremely-low-birth-weight infants: National Institute of Child Health and Human Development Neonatal Research Network. N Engl J Med 2001;344:95–101.
29. Lucas A, Fewtrell MS, Morley R, et al. Randomized outcome trial of human milk fortification and developmental outcome in preterm infants. Am J Clin Nutr 1996;64:142–151.
30. Hylander MA, Strobino DM, Dhanireddy R. Human milk feedings and infection among very low birth weight infants. Pediatrics 1998;102:e38.
31. Lucas A, Cole TJ. Breast milk and neonatal necrotizing enterocolitis. Lancet 1990;336:1519–1523.
32. Reis BB, Hall RT, Schanler RJ, et al. Enhanced growth of preterm infants fed a new powdered human milk fortifier: a randomized, controlled trial. Pediatrics 2000;106:581–588.
33. Kamitsuka MD, Horton MK, Williams MA. The incidence of necrotizing enterocolitis after introducing standardized feeding schedules for infants between 1250 and 2500 grams and less than 35 weeks of gestation. Pediatrics 2000;105:379–384.

34. Schanler RJ, Shulman RJ, Lau C. Feeding strategies for premature infants: beneficial outcomes of feeding fortified human milk versus preterm formula. Pediatrics 1999;103:1150–1157.

35. American Academy of Pediatrics Task Force on Breastfeeding. Breastfeeding and the use of milk. Pediatrics 1997;100:1035–1039.

36. Worrell LA, Thorp JW, Tucker R, et al. The effects of the introduction of a high-nutrient transitional formula on growth and development of very-low-birth-weight infants. J Perinatol 2002;22:112–119.

37. Carver JD, Wu PY, Hall RT, et al. Growth of preterm infants fed nutrient-enriched or term formula after hospital discharge. Pediatrics 2001;107:683–689.

38. Bishop NJ, King FJ, Lucas A. Increased bone mineral content of preterm infants fed with a nutrient enriched formula after discharge from hospital. Arch Dis Child 1993;68:573–578.

39. Griffin IJ. Postdischarge nutrition for high risk neonates. Clin Perinatol 2001;29:327–344.

40. Lucas A, Fewtrell MS, Morley R, et al. Randomized trial of nutrient-enriched formula versus standard formula for postdischarge preterm infants. Pediatrics 2001;108:703–711.

41. Committee on Nutrition, American Academy of Pediatrics. Calcium requirements of infants, children, and adolescents. Pediatrics 1999;104:1152–1157.

42. Specker, BL, Beck A, Kalfwarf H, Ho M. Randomized trial of varying mineral intake on total body bone mineral accretion during the first year of life. Pediatrics 1997;99:E12.

43. Abrams SA, Griffin IJ, Davila PM. Calcium and zinc absorption from lactose-containing and lactose-free infant formulas. Am J Clin Nutr 2002;76:442–446.

44. Lifschitz CL, Abrams SA. Addition of rice cereal to formula does not impair mineral bioavailability. J Pediatr Gastroenterol Nutr 1998;26:175–178.

45. Jones G, Riley M, Dwyer T. Breastfeeding in early life and bone mass in prepubertal children: A longitudinal study. Osteoporosis Int 2000;11:146–152.

46. Gafni RI, McCarthy EF, Hatcher T, et al. Recovery from osteoporosis through skeletal growth: Early bone mass acquisition has little effect on adult bone density. FASEB J 2002;16:736–738.

47. Abrams SA, Wen J, Stuff JE. Absorption of calcium, zinc, and iron from breast milk by five- to seven-month-old infants. Pediatr Res 1997;41:384–390.

48. Kooh SW, Graser D, Reilly BJ, Hamilton JR, Gall DG, Bell L. Rickets due to calcium deficiency. N Eng J Med. 1977;297:1264–1266.

49. Legius E, Proesmans W, Eggermont E, Vandamme-Lombaerts R, Bouillon R, Smet M. Rickets due to dietary calcium deficiency. Eur J Pediatr 1989;148:784–785.

50. Pettifor JM, Ross P, Moodley G, Shuenyane E. Calcium deficiency in rural black children in South Africa—a comparison between rural and urban communities. Am J Clin Nutr 1979;32:2477–2483.

51. Thatcher TD, Fischer PR, Pettifor JM, Lawson JO, Isichei CO, Chan GM. Case-control study of factors associated with nutritional rickets in Nigerian children. J Pediatr 2000;137:367–373.

52. Okonofua F, Gill DS, Alabi ZO, Thomas M, Bell JL, Dandona P. Rickets in Nigerian children: a consequence of calcium malnutrition. Metabolism 1991;40:209–213

53. Pfitzner MA, Thacher TD, Pettifor JM, et al. Absence of vitamin D deficiency in young Nigerian children. J Pediatr 1998;133:740–744

54. Thatcher TD, Fischer PR, Pettifor JM, et al. A comparison of calcium, vitamin D, or both for nutritional rickets in Nigerian children. N Engl J Med 1999;341:563–568

55. Lawson DE, Cole TJ, Salem S, et al. Etiology of rickets in Egyptian children. Hum Nutr Clin Nutr. 1987;41:199–208

56. Oginni LM, Worsfold M, Oyelami OA, Sharp CA, Powell DE, Davie MWJ. Etiology of rickets in Nigerian children. J Pediatr 1996;128:692–694.

57. Ames SK, Gorham BM, Abrams SA. Effects of high vs low calcium intake on calcium absorption and red blood cell iron incorporation by small children. Am J Clin Nutr 1999;70:44–48.

58. Johnston CC. Miller JZ, Slemenda CW, et al. Calcium supplementation and increases in bone mineral density in children. N Engl J Med. 1992, 327:82–87.

59. Abrams SA, Griffin IJ, Davila P, Liang L. Calcium fortification of breakfast cereal enhances calcium absorption in children without affecting iron absorption. J Pediatr 2001;139:522–526.

60. Bonjour JP, Chevalley T, Ammann P, Slosman D, Rizzoli R. Gain in bone mineral mass in prepubertal girls 3.5 years after discontinuation of calcium supplementation: a follow-up study. Lancet 2001;358:1208–1212.

17 Prepuberty and Adolescence

Connie M. Weaver

KEY POINTS

- Adolescence is an especially important period for adequate calcium intakes, because 25–50% of peak bone mass is accumulated during this period. The minimal calcium intake that allows maximal calcium retention is 1300 mg/d.
- Calcium intake shows a moderate degree of tracking.
- All randomized, controlled trials in children show a benefit of calcium supplementation from any source to one or more skeletal sites.
- Children with low milk intake have greater risk for fracture later in life.

1. INTRODUCTION

Adequate intake of calcium in prepuberty and adolescence is very important while peak bone mass is being acquired. The rate of calcium accretion during growth was determined from gains in bone mineral content (BMC) taken annually in a longitudinal study of a cohort of Caucasian Canadian boys and girls *(1)*. Because calcium is a constant component of BMC, profiles of gains in BMC as shown in Fig. 1 also reflect calcium accretion. It is clear from this figure that rates of calcium retention are not uniform across childhood. The curve has a rather sharp peak; approximately one-fourth of adult BMC is acquired in 2 yr bracketing the peak accretion rate. Likely regulators of pubertal growth spurt and skeletal maturation include insulin-like growth factor-1 and sex steroid hormones *(2)*. The figure further shows that boys have a higher mean peak rate of BMC accretion than girls (409 vs 325 g/yr) and the peak occurs later in boys than girls (age 14 vs 12.5 yr). A nonparametric function of age using weighted and mean averages of longitudinal data in white females showed maximum bone growth occurs at age 12 yr (11–12, 90% confidence interval [CI]) for the spine and femoral neck (10–14, 90% CI), whereas cessation of growth at the spine occurred at age 36 yr (32–44, 90% CI) and at age 24 yr (19–34, 90% CI) for the femoral neck *(3)*. Estimates of the percent of peak BMC for selected sites are illustrated in Fig. 2 taken from data reported by Teegarden *(4)* and Lin *(5)*. The age of attaining peak spine BMC was beyond the age of the cohort studied by Lin et al. *(5)*, but the age at which 90% of peak spine BMD was achieved was 15.2 yr, and 17.6 yr for 95%. Bone accretion rates with age are not available for other races and ethnic groups.

From: *Calcium in Human Health*
Edited by: C. M. Weaver and R. P. Heaney © Humana Press Inc., Totowa, NJ

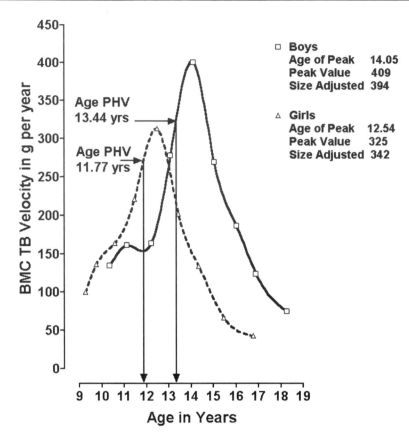

Fig. 1. Total body (TB) peak bone mineral conten (BMC) velocity curve illustrating velocity at peak and ages at peak BMC and peak health velocities (PHV) by chronological age for boys and girls. (Reproduced from ref. *1*, with permission of the American Society of Bone and Mineral Research.)

In this chapter, trends in calcium intake of school-age children, calcium metabolism, calcium requirements, and relationships of calcium to development of peak bone mass are discussed. In some ways, the phase of pubertal growth dominates over other influences such as modifiers of calcium absorption, but in other ways, such as gender and race, this period enables strong differences to emerge.

2. DIET

The diet of children is largely influenced by caregivers until the transition begins between dependence and independence. During puberty, peer influence and preoccupation with physical appearance can influence food choices and eating habits. Consequently, on average, intakes of calcium meet requirements up until approximately age 11 yr, after which only Caucasian boys consume intakes that meet or exceed recommended intakes (*see* Chapter 8).

2.1. Trends in Calcium Intake

Consistent with the trends of declining milk intake and increasing soft-drink consumption for all Americans over several decades, depicted in Fig. 4 in Chapter 9, are intake

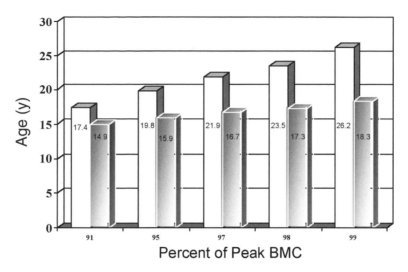

Fig. 2. Estimates of ages at which selected percentages of peak bone mineral content is achieved for total body (light bars) and femoral neck (dark bars). (Data from refs. *4* and *5*.)

trends specific to children. In the Bogalusa Heart Study, from 1972 to 1994 the proportion of 10-yr-old children consuming milk declined over time, whereas those consuming sweetened beverages including soft drinks, sweetened coffee, and sugar- and fruit-flavored drinks, increased *(6)*. Average milk consumption decreased by 64 g during these two decades, although cheese consumption increased slightly by 18 g during this same period. Total calcium intakes increased despite declining milk consumption through a wider variety of foods, although intakes did not achieve recommended levels. Students who participate in school lunch and breakfast programs have higher intakes of calcium and other nutrients *(7)*.

Increased soft-drink consumption and decreased milk consumption in childhood and adolescence have been associated with decreased quality of the overall diet *(8,9)*. The average daily consumption of soda is almost as high as that for milk *(7)*. In a summer day camp, when children aged 6–13 yr consumed more than three glasses (>16%) of sweetened drinks per day, they drank significantly less milk by 247 g or 1 c/d than when they consumed no sweetened drinks *(10)*. This also resulted in lower intakes of protein, calcium, phosphorus, magnesium, and zinc. Two studies evaluated the consequences of soft-drink consumption on bone gain. One was a cross-sectional study of heel bone mineral density in 591 boys and 744 girls either 12 or 15 yr old *(11)*. The other was longitudinal study in Canadian children using one-tenth as many subjects, but a stronger measure of bone accrual, total body BMC, and bone mineral density (BMD) over the 2 yr of maximal bone gain *(12)*. Soft-drink intake negatively impacted the bone mineral accrual of adolescent girls, but not of boys, in both studies, even though fluid milk consumption was negatively related to soft-drink consumption in both boys and girls.

2.2. Tracking of Calcium Intake

Because in the 20th century, most dietary calcium comes from dairy foods, calcium intakes show a moderate degree of tracking *(13–15)*. Consumption of milk during childhood persisted into adolescence with an association of $r = 0.66$, $p < 0.0001$ *(15)*. The associations between childhood and adolescent milk intakes and current calcium intake as young adults were $r = 0.26$, $p < 0.0001$ and $r = 0.33$, $p < 0.0001$, respectively. In a 15-yr study of a cohort begun as adolescents-tracking for calcium intake over time, the coefficient of correlation was $r = 0.43$ for males and $r = 0.38$ for females *(16)*. One study reported that dairy food intakes are largely established by the age of 5 yr *(17)*.

The type of dairy products consumed over time changes with age, according to some studies. In the Bogalusa Heart Study cohort, mean consumption of milk decreased as children became young adults, whereas cheese consumption increased *(6)*.

Tracking of obesity is at least as strong as tracking of calcium intake. Thus, for several reasons, the importance of nutrition guidance during the formative years should be emphasized.

3. METABOLISM

Calcium metabolism alters through the pubertal growth spurt to accomplish the bone gains illustrated in Fig. 1. Calcium retention in Caucasian adolescent girls was in strikingly more positive calcium balance than that of young adults in the same study *(18)*. Calcium retention was strongly negatively correlated with years postmenarche ($r = 0.788$, $p < 0.001$). The peak in calcium retention corresponds to the onset of menses. The higher retention during puberty compared with young adults was accomplished because adolescents were more efficient at absorbing calcium, conserving it at the kidney, and making it available for bone deposition *(19)*. Extravascular pool sizes were larger in adolescents because of slower pool turnover rates; in adults, calcium was returned to plasma where it was excreted, whereas in adolescents, it was directed to extravascular pools where it was available for bone deposition. Figure 3 illustrates that black girls use calcium much more efficiently than white girls *(20)*. Blacks had greater calcium retention, resulting from increased calcium absorption and decreased urinary output compared with whites. Blacks had greater bone formation rates relative to bone resorption rates compared with whites. The bone is moving much more calcium in and out for blacks than for whites, and appears to be driving increased intestinal calcium absorption and more efficient conservation at the kidney. We previously modeled the rapid decline in calcium retention with postmenarcheal age (PMA) and projected the racial differences in bone mass that would be observed at 20 yr PMA (Fig. 4). We assumed that the prestudy calcium intakes were maintained through this period. Racial differences in adult bone mass predicted in this manner would be approx 12%, a difference consistent with the differences in adult bone mass observed between blacks and whites *(21)*.

In contrast, calcium absorption and urinary excretion were similar between prepubertal Mexican-American and Caucasian girls *(22)*.

4. DIETARY REQUIREMENTS

Calcium retention increases with calcium intake up to a point, after which it plateaus. Evidence for threshold behavior was proposed by Matkovic and Heaney *(23)*. To determine the intake associated with maximal retention, 35 adolescent girls aged 12–14 yr were studied at eight calcium intake levels between 800 and 2100 mg/d *(24)*. Subjects were assigned to one of four groups in an attempt to equalize mean serum osteocalcin levels and PMA. Each group was studied at two levels of calcium intake using a crossover

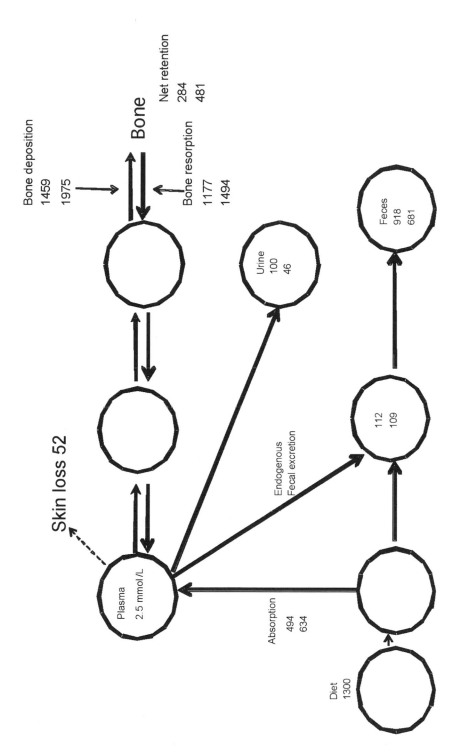

Fig. 3. Calcium metabolism. Daily mass transfer (mg/day) in Caucasian adolescent girls (upper values) and African-American girls (lower values). Circles represent compartments determined from kinetic modeling and do not necessarily represent discreet physiological or anatomical entities. Numbers in compartments represent mass (mg) of compartments. (Data taken from Wastney et al. [19] and Bryant et al. [20].)

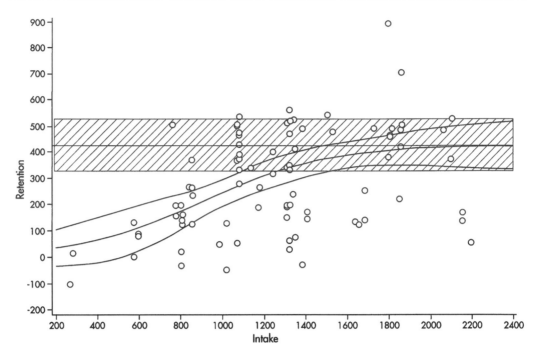

Fig. 4. Nonlinear regression of calcium intake and calcium retention in adolescent females. The three lines represent the mean and 95% confidence interval (CI) of the regression. The shaded area depicts the mean maximal retention and the 95% CI (Data from refs. *23* and *24*; reproduced from ref. *25*, with permission from, Springer-Verlag, Germany.)

design. Each period lasted 3 wk, with a 1-mo washout period in between. A nonlinear regression model was developed from data collected in adolescent girls (Fig. 4). The average calcium requirement based on maximal calcium retention can be determined from this relationship, as shown in Fig. 5. The lowest intake that permitted achievement of the maximal calcium accretion of 423 mg/d within the 95% confidence interval of the estimate was 1300 mg/d. To determine Dietary Reference Intakes for the United States and Canada, this level was used by the Institute of Medicine panel as the Adequate Intake of calcium for 9- to 18-yr-olds *(26)*.

When the nonlinear regression model was modified to include PMA (Fig. 6), it was found that although maximal calcium retention decreased with age, the calcium intake required to achieve maximal retention remained unchanged *(24)*. Declines in calcium absorption efficiency with PMA accounted for the decrease in calcium retention. Comparison of biochemical markers of bone turnover on high- (1900 mg/d) and low- (860 mg/d) calcium diets showed that biochemical markers did not change with calcium intake, although Vo⁻ decreased to produce a much higher calcium retention on higher calcium intakes *(27)*. Very low calcium intakes (<400 mg/d) lead to an upregulation in calcium absorption efficiency compared with recommended intake levels of approx 1300 mg/d, that is, 63.4 ± 1.7 vs 44.9 ± 1.9%, respectively *(28)*. Furthermore, endogenous fecal excretion and urinary calcium excretion were also reduced under low calcium intakes. However, the homeostatic adjustments were insufficient to restore optimal calcium retention. Despite adaptation, net calcium balance was much lower on the low calcium intakes, 131 ± 14 vs 349 ± 32 mg/d, $p < 0.001$).

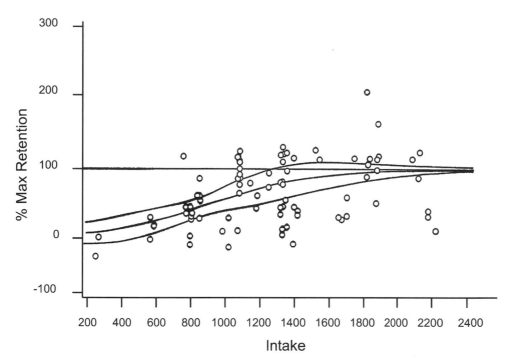

Fig. 5. Maximal calcium retention as a function of intake (mean and 95% CI) in female adolescents when the y axis is expressed as % maximal retention. (Reproduced from ref. 25, with permission from, Springer-Verlag, Germany.)

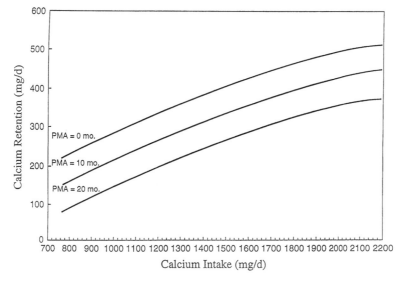

Fig. 6. Relationship of calcium intake and calcium retention as a function of postmenarcheal age (PMA) (in months) in adolescent females. (Reproduction from Jackman et al. (24), with permission from the American Society of Clinical Nutrition.)

5. DIETARY CALCIUM AND DEVELOPMENT OF PEAK MASS

The role of dietary calcium and other lifestyle factors in development of peak bone mass was reviewed by several authors in this book *(29)*. The profiles of calcium accrual as measured by bone mineral gains in Fig. 1 are undoubtedly influenced by dietary calcium through this period. Dietary calcium estimated from 24-h recalls averaged 1113 mg/d in girls and 1140 mg/d in boys in the children profiled in Fig. 1 *(1)*. Dietary calcium explained less than 1% of the variance in peak calcium accretion rates in this study. In contrast, increasing calcium intakes in a group of adolescent girls participating in a metabolic balance study from their prestudy mean intakes of approx 900 mg/d to an intake above the threshold of approx 1900 mg/d increased calcium retention by 452 mg/d *(27)*. If this increase was sustained for 1 yr, it would represent an increase in skeletal bone mass of 4%. If retained into adulthood, risk of fracture could be decreased considerably.

6. CHILDHOOD FRACTURE RISK

Fractures are common in childhood and adolescence (Fig. 7). One report estimates that 42% of girls and 54% of boys suffer a fracture by the age of 18 yr *(31)*. Peak height is achieved before peak bone mass (Table 1). Thus, a lag period of reduced bone density occurs, which may increase vulnerability to fracture. Low bone density is associated with increased risk of fracture even in children. In 3- to 15-yr-old girls, the odds ratios of fracture associated with low bone density for radius, spine, and hip were 2.3, 2.4, and 2.0, respectively *(33)*. The transient increase in porosity occurs in cortical bone in response to an enhanced bone turnover in response to greater calcium demand during puberty *(34)*. If the demand for BMC cannot be met from diet, cortical bone becomes the source of the raw materials for newly formed bone.

The incidence of forearm fracture in Rochester, Minnesota has increased over three decades (Fig. 8). From 1969–1971 to 1999–2001, age-adjusted fracture rates increased 32% among males and 56% among females; the peak incidence and greatest increase was observed in boys aged 11–14 yr and girls aged 8–11 yr *(35)*. This increase was partially explained by the increase in recreational activities. Part of the explanation for the increase in fractures may also be related to decline in consumption of milk. Milk consumption in children has been inversely associated with fracture risk *(33,36)*. Milk avoiders under age 10 yr had low total skeletal BMC (average z scores of –0.53) and were shorter *(36)*. An examination of National Health and Nutrition Examination Survey (NHANES)-III data showed that low milk consumption in childhood was associated with fewer fractures before puberty and a twofold greater risk of fracture in later adult life than those who drank milk regularly as children *(37)*. This greater risk of fracture resulting from low milk intake explained 11% of osteoporotic fractures.

6.1. Randomized, Controlled Trials

The primary line of evidence for the importance of sufficient dietary calcium to maximize peak bone mass, within the genetic potential, comes from randomized, controlled trials (Table 2). All of the published trials in children resulted in higher BMC or BMD, with increasing calcium intakes from either supplements, fortified foods, or dairy products at one or more skeletal sites; however, there is some discrepancy as to what age is most receptive to dietary calcium. The intervention in the oldest children was a 1-yr study

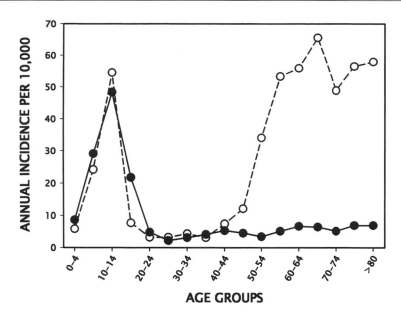

Fig. 7. Age-specific incidence of limb fracture in males (●) and females (○) from southern Sweden. (Adapted from Alffram and Bauer *[30]*.)

Table 1
Vulnerable Fracture Period at Puberty

	Age at peak height velocity (yr)	Age at peak BMC velocity (yr)	Lag in peak Calcium accretion behind peak height velocity (yr)	Age of increased fracture
Girls	11.8	12.4	0.7	11.5–12.5
Boys	13.4	14.1	0.6	13.5–14.5

BMC, bone mineral content.(From Bailey et al. *[32]*.)

in 100 girls aged 14 ± 0.5 yr, which showed 1 g calcium per day increased the gain in total body BMD and lumbar spine BMD, but not BMC, over the control group *(46)*. Lloyd et al. *(39)* reported a significantly greater increase in vertebral BMD, spine BMC, and total body BMD over 18 mo in 94 girls aged 11.9 ± 0.5 yr in a placebo-controlled trial with a 500 mg calcium supplement. Calcium intakes averaged 1370 and 935 mg/d for the supplemented and placebo groups, respectively. Thus, even a modest increase in calcium intake had a positive influence on mineral retention during adolescence. Johnston et al. *(38)* studied a wider age range (6–14 yr) in boys and girls using the monozygotic twin model. In prepubertal, but not pubertal twins, the calcium-supplemented (average 1600 mg calcium per day) twins' spine and radial BMDs were significantly higher than that of placebo-treated twins who averaged 900 mg calcium per day. The greatest increase in bone mass with calcium supplementation occurred in children who originally had the lowest dietary calcium intakes *(44)*. When Wosje and Specker *(48)* compared trials by

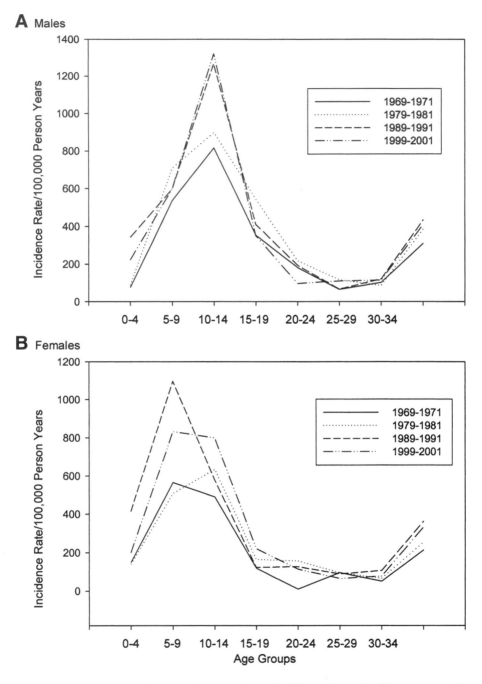

Fig. 8. Incidence rate of distal forearm fractures in males (**A**) and females (**B**) among residents of Rochester, Minnesota in four time periods between 1960 and 2001 *(35)*.

expressing the changes in BMD as the annualized percent changes in BMD, they concluded that increases in BMD occurred primarily in cortical bone sites and that spine BMD increased more in pubertal than prepubertal children.

Follow-up observations after calcium supplementation was withdrawn indicated that the increase in skeletal mass, attributed to calcium supplementation, was maintained in some studies *(43,44)*, but not others *(49,50)*. The failure of several follow-up studies to show sustained differences following discontinuation of calcium intervention has led some to question the importance of achieving adequate calcium during development of peak bone mass. It can be expected that some remodeling would occur following cessation of the intervention. These studies were not powered to determine residual group differences. Continued supplementation in a randomized, controlled trial of 1 g of calcium per day in girls from age 10.8 ± 0.8 to age 18 ± 0.8 yr showed higher BMD of the forearm, but not the spine, in the treated group than in the placebo group *(51,52)*. The question has been addressed more definitively in studies of rats on controlled diets. Rats were given a range of calcium intakes during the first 8 or 20 wk of life followed by re-randomization to low, medium, and high calcium intakes until 37 wk *(52)*. Low calcium intakes during pubertal growth had a nonreversible, deleterious effect on peak bone mass, regardless of later calcium intakes. This suggests that adolescence is a critical period for developing lifestyle choices conducive to optimal skeletal growth and that calcium deprivation through this period cannot be corrected later.

Some researchers have suggested that the benefits of milk consumption exceed calcium supplementation alone in augmenting development of peak bone mass and in persistence of the advantage. Bone size and height were increased in the dairy calcium-fortified food interventions *(43)*, but not the supplemented trials. Biochemical markers of bone formation remained higher with milk than with calcium *(54)*. A milk advantage could be due to different hormonal response, or to dairy constituents such as cytokines, or other bone-important nutrients including phosphorus, protein, magnesium, and vitamin D *(55)*. However, milk and calcium supplements have not been compared in the same study for their effects on bone health. A recent report of a comparison between cheese (100 g/d) and calcium carbonate (both at 1 g calcium per day) in 10- to 12-yr-old Finnish girld showed a significant advantage in total body bone mass gain over 2 yr in the girls receiving cheese if the girls were at Tanner stage 1, but not Tanner stage 2, at baseline *(56)*.

6.2. Retrospective Studies

Another line of evidence that suggests that childhood calcium and milk consumption influence bone mass comes from retrospective studies *(15,57–60)*. In retrospective studies, adjusting for current calcium intake is necessary in order to separate the independent effects of childhood and adolescent calcium intake. One study reported that childhood milk consumption predicted spine and hip BMD in women aged 45–49 yr *(59)*. Similarly, another study found that childhood and adolescent milk intake was associated with bone mass in postmenopausal women *(60)*. The cumulative effect of calcium and milk intake from childhood to young adulthood on BMC and BMD was evaluated by Teegarden et al. *(15)*. Milk intake during adolescence, but not childhood, was associated with total body and radius BMD, but there was no association with spine and hip BMD as young women. Teenage calcium intake was associated with hip BMD, but not with spine or radial BMD in 30- to 39-yr-old women *(58)*. In a large national representation of 3251 women surveyed in NHANES-III, there was a significant ($p < 0.04$) association between

Table 2
Differences in Mean Changes in Bone Mineral Content (BMC) and Bone Mineral Density (BMD) in Calcium-Treated vs Placebo Groups in Randomized, Controlled Trials in Adolescents

Source	Ref. no.	Subj. no	Age (yr)	Sex	Race/location	Length study (mo)	Calcium intake controls (mg/d)	Calcium intake treatment (mg/d)	Site	Measure	Group mean in % increase Treatment (T)	Placebo (P)
Johnston et al., 1992	38	140	6–14	F/M	white, IN	36	908	1612	Midshaft radius	BMD	17.7	15.2
									Distal radius	BMD	21.5	18.2
									Lumbar spine	BMD	20.1	19.5
									Femoral neck	BMD	15.3	14.9
									Ward's triangle	BMD	15.4	14.2
									Greater trochanter	BMD	18.1	17.11
Lloyd et al., 1993	39	94	11.9 ± 0.5	F	white, PA	18	960	1314	Total Body	BMC	9.6	8.3, $p = 0.003$
									Spine	BMC	2.9, $p = 0.03$	4.7, $p = 0.05$
Chan et al., 1995	40	48	9–13	F	white, UT	12	728	1437	Total body	BMC	14.2 ± 7.0	7.6 ± 6.0 $p < 0.001$
									Lumbar spine	BMD	22.8 ± 6.9%	12.9 ± 8.3, $p < 0.001$
Lee et al., 1995	41	109	7	F/M	Asian, China	18	571	1363	Distal radius	BMC	15.92 (T) vs 14.95% (P) gain, $p = 0.53$	
										Area	7.74 (T) vs 6.00% (P) gain, $p = 0.081$	
									Lumbar spine	BMC	20.92 (T) vs 16.34% (P) gain, $p = 0.035$	
										Area	11.16 (T) vs 8.71% (P) gain, $p = 0.049$	
									Proximal femoral neck	BMC	24.19 (T) vs 23.42% (P) gain, $p = 0.37$	
Cadogan et al., 1997	42	82	12.2	F	white, Sheffield UK	18	753	1125	Total body	BMD	9.6 (T) vs 8.5% (P), $p = 0.017$	

Reference		n	Age	Sex	Population			Site		Result
Bonjour et al., 1997	43	149	7.9 ± 0.1	F	white, Geneva, CH	1723	916	Radial meta-physics	BMC	27.0% (T) vs 24.1% (P $p = 0.009$
								Femoral neck	BMD	16 ± 3 g/cm² (T) vs 9 ± 2 g/cm² (P), $p < 0.08$
									BMD	22 ± 4 g/cm² (T) vs 13 ± 4 g/cm² (P)
								Femoral dia-physis	BMD	66 ± 3 g/cm² (T) vs 54 ± 4 g/cm² (P) $p < 0.01$
								Lumbar spine	BMD	25 ± 3 g/cm² (T) vs 23 ± 3 g/cm² (P)
Dibba et al., 2000	44	160	8.3–11.9	F/M	black, Gambia	1056	342	Midshaft radius	BMC	3.0 ± 1.4% (T-P), $p = 0.034$
									BMD	4.5 ± 0.9% (T-P), $p < 0.0001$
Moyer-Mileur et al., 2003	45	71	12	F	white, UT	1524	865	pQCT of Distal tibia	BMC	4.1% (T) vs 1.6% (P), $p < 0.006$
									vBMD	1.0% (T) vs −2.0% (P), $p < 0.006$
Rozen et al., 2003	46	100	14 ± 0.5	F	85 Jewish/ 26 Arab, Haifa, Israel	1110	480	Total body	BMC	4.63 ± 0.42% (T) vs 4.65 ± 0.54%, NS
								Lumbar spine	BMD	3.80 ± 0.30% (T) vs 3.07 ± 0.29%, (P), $p < 0.05$
									BMD	4.52 ± 0.48% (T) vs 3.95 ± 0.58% (P), NS
									BMC	3.66 ± 0.35% vs 3.00 ± 0.43%, $p < 0.05$
								Femoral neck	BMC	4.30 ± 0.86% (T) vs 3.00 ± 0.81%, NS
									BMD	2.00 ± 0.51% (T) vs 1.39 ± 0.42%, (P), NS
Stear et al., 2003	47	144	17.3 ± 0.3	F	Cambridge, UK	+1 g Ca supplement	928	Whole body	BMC	0.8 ± 0.5% (T vs P), $p < 0.01$
								Lumbar spine	BMC	0.9 ± 0.8% (T vs P), $p < 0.001$
								Hip	BMC	5.3 ± 1.0% (T vs P), $p < 0.001$

pQCT, peripheral quantitative computed tomography; vBMD, volumetric bone mineral density.

milk intake during both childhood and adolescence and hip BMC and BMD of women <50 yr of age *(37)*. Milk intake during childhood, but not during adolescence, was also positively associated with bone area. The authors interpreted the association of low milk intake during growth with low BMD and BMD of the hip in adulthood as a persistent negative effect of low milk consumption during accumulation of peak bone mass. This relationship is not ameliorated by current calcium intake, because this was adjusted for in their model. In contrast, there was no association between milk intake in youth and later BMD in black women in NHANES-III *(61)*.

7. CONCLUSION AND FUTURE DIRECTIONS

Much information has been accumulated about calcium intake, metabolism, and requirements for optimizing development of peak bone mass during prepubertal and pubertal growth. This period is characterized by upregulated calcium absorption, decreased excretion, high rates of bone turnover, and very high calcium retention. Between 25 and 50% of adult peak bone mass is accumulated during adolescence.

Our understanding of calcium metabolism and calcium accretion in adolescence is well developed for Caucasians. Some racial comparisons have been made for calcium absorption and excretion. However, calcium accretion rates and underlying differences in various racial and ethnic groups is incomplete. Current calcium intakes fall short of recommended intakes for development of maximal peak bone mass. The trend of replacing milk with soft drinks as a beverage of choice is detrimental to bone gain, at least in girls, who have lower total calcium intakes than boys *(62)*. Behavior modification to improve dietary habits is critical, not only for bone health, but to prevent obesity (*see* Chapter 21). It is important to establish dietary habits that include sufficient calcium intakes, because there is much evidence that calcium intake shows tracking behavior from childhood until later life.

REFERENCES

1. Bailey DA, Martin AD, McKay AA, Whiting S, Miriwald R. Calcium accretion in girls and boys during puberty: A longitudinal analysis. J Bone Miner Res 2000;15:2245–2250.
2. Weaver CM. Adolescence, the period of dramatic bone growth. Endocrine 2002;17:43–48.
3. Hui SL, Zhou L, Evans R, et al. Rates of growth and loss of bone mineral in the spine and femoral neck in white females. Osteoporosis Int 1999;9:200–205.
4. Teegarden D, Proulx WR, Martin BR, et al. Peak bone mass in young women. J Bone Miner Res 1995;10:711–715.
5. Lin Y-C, Lyle RM, Weaver CM, McCabe GP, Johnston CC Jr, Teegarden D. Peak spine and femoral neck bone mass in young women. Bone 2003;32:546–553.
6. Nicklas TA. Calcium intake trends and health consequences from childhood through adulthood. J Am Coll Nutr 2003;22:340–356.
7. Nutrition Assistance Program Report Series. The Office of Analysis, Nutrition and Evaluation. Children's Diets in the Mid-1990s: Dietary Intake and its Relationship with School Meal Participation. Special Nutrition Programs Report No. CN-01-CD1, 2001. United States Department of Agriculture, Food and Nutrition Service, Washington, DC: January, 2001.
8. Johnson RK, Frary C, Wang MQ. The nutritional consequences of flavored-milk consumption by school-aged children and adolescents in the United States. J Am Diet Assoc 2002;102:853–856.
9. Ballow C, Kuester S, Gillespie C. Beverage choices affect adequacy of children's nutrient intakes. Arch Pediatr Adolesc Med 2000;154;1148–1152.

10. Mrdjenovic G, Levitsky DA. Nutritional and energetic consequences of sweetened drink consumption in 6- to 13-year old children. J Pediatr 2003;142:604–610.

11. McGartland C, Robson PJ, Murray L, et al. Carbonated soft drink consumption and bone mineral density in adolescence: the Northern Ireland Young Hearts project. J Bone Miner Res 2003;18:1563–1569.

12. Whiting SJ, Healey A, Psiuk S, Mirwald R, Kowalski K, Bailey DA. Relationship between carbonated and other low nutrient dense beverages and bone mineral content of adolescents. Nutr Res 2001;21:1107–1115.

13. Welton DC, Kemper HC, Post GB, Van Staveren WA, Twisk JW. Longitudinal development and tracking of calcium and diary intake from teenager to adult. Eur J Clin Nutr 1997;51:612–618.

14. Dwyer JT, Gardner J, Halvorsen K, Krall EA, Cohen A, Valadian I. Memory of food intake in the distant past. Am J Epidemiol 1989;130:1033–1046.

15. Teegarden D, Lyle RM, Proulx WR, Johnston CC Jr, Weaver CM. Previous milk consumption is associated with greater bone density in young women. Am J Clin Nutr 1999;69:1014–1017.

16. Lytle LA, Seifert S, Greenstein J, McGovern P. How do children's eating patterns and food choices change over time? Results from a cohort study. Am J Health Promot 2000;14;222–228.

17. Skinner JD, Bounds W, Carruth BR, Ziegler P. Longitudinal calcium intake is negatively related to children's body fat indices. J Am Diet Assoc 2003;103:1026–1031.

18. Weaver CM, Martin BR, Plawecki KL, et al. Differences in calcium metabolism between adolescent and adult females. Am J Clin Nutr 1995;61:577–581.

19. Wastney ME, Ng J, Smith D, Martin BR, Peacock M, Weaver CM. Differences in calcium kinetics between adolescent girls and young women. Am J Physiol 1996;271:R208–R216.

20. Bryant RJ, Wastney ME, Martin BR, et al. Racial differences in bone turnover and calcium metabolism in adolescent females. J Clin Endocrinol Metab 2003;88(3):1043–1047.

21. Looker AC, Wahner HW, Dunn WL, et al. Updated data on proximal femur bone mineral levels of U.S. Adults. Osteoporos Int 1998;8:468–489.

22. Abrams SA, Copeland KC, Gunn SK, Staff JE, Clarke LL, Ellis KJ. Calcium absorption and kinetics are similar in 7- and 8-year old Mexican-American girls despite hormonal differences. J Nutr 1999;129:666–671.

23. Matkovic V, Heaney RP. Calcium balance during human growth: evidence for threshold behavior. Am J Clin Nutr 1992;55:992–996.

24. Jackman LA, Millane SS, Martin BR, et al. Calcium retention in relation to calcium intake and postmenarcheal age in adolescent females. Am J Clin Nutr 1997;66:327–333.

25. Weaver CM, McCabe GP, Peacock M. Calcium intake and age influence calcium retention in adolescence. In: Burckhardt P, Dawson-Hughes B, Heaney RP, eds. Nutritional Aspects of Osteoporosis. Serono Symposium, Springer-Verlag, New York: 1998; pp. 3–10.

26. Dietary Reference Intakes for Calcium, Phosphorus, Magnesium, Vitamin D, and Fluoride. Standing Committee on the Scientific Evaluation of Dietary Reference Intakes, Food and Nutrition Board, Institute of Medicine. National Academy Press, Washington, DC: 1997.

27. Wastney ME, Martin BR, Peacock M, et al. Changes in calcium kinetics in adolescent girls induced by high calcium intake. J Clin Endocrinol Metab 2000;85:4470–4475.

28. Abrams S, Griffin IJ, Hicks PD, Gunn SK. Pubertal girls only partially adapt to low calcium intakes. J Bone Miner Res 2004;19:759–762.

29. Heaney RP, Abrams S, Dawson-Hughes B, et al. Peak bone mass. Osteoporos Int 2000;11:985–1009.

30. Alffram PA, Bauer GCH. Epidemiology of fractures of the forearm. J Bone Joint Surg Am 1962;44:105–114.

31. Jones IE, Williams SM, Dow N, Goulding A. How many children remain fracture-free during growth? A longitudinal study of children and adolescents participating in the Dunedin Multidisciplinary Health and Development Study. Osteoporos Int 2002;13:990–995.

32. Bailey DA, Wedge JH, McCullough RG, Martin AD, Bernhardson SC. Epidemiology of fractures of the distal end of the radius in children as associated with growth. J Bone Joint Surg 1989;71A:1225–1231.

33. Goulding A, Cannan R, Williams SM, Gold EJ, Taylor RW, Lewis-Barned NJ. Bone mineral density in girls with forearm fractures. J Bone Miner Res 1998;13:143–148.

34. Parfitt AM. The two faces of growth: benefits and risks to bone integrity. Osteoporos Int 1994:4:382–298.

35. Khosla S, Melton III LJ, Delutoski MB, Achenbach SJ, Oberg AL, Riggs BL. Incidence of childhood distal forearm fractures over 30 years. JAMA 2003;290:1479–1485.

36. Black RE, Williams SM, Jones IE, Goulding A. Children who avoid drinking cow milk have low dietary calcium intakes and poor bone health. Am J Clin Nutr 2002;76:675–680.

37. Kalkwarf HJ, Khoury JC, Lanphear BP. Milk intake during childhood and adolescence, adult bone density, and osteoporotic fractures in US women. Am J Clin Nutr 2003;77:257–265.
38. Johnston CC Jr, Miller JZ, Slemenda CW, et al. Calcium supplementation and increases in bone mineral density in children. N Engl J Med 1992;327:82–87.
39. Lloyd T, Andon MB, Rollings N, et al. Calcium supplementation and bone mineral density in adolescent girls. JAMA 1993;270:841–844.
40. Chan GM, Hoffman K, McMurry M. Effects of dairy products on bone and body composition in pubertal girls. J Pediatr 1995;126(4):551–556.
41. Lee WTK, Leung SSF, Wang SH, et al. Double-blind controlled calcium supplementation and bone mineral accretion in children accustomed to low calcium diet. Am J Clin Nutr 1994;60:744–752.
42. Cadogan J, Eastell R, Jones N, Barker ME. Milk intake and bone mineral acquisition in adolescent girls: Randomized, controlled intervention trial. Br Med J 1997;315:1255–1260.
43. Bonjour JP, Carrie AL, Ferrari S, et al. Calcium-enriched foods and bone mass growth in prepubertal girls—a randomized, double-blind, placebo-controlled trial. J Clin Invest 1997;99:1287–1294.
44. Dibba B, Prentice A, Ceesay M et al. Effect of calcium supplementation on bone mineral accretion in gambian children accustomed to a low-calcium diet. Am J Clin Nutr 2000;71(2):544–549.
45. Moyer-Mileur LJ, Xie B, Ball SD, Pratt T. Bone mass and density response to a 12-month trial of calcium and vitamin D supplementation preadolescent girls. J Musculoskel Neuron Interact 2003;3:63–70.
46. Rozen GS, Rennert G, Dodiuk-Gad R, et al. Calcium supplementation provides an extended window of opportunity for bone mass accretion after menarche. Am J Clin Nutr 2003;78:993–998.
47. Stear SJ, Prentice A, Jones SC, et al. Effect of a calcium and exercise intervention on the bone mineral status of 16-18 year-old adolescent girls. Am J Clin Nutr 2003;77(4):985–992.
48. Wosje KS, Specker BL. Role of calcium in bone health during childhood. Nutr Rev 2000;58(9):253–268.
49. Slemenda CW, Peacock M, Hui S, Zhou L, Johnston CC. Reduced rates of skeletal remodeling are associated with increased bone mineral density during the development of peak skeletal mass. J Bone Miner Res 1997;12:676–82.
50. Lee WTK, Leung SSF, Leung DMY, Cheng JCY. A follow-up study on the effect of calcium-supplement withdrawal and puberty on bone acquisition of children. Am J Clin Nutr 1996;64:71–77.
51. Matkovic V, Badenhop-Stevens NE, Landoll JD, Nagode LA, Goel P. Effect of calcium on bone mass of young females from childhood to young adulthood. Fifth International Symposium: Clinical Advances in Osteoporosis, National Osteoporosis Foundation, March 6–9, 2002. Abstract #1.
52. Matkovic V, Landoll JD, Badenkop-Stevens NE, et al. Nutrition influences skeletal development from childhood to adult: a study of hip, spine, and forearm in adolescent females. J Nutr 2004;134:701S–705S.
53. Peterson CA, Earell JAC, Erdman JW. Alterations in calcium intake on peak bone mass in the female rat. J Bone Miner Res 1995;10:81–95.
54. Eastell R, Lambert H. Diet and healthy bones. Calcif Tissue Int 2002;70:400–404.
55. Goulding A. Milk components and bone health. Aust J Dairy Technol 2003;58:73–78.
56. Lyytikäinen A, Nawa M, Kopela R, et al. Cheese as a source of calcium and its effects on body composition in pubertal Finnish girls. J Bone Miner Res 2003;18:S183, Abst# SU 010.
57. Haliorua L, Anderson JJ. Lifetime calcium intake and physical activity habits: independent and combined effects on the radial bone of healthy premenopasual Caucasian women. Am J Clin Nutr 1989;49:534–541.
58. Nieves JW, Golden AL, Siris E, Kelsey JL, Lindsay R. Teenage and current calcium intake are related to bone mineral density of the hip and forearms in women aged 30–39 years. Am J Epidemiol 1995;141:342–251.
59. New SA, Bolton-Smith C, Grubb DA, Reid DM. Nutritional influence on bone mineral density, a cross-sectional study in pre-menopausal women. Am J Clin Nutr 1997;65:1831–1839.
60. Sandler RB, Slemenda CW, La Porter RE, et al. Postmenopausal bone density and milk consumption in childhood and adolescence. Am J Clin Nutr 1985;42:270–274.
61. Opotowsky AR, Bilezikian JP. Racial differences in the effect of early milk consumption on peak and postmenopausal bone mineral density. J Bone Miner Res 2003;18:1978–1988.
62. Whiting SJ, Vatanparast H, Baxter-Jones A, Faulkner RA, Miriwald R, Bailey DA. Factors that affect bone mineral accrual in the adolescent growth spurt. J Nutr 2004;134–696S–700S.

18 Calcium in Pregnancy and Lactation

Heidi J. Kalkwarf

KEY POINTS

- Pregnancy and lactation are times of high calcium demand. Different physiological adaptations in maternal calcium metabolism are invoked to secure calcium for fetal bone and breast milk production.
- During pregnancy, additional calcium is obtained by an increase in intestinal calcium absorption and, in the third trimester, by mobilization of calcium from bone.
- During lactation, significant demineralization of maternal bone occurs to meet the increased calcium demand of the neonate. This bone loss is transient as bone mass and density increase after lactation ceases.
- Epidemiological evidence suggests that pregnancy and lactation do not increase risk of osteoporotic fracture.

1. INTRODUCTION

1.1. Calcium Transferred During Pregnancy and Lactation

Pregnancy and lactation are times of high calcium demand. Approximately 25 to 30 g of calcium are transferred to the fetal skeleton by the end of pregnancy. The fetus accumulates 2–3 mg/d of calcium during the first trimester, increasing to 250 mg/d during the third trimester *(1)*. Maternal calcium losses to breast milk are approx 200–240 mg/d *(2)*. Considering that the maternal skeleton contains about 900 g of calcium, the loss of calcium during pregnancy and 6 mo of lactation are equivalent to 3 and 5%, respectively, of a mother's total skeletal calcium content.

1.2. Recommended Calcium Intakes for Pregnant and Lactating Women Over Time

It has long been assumed that pregnant and lactating women need to consume greater amounts of calcium to compensate for the loss of calcium from the mother to the fetus and infant. Since the inception of the Recommended Dietary Allowances (RDAs) in the early 1940s, the recommended calcium intakes have been higher for pregnant and lactating women as compared with those for nonpregnant, nonlactating women (Fig. 1). Recommended calcium intakes have been as high as 1500 mg/d for pregnant women and

From: *Calcium in Human Health*
Edited by: C. M. Weaver and R. P. Heaney © Humana Press Inc., Totowa, NJ

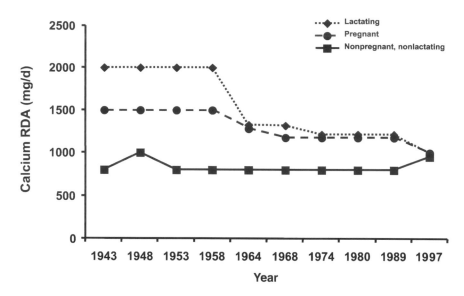

Fig. 1. Recommended calcium intakes for pregnant and lactating women, 1943–1997. The values for 1943–1989 are Recommended Dietary Intakes (RDAs), whereas the value for 1997 is an adequate intake and does not have the same meaning as an RDA (adequate intake [AI]).

2000 mg/d for lactating women. The 1997 Dietary Reference Intake (DRI) represents the first time that recommended calcium intakes for pregnant and lactating women were the same as those for nonpregnant, nonlactating women—1000 mg/d *(3)*. Although the 1997 DRI for calcium was an adequate intake, which differs conceptually from an RDA, the similarity in requirement for dietary calcium by pregnant, lactating and nonpregnant women remains salient. These recent recommendations are based on the recognition that there are physiological adaptations in maternal calcium homeostasis to compensate for the transfer of calcium to the fetus and infant, while maternal circulating calcium concentrations are still maintained within a narrow range. Much has been learned in the last 10 yr regarding adaptations in calcium homeostasis during pregnancy and lactation. Prior to the development of the 1997 DRI, there were very little experimental data on humans from which to determine dietary calcium requirements of pregnant and lactating women.

2. PREGNANCY

2.1. Changes in Calcium Metabolism During Pregnancy

Parathyroid hormone (PTH) and 1,25 dihydroxyvitamin D (1,25[OH]$_2$D), the active form of vitamin D, are the classical regulators of calcium homeostasis, and function together to maintain serum calcium concentrations within a narrow range via three mechanisms: (1) stimulating renal calcium reabsorption, (2) increasing intestinal calcium absorption, and (3) mobilizing calcium from bone. Serum concentrations of intact PTH have been reported to decrease or not change over the course of pregnancy *(4–6)*, whereas circulating concentrations of 1,25(OH)$_2$D are markedly increased. Compared with prepregnant values, serum concentrations of 1,25(OH)$_2$D increase by 50–100% in the second trimester of pregnancy and by 100% in the third trimester *(7,8)*. The signal to increase 1,25(OH)$_2$D synthesis is not clear because PTH concentrations are not elevated. Vitamin D-binding protein concentrations increase in pregnancy, which may explain some of the increase *(8,9)*. However, the amount of free 1,25(OH)$_2$D also is elevated. Some of the circulating 1,25(OH)$_2$D may be of placental origin, because maternal 1,25(OH)$_2$D concentrations rapidly decrease within a few days after delivery of the fetus *(10)*.

Intestinal calcium absorption is increased during pregnancy as would be predicted by the increase in 1,25(OH)$_2$D concentrations. The increase in maternal intestinal calcium absorption is an important physiological adaptation to secure additional calcium. Fractional calcium absorption increases by 50–56% over prepregnant levels in the second trimester of pregnancy and by 54–62% in the third trimester *(7,8)*. Assuming a dietary intake of 1000 mg/d of calcium and a baseline fractional absorption of 33%, this increase in absorption efficiency would result in an additional 165–205 mg/d of calcium for the fetus. In contrast with expectations considering the increased need for calcium, urinary calcium excretion increases over the course of pregnancy by 30–125% depending on dietary calcium intake *(6,8)*. The increased urinary excretion is most likely caused by the marked increase in glomerular filtration rate (GFR) and increased absorptive load. This increased loss of calcium in the urine during pregnancy has been estimated to be 80–136 mg/d and negates some of the potential gain from increased intestinal calcium absorption *(6,8)*.

Pregnancy appears to be a time of increased bone turnover. Serum concentrations of bone-specific alkaline phosphatase and the propeptide of type 1 collagen, two biochemical markers of bone formation, are elevated in the third trimester with a steep peak in the last month of pregnancy *(4,6)*. There have been conflicting reports as to whether there are changes in these markers in the first two trimesters of pregnancy. Concentrations of osteocalcin, which is synthesized by osteoblasts and which also may signify bone formation, have been found to decrease, decrease then increase, or not change during pregnancy *(6,8,10)*. Markers of bone resorption also are elevated during pregnancy. Concentrations of the breakdown products of collagen, such as pyridinoline, deoxypyridinoline, and *N*-telopeptide cross-links, increase throughout pregnancy reaching a peak at the end of pregnancy *(4,6,8)*. Increases in insulin-like growth factor (IGF)-1 and placental lactogen have been suggested as the possible mechanisms behind increased bone turnover during pregnancy *(4,6)*. However, the increase in IGF-1 concentrations precedes the increase in bone formation markers, and IGF-1 concentrations correlate more strongly with markers of bone formation than bone resorption. Although bone turnover may be elevated, it is difficult to predict whether there is a net loss of maternal bone during pregnancy using biochemical markers alone. Factors such as whether the markers are of maternal, placental, or fetal origin, and the effects of pregnancy on the metabolic clearance of these proteins by the liver and kidney, confound the interpretation of biochemical markers of bone turnover during pregnancy. It also has been speculated that some of the increase in bone resorption markers is due to increased turnover of soft tissue collagen of the uterus and skin *(6)*. Heaney and Skillman *(11)* performed a stable isotopic study to evaluate calcium kinetics during pregnancy. They found that calcium accretion increased throughout pregnancy, beginning prior to significant fetal bone accretion, and that bone resorption increased above non-pregnant levels at the end of pregnancy.

2.2. Bone Mass and Density During Pregnancy

Data on bone mineral density (BMD) assessed by dual energy x-ray absorptiometry on women throughout pregnancy are sparse as a result of concern about potential risks associated with radiation exposure to the fetus. To circumvent this potential risk, different approaches have been used to evaluate the impact of pregnancy on maternal bone. One approach has been to measure BMD before conception and shortly after delivery. Results of studies using this approach have been inconsistent. Some studies have found no significant loss of bone density *(7,8,12,13)*, whereas other studies report losses of –2 to –2.6% at the ultradistal radius *(14,15)*, –2 to –4% at the spine *(4,6,16)*, and –2.4 to –3.6% at the hip *(4,17)*. Part of the inconsistency in the findings may be attributable to the fact that in some of the studies, bone density was measured as late as 6 wk postpartum, making interpretation of the results difficult because significant losses of bone may occur within the immediate postpartum period. The change in bone density during pregnancy may vary according to skeletal site. In one study, bone density at trabecular-rich sites (pelvis and spine) decreased by 3 to 4%, whereas bone density at cortical sites (arms and legs) increased by 2% *(6)*.

Ultrasound also has been used to investigate changes in bone during pregnancy because it does not involve radiation exposure. Speed of sound (SOS) and bone ultrasound attenuation (BUA) are strongly correlated with bone density measured at the same skeletal site. Longitudinal studies with repeated measurements over the course of pregnancy have found decreases in SOS and BUA at the os calcis and phalanges in the latter half of pregnancy *(18–21)*. The decrease is the most pronounced in the third trimester, the time when the fetus is accreting bone mineral most rapidly. Thus, it is likely that calcium from the maternal skeleton is mobilized at the end of pregnancy to meet some of the fetal need for calcium. In keeping with this, longitudinal studies of BMD in women who do not lactate after delivery show that bone density at the spine and hip increase by about 2% in the first year postpartum *(22–24)*. It is possible that this increase in BMD may compensate for that lost during pregnancy.

Whether or not dietary calcium intake modifies the pregnancy-induced changes in calcium homeostasis and bone turnover is largely unknown. Theoretically, women with very low calcium intakes may have a greater increase in intestinal calcium absorption, less urinary calcium excretion, and greater bone loss during pregnancy, whereas these changes may be blunted in women with very high calcium intakes. In contrast with the pregnancy-induced increase in urinary calcium excretion observed in women with calcium intakes around 1200 mg/d, Bezerra and co-workers found no pregnancy-induced increase in urinary calcium excretion in women with calcium intakes around 400–500 mg/d *(25)*. In addition, another study reported that the increase in markers of bone resorption during pregnancy was inversely related to calcium intake *(26)*. Detailed studies of calcium homeostasis and bone mass during pregnancy and postpartum are needed, especially those involving women with differing calcium intakes.

2.3. Maternal Calcium Intake and Fetal Bone

Little is known about the effects of maternal calcium intake during pregnancy on fetal bone mineral accretion, because only two calcium supplementation studies that also evaluated neonatal bone mass have been conducted among pregnant women. In a study of undernourished Indian women, infants born to women who received an additional

300 mg/d or 600 mg/d of calcium had greater bone mass than infants born to unsupplemented women *(27)*. A randomized calcium-supplementation trial of pregnant women in the United States showed that supplemental calcium intake resulted in an increase in newborn bone mass only among women whose dietary calcium intake was below 600 mg/d *(28)*. Chang and co-workers *(29)* evaluated the relation between dairy intake among pregnant adolescent African Americans and fetal femur length measured by ultrasound between 20 and 34 wk gestation. Fetal femur length among pregnant adolescents who consumed less than two servings of dairy products daily was lower than the fetal femur length of pregnant adolescents consuming more than three servings of dairy products daily. Thus, fetal bone mineralization and bone growth may be compromised when maternal dietary calcium intake is very low.

3. LACTATION

3.1. Calcium Metabolism During Lactation

Physiological compensations to secure additional calcium for lactation differ from those invoked during pregnancy. In contrast with pregnancy, there is no increase in circulating concentrations of $1,25(OH)_2D$ *(30,31)* or intestinal calcium absorption in lactating as compared with nonlactating postpartum women *(8,32–34)*. Furthermore, serum concentrations of PTH are lower in lactating as compared with nonlactating women in the first 3 mo postpartum *(30,31,35)*.

The lower PTH concentrations during early lactation are likely to be a consequence of bone resorption caused by hypoestrogenemia and elevated circulating concentrations of parathyroid hormone-related peptide (PTHrP) *(36–38)*. Lactation results in prolonged postpartum amenorrhea and hypoestrogenemia as a result of suppression of the hypothalamic–pituitary–gonadal axis. Hypoestrogenemia results in bone resorption in a variety of situations. PTHrP is made in the mammary gland, is present in very high concentrations in breast milk, and circulating concentrations are elevated in lactating women *(39)*. Circulating PTHrP has actions similar to PTH *(40)*. PTHrP stimulates bone resorption, and administration of PTHrP results in an immediate increase in serum calcium concentrations *(41)*. Evidence for the potential physiological role of PTHrP in calcium metabolism during lactation comes from the fact that serum concentrations of calcium are more highly correlated with PTHrP than with PTH among lactating women *(37)*.

The effects of lactation on urinary calcium conservation are unclear. Some studies have found a 20 to 50% decrease in urinary calcium excretion during lactation *(8,42–46)*. However, other studies have found no difference in urinary calcium between lactating and nonlactating postpartum women *(30,31,34,35)*. One possible explanation for this discrepancy is that urinary calcium may be decreased in all postpartum women, regardless of lactation, to compensate for calcium lost during pregnancy.

Alterations in the calcium economy also occur after weaning when lactation has ceased. Within 2 to 3 mo after weaning, serum concentrations of $1,25(OH)_2D$ are higher in previously lactating women as compared to nonlactating postpartum women. This is accompanied by a slight increase (39% vs 31%) in fractional absorption of calcium by the intestine *(32)*. The increase in intestinal calcium absorption is one mechanism by which additional calcium is secured for reconstitution of bone after weaning (discussed later). The increase in intestinal absorption is also seen in lactating women who have resumed menses. Thus, it is likely that changes in intestinal calcium absorption are secondary to effects of estrogen on calcium and bone metabolism.

3.2. Changes in Bone Mass and Density During Lactation and After Weaning

There have been more than two dozen longitudinal studies that have examined changes in bone mass and density over the course of lactation. Despite differences in study design and population studied, all of them have found bone loss at one or more skeletal sites during lactation. Decreases within the range of −2 to −7% in bone mass and density of the lumbar spine and femoral neck during lactation consistently have been found across studies (15,22–24,47–49). The decrease in bone density occurs rapidly within the first 3 to 6 mo of lactation, and bone density remains lower with continued lactation (49,50). Changes in bone density of the forearm at the trabecular-rich ultra-distal site and the cortical bone at the shaft have been less consistent with some studies finding decreases during lactation (24,42,51) than with others finding no change (15,23,49).

Although there is a decrease in bone mass and density during lactation, this loss is transient and there is a compensatory increase in bone density shortly after weaning (23,24,49,52). Recovery of bone mass and density after weaning occurs earlier for the spine than for the femoral neck. Most studies have found complete recovery of bone density at the spine 6 mo after weaning. However, it is not clear if there is complete recovery of bone density at the femoral neck. Although most studies show an increase in bone density at this skeletal site after weaning, in several studies a deficit in bone density was still evident at the end of the follow-up period (15,48,50). It is possible that a greater increase in bone density would have been evident had the women been followed for a longer period.

The amount of bone lost during lactation and the time-course of recovery of bone after weaning is strongly related to the duration of postpartum amenorrhea. The length of postpartum amenorrhea is as good as the length of lactation in predicting change in bone density (15,24,49). Although the length of postpartum amenorrhea is correlated with the length of lactation, some women do resume menses while breast-feeding. Examination of the pattern of change in bone density in these women has enabled better understanding of the role of hypoestrogenemia in modulating bone loss during lactation. Polatti et al found less of a deficit in bone density in lactating women who resumed menses by 5 mo postpartum than in those who remained amenorrheaic (−3.0% vs −5.8%) (24).

3.3. Calcium Intake and Bone Changes During Lactation and After Weaning

Bone loss during lactation and recovery after weaning are relatively independent of dietary calcium intake. Lactation-induced bone loss at the femoral neck and spine have been reported for women with high (>1500 mg/d) dietary calcium intakes (15,35,50,53). Three randomized calcium-supplementation trials also have shown that calcium supplementation does not prevent bone loss during lactation. Kalkwarf et al. randomized 83 lactating women and 81 nonlactating postpartum women whose dietary calcium intake averaged 735 mg/d to receive 1 g/d calcium or placebo for 6 mo (23). When considering all women, there was a small effect of calcium supplementation on bone density (+1.2%) (Fig. 2). However, there was no effect of calcium supplementation on lactation-induced bone loss at the spine; bone loss did not significantly differ between lactating women who

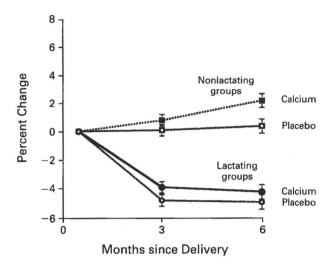

Fig. 2. Effects of calcium supplementation (1/g) and lactation on percent change in bone density of the lumbar spine during the first 6 mo postpartum. (Reprinted from ref. *23*.)

received the calcium supplement and those that received the placebo –4.2% vs –4.9%). Nonlactating women benefited from calcium supplementation as much as or more than did lactating women. Polatti et al. conducted a 6-mo randomized supplementation trial involving 139 lactating women who received 1 g/d of calcium and 135 lactating women who received a placebo *(24)*. There was no difference between groups in the amount of bone loss at the lumbar spine (–4.0% vs –4.4%) and ultra-distal radius (–2.0% vs –2.2%) over the 6-mo intervention period. Prentice et al. randomized 60 lactating women in the Gambia who had a very low calcium intake (283 mg/d) to receive a supplement averaging 714 mg/d of calcium or a placebo for 12 mo *(42)*. Although there was a significant decrease in bone mass at the radial shaft during lactation, there was no difference in bone loss between lactating women who received the calcium supplement and those who received the placebo. One would hypothesize that women with very low calcium intakes, such as the women in the Gambia, would be the most likely to benefit from calcium supplementation. Bone density measurements were only obtained at the forearm in this study, and it is unknown whether calcium supplementation would reduce lactation-induced bone loss at other skeletal sites in women with very low calcium intakes.

The increase in bone density after weaning occurs in women across a wide range of dietary calcium intakes. The rate of recovery of bone density after weaning may be faster in women who received 1 g/d of supplemental calcium after weaning *(23)* (Fig. 3). However, by 12 mo after weaning, there was no difference in bone density between women who received a calcium supplement during lactation and those who did not *(24)*.

3.4. Dietary Calcium Intake and Breast Milk Calcium Concentrations

There is significant variability in calcium concentrations of breast milk among women, but the factors that account for this variation remain uncertain. Maternal calcium intake during lactation appears to have very little effect on breast milk calcium concentrations. Populations with low dietary calcium intake have been found to have both low and high

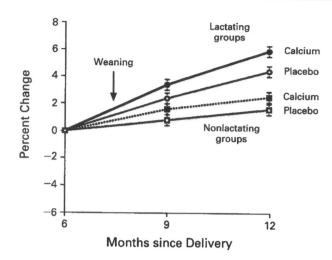

Fig. 3. Effects of calcium supplementation (1 g/d) and weaning on percent change in maternal bone density of the lumbar spine from 6 to 12 mo postpartum. (Reprinted from ref. *23*.)

breast milk calcium concentrations. Furthermore, two randomized, double-blinded calcium supplementation trials failed to find an effect of supplemental calcium on breast milk calcium concentration *(23,42)*.

4. PREGNANCY, LACTATION, AND RISK OF OSTEOPOROTIC FRACTURE

Because of the significant transfer of calcium into the fetus and the decrease in maternal bone density during pregnancy and lactation, there has been concern that pregnancy and lactation may increase a woman's risk of osteoporotic fracture in her later years. Most studies have focused on risk of hip fracture because of its high morbidity and mortality. In general, it appears that pregnancy and lactation do not affect long-term risk of hip fracture. Several large epidemiological studies have found that parity or ever having been pregnant are not associated with risk of hip fracture *(54)*. Contrary to expectations, other studies have shown that pregnancy is associated with a lower, not higher, risk of hip fracture *(55–58)*. One possible explanation for this is that some nulliparous women may have a compromised endocrine profile that also adversely affects their bone density, and thus infertility may result in increased risk of osteoporotic hip fracture *(56,59,60)*.

Several studies have shown that ever having lactated, lactating for long periods, breastfeeding several infants, or a long cumulative duration of lactation also do not appear to increase risk of hip fracture *(55,57,61–64)*. Because of the inverse association between parity and hip fracture, it is necessary to examine the effects of lactation on fracture risk only among parous women. In a case–control study of 664 elderly women with hip fracture and 1848 controls, there was no association between lactation and risk of hip fracture among parous women. The odds ratios (95% confidence interval) for hip fracture associated with breastfeeding for 6–10 mo, 11–16 mo, and more than16 mo were 0.90 (0.7–1.15), 0.95 (0.72–1.26), and 1.01 (0.75–1.15), respectively *(58)*. Although the results from studies to date do not indicate that lactation affects risk of osteoporotic fracture in general, no studies have addressed this question in subgroups of women who have characteristics that, theoretically, may place them at higher risk, such as women who lactate close to the onset of menopause, or those with very low calcium intakes.

5. CALCIUM HOMEOSTASIS AND BONE MASS DURING HUMAN REPRODUCTION: AN EVOLUTIONARY PERSPECTIVE

From an evolutionary standpoint, it is highly advantageous that the maternal calcium regulatory system is able to invoke multiple mechanisms by which to secure the necessary calcium for the fetus and for breast milk production in lieu of depending on abundant availability of dietary calcium. The availability of sufficient amounts of dietary calcium to meet the needs of reproduction among hunters and gathers was likely to have been unreliable. A calcium-securing strategy that is more reliable, and therefore safer for the survival of the fetus and infant, is for the mother to invoke compensatory calcium regulatory mechanisms.

At the outset, it would seem that the dependence on maternal calcium stored in bone for the support pregnancy and lactation would undermine the structural integrity of the maternal skeleton and place the mother at an immediate increased risk of fracture. If this were the case, it would likely compromise infant survival and, thus, would not be desirable evolutionarily. However, it is now becoming evident that women of reproductive age may have a surfeit of bone mineral relative to that needed for structural and locomotive functions *(65)*. There is a strong relationship between bone mass and muscle mass, which reflects their functional and interrelated roles in locomotion and performing other types of work. This relation has been demonstrated across a wide range of populations of varying ages, genders, races, and geographic regions. Ferretti and co-workers demonstrated that the ratio of bone mass to muscle mass was greater for premenopausal women than for men, prepubertal children, and postmenopausal women *(66)*. From a biomechanical efficiency perspective, it is desirable to have the minimum amount of bone mineral necessary to provide its structural function. Thus, the additional bone mineral per muscle mass in premenopausal women is likely there to support reproduction. The loss of bone mineral after menopause may be a consequence of the fact that the surfeit of bone is no longer necessary to support potential reproductive needs. However, women today live several decades longer than did women thousands of years ago. Postmenopausal bone loss, coupled with age-related bone loss, is associated with a high rate of osteoporotic fracture in older women. Thus, adoption of a lifestyle that maximizes bone mass and density is important for decreasing fracture risk in the later years.

6. CONCLUSIONS

Pregnancy and lactation are times of high calcium demand. Approximately 25–30 g of calcium are transferred to the fetus during pregnancy, and 200–240 mg/d of calcium are secreted in breast milk. Different physiological adaptations in maternal calcium metabolism are invoked to secure sufficient calcium for fetal bone mineral accretion and breast milk production. During pregnancy, the primary adaptation to secure additional calcium is an increase in maternal intestinal calcium absorption. Additional calcium may come from demineralization of maternal bone in the last trimester of pregnancy, when the fetus is accreting bone most rapidly. Urinary calcium excretion is increased during pregnancy as a result of increased GFR, but this increase may not occur in women with low calcium intakes.

The primary mechanism by which to secure calcium for the support of breast milk production is reduction of maternal bone mass. Urinary calcium conservation also may occur during lactation, although the results from studies are conflicting. Bone loss during lactation is related to the length of postpartum amenorrhea and is not affected by maternal calcium intake. The bone loss during lactation is transient, because bone density increases after weaning. Recovery of bone density after pregnancy and lactation appears to be complete, and previous pregnancy and lactation are not associated with increased risk of hip fractures among elderly women.

REFERENCES

1. Widdowson EM. Changes in body composition during growth. In: Davis JA, Dobbings J, eds. Scientific Foundations of Paediatrics. William Heinemann Medical Books Ltd., London: 1981: pp. 330–342.
2. Laskey MA, Prentice A, Hanratty LA, et al. Bone changes after 3 mo of lactation: Influence of calcium intake, breast-milk output, and vitamin D-receptor genotype. Am J Clin Nutr 1998;67:685–692.
3. Standing Committee on the Scientific Evaluation of Dietary Reference Intakes. Dietary reference intakes for calcium, phosphorus, magnesium, vitamin D, and fluoride. National Academy Press, Washington, DC: 1997.
4. Black A, Topping J, Durham B, Farquharson R, Fraser W. A detailed assessment of alterations in bone turnover, calcium homeostasis, and bone density in normal pregnancy. J Bone Miner Res 2000;15:557–564.
5. Gallacher SJ, Fraser WD, Owens OJ, et al. Changes in calciotrophic hormones and biochemical markers of bone turnover in normal human pregnancy. Eur J Endocrinol 1994;131:369–374.
6. Naylor KE, Iqbal P, Fledelius C, Fraser RB, Eastell R. The effect of pregnancy on bone density and bone turnover. J Bone Miner Res 2000;15:129–137.
7. Cross NA, Hillman LS, Allen SH, Krause GF, Vieira NE. Calcium homeostasis and bone metabolism during pregnancy, lactation, and postweaning: a longitudinal study. Am J Clin Nutr 1995;61:514–523.
8. Ritchie LD, Fung EB, Halloran BP, et al. A longitudinal study of calcium homeostasis during human pregnancy and lactation and after resumption of menses. Am J Clin Nutr 1998;67:693–701.
9. Bikle DD, Gee E, Halloran B, Haddad JG. Free 1,25-Dihydroxyvitamin D levels in serum from normal subjects, pregnant subjects, and subjects with liver disease. J Clin Invest 1984;74:1966–1971.
10. Uemura H, Yasui T, Kiyokawa A, et al. Serum osteoprotegerin/osteoclastogenesis-inhibitory factor during pregnancy and lactation and the relationship with calcium-regulating hormones and bone turnover markers. J Endocrinol 2002;174:353–359.
11. Heaney RP, Skillman, TG. Calcium metabolism in normal human pregnancy. J Clin Endocrinol 1971;33:661–669.
12. Matsumoto I, Kosha S, Noguchi S, et al. Changes of bone mineral density in pregnant and postpartum women. J Obstet Gynaecol 1995;21:419–425.
13. Sowers M, Crutchfield M, Jannausch M, Updike S, Corton G. A prospective evaluation of bone mineral change in pregnancy. Obstet Gynecol 1991;77:841–845.
14. Bjorklund K, Naessen T, Nordstrom ML, Bergstrom S. Pregnancy-related back and pelvic pain and changes in bone density. Acta Obstet Gynecol Scand 1999;78:681–685.
15. Kolthoff N, Eiken P, Kristensen B, Nielsen SP. Bone mineral changes during pregnancy and lactation: a longitudinal cohort study. Clin Sci 1998;94:405–412.
16. Shefras J, Farquharson R. Bone density studies in pregnant women receiving heparin. Eur J Obstet Gynecol Reproductive Biol 1996;65:171–174.
17. Drinkwater BL, Chesnut CH, III. Bone density changes during pregnancy and lactation in active women: a longitudinal study. Bone Miner 1991;14:153–160.
18. Paparella P, Giorgino R, Maglione A, et al. Maternal ultrasound bone density in normal pregnancy. Clin Experimental Obstet Gynecol 1995;22:268–278.

19. Gambacciani M, Spinetti A, Gallo R, Cappagli B, Teti GC, Facchini V. Ultrasonographic bone characteristics during normal pregnancy: longitudinal and cross-sectional evaluation. Am J Obstet Gynecol 1995;173:890–893.

20. Yamaga A, Taga M, Minaguchi H, Sato K. Changes in bone mass as determined by ultrasound and biochemical markers of bone turnover during pregnancy and puerperium: a longitudinal study. J Clin Endocrinol Metab 1996;81:752–756.

21. Aguado F, Revilla M, Hernandez ER, et al. Ultrasonographic bone velocity in pregnancy: A longitudinal study. Am J Obstet Gynecol 1998;178:1016–1021.

22. Hopkinson JM, Butte NF, Ellis K, Smith EO. Lactation delays postpartum bone mineral accretion and temporarily alters its regional distribution in women. J Nutr 2000;130:777–783.

23. Kalkwarf HJ, Specker BL, Bianchi DC, Ranz J, Ho M. The effect of calcium supplementation on bone density during lactation and after weaning. N Engl J Med 1997;337:523–528.

24. Polatti F, Capuzzo E, Viazzo F, Colleoni R, Klersy C. Bone mineral changes during and after lactation. Obstet Gynecol 1999;94:52–56.

25. Bezerra FF, Laboissiere FP, King JC, Donangelo CM. Pregnancy and lactation affect markers of calcium and bone metabolism differently in adolescent and adult women with low calcium intakes. J Nutr 2002;132:2183–2187.

26. Zeni SN, Ortela Soler CR, Lazzari A, et al. Interrelationship between bone turnover markers and dietary calcium intake in pregnant women: a longitudinal study. Bone 2003;33:606–613.

27. Raman L, Rajalakshmi K, Krishnamachari KAVR, Gowrinath Sastry J. Effect of calcium supplementation to undernourished mothers during pregnancy on the bone density of the neonates. Am J Clin Nutr 1978;31:466–469.

28. Koo W, Walters J, Esterlitz J, Levine R, Bush A, Sibai B. Maternal calcium supplementation and fetal bone mineralization. Obstetrics Gynecology 1999;94:577–582.

29. Chang S-C, O'Brien KO, Nathanson MS, Caulfield LE, Mancini J, Witter FR. Fetal femur length is influenced by maternal dairy intake in pregnant African American adolescents. Am J Clin Nutr 2003;77:1248–1254.

30. Kalkwarf HJ, Specker BL, Ho M. Effects of calcium supplementation on calcium homeostatis and bone turnover in lactating women. J Clin Endocrinol Metab 1999;84:464–470.

31. Krebs NF, Reidinger CJ, Robertson AD, Brenner M. Bone mineral density changes during lactation: maternal, dietary, and biochemical correlates. Am J Clin Nutr 1997;65:1738–1746.

32. Kalkwarf HJ, Specker BL, Heubi JE, Vieira NE, Yergey AL. Intestinal calcium absorption of women during lactation and after weaning. Am J Clin Nutr 1996;63:526–531.

33. Fairweather-Tait S, Prentice A, Heumann KG, et al. Effect of calcium supplements and stage of lactation on the calcium absorption efficiency of lactating women accustomed to low calcium intakes. Am J Clin Nutr 1995;62:1188–1192.

34. Moser-Veillon PB, Mangels AR, Vieira NE, et al. Calcium fractional absorption and metabolism assessed using stable isotopes differ between postpartum and never pregnant women. J Nutr 2001;131:2295–2299.

35. Affinito P, Tommaselli GA, Di Carlo C, Guida F, Nappi C. Changes in bone mineral density and calcium metabolism in breastfeeding women: a one year follow-up study. J Clin Endocrinol Metab 1996;81:2314–2318.

36. Sowers MF, Hollis BW, Shapiro B, et al. Elevated parathyroid hormone-related peptide associated with lactation and bone density loss. JAMA 1996;276:549–554.

37. Dobnig H, Kainer F, Stepan V, et al. Elevated parathyroid hormone-related peptide levels after human gestation: relationship to changes in bone and mineral metabolism. J Clin Endocrinol Metab 1995;80:3699–3707.

38. Lippuner K, Zehnder H-J, Casez J-P, Takkinen R, Jaeger P. PTH-related protein is released into the mother's bloodstream during lactation: evidence for beneficial effects on maternal calcium-phosphate metabolism. J Bone Miner Res 1996;11:1394–1399.

39. Seki K, Kato T, Sekiya S, et al. Parathyroid-hormone-related protein in human milk and its relation to milk calcium. Gynecologic Obstet Invest 1997;44:102–106.

40. Fraher LJ, Klein K, Marier R, et al. Comparison of the pharmacokinetics of parenteral parathyroid hormone-(1-34) [PTH-(1-34)] and PTH-related peptide-(1-34) in healthy young humans. J Clin Endocrinol Metab 1995;80:60–64.

41. Fraher LJ, Hodsman AB, Jonas K, et al. A comparison of the in vivo biochemical responses to exogenous parathyroid hormone-(1-34) [PTH-(1-34)] and PTH-related peptide-(1-34) in man. J Clin Endocrinol Metab 1992;75:417–423.

42. Prentice A, Jarjou LMA, Cole TJ, Stirling DM, Dibba B, Fairweather-Tait S. Calcium requirements of lactating Gambian mothers: effects of a calcium supplement on breast-milk calcium concentration, maternal bone mineral content, and urinary calcium excretion. Am J Clin Nutr 1995;62:58–67.

43. Kent GN, Price RI, Gutteridge DH, et al. Human lactation: Forearm trabecular bone loss, increased bone turnover, and renal conservation of calcium and inorganic phosphate with recovery of bone mass following weaning. J Bone Miner Res 1990;5:361–369.

44. Klein CJ, Moser-Veillon PB, Douglass LW, Ruben KA, Trocki O. A longitudinal study of urinary calcium, magnesium, and zinc excretion in lactating and nonlactating postpartum women. Am J Clin Nutr 1995;61:779–786.

45. Specker BL, Vieira NE, O'Brien KO, et al. Calcium kinetics in lactating women with low and high calcium intakes. Am J Clin Nutr 1994;59:593–599.

46. Donangelo CM, Trugo NMF, Melo GJO, Gomes DD, Henriques C. Calcium homeostasis during pregnancy and lactation in primiparous and multiparous women with sub-adequate calcium intakes. Nutr Res 1996;16:1631–1640.

47. Honda A, Kurabyashi T, Yahata T, Tomita M, Takakuwa K, Tanaka K. Lumbar bone mineral density changes during pregnancy and lactation. Int J Gynecol Obstet 1998;63:253–258.

48. Karlsson C, Obrant KJ, Karlsson M. Pregnancy and lactation confer reversible bone loss in humans. Osteoporos Int 2001;12:828–834.

49. Laskey M, Prentice A. Bone mineral changes during and after lactation. Obstet Gynecol 1999;94:608–615.

50. Sowers MF, Corton G, Shapiro B, et al. Changes in bone density with lactation. JAMA 1993;269:3130–3135.

51. Chan GM, McMurry M, Westover K, Engelbert-Fenton K, Thomas MR. Effects of increased dietary calcium intake upon the calcium and bone mineral status of lactating adolescent and adult women. Am J Clin Nutr 1987;46:319–323.

52. Lopez JM, Gonzalez G, Reyes V, Campino C, Diaz S. Bone turnover and density in healthy women during breastfeeding and after weaning. Osteoporos Int 1996;6:153–159.

53. Hayslip CC, Klein TA, Wray HL, Duncan WE. The effects of lactation on bone mineral content in healthy postpartum women. Obstet Gynecol 1989;73:588–592.

54. Parazzini F, Tavani A, Ricci E, La Vecchia C. Menstrual and reproductive factors and hip fractures in post menopausal women. Maturitas 1996;24:191–196.

55. Cummings SR, Nevitt MC, Browner WS, et al. Risk factors for hip fracture in white women. N Engl J Med 1995;332:767–773.

56. Nguyen TV, Jones G, Sambrook PN, White CP, Kelly PL, Eisman JA. Effects of estrogen exposure and reproductive factors on bone mineral density and osteoporotic fractures. J Clin Endocrinol Metab 1995;80:2709–2714.

57. Jacobsen BK, Nilssen S, Heuch I, Kvale G. Reproductive factors and fatal hip fractures. A Norwegian prospective study of 63,000 women. J Epidemiol Community Health 1998;52:645–650.

58. Michaelsson K, Baron JA, Farahmand BY, Ljunghall S. Influence of parity and lactation on hip fracture risk. Am J Epidemiol 2001;153:1166–1172.

59. Tuppurainen R, Honkanen H, Kroger H, Saarikoski S, Alhava E. Osteoporosis risk factors, gynaecological history and fractures in perimenopausal women—the results of the baseline postal enquiry of the Kuopio Osteoporosis Risk Factor and Prevention Study. Maturitas 1993;17:89–100.

60. Petersen HC, Jeune B, Vaupel JW, Christensen K. Reproduction life history and hip fractures. Ann Epidemiol 2002;12:257–263.

61. Kreiger N, Kelsey JL, Holford TR, O'Connor T. An epidemiologic study of hip fracture in postmenopausal women. Am J Epidemiol 1982;116:141–18.

62. Alderman BW, Weiss NS, Daling JR, Ure CL, Ballard JH. Reproductive history and postmenopausal risk of hip and forearm fracture. Am J Epidemiol 1986;124:262–267.

63. Cumming RG, Klineberg RJ. Breastfeeding and other reproductive factors and the risk of hip fractures in elderly women. Int J Epidemiol 1993;22:684–691.
64. Hoffman S, Grisso JA, Kelsey JL, Gammon MD, O'Brien LA. Parity, lactation and hip fracture. Osteoporos Int 1993;3:171–176.
65. Jarvinen TL, Kannus P, Sievanen H. Estrogen and bone—a reproductive and locomotive perspective. J Bone Miner Res 2003;18:1921–1931.
66. Ferretti JL, Capozza RF, Cointry GR, et al. Gender-related differences in the relationship between densitometric values of whole-body bone mineral content and lean body mass in humans between 2 and 87 yeas of age. Bone 1998;22:683–690.

VI   CALCIUM AND DISEASE

19 Calcium in Systemic Human Health

Robert P. Heaney

KEY POINTS

- Low calcium intake affects multiple body systems through three basic mechanisms: reduction in the size of the calcium nutrient reserve, reduction of complexation of potentially harmful byproducts of digestion because of low calcium content in the food residue, and inappropriate second messenger action of calcium ions as a result of high calcitriol levels evoked in response to low calcium intake.
- Although the resulting diseases are multi-factorial, improving calcium intake at a population level will nevertheless reduce national disease burden and health care costs substantially.

Low calcium intakes have been linked to a bewildering array of different diseases. In the chapters of this section, we describe the pathogenesis of the best attested of these disorders and review the evidence for the role of variations in calcium intake in their causation, prevention, and treatment. First, however, it is useful to establish the broad functional context in which calcium operates.

Regulation of extracellular fluid (ECF) [Ca^{2+}], especially when that involves adapting to chronically low calcium intakes, produces effects that are not confined to bone health. Adaptation, although obviously a necessary capacity to tide the organism over fluctuating and uncontrolled inputs, may nevertheless exert harmful collateral effects when constantly invoked. Examples for nonskeletal systems include effects on blood pressure regulation and body fat metabolism. Medical science is familiar with this phenomenon in the case of stress—with its high adrenergic hormone levels and high secretion of adrenal glucocorticoids—useful in emergencies, but harmful when sustained.

The mechanisms that underlie the collateral effects flowing from maintenance of the constancy of ECF [Ca^{2+}] are less well understood, but are gradually becoming clearer. Most direct is an increase in parathyroid cell mass itself *(1)*. Associated with this phenomenon is an age-specific increase in incidence of hyperparathyroidism among postmenopausal women *(2)*. Whether the two phenomena are causally related is not settled, but it is true for other organ systems that constant stimulation promotes development of

From: *Calcium in Human Health*
Edited by: C. M. Weaver and R. P. Heaney © Humana Press Inc., Totowa, NJ

Table 1
Classification of Disorders Related to Low Calcium Intake

As a result of: Decreased Ca nutrient reserve	Low food residue Ca in chyme	Adaptive mechanisms maintaining ECF [Ca²⁺]
Osteoporosis	Colon cancer Renolithiasis	Hypertension Pre-eclampsia Premenstrual syndrome Obesity Polycystic ovary syndrome Hyperparathyroidism

autonomous cell clones or frank neoplasia, and it would be surprising if this same relationship were not true for the parathyroid glands as well.

Pathogenesis of all of the other disorders currently linked to low calcium intake can be reduced to only three basic mechanisms: (1) decrease in the size of the calcium reserve; (2) decrease in residual calcium in the intestinal contents as they reach the lower bowel; and (3) nonskeletal responses to the hormones mediating adaptation to low calcium intake. The principal disorders associated with low calcium intakes are classified on this mechanistic basis in Table 1, and can be briefly characterized as follows:

- Osteoporosis is the disorder that results when the size of the calcium reserve (the skeleton) is depleted for nutritional reasons (*see* Chapter 2). The hormonal responses to insufficient intake succeed in maintaining ECF [Ca²⁺], but they often end up doing so by depleting the nutrient reserve (bone mass).
- The risk of both colon cancer and kidney stones rises as the calcium content of the diet residue falls, both for the same basic reason: insufficient calcium in the food residue to complex potentially harmful byproducts of digestion.
- The best available explanation for at least some of the remaining disorders lies in the fact that, in addition to its classical effects regulating ECF [Ca²⁺], parathyroid hormone (PTH) induces a high level of production of 1,25 dihydroxyvitamin D (1,25[OH]₂D), which not only optimizes intestinal calcium absorption, but elevates cytosolic calcium ion concentrations in many tissues unrelated to the operation of the calcium economy, thereby altering their basal level of functional activity. (*See* Chapter 3 for a detailed exposition of the actions and regulation of calcium ion levels in the cell interior.)

The first two mechanisms are straightforward. They are both reflections of the reduction in calcium mass—the less mass ingested, the less mass absorbed, and the less residual calcium mass in the intestine left over from the diet. All are inescapable aspects of low intake.

The other disorders have been termed "calcium paradox" diseases *(3)* because of the seeming paradox of reduced calcium intakes and elevated cytosolic [Ca²⁺]. The mechanisms that underlie these disorders are more subtle and are set forth schematically in Fig. 1. Whereas expression of the disorders in the first two groups is an immediate, direct consequence of low calcium intake, expression of the calcium paradox diseases

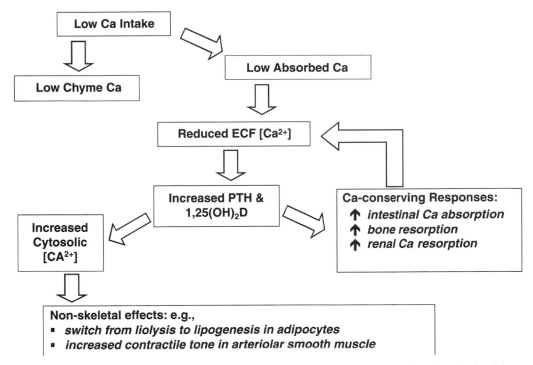

Fig. 1. Schematic depiction of the consequences of low levels of ingested and/or absorbed calcium. The primary hormonal response (i.e., increased parathyroid hormone secretion) initiates not only the well described calcium-conserving responses that are a part of the negative feedback loop regulating extracellular fluid [Ca^{2+}], but also elevates cytosolic [Ca^{2+}] in certain tissues, thereby falsely signaling responses in cells that are not a part of the calcium homeostatic control loop. (Copyright Robert P. Heaney, 1999. Reproduced with permission.)

almost certainly requires interaction of multiple defects and triggering mechanisms. At least three such factors can be identified for most of them: (1) the low calcium intake that leads to increased circulating 1,25(OH)$_2$D, which produces a leak of calcium into the cytosol; (2) a genetic sensitivity that renders certain cell types (or individuals) more than usually sensitive to the leak of calcium ions into their cytosol (as, for example, by weak mechanisms for extruding the unneeded calcium); and (3) an environmental trigger. Such triggers might include high salt intakes for hypertension or an abundance of food energy for obesity.

In brief, for the calcium paradox diseases, the constant high serum 1,25(OH)$_2$D level of low calcium intake stresses the system beyond the reserve capacity of sensitive tissues or individuals. An instructive parallel is seen in hemolytic anemia that develops, for example, on exposure to certain drugs or to ingestion of fava beans in individuals with erythrocyte glucose-6-phosphate dehydrogenase deficiency (known in the medical literature as "favism"). In the absence of the trigger (e.g., eating fava beans), little or no clinical evidence of anemia is present. As with favism, the disorders that follow upon a hypersensitivity to 1,25(OH)$_2$D manifest themselves in individuals who lack sufficient redundancy in the cell control mechanisms to neutralize the unsignaled elevation in cytosolic calcium ion concentration.

At the same time, it must also be emphasized that all of the disorders in all three categories are, in their own right, multi-factorial. For example, there are many ways to have a reduced skeletal mass in addition to inadequate nutrient intake, and there are many ways to have elevated blood pressure in addition to high endogenous PTH production. Thus low calcium intake is only one factor in the genesis of these disorders, and if one could optimize calcium intake in the entire population, it is virtually certain that none of the diseases concerned would be totally eradicated. Nevertheless, altering calcium intake will reduce the total disease burden for all of these disorders. Furthermore, doing so is a cost-effective intervention within society's grasp, and one that therefore demands attention *(4)*.

Given the involvement of inadequate calcium intake in so many different diseases, McCarron and Heaney *(4)* undertook to analyze the health system cost savings associated with a group of nine disorders for which there is solid evidence of a calcium benefit. Their thesis was that, even if an adequate calcium intake were to reduce a particular disease burden by only a few percentage points, such savings, aggregated over several disorders, would nevertheless result in substantially reduced costs. Moreover, if the disease itself were very common or very expensive to treat, then even a small percent reduction would still be a lot of dollars. Finally, once one has increased the population level of calcium intake for disease A, the cost of doing so for diseases B, C, and D is zero. Hence, the more diseases involved, the more favorable the cost–benefit relationship.

McCarron and Heaney took a conservative approach to calculating cost savings. The chapters that follow present data indicating, for example, in osteoporosis, a 40–55% reduction in fracture risk; by contrast McCarron and Heaney based their calculation of savings on only a 20% reduction in fractures. Similarly high calcium intake (particularly from dairy sources) could produce substantial reduction in prevalence of obesity; yet McCarron and Heaney calculated only a 5% reduction. However, obesity is such an expensive problem (estimated at $60 to more than $100 billion each year), that even a 5% reduction results in huge savings.

Figure 2 summarizes the 5-yr savings for the nine groups of disorders analyzed. It is immediately apparent, for example, that although calcium is traditionally associated with reduction in osteoporotic fractures, the actual savings from reduced fracture risk ($14 billion), although substantial, are dwarfed by the much larger savings from even a modest reduction in cardiovascular disease ($106.5 billion) and in obesity and type 2 diabetes ($75 billion). Figure 2 also illustrates forcefully the total body involvement of calcium in health and disease.

In conclusion, calcium is important for many body systems, and low calcium intakes contribute to the disease burden of many chronic diseases, several of which are described in ensuing chapters. The mechanisms behind all these effects are just threefold: depletion of the nutrient reserve (osteoporosis); inadequate intraintestinal neutralization of potentially harmful byproducts of digestion (colon cancer and kidney stones); and collateral effects on many tissues, produced by the hormones evoked to sustain plasma calcium homeostasis (hypertension, obesity, polycystic ovary syndrome, and others). Raising national calcium intakes to currently recommended values, by reducing the disease burdens of these disorders, can be shown to produce aggregate savings of more than $200 billion within 5 yr.

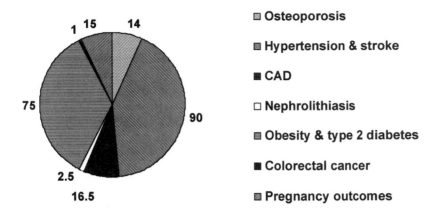

Fig. 2. Five-year cost savings ($ billions) for the nine groups of disorders for which adequate calcium intake has been shown to reduce disease burden or severity. CAD, coronary artery disease. *See* ref. *28* for details. (Copyright, Robert P. Heaney, 2003. Used with permission.)

REFERENCES

1. McKane WR, Khosla S, Egan KS, Robins SP, Burritt MF, Riggs BL. Role of calcium intake in modulating age-related increases in parathyroid function and bone resorption. J Clin Endocrinol Metab 1996;81:1699–1703.
2. Heath H III, Hodgson SF, Kennedy MA. Primary hyperparathyroidism. Incidence, morbidity, and potential economic impact in a community. N Engl J Med 1980;302:189–193.
3. Fujita T, Palmieri GMA. Calcium paradox disease: calcium deficiency prompting secondary hyperparathyroidism and cellular calcium overload. J Bone Miner Metab 2000;118:109–125.
4. McCarron DA, Heaney RP. Estimated healthcare savings associated with adequate dairy food intake. Am J Hypertension 2004;17:88–97.

20 Calcium and Oral Health

Elizabeth A. Krall

KEY POINTS

- Prior to tooth eruption, deficiency of calcium can adversely affect tooth enamel mineralization, tooth size, and timing of eruption.
- After tooth eruption, deficiency of calcium produces osteoporosis in the alveolar bone of animals, which is reversible upon calcium replenishment.
- Clinical and epidemiological studies of the effects of calcium nutrition on teeth and oral bone suggest it is one of several important factors that aids in maintaining periodontal health and retaining teeth among adults.
- These findings need to be investigated further with randomized clinical trials.

1. MINERALIZED TISSUES IN THE ORAL CAVITY

Calcium is vital for the proper development and maintenance of calcified oral tissues. These include tissues incorporated into the structure of the teeth themselves and the bone in which they are embedded. The mineralized tissues of the tooth, enamel, cementum and dentin, have characteristics that are distinct from bone. The enamel covering of the coronal portion of the tooth is composed of large, densely packed hydroxyapatite crystals (Fig. 1). Compared with bone, enamel has a higher ratio of mineral to water and organic material (96% mineral, 3% water, and <1% collagen). Enamel has no vascular or nerve supply after the tooth has been formed, and does not undergo remodeling. Demineralization and remineralization occur only in localized areas on the tooth surface.

Cementum is the calcified layer that extends from the coronal enamel to cover the exterior of the root surfaces. However, the composition of cementum is approx 50% mineral and 50% organic.

Beneath the enamel or cementum layers and directly surrounding the pulpal cavity is the dentin. Dentin is 70% mineral, 10% water, and 20% organic material, mostly collagen. Like enamel, it has no vascular system but it does allow limited transport of nutrients from the pulp via dentinal tubules.

Sockets in the alveolar bone anchor the tooth roots and provide support. Alveolar bone is primarily trabecular and, unlike mineralized tissues of the teeth, does undergo remodeling. In the healthy jaw, the height of the alveolar bone crest completely encases the tooth root as it reaches approximately to the level of the juncture of the coronal enamel and root cementum.

From: *Calcium in Human Health*
Edited by: C. M. Weaver and R. P. Heaney © Humana Press Inc., Totowa, NJ

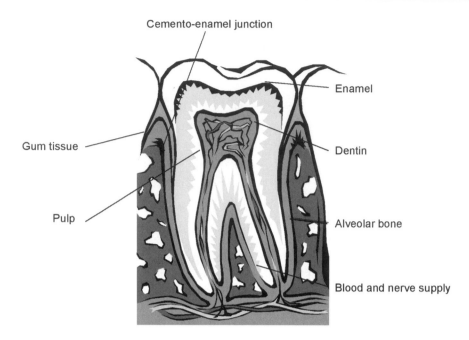

Fig.1. Diagram of the structure of a tooth. (Copyright Microsoft Corp., 2004.)

2. PRE-ERUPTIVE EFFECTS OF CALCIUM

Mineralization of the primary teeth begins around 4 mo *in utero*. Mineralization of the permanent teeth begins around birth and continues until they erupt, between the ages of 6 and 13 yr. During formation, the enamel and cementum have a vascular system to supply nutrients for mineralization, but this system is severed at the time of eruption. As a result, the time when an imbalance in calcium nutrition will have its major effect on tooth structure is during gestation and childhood. Data from animal experiments indicate that diets deficient in calcium, or diets with a low calcium to phosphorus ratio (1:3) will result in hypomineralization defects in enamel and dentin *(1,2)*, small tooth size *(3)*, and delayed eruption *(4)*. Restriction of both calcium and vitamin D results in a reduced quantity of cementum in the rat tooth *(5)*, and lower weight of ash and total tooth weight *(6)*.

3. EFFECTS OF CALCIUM ON ALVEOLAR BONE

In the adult, the primary impact of calcium nutrition on oral tissues is on alveolar bone. Many animal studies have manipulated the calcium content of the diet, or the calcium to phosphorus ratio to induce secondary hyperparathyroidism, in order to study the effects on alveolar bone. Findings from these studies consistently show that a calcium imbalance will produce signs of osteoporosis in the jaw and alveolar crest *(5,7–9)*. The alveolar porosity and thinning of the trabeculae parallel those seen in the long bones of the same animals *(8,9)*. Replenishing calcium intake to adequate levels reverses these signs throughout the skeleton *(8)*. It has been suggested that the jaws exhibit osteoporotic changes first *(9,10)*, before osteoporosis becomes evident in the spine or peripheral sites but this has been disputed *(8)*.

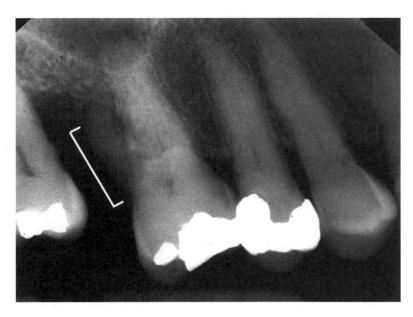

Fig. 2. Radiograph of upper molar showing alveolar bone loss, indicated by the bracket. In comparison, the right side of the tooth shows minimal bone loss from the cemento-enamel junction to the alveolar crest.

3.1. Early Studies of Calcium and Periodontal Disease

In addition to systemic influences such as calcium deprivation, alveolar bone is subject to local factors that affect resorption and formation. In periodontal disease, inflammatory factors released by oral bacteria and the host response to infection destroy both soft (gum and periodontal ligament) and calcified tissues (alveolar bone) of the periodontium. Alveolar bone loss is a key diagnostic feature of periodontal disease, however the bone loss is manifested primarily as loss of alveolar bone height around the tooth socket (Fig. 2). Consequences of the loss of bone support include increased tooth mobility and risk of tooth loss. Other clinical indicators of periodontal bone loss include loss of attachment of the gum tissue and deep pockets forming around the tooth roots. More than one-half of the adult population in developed countries has some form of periodontal disease, and the prevalence increases with age *(11,12)*. In the majority of patients, the disease is mild or limited to a few teeth but approx 10–25% of adults have moderate to severe forms that place the affected teeth at an increased risk of tooth loss. In the elderly, more than 25% of missing teeth were extracted because of periodontal disease *(13)*.

The role of calcium intake in periodontal disease has been the subject of controversy for many years. A series of papers by Henrikson, Krook, and colleagues described the effects of diet-induced secondary hyperparathyroidism in beagle dogs and low calcium intake in humans and attributed radiological and clinical signs of periodontal disease to low dietary calcium *(10,14–16)*. The findings prompted them to suggest that calcium deficiency, not inflammation, may be the primary cause of periodontal disease. In a repeat of the experiment in beagles, Svanberg *(17)* observed demineralization of the alveolar crest but no reduction in alveolar bone height. The calcium-deficient animals showed a tendency to more loss of attachment, deeper periodontal pockets and decreased radiographic density of alveolar bone but with six animals, the study may not have had sufficient statistical power. Other investigators also failed to see decreases in alveolar bone height in animals on low-calcium diets even though, as noted previously, the diets produced signs of osteoporosis in alveolar bone (5,7–9).

Krook et al. conducted a 6-mo study of ten periodontal disease patients in which their low usual dietary calcium intakes were supplemented with 1 g of calcium per day (16). They reported that alveolar height loss was restored, pocket depths were reduced and tooth mobility was reduced or eliminated. However, the study had no control group, and no quantitative measures of bone, pocket depth, or mobility were presented. Urbohm and Erickson attempted to repeat the clinical study with a larger study cohort but failed to see any statistically significant differences in outcomes between the treated patients and a control group (18).

Although the view that calcium deficiency initiates periodontal disease has been discounted, it has been proposed that chronic nutritional imbalances that result in alveolar osteoporosis may affect the course of periodontal disease, so that if bacterial infection does occurs, periodontal disease will progress more rapidly than if the bone had normal density. The previous clinical studies, with follow-up times of 6 mo to 1 yr may not have been of sufficient length to detect real differences in periodontal disease progression by calcium supplementation status.

Alveolar bone grows in response to tooth eruption and is resorbed when the teeth are lost. Alveolar ridge resorption can be severe in patients who wear full dentures to replace all teeth. Calcium intakes tend to be lower among edentulous patients with severe erosion compared to patients with minimal erosion (19,20). Supplementation with 750 mg calcium and 375 international units (IU) vitamin D shortly after tooth extraction resulted in less alveolar bone loss 1 yr later among denture patients (21).

3.2. Recent Studies of Calcium Intake, Periodontal Disease, and Tooth Loss

The similarities of alveolar and peripheral bone with respect to histology and response to calcium undernutrition have led to numerous investigations of the correlation of bone density at systemic sites with oral bone, clinical indicators of periodontal disease, and tooth loss. The majority of studies have been cross-sectional in design with small sample sizes, but although results have been mixed, the overall evidence tends to support associations between low systemic bone density and increased risks of periodontal disease and tooth loss (22). One of the few prospective studies followed 38 postmenopausal women with periodontal disease for 2 yr and found that women with osteoporosis or osteopenia of the spine exhibited more loss of alveolar bone height than women with normal spine bone mineral density (23). These associations, along with the wealth of data showing that calcium nutrition is important to maintenance of the systemic skeleton, have renewed interest in the role of calcium in periodontal disease.

3.2.1. CALCIUM INTAKE AND ALVEOLAR BONE LOSS

A series of prospective analyses of alveolar bone loss and other periodontal disease measures was conducted in a cohort of older men participating in a longitudinal study of aging and oral health (24). In the first study, which had a maximum follow-up time of 7 yr, alveolar bone loss was the outcome measurement. A total of 550 men had repeated radiographic measurements of alveolar bone height on all teeth present during this time interval. Rapid progression of alveolar bone loss at each tooth was defined as a change from minimal bone loss (80% or more of alveolar bone remaining around the tooth) to high bone loss (<80% of bone remaining). Usual calcium intake was estimated from repeated food frequency questionnaires and intake was dichotomized at 1000 mg/d. After adjustment for age, initial number of teeth, smoking status, vitamin D intake, caries status, bleeding on probing, clinical attachment loss, and probing pocket depth, the percent of teeth with alveolar bone loss progression of alveolar bone loss was compared between men with low calcium intakes and high calcium intakes. Men whose calcium intakes were below 1000 mg/d had 30% more teeth with rapid progression of alveolar bone loss compared with men who had calcium intakes above this level.

In a further analysis of this male cohort that extended the follow-up period to 17 yr, additional periodontal measures and tooth loss were also examined *(25)*. Progression of alveolar bone loss, clinical attachment loss and tooth loss were examined by quartile of calcium intakes and adjusted for age, smoking status, dental variables associated with periodontal disease (discussed previously), and mean intakes of vitamin D and phosphorus. The mean number of teeth with alveolar bone loss progression in men in the highest calcium intake quartile (990 mg/d) was 23% less than in men with intakes below 990 mg. The clinical attachment loss and tooth loss data showed similar trends. Men in the highest quartile of calcium intake had 25% less progression of clinical attachment loss and lost 31% fewer teeth than men with lower calcium levels.

3.2.2. Calcium Intake and Clinical Attachment Loss

A cross-sectional analysis of data from more than 12,000 adults who participated in the third National Health and Nutrition Examination Survey found that intakes of calcium of 800 mg or more were associated with lower prevalence of clinical attachment loss *(26)*. Calcium from food sources was computed and categorized into three levels: the reference group that consumed 800 mg or more, moderate calcium (500–800 mg/d), and low calcium (<500 mg/d). Average clinical attachment loss of 1.5 mm or more was defined as periodontal disease. After controlling for smoking, age, and gingival bleeding, the odds ratios for periodontal disease were 30% higher in individuals with moderate calcium intake compared to the reference group, and 30% higher (in men) to 60% higher (in women) in those with low calcium intakes.

3.2.3. Calcium Intake and Tooth Loss

Calcium intake and tooth loss over a period of 5 yr were examined in 145 healthy men and women age 65 yr and older *(27)*. In the first phase of the study, a 3-yr randomized, controlled clinical trial, subjects took either placebos or supplements containing 500 mg of calcium and 700 IU of vitamin D per day. During a 2-yr follow-up phase in which study supplements were discontinued, total calcium and vitamin D intakes were self-selected. During the randomized trial, the odds of losing any teeth were significantly reduced in the supplemented group (odds ratio [OR] = 0.4, 95% confidence interval [CI] = 0.2–0.9) relative to the placebo group. During the uncontrolled follow-up phase, the odds of tooth loss were also significantly lower in subjects with calcium intake greater than or equal to 1000 mg/d compared to those who consumed less than 1000 mg (OR = 0.5, 95% CI = 0.2–0.7). Tooth loss was not the primary purpose of this trial and there were no measures of alveolar bone to add support to the findings.

4. CONCLUSIONS

Defects in tooth mineralization, periodontal disease, and tooth loss are multi-factorial oral conditions that are largely preventable. Inadequate calcium nutrition is one contributing factor to these oral diseases. A limited number of earlier clinical studies of calcium intake levels or supplements in relation to periodontal disease and tooth loss reached contradictory conclusions. Recent large, well-controlled studies show consistent support for the hypothesis that calcium status influences the progression of oral bone loss, clinical measures of periodontal disease, and the risk of tooth loss. These findings must be confirmed with randomized, controlled trials.

REFERENCES

1. Mellanby M. The effect of diet on the structure of teeth. The interrelationship between the calcium and other food factors. Brit Dent J 1923;44:1031–1049.
2. Larsen MJ, Fejerskov O, Jensen SJ. Effects of fluoride, calcium, and phosphate administration on mineralization in rats. Calcified Tiss Int 1980;31:225–230.
3. Paynter KJ, Grainger RM. The relation of nutrition to the morphology and size of the rat molar teeth. J Can Dent Assn 1956;22:519–531.
4. Mellanby M. The chief dietetic and environmental factors responsible for the high incidence of dental caries: correlation between animal and human investigations. Brit Dent J 1928;49:769–792.
5. Ferguson HW, Hartles RL. The effects of diets deficient in calcium or phosphorus in the presence and absence of supplements of vitamin D on the secondary cementum and alveolar bone of young rats. Arch. Oral Biol. 1964;9: 647–58.
6. Harrand RB, Hartles RL. The effect of vitamin D in rats maintained on diets with different mineral content but with the same calcium to phosphorus ratio of unity. Brit J Nutr 1970;24:929–942.
7. Bissada NF, DeMarco TJ. The effect of a hypocalcemic diet on the periodontal structures of the adult rat. J. Periodontol 1974;45, 739–745.
8. Messer HH, Goebel NK, Wilcox L. A comparison of bone loss from different skeletal sites during acute calcium deficiency in mice. Arch Oral Biol 1981;26: 1001–1004.
9. Ericsson Y, Ekberg O. Dietetically provoked general and alveolar osteopenia in rats and its prevention or cure by calcium and fluoride. J Periodont Res 1975;10:256–269.
10. Krook L, Whalen JP, Lesser GV, Lutwak L. Human periodontal disease and osteoporosis. Cornell Vet 1972;62:371–391.
11. Benigeri M, Brodeur JM, Payette M, Charbonneau A, Ismail AI. Community periodontal index of treatment needs and prevalence of periodontal conditions. J Clin Periodontol 2000;27: 308–312.
12. Albandar JM, Brunelle JA, Kingman A. Destructive periodontal disease in adults 30 years of age and older in the United States, 1988–1994. J Periodontol 1999;70:13–29.
13. Brown LJ, Brunelle JA, Kingman A. Periodontal status in the United States, 1988–1991: prevalence, extent, and demographic variation. J Dent Res 1996;75(Spec No):672–683.
14. Henrikson PA. Periodontal disease and calcium deficiency. An experimental study in the dog. Acta Odontol Scand 1968;26(Suppl 50):1–132.
15. Krook L, Lutwak L, Henrikson PA, Kallfelz F, Hirsch C, Romanus B, Marier JR, Sheffey BE. Reversibility of nutritional osteoporosis;physicochemical data on bones from and experimental study in dogs. J Nutr 1971;101:233–246.
16. Krook L, Lutwak L, Whalen JP, Henrikson PA, Lesser GV, Uris R. Human periodontal disease. Morphology and response to calcium therapy. Cornell Vet 1972;62: 32–53.
17. Svanberg G, Lindhe J, Hugoson A, Grondahl HG. Effect of nutritional hyperparathyroidism on experimental periodontitis in the dog. Scand J Dent Res 1973;81:1551–1562.
18. Uhrbom E, Jacobson L. Calcium and periodontitis: clinical effect of calcium medication. J Clin Periodontol 1984;11:230–241.

19. Kribbs PJ, Smith DE, Chesnut CH III. Oral findings in osteoporosis. Part II: Relationship between residual ridge and alveolar bone resorption and generalized skeletal osteopenia. J Prosthet Dent 1983;50:719–724.

20. Wical KE, Swoope CC. Studies of residual ridge resorption. Part II. The relationship of dietary calcium and phosphorus to residual ridge resorption. J Prosthet Dent 1974;32:13–22.

21. Wical KE, Brussee P. Effects of a calcium and vitamin D supplement on alveolar ridge resorption in immediate denture patients. J Prosthet Dent 1979;41:4–11.

22. Wactawski-Wende J. Periodontal diseases and osteoporosis: association and mechanisms. Annals Periodontol 2001;6:197–208.

23. Payne JB. Reinhardt RA. Nummikoski PV. Patil KD. Longitudinal alveolar bone loss in postmenopausal osteoporotic/osteopenic women. Osteoporosis Int 1999;10:34–40.

24. Krall EA. The periodontal-systemic connection: implications for treatment of patients with osteoporosis and periodontal disease. Annals Periodontol 2001;6:209–213.

25. Krall EA. Nutrition and teeth. In: Burckhardt P, Dawson-Hughes B, Heaney RP, eds. Nutritional Aspects of Osteoporosis, 2nd ed. Elsevier Academic Press, London, 2004, pp. 153–162.

26. Nishida M, Grossi SG, Dunford RG, Ho AW, Trevisan M, Genco RJ. Calcium and the risk for periodontal disease. J. Periodontol 2000;71:1057–1066.

27. Krall EA, Wehler C, Harris SS, Garcia RI, Dawson-Hughes B. Calcium and vitamin D supplements reduce tooth loss in the elderly. Am J Med 2001;111:452–456.

21 Dietary Calcium and Obesity

Dorothy Teegarden

KEY POINTS

- Substantial epidemiological evidence supports an association between higher dairy product intakes and lower body weight or body fat mass; however, the role of calcium intake remains unsettled.
- There is evidence to support several mechanisms proposed to mediate a calcium-specific effect on change in body weight, including the formation of calcium/fatty acid soaps in the intestine and modulation of lipolysis and lipid oxidation through dietary calcium regulation of serum parathyroid hormone and 1,25 dihydroxyvitamin D levels.

1. DIETARY CALCIUM INTAKE AND OBESITY

The incidence of obesity in the United States is reaching epidemic proportions, and it is estimated that 97 million adults are overweight or obese (1). Obesity substantially increases morbidity from a variety of diseases, including hypertension, dyslipidemia, type 2 diabetes, and stroke. Recent studies also support an association between obesity and increased risk of several types of cancers including endometrial, breast, prostate, and colon (1). Despite efforts to reduce the prevalence of obesity, the incidence has risen since 1960, and in the last decade 55% of adults age 20 yr or older are overweight and obese. Clearly, obesity is a multifactorial disease that involves interactions with genetics and environment; its rapid rise in the last several decades demonstrates that environmental factors play a substantial role in the recent development and increase in the incidence of this disease.

Controversy remains as to the ideal dietary guidelines for macronutrients to both prevent obesity and reduce weight, but it is not surprising that bioactive components of the diet, such as calcium, may play a role in regulation of energy metabolism. There is substantial evidence that calcium or dairy products, the primary source of calcium in the US diet (see Chapter 9), may contribute to regulation of weight and body fat. Minimally, increased intake of dairy products does not lead to increased weight gain, but not all studies support a relationship between calcium or dairy intake and changes in weight. The mechanisms by which calcium (or dairy products) modulate weight are likely to be multifactorial, leading to a shift in overall energy balance that may contribute to weight maintenance or enhanced weight loss.

From: *Calcium in Human Health*
Edited by: C. M. Weaver and R. P. Heaney © Humana Press Inc., Totowa, NJ

2. HUMAN STUDIES LINKING CALCIUM WITH WEIGHT REGULATION

An association between higher calcium intakes and lower body weight was noted in a few publications the late 1980s *(2,3)*, but it was not until the late 1990s that the relationship has been more thoroughly explored. McCarron et al. *(2)* reported an inverse association between calcium intake (of which dairy products are the predominant dietary source) and body weight based on data from the first National Health and Nutritional Examination Survey (NHANES-I). This association was subsequently confirmed by Zemel et al., who re-analyzed data collected for the NHANES-III and showed that the highest quartile of calcium or dairy product intake reduced the odds ratio of being in the highest fat quartile to 0.16 *(4)*. In 1988, Metz et al. demonstrated a reduction in body fat mass in two strains of hypertensive rats with higher calcium intakes (in conjunction with a higher sodium intake) *(3)*. Furthermore, a study by Lin et al. demonstrated that higher calcium intakes in young (aged 18–31 yr) women predicted a negative relationship with body weight, specific to changes in body fat mass over 2 yr when analyses were corrected for energy intakes *(5)*.

The early studies prompted investigators to mine existing datasets to test for a relationship between dietary calcium intake and measures of body weight or body fat. A variety of studies, as discussed later, have shown this relationship, but a number of issues must be considered when reviewing this literature. Because the primary source of dietary calcium in the US diet is dairy products, in epidemiological studies dairy product intake is often used as a surrogate measure for calcium intake. However, it is possible that components of dairy products other than calcium may have a synergistic effect with calcium, or even an independent effect that may be obscured in many of the studies to date. Second, low dietary calcium intake is associated with a less healthy lifestyle or diet *(6)*, and thus, a cause-and-effect relationship cannot be established in the epidemiological investigations. Third, it is unlikely that an effect of dietary calcium on body composition is independent of energy intake. Higher energy intakes are likely to obscure any effects of dietary calcium on body composition. Dietary energy intake is very difficult to assess even when attempted (*see* Chapter 4), but in many of the studies available, a measurement of energy intake is not available. In some cases, either energy intake or a component of energy intake, protein, is utilized in the analysis to address this confounding issue. Fourth, dietary calcium intake may have an effect only under certain circumstances, such as during weight loss, or in obese individuals, or in individuals who are vitamin D-sufficient. Finally, many of the human trials to date were not designed to study the impact of calcium on body composition or weight—rather, these are secondary analyses of trials.

2.1. Cross-Sectional Studies

A variety of cross-sectional studies across adult ages have suggested a relationship between higher calcium intakes and reduced body weights, body fat, or body mass index (BMI). Evidence from the HERITAGE Family Study ($N = 824$), including both men and women, demonstrates an inverse relationship between tertiles of calcium intake adjusted for calorie intake with fat mass, BMI, and waist circumference *(7)*. In a study of women aged 18–28 yr, in which baseline data from two studies were combined ($N = 348$), calcium/protein (mg/g) ratio negatively predicted BMI *(8)*. An analysis from the Quebec Family Study, a cohort of 470 men and women aged 20–65 yr, shows that the lowest calcium intake group (less than 600 mg/d) had significantly higher body weight, percent body fat mass, BMI, waist circumference, and total abdominal adipose tissue area than other groups categorized by calcium intake *(9)*. In contrast, analyses of a large adult cohort (9252 men and 9662 women) show that calcium intake is significantly positively correlated with BMI in men when corrected for age, but no association is noted in women *(10)*. Thus, several cross-sectional studies, but not all, demonstrate a relationship between calcium or dairy product intake and lower measures of body composition such as weight, fat mass, or BMI. However, the specific role of calcium intake in this association cannot be determined from these studies.

The impact of calcium on body fat or weight has been noted in both white and African Americans, although the results remain mixed. At the end of the year-long intervention, African-American obese, hypertensive subjects who consumed yogurt to achieve calcium intakes of 1029 ± 74 mg/d had significantly less body fat than the low calcium-intake group (calcium intake 447 ± 126 mg/d) *(4)*. In addition, Buchowski et al., in a study investigating the impact of lactose intolerance and maldigestion on calcium intakes in 50 premenopausal African-American women *(11)*, demonstrated that calcium intakes adjusted for energy intakes is negatively associated with BMI in the lactose-tolerant individuals (mean calcium intake 781 (305 mg/d; mean (SD) compared with the lactose-intolerant group (388 ± 150 mg/d). Thus, the evidence suggests that with sufficient dietary intakes of calcium (mean intakes in cohort >700) epidemiological studies support an impact of dietary calcium intake on body weight. In addition, a cross-sectional analysis of 149 premenopausal women, a negative correlation between calcium intakes and percent body fat was specific to the white women *(12)*. The white women consumed significantly more calcium (758 ± 25 mean; SEM) compared with the African-American women (518 ± 34). The African Americans in this study may not have achieved dietary calcium levels that impact body fat. Thus, it is important to consider the level of calcium intake when comparing racial differences, because dairy consumption, and thus usually calcium intake, is generally lower in African Americans compared with whites. The evidence in studies in which calcium intakes are likely to be sufficient to demonstrate an effect *(4,11)* are supportive of the fact that increased calcium or dairy intakes may have an impact in reducing body weight or body fat mass in African Americans.

Gender is also an important consideration in determining the impact of calcium intake on body fat mass. Many of the epidemiological studies employ both men and women in their analysis, whereas intervention studies are primarily in women. The analysis of NHANES-III by Zemel et al. *(4)*, utilizing data from 380 women and 7114 men, shows a negative relationship in both men and women separately, though analysis by Barr et al., employing a larger number of subjects from the NHANES-III dataset, does not support these results *(13)*. In contrast, cross-sectional analysis of 470 men and women aged 20–65 yr demonstrated that low daily calcium intake was associated with greater adiposity in women, but not men, when analyses were corrected for factors including age and energy intake *(9)*. Another cross-sectional analysis of 204 men and women, mixed race, shows that calcium intake or calcium/protein negatively associated with BMI ($r = -0.22$) and body fat ($r = -0.35$) specific to the women *(14,15)*. Thus, data suggest that higher calcium/dairy intakes are associated with reduced fat mass in women, but the results are not as consistent for men.

One confounding factor in analyzing results of studies investigating the relationship of calcium intake and body weight is the adiposity of the cohorts. This difference is specifically addressed by the results of the CARDIA study *(16)*, in which subjects ($N =$ 3157) aged 18–30 yr were followed for 10 yr. Increased dairy intake in overweight individuals was associated with reduced risk of developing obesity, with a nonsignificant association in nonobese individuals. The reduction in odds ratio of the highest dairy intake category ($\geq$35 times per week) was 70% compared with the lowest dairy intake category ($\leq$10 times per week)

Several other prospective studies also support the relationship between weight and body composition. Prospective analysis of women by Lin et al. *(5)* shows that calcium, adjusted for energy intake, negatively predicted a 2-yr change in body weight and body fat mass in normal-weight young women (aged 18–30 yr). Two observational studies in women with bone as the primary outcome were combined and the dietary calcium/protein ratio negatively predicted weight change ($N = 216$, ages 35–58 yr) *(8)*. Contrary to other prospective studies, milk intake was associated with increased obesity in 24,604 men and women aged 25–64 yr studied over a 15-yr period; however, correction for total energy intake was not used in these analyses *(17)*. Although most of the prospective studies suggest an association between milk intake, particularly when energy consumption is considered, the independent effect of calcium vs dairy products cannot be ascertained in these study designs.

Clearly, the only way to determine a specific effect of calcium on body composition is by intervention studies utilizing calcium supplements. Far fewer intervention studies designed to investigate dietary calcium's effect on body mass are currently available. Barr *(18)* reviewed the literature of randomized calcium ($N = 17$ trials) or dairy product ($N = 9$ trials) intervention. The endpoint of these trials was primarily bone status, and the cohorts were of mixed ages and primarily women were included in the trials. Of the dairy trials, either no difference in weight ($n = 7$) or an increase in weight ($n = 2$) was noted, but compensation for individual energy intake was not controlled because body mass was not the primary endpoint. In a randomized, controlled dairy trial that specifically analyzed energy intakes, healthy men and women (aged 55–85 yr, $N = 204$), in which one group was advised to increase milk intake from low fat sources by 3 c/d or maintain usual diet for 12 wk *(19)*, the milk intake group gained more than the control group. However, the gain was less than predicted, suggesting dietary or metabolic compensation for the increased intake of dairy.

2.2. Intervention Studies

Of the 17 calcium intervention studies reviewed by Barr *(18)*, only one showed greater weight loss in the calcium supplemented group compared with the controls *(20)*. When authors reported energy intakes, they were not different between groups, but none of these analyses was corrected for individual energy intakes. In three trials of 3- to 4-yr duration in postmenopausal *(21,22)* or perimenopausal women *(23)*, no difference in weight changes were noted in the calcium supplement compared with placebo control groups. The best evidence to date to support an independent effect of calcium intake on prevention of body fat mass accumulation is a randomized, placebo-controlled trial in women (aged 59–89 yr), again with bone as the primary endpoint *(24)*. The intervention of 1500 mg calcium per day was maintained for a mean of 3.89 yr duration ($n = 52$). The placebo-control group gained significantly more body fat mass than the calcium supplemented group. It should be noted that the difference in the two groups was approx 5–6% body fat at the end of the 3-yr period. This demonstrates a small, but significant effect, and small effects over the years can have a substantial impact on obesity. In addition, this small effect represents a 1 or 2% difference in 1 yr; thus, the length of this trial may have enhanced the ability to measure these small changes. Trials of shorter duration or small numbers may not have sufficient power to detect small changes in body fat that dietary calcium may elicit.

Another study demonstrates that a 1-yr, dairy product, randomized, controlled intervention trial specifically designed to test changes in body fat mass showed no significant impact in healthy young (aged 18–30 yr) normal-weight women *(25)*. In this trial, participants substituted dairy products for other elements of their diets to maintain isocaloric intakes. The women in this randomized, controlled trial were younger and more active, and the trial was of shorter duration (1 yr), compared with the prospective analysis of Lin et al. *(5)* from the same laboratory where an effect of calcium intake was seen. In general, the women with low calcium intakes in the prospective study gained weight, whereas the controls in the randomized, controlled study did not, consistent with the differences in the cohorts. Thus, other factors that play a role in body weight maintenance, including age and physical activity, must be considered when expecting responses to dietary intakes of calcium or dairy products.

3. WEIGHT LOSS

Weight loss represents a period of changing energy balance during which calcium intake may have a greater impact, thus making it easier to assess differences in a short period of time. Elemental calcium intake increased weight loss by 26% in individuals during a 500-kcal deficit, intentional 24-wk weight-loss diet ($N = 32$) compared with the low calcium-intake group, with an even greater enhancement of 70% increased weight loss with dairy products incorporated into the diet *(26)*. In contrast, the results of a similar study design did not show an improved weight loss with calcium supplements in postmenopausal women *(26a)*. Dairy products were not tested in this study. In another 16-wk, randomized, controlled intentional weight-loss study, participants who consumed an isoenergetic milk-only diet lost significantly more weight (11.2 ± 5.2 kg) compared with the conventional diet (2.6 ± 4.1 kg) *(27)*. Furthermore, overweight and obese women aged 25–45 yr participated in a 6-mo behavioral modification weight-loss trial with self-selected intakes of calcium. As might be expected, calcium intakes decreased during the intervention from 833 ± 303 to 681 ± 207 mg/d. On average, those in the highest quartile of calcium intake during treatment had significantly greater weight loss. Overall, the studies on weight loss suggest that dairy intake enhances weight loss.

The results of a multi-site trial strongly support that dairy product, but not increased calcium intake, enhances weight loss *(28)*. The protocol for this trial was modeled on the trial by Zemel et al., as a 500-kcal deficit, intentional weight loss in overweight and obese individuals. Subjects were randomized into one of three groups: placebo control with low calcium intake, low dairy intake with supplemental calcium, or placebo and high dairy product intake incorporated into the diet. The multisite trial was 12 wk compared with the prior 24-wk trial, and the participants were significantly lower in weight, because the weight range acceptable for admission to the study ($\geq$25 BMI) was lower than the previous trial ($\geq$30 BMI). This multisite trial demonstrated that high dairy product intake in the diet enhanced fat mass loss twofold compared with both the placebo-controlled and calcium-supplemented group. These results suggest that if elemental calcium has an effect on weight loss, it may be small enough that a short trial or inclusion of overweight (compared to obese) may make the effect harder to detect than a trial confined to obese individuals.

4. CHILDREN

The incidence of obesity in children is growing at a rapid rate. According to results from the 1999–2000 NHANES, using measured heights and weights, approx 15% of children and adolescents aged 6–19 yr are overweight, a 4% increase from the overweight estimates obtained from NHANES-III (1988–1994) *(29)*. Thus, determining the relationship between calcium intakes and body composition changes in children is critical for the development of strategies to improve more than just bone status, and doing so may also potentially reduce the growing incidence of obesity in adults.

Several cross-sectional analyses suggest a relationship between higher dairy intakes and lower body weight or BMI in children. Cross-sectional analyses of 323 girls aged 9–14 yr showed that calcium or dairy product intake was a significant component, with energy intake in the model, of a regression model to predict iliac skinfold thickness and body weight *(30)*. Furthermore, a case-controlled study comparing obese (BMI $\geq$85th percentile [$n = 29$]) or controls (BMI $\leq$85th percentile [$n = 24$]) prepubertal Puerto Rican children (aged 7–10 yr) *(31)* showed lower dairy product intake was associated with the higher BMI levels ($R = -0.38$). Thus, the cross-sectional studies in children support a role for dairy calcium in reducing body fat mass or BMI.

Several prospective analyses have been completed that also suggest a relationship between calcium intake and body composition in children. Carruth et al. *(32)* determined food consumption in 53 white children between the ages of 24 and 60 mo, and measured body composition at the age of 70 mo. Multiple regression analysis showed that dietary calcium or dairy were negatively associated with body fat mass. A follow-up study showed that for these children, at approx 8 yr of age, calcium intake negatively predicted percent body fat mass *(33)*. In contrast, a longitudinal study employing 196 nonobese girls aged 8–12 until 4 yr postmenarche showed no relationship between BMI or percent body fat and measures of dairy food or calcium consumption *(34)*. The model contained many factors, including parental overweightness, that may confound the analyses. In summary, there is substantial epidemiological evidence that higher intakes of dairy product are associated with lower body weights or body fat mass in children. However, the design of the available studies does not allow the establishment of a cause-and-effect relationship. If there is an effect, the identity of the bioactive component(s) in dairy products that may affect (or enhance the impact of calcium on) body fat remains to be elucidated.

None of the intervention trials in children that employed elemental calcium has demonstrated a significant effect of calcium intake on body weight or body fat mass; however, no trials have been undertaken to specifically address the impact of calcium on body composition as the primary outcome. For example, randomized, controlled intervention of 1000 mg/d calcium in 3- to 5-yr-olds *(35)* did not show a significant effect on change in BMI or body composition. However, the initial intakes of calcium (1017 mg/d) may have been sufficient to obscure effects of further increases in calcium or dairy intake. On the other hand, several studies of dairy product intervention in female children showed that they did not gain more weight with the addition of the supplement, without controlling or attempting to manipulate the overall caloric intake. For example, Cadogan et al. *(36)* studied 82 white girls aged 12.2 ± 0.3 SD years who were supplemented with two servings of milk per day for 18 mo, and these results show a nonsignificant trend toward greater gain in weight and lean body mass, with a reduction in percent body fat mass. In addition, in a 12-mo dairy food intervention in 48 nonobese children with a mean age of 11 yr, there was no difference in weight or body fat between the controls and the dairy-supplemented participants *(37)*. All of the intervention studies to date have not included obese children, and thus, this population has not been examined. To definitively answer the question of the role of calcium in regulating body fat mass in children, where analyses are also confounded by issues related to growth, it is critical to undertake long-term studies specifically with body fat mass as the endpoint.

5. ANIMAL STUDIES

Whereas the human trials often show inconsistent results, studies in rodent models support a role of calcium specifically in preventing weight gain and enhancing body weight loss *(2–4,38)*. Although animal models are not completely representative of human models, studies in appropriate animal and cell models can provide insights and aid in designing studies in humans. Studies in genetically obese *agouti* mice, which have adipocyte-specific expression of the *agouti* gene product and are a model for diet-induced obesity, show a specific effect of calcium in preventing weight gain *(4)* and enhancing weight loss *(38)*. Consistent with the trials in humans, the effect is increased when dairy product is included in the diet. In addition, increased dietary calcium suppressed weight gain in several rat models, both lean and obese *(2,39)*. Thus, studies in animal models support the effect of dietary calcium, specifically, in negatively regulating body fat.

6. MECHANISMS OF BODY WEIGHT REGULATION

To decrease body weight, there must be a shift in the balance between available energy and energy utilization leading to a net energy deficit. Dietary calcium intake has been proposed to affect both components (Fig. 1). The proposed mechanisms for reducing energy availability include increasing satiety and decreasing the absorption of fatty acids through the formation of calcium soaps in the intestine.

On the other side of the energy equation, there is evidence to suggest that increased calcium intake is associated with an increase in energy utilization. To achieve an increase in energy utilization, several processes may be affected (Fig. 1), with several organs playing important roles. For example, in a fasting state, increased lipolysis from the adipocytes to release free fatty acids from their storage depot may provide substrate for increased lipid oxidation (Fig. 1). In the fasting or fed state, the activity of enzymes may be increased to facilitate increased lipid oxidation, with the most active tissues being the

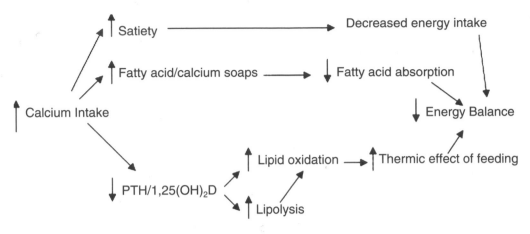

Fig. 1. Proposed mechanisms for calcium effects on energy balance.

muscle followed by the liver (Fig. 1). Increased glucose disposal may also contribute, though little evidence is available to support this mechanism in response to dietary calcium. In both cases, the increase in energy production must be accompanied with an increase in energy utilization. The mechanism(s) by which dietary calcium regulates energy utilization has not been determined, however, a hormonal control is being investigated. Increased dietary calcium is known to suppress levels of parathyroid hormone (PTH) and 1,25 dihydroxyvitamin D (1,25[OH]$_2$D), hormones that regulate calcium homeostasis. As described below, there is evidence that suppression of these hormones may contribute to decreased fatty acid synthesis, increased lipolysis in adipocytes, and increased fat oxidation.

6.1. Fatty Acid Soaps

One mechanism that potentially contributes to the effect of dietary calcium on body fat and which has received little attention is decreased energy absorption through formation of indigestible calcium-fatty acid soaps in the gastrointestinal tract. High concentrations of calcium can inhibit absorption of dietary fatty acids. For example, fecal fat was increased from 6 to 13% from a low (410 mg/d) to a high (2200 mg/d) diet in a randomized trial of 13 healthy men *(40)*. On the other hand, when calcium intake is doubled, the average ratio of fecal fat to calcium in adolescent children participating in a metabolic study is similar, 2.94 vs 2.34 g/g, although the range by individuals was great from 0.74 to 3.83 *(41)*. Results in a rat model demonstrate that increased fecal calcium with higher intakes of calcium accounted for the differences in weight gain noted in the animals *(39)*. Clearly, calcium soaps do form; however, the impact of the increase with high calcium intakes on changes in weight is unsettled.

6.2. Satiety

Another mechanism that has been proposed to regulate available energy is satiety. At this time, little evidence is available to support or refute the impact of calcium or dairy product intake on satiety and, ultimately, the role of calcium- or dairy-mediated satiety on changes in body composition. Barr et al. *(19)* found that elderly people compensated well for the energy contained in three daily servings of milk by reducing food intake from other sources. The satiety value of yogurt and cheese has been determined empirically to be higher than many similar foods *(42)*. However, Almiron-Roig, et al. demonstrated that intake of milk was not associated with compensation for the energy contained in milk consumed *(43)*.

The response of specific regulators of satiety to dietary calcium can also provide insights that can be applied to the overall response in humans. For example, cholecysto-kinin (CCK) mediates meal termination and possibly early phase satiety through its effects on gastric emptying *(44)*. Intake of meals containing dairy products increased CCK levels more than non-dairy product meals, however, the non-dairy product meals were more satiating than the dairy product meals in a randomized crossover design in 24 young adults *(45)*. Thus, satiety may play a role particularly by dairy products, but this issue remains unsettled and the role of calcium on satiety is still to be fully explored.

7. CALCIUM INTAKE AND ENERGY UTILIZATION

7.1. Lipid Oxidation

Energy utilization is a sum of resting metabolism, thermic effect of a meal, and activity. It has been proposed that calcium or dairy product intake influence each of these factors. A cross-sectional study by Melanson, et al. showed that higher self-selected acute intakes of calcium, corrected for calorie intake, are associated with increased whole-body lipid oxidation throughout a 24-h period ($N = 35$) *(46)*. Total calcium intake was a stronger predictor of 24-h fat oxidation than dairy calcium intake. Habitual (but not acute) calcium intake, as assessed by 4-d food records, was not associated with lipid oxidation. In addition, in a 1-yr randomized dairy calcium dietary intervention trial in young women (aged 18–20 yr, $N = 19$), lipid oxidation as assessed by indirect calorimetry was increased in the intervention group compared with the low dairy intake group following a meal challenge *(47)*. These results, in contrast with those of Melanson et al. *(46)*, suggest a long-term effect of habitual higher dairy product intakes. A similar mechanism was studied in 15 healthy, overweight premenopausal women (BMI 25–32) on a 1500 mg/d supplement for 3 mo. In this small sample and uncontrolled study, there were no changes in lipolysis or fat oxidation over the 3-mo period *(48)*. Thus, there is evidence in clinical trials that increased dairy intakes elevate overall body lipid oxidation. However, these study designs, either cross-sectional using self-selected intakes *(46)* or dairy product intervention *(47)*, do not allow assessment of calcium-specific effects on lipid oxidation.

7.2. Hormonal Regulation

The mechanism most often cited to explain a specific effect of dietary calcium on energy utilization is the ability of calcium to regulate, at least acutely, levels of the hormones PTH and $1,25(OH)_2D$. With low dietary calcium intakes, serum calcium is reduced. This reduction is sensed by a calcium receptor on the parathyroid gland, stimulating the release of PTH. PTH acts to activate the renal 1α-hydroxylase, which converts 25 hydroxyvitamin D (25[OH]D) to the active metabolite, $1,25(OH)_2D$. PTH and $1,25(OH)_2D$ coordinately act on the intestine, kidneys, and bone to increase the levels of serum calcium (*see* Chapter 10).

In addition to these classical functions of PTH and $1,25(OH)_2D$ in maintaining serum calcium homeostasis, a variety of other functions have been credited to these hormones. For example, increased levels of fasting PTH are hypothesized to influence increased levels of body fat mass (49). Fasting serum PTH levels positively correlate with body fat mass at baseline ($n = 155$) and change in serum PTH predicted the change in body fat mass over 1 yr in a cohort of normal-weight young women (50). Another link between serum PTH levels and body composition is shown in a study of 302 adults of mixed race, both obese and nonobese, in which PTH positively correlated with BMI and body fat mass (51). In contrast, serum $25(OH)D$ and $1,25(OH)_2D$ were negatively correlated with BMI and body fat mass, and serum $1,25(OH)_2D$ was lower in the obese than in nonobese subjects. These results indicate that there is substantial evidence, albeit associative, that fasting serum PTH levels correlate with increased body weight and body fat. However, the limited data reported suggest that $1,25(OH)_2D$ and $25(OH)D$ may have the opposite effect on body fat. If PTH is the primary mediator of changes in body fat this may be due to the impact of $25(OH)D$ in suppressing serum PTH levels (Fig. 1) (52).

More direct evidence linking dietary calcium and hormonal regulation of body composition is provided in studies employing the *agouti* mouse model for diet-induced adult onset obesity (4,38). Increased dietary calcium intake in this model causes reduced fat mass accumulation with reduced activity and expression of fatty acid synthase, as well as increased lipolysis in fat tissue. $1,25(OH)_2D$ (4) and PTH (4,53) stimulated increased intracellular calcium in adipocytes; changes in intracellular calcium in turn regulate fatty acid synthase (4). Furthermore, $1,25(OH)_2D$ inhibits lipolysis in cultured human adipocytes (4). These results suggest that the regulation of these hormones by dietary calcium may play a role in the response at the level of the adipocyte following dietary intervention.

Although the adipocyte is the primary storage tissue for fat, it is important to determine the impact of the dietary calcium-regulated hormones on energy metabolism in the primary energy-consuming tissues, such as muscle. This is particularly true in light of evidence demonstrating a role of calcium in regulating lipid oxidation, because muscle and liver are the most highly oxidative tissues. Studies support a direct role for PTH in suppressing lipid oxidation in muscle. Smogorzewski et al. (54) demonstrated that lipid oxidation of muscle tissue is suppressed in chronic renal failure rats (which are hyperparathyroid) and in rats treated with PTH. Furthermore, the activity of carnitine palmitoyl tranferase-1, the mitochondrial transfer protein that is the rate-limiting step in mitochondrial β-oxidation, is reduced in the chronic renal failure and PTH-treated rats (54). These results suggest that PTH may be a mediator of regulation of lipid oxidation by dietary calcium, but do not eliminate a role for $1,25(OH)_2D$.

In contrast, vitamin D status and $1,25(OH)_2D$ may have opposing effects to PTH in regulating fat mass in humans. Both the biomarker of vitamin D status, $25(OH)D$ the active metabolite, and $1,25(OH)_2D$, negatively correlated with BMI and body fat mass in a study by Parikh (51). Furthermore, $1,25(OH)_2D$ levels are lower in obese than in nonobese (51). Finally, in the Quebec Family Study, vitamin D intake negatively correlated with BMI in both men and women when analyses were corrected for age. It is clear that a key regulator of fasting serum PTH levels is improvement of vitamin D status (52). Thus, it is intriguing to consider that the suppression of PTH levels by improved vitamin D status may also contribute to regulation of fat mass accumulation.

8. CONCLUSIONS

In summary, substantial data in humans support an association of dairy product intake on body fat mass. The relative roles of elemental calcium and dairy product intake in controlling body weight remain unclear. When the mechanisms underlying effects noted in epidemiological studies are explored, nutritionists traditionally investigate individual nutrient effects on biological functions. However, the overall impact of all the components of a food is important to consider. This is particularly important when discussing calcium, because in the United States, approx 70% of dietary calcium is obtained from dairy products. The data suggest that although calcium may play a role in reducing body weight and body fat, this effect may be enhanced by dairy products. It is not clear what component(s) of dairy enhance the effect of calcium, but they may include the protein source *(53)*.

On the other hand, limited data in humans and animal models demonstrate a specific impact, though potentially small, of dietary calcium on reducing body fat accumulation and enhancing weight loss. Overall balance between energy intake and utilization controls the level of body weight and body fat, and increased calcium intake may shift the balance. A small shift in the balance of energy, which might occur with increased dietary intakes of calcium, may substantially contribute to weight changes over the long term. Dietary calcium may mediate an increase in lipid oxidation and the situation (adiposity, weight loss, weight gain, physical activity) may determine if this alteration translates to changes in body composition.

The effect of dietary calcium (either elemental or from dairy) in reducing fat mass has been observed at the recommended levels of intake. However, calcium intakes in the United States are currently far below the recommended levels. Heaney utilized his study population to estimate the potential impact of doubling dietary calcium intake in this cohort *(54)*. If women in the 25th percentile of calcium intakes increased their intakes to recommended values, the fraction of young women who were overweight would decrease from 15 to 4%, and the rate of weight gain in women in midlife would change from +0.42 kg/yr to 0.01 kg/yr. Thus, although the impact of calcium or dairy intake may be small, over time an increase in dietary intake would predict a substantial change in overweight and obesity prevalence by as much as 60–80% *(54)*. Thus, it is critical to design intervention studies specifically to address the role of dietary calcium in modulating fat mass and to identify the mechanisms and the populations in which alterations in dietary calcium intake may lead to changes in fat mass, so that recommendations for reducing the incidence of obesity can be developed.

REFERENCES

1. National Institute of Health; Clinical guidelines on the identification, evaluation and treatment of overweight and obesity in adults: Executive Summary. National Heart, Lung, and Blood Institute; Obesity Education Initiative.
2. McCarron DA, Morris CD, Henry HJ, Stanton JL. Blood pressure and nutrient intake in the United States. Science 1984;224:1392–1398.
3. Metz JA, Karanja N, Torok J, McCarron DA. Modification of total body fat in spontaneously hypertensive rats and Wistar-Kyoto rats by dietary calcium and sodium. Am J Hypertens 1988;1:58–60.
4. Zemel MB, Shi H, Greer B, DiRienzo D, Zemel PC. Regulation of adiposity by dietary calcium. FASEB J 2000;14:1132–1138.

5. Lin, Y-C, Lyle R.M, McCabe LD, McCabe GP, Weaver CM, Teegarden D. Calcium intake effects on two year changes in body composition in young women. J Am Coll Nutr 2000;19:754–760.

6. Barger-Lux MJ, Heaney RP, Packard PT, Lappe JM, Recker RR. Nutritional correlates of low calcium intake. Clin Appl Nutr 1992;2:39–44.

7. Loos R, Rankinen T, Leon A, Rao DC, Skinner J, Wilmore J, Bouchard C. Calcium intake and body composition in the HERITAGE Family Study. Am J Clin Nutr 2003;76:A145.

8. Davies KM, Heaney RP, Recker RR, et al. Calcium intake and body weight. J Clin Endo Metab 2000;85:4635–4638.

9. Jacqmain M, Doucet E, Despres J-P, Bouchard C, Tremblay A. Calcium intake, body composition and lipoprotein-lipid concentrations in adults. Am J Clin Nutr 2003;77:1448–1452.

10. Kamycheva E, Joakimsen RM, Rolf J. Intakes of calcium and vitamin D predict body mass index in the population of Northern Norway. J Nutr 2002;132:102–106.

11. Buchowski MS, Semenya J, Johnson AO. Dietary calcium intake in lactose maldigesting intolerant and tolerant African-American women. J Am Coll Nutr 2002;21:47–54.

12. Lovejoy JC, Champagne CM, Smith SR, de Longe L, Xie H. Ethnic differences in dietary intakes, physical activity and energy expenditure in middle-aged, premenopausal women: the Healthy Transitions Study. Am J Clin Nutr 2001;74:90–95.

13. Barr S, Fulgoni V, Pereira MA. Relationship of calcium or dairy product intakes on percent body fat, BMI, and anthropometric measures in NHANES-III. FASEB J 2004;8:A873.

14. Parikh SJ and Yanovski JA. Calcium intake and adiposity. Am J Clin Nutr 2003;77: 281–287.

15. Parikh S, Denkinger B, Sebring N, et al. Calcium intake is negatively correlated to measures of adiposity in women but not in men. Am J Clin Nutr 2003;77:A276.

16. Pereira MA, Jacobs DR Jr., Van Horn L, Slattery ML, Kartashov AI, Ludwig DS. Dairy consumption, obesity and the insulin resistance syndrome in young adults: The CARDIA study. JAMA 2002; 287:2081–2089.

17. Lahti-Koski M, Pietinen, Heliovaara M, Vartiainen E. Associations of body mass index and obesity with physical activity, food choices, alcohol intake and smoking in the 1982–1997 FINRISK Studies. Am J Clin Nutr 2002;75:809–187.

18. Barr SI. Increased dairy product or calcium intake: is body weight or composition affected in humans? J Nutr 2003;133:245S–248S.

19. Barr SI, McCarron DA, Heaney RP, et al. Effects of increased consumption of fluid milk on energy and nutrient intake, body weight, and cardiovascular risk factors in healthy older adults. J Am Diet Assoc 2000;100:810–817.

20. Recker RR, Hinders S, Davies KM, et al. Correcting calcium nutritional deficiency prevents spine fractures in elderly women. J Bone Miner Res 1996;11:1961–1966.

21. Riggs BL, O'Fallon WM, Muhs J, O'Conner MK, Melton LJ III. Long-term effects of calcium supplementation on serum parathyroid level, bone turnover, and bone loss in elderly women. J Bone Miner Res 1998;13:168–174.

22. Dawson-Hughes B, Harris S, Krall EA, Dallal GE. Effect of calcium and vitamin D supplementation on bone density in men and women 65 years of age or older. N Engl J Med 1997;337:523–529.

23. Elders PJM, Lips P, Netelenbos JC, et al. Long-term effect of calcium supplementation on bone loss in perimenopausal women. J Bone Miner Res 1994;9:963–970.

24. Barger-Lux MJ, Davies KM, Heaney RP, Chin BK, Rafferty K. Calcium supplementation may attenuate accumulation of fat in young women. J Bone Min Res 2001;16:S219.

25. Gunther CW, Legowski PA, Lyle RM, et al. Dairy products do not lead to alterations in body weight and fat mass in young women in a one year intervention. Am J Clin Nutr 2005;81:751–756.

26. Zemel MB, Thompson W, Milstead A, Morris K, Campbell P. Calcium and dairy acceleration of weight and fat loss during energy restriction in obese adults. Obes Res 2004;12:582–590.

26a. Shapses SA, Heshka S, Heymsfield SB. Effect of calcium supplementation on weight and fat loss in women. J Clin Endocrinol Metab 2004;89:632–637.

27. Summerbell CD, Watts C, Higgins JPT, Garrow JS. Randomised controlled trial of novel, simple, and well supervised weight reducing diets in outpatients. BMJ 1998;317:1487–1489.

28. Zemel M, Teegarden D, Van Loan M, et al. Role of dairy products in modulating weight and fat loss: A multi-center trial. FASEB J 2004b;15:A845.

29. Center for Disease Control. http://www.cdc.gov/nccdphp/dnpa/obesity/. Accessed May 2005.
30. Novotny R, Daida YG, Acharya S, Grove JS, Vogt TM. Dairy intake is associated with lower body fat and soda intake with greater weight in adolescent girls. J Nutr 2004;134:1905–1909.
31. Tanasescu M, Ferris AM, Himmelgreen DA, Rodriguez N, Perez-Escamilla R. Biobehavioral factors are associated with obesity in Puerto Rican children. J Nutr 2000;130:1734–1742.
32. Carruth BR and Skinner JD. The role of dietary calcium and other nutrients in moderating body fat in preschool children. Int J Obesity 2001;25:559–566.
33. Skinner JD, Bounds W, Carruth BR, Ziegler P. Longitudinal calcium intake is negatively related to children's body fat indexes. J Am Diet Assoc 2003;103:1626–1631.
34. Phillips SM, Bandini LG, Cyr H, Colclough-Douglas S, Naumova E, Must A. Dairy food consumption and body weight and fatness studied longitudinally over the adolescent period. Int J Obes 2003;27:1106–1113.
35. Englert AD, Specker BL, Binkley TL, Kattelman K. Calcium intake does not influence change in % body fat in children. FASEB J 2004;18:A179.
36. Cadogan J, Eastell R, Jones N, Barker M. Milk intake and bone mineral acquisition in adolescent girls: randomized, controlled intervention trial. BMJ 1997;315:1255–1260.
37. Chan GM, Hoffman K, McMurry M. Effect of dairy products on one and body composition in pubertal girls. J Pediatr 1995;126:551–556.
38. Shi H, DiRienzo D, Zemel MB. Effects of dietary calcium on adipocyte lipid metabolism of body weight regulation in energy-restricted a P2-agouti transgenic mice. FASEB J 2001;15:291–293.
39. Papakonstantinou E, Flatt WP, Huth PJ, Harris RB. High dietary calcium reduces body fat content, digestibility of fat, and serum vitamin D in rats. Obes Res 2003;11:387–394.
40. Denke MA, Fox MM, Schulte MC. Short-term dietary calcium fortification increases fecal saturated fat content and reduces serum lipids in men. J Nutr 1993;123:1047–1053.
41. Lutwak L, Laster L, Gitelman HJ, Fox M., Whedon D. Effects of high dietary calcium and phosphorus on calcium, phosphorus, nitrogen and fat metabolism in children. Am J Clin Nutr 1964;14:76–82.
42. Holt SH, Miller JC, Petocz P, Farmakalidis E. A satiety index of common foods. Eur J Clin Nutr 1995;49:675–690.
43. Almiron-Roig E, Drewnowski A. Hunger, thirst, and energy intakes following consumption of caloric beverages. Physiol Behav 2003;79:767–773.
44. Scarpignato C, Varga G, Corradi C. Effect of CCK and its antagonists on gastric emptying. J Physiol Paris 1993;87:291–300.
45. Schneeman BO, Burton-Freeman B, Davis P. Incorporating dairy foods into low and high fat diets increases the postprandial cholecystokinin response in men and women. J Nutr 2003;133:4124–4128.
46. Melanson EL, Sharp TA, Schneider J, Donahoo WT, Grunwald GK, Hill JO. Relation between calcium intake and fat oxidation in adult humans. Int J Obes Relat Metab Disord 2003;27:196–203.
47. Gunther CW, Legowski PA, James JM, Lyle RM, Teegarden D. Lipid oxidation increases in women following 1 year dairy calcium intervention FASEB J 2002;LBA:58.
48. Sampath V, King JC, Christiansen M, Havel PJ. Effects of calcium (Ca) supplementation on lipid metabolism in overweight women. FASEB J 2003;17:A1088.
49. McCarty MF, Thomas CA. PTH excess may promote weight gain by impeding catecholamine-induced lipolysis—implications for the impact of calcium, vitamin D, and alcohol on body weight. Med Hypotheses 2003;61:535–542.
50. Gunther CW, Lyle RM, Teegarden D. One year change in log parathyroid hormone negatively predicts one year change in postprandial lipid oxidation in young women on dairy calcium intervention. FASEB J 2004;18:A924.
51. Parikh SJ, Edelman M, Uwaifo GI, et al. The relationship between obesity and serum 1,25-dihydroxy vitamin D concentrations in healthy adults. J Clin Endocrinol Metab 2004;89:1196–1199.
52. Dawson-Hughes B, Dallal GE, Krall EA, Harris S, Sokoll LJ, Falconer G. Effect of vitamin D supplementation on wintertime and overall bone loss in healthy postmenopausal women. Ann Int Med 1991;115:505–512.
53. Layman DK. The role of leucine in weight loss diets and glucose homeostasis. J Nutr 2003;133:261S–267S.
54. Heaney RP. Normalizing calcium intake: projected population effects for body weight. J Nutr 2003;133:268S–270S.

22 Polycystic Ovary Syndrome and Reproduction

Susan Thys-Jacobs

KEY POINTS

- Polycystic ovary syndrome (PCOS) is an extremely common disorder characterized by chronic anovulation, hyperandrogenism, and follicular arrest.
- Calcium is an important primary intracellular signal in invertebrates, amphibians, and mammals, involved in the maturation and differentiation of the oocyte and the initiation of the development of the egg at fertilization and in egg activation.
- Calcium and vitamin D dysregulation may ultimately be responsible for the arrested follicular development and menstrual disturbances associated with PCOS.

1. INTRODUCTION

In 1921, Achard and Thiers published their classic description of a bearded woman with diabetes, linking androgen excess and insulin resistance *(1)*. Subsequently, in 1935, Stein and Leventhal reported the association of enlarged polycystic ovaries with the clinical triad of amenorrhea, hirsutism, and obesity *(2)*. Polycystic ovary syndrome (PCOS), or Stein–Leventhal syndrome has since been recognized to be one of the most common female endocrine disorders characterized by two major features: hyperandrogenism and chronic anovulation *(3)*. PCOS has been associated with an increased incidence of endometrial cancer and has many serious consequences, such as insulin resistance, diabetes mellitus, and increased cardiovascular and metabolic risks. PCOS affects approx 5–10% of women of reproductive age and is a major cause of infertility.

Interestingly, despite its prevalence among young women, PCOS is virtually unknown in the animal kingdom, although the importance of calcium in follicular development has been extensively investigated over the past 30 yr in many animal studies. Calcium appears to be an essential primary signal and universal messenger in egg activation *(4)*. It has a critical role in the regulation and resumption of meiosis and in mitosis as well as in the maturation of mammalian and nonmammalian oocytes. Recent preliminary evidence similarly suggests that in humans, abnormalities in calcium homeostasis and vitamin D metabolism may underlie the pathogenesis of PCOS. Disordered calcium regulation may

From: *Calcium in Human Health*
Edited by: C. M. Weaver and R. P. Heaney © Humana Press Inc., Totowa, NJ

Table 1
Criteria for the Clinical Diagnosis of Polycystic Ovarian Syndrome

- Chronic anovulation
  – irregular menses, oligomenorrhea, amenorrhea
- Hyperandrogenism
  – acne, hirsutism, alopecia, infertility
- Exclusion of other androgen disorders
- Ultrasonographic evidence of polycystic ovaries may or may not be present

be responsible for the arrested follicular development and immature oocytes, predisposing susceptible women to the reproductive and menstrual disturbances that have been identified as PCOS.

2. DIAGNOSIS AND DEFINITION

The diagnosis of PCOS is usually made on the basis of clinical and biochemical criteria. In 1990, a National Institutes of Health consensus panel proposed chronic anovulation or menstrual irregularity with evidence of either clinical or biochemical hyperandrogenism as minimal criteria for diagnosis (Table 1) (5). Other causes of androgen excess must be excluded before a diagnosis is made. The typical woman with PCOS commonly presents with oligomenorrhea dating from menarche and complaints of progressive hirsutism, obesity, infertility, and inability to lose weight. The cardinal features of androgen excess may include acne, temporal balding, acanthosis nigricans, and hirsutism. Hirsutism is characterized by increased numbers of terminal hairs in certain areas such as the chin, upper lip, neck, or upper back, where terminal hairs are not normally found. Often, there is a strong family history of PCOS or menstrual irregularity. The chronic anovulation is usually reported as amenorrhea or irregular menstrual cycles with cycles more than 35–40 d in length (approximately eight or fewer menstrual cycles a year). Some women do have regular cycles and not all women are obese, with approx 30% of women being lean. An abnormally elevated androgen level is not necessary to confirm the diagnosis, although an elevated free testosterone is a very common finding. Alternative causes of menstrual dysfunction and hyperandrogenism must be excluded before a diagnosis of PCOS is confirmed. This requires an evaluation for thyroid disease, late-onset adrenal hyperplasia, hyperprolactinemia, Cushing's syndrome, and androgen-secreting tumors. Late-onset adrenal hyperplasia owing to 21 hydroxylase deficiency can be screened for with the measurement of a serum 17 hydroxyprogesterone (17OHP) level. Concentrations of serum 17OHP less than 250 ng/dL are considered normal; above this, an adrenocorticotropic hormone stimulation should be performed for possible confirmation of late-onset adrenal hyperplasia. Total testosterone concentrations are occasionally elevated and usually less than 100 ng/dL, whereas free testosterone concentrations are more frequently elevated. An elevated serum total testosterone concentration greater than 200 ng/dL suggests an androgen-secreting tumor and warrants further investigation. The ratio of luteinizing hormone (LH) to follicle stimulating hormone (FSH) may be abnormally elevated, at levels of 2.5–3.0. Although multiple ovarian cysts as imaged with pelvic ultrasound are helpful and noted in more than 50% of women with PCOS, many with PCOS do not demonstrate this feature. Abnormal ovarian morphology alone does not establish the diagnosis, because 25% of normal women have cysts on their ovaries, and the absence of polycystic ovaries does not exclude the diagnosis.

3. ETIOLOGY

The precise pathophysiological mechanisms resulting in the endocrinological disturbances of PCOS are not known. The most widely accepted theory proposes that PCOS is a self-perpetuating cycle of hormonal events with increased intra-ovarian concentrations of androgens resulting in polycystic ovaries, theca cell hyperplasia, and arrested follicular cell development *(6,7)*. A number of biochemical endocrine abnormalities have been identified, including a chronically elevated LH with an elevated LH to FSH ratio, elevated serum androgens that may include androstenedione, dehydroepiandrosterone sulfate, and total/free testosterone concentrations, increased estrone and normal estradiol concentrations, and, most recently identified, hyperinsulinemia *(8)*. The serum free testosterone concentration appears to be the best single marker of hyperandrogenism. A number of women with PCOS (both lean and overweight) have insulin resistance and hyperinsulinemia. Insulin enhances ovarian steroidogenesis, stimulating estrogen, testosterone, and progesterone secretion *(9)*. Insulin may also enhance the release of LH and may affect follicular maturation. Many of the late complications of PCOS appear to be related to insulin resistance *(10)*. It has been proposed by some that hyperinsulinemia is the primary event in the pathogenesis of PCOS and causes the hyperandrogenism *(11)*, whereas others support the theory that hyperandrogenism is the primary defect initiating menstrual dysfunction and hyperinsulinemia *(12)*. Whether hyperandrogenism or insulin resistance are primary or secondary events in the etiology of PCOS remains a controversial and unsettled issue.

Evidence now suggests that abnormalities in calcium regulation may comprehensibly explain the clinical presentation of PCOS, including the reproductive abnormalities and insulin resistance. This evidence is supported by several facts: (1) the importance of calcium in egg activation and in triggering meiotic resumption, (2) the role of calcium in LH-induced meiotic maturation, (3) the role of calcium and vitamin D in insulin resistance, and (4) the clinical evidence of abnormalities in calcium homeostasis in reproductive disturbances and in women with PCOS.

4. CALCIUM AND OOCYTE MATURATION: ANIMAL INVESTIGATIONS

The development of the female mammalian oocyte begins early in fetal life. Mitosis determines the finite number of gametes; whereas oocyte maturation is dependent on the progressive stages of meiosis affected by various growth factors and steroid hormones. At birth, the mammalian oocyte is arrested in its meiotic maturation at prophase of meiosis I, released from meiotic arrest by the preovulatory LH surge, only to be arrested again at metaphase II, awaiting fertilization and meiosis completion. In many species, progression from one meiotic or mitotic phase to the next appears to be determined by intracellular calcium changes or transients *(13)*. In mammals, resumption of meiosis and maturation of the oocyte, as well as fertilization, appear to require a series of intracellular calcium changes.

4.1. Calcium in Egg Activation and Fertilization

In fertilization, a rise in intracellular calcium ions is believed to be the primary signal responsible for the initiation of egg development (*see also* Chapter 3). This is widely supported by the observations in many species demonstrating increases in intracellular calcium at fertilization and conversely demonstrating that inhibition of the rise in intracellular calcium prevented calcium oscillations and blocked both resumption of meiosis and progression in cell development. In 1974, Steinhardt and colleagues activated sea urchin eggs parthenogenetically using a divalent calcium-transporting ionophore A23187 *(14)*. Membrane conductance measurements, respiration, and DNA synthesis, all normally activated by sperm, were similarly noted to be activated by the divalent ionophore. Steinhardt proposed that the ionophore acted by mediating calcium fluxes and releasing intracellular calcium ions, and that calcium may have a universal role in egg activation *(15)*. Since then, the importance of calcium in the regulation of both meiotic and mitotic cell division cycles in mammalian and nonmammalian oocytes has been of considerable interest *(4)*. Eggs of the medaka fish were found to be naturally activated by a huge pulse of free cytosolic calcium and the calcium from the pulses emanated from the internal stores of endoplasmic reticulum. Similarly, sea urchin eggs, when activated, were noted to be accompanied by a calcium "explosion" *(16)*. In amphibian and nonmammalian eggs, the main initial source of egg activation is a propagated wave or pulse of calcium ions in the cytosol (*see* Chapter 3). Collas and colleagues electrically induced activation of mammalian bovine oocytes in the parthenogenetic development of these oocytes and demonstrated elevations in intracellular calcium concentrations as measured by fluorescence *(17)*. They noted that the intracellular calcium response to a given electrical stimulus was variable and regulated by incubation conditions, pulse duration, and electrical field strength. The presence of extracellular calcium was required to obtain high rates of activation and development of these mammalian oocytes. In mouse oocytes, sperm elicit a large transient increase in intracellular calcium lasting approx 2 min, followed by repetitive calcium transients lasting half a second. Incubation of denuded mouse oocytes with the calcium chelator 1,2 *bis* O-aminophenoxyethane-*N,N,N′,N′*-tetraacetic acid (BAPTA) inhibited all calcium transients (*see* Fig. 1) *(18)*. Calcium oscillations during fertilization in the activation of both nonmammalian and mammalian oocytes have been widely studied and appear to be firmly established. Changes in intracellular calcium have been demonstrated to occur at fertilization in mouse and hamster ooytes. Artificially increasing intracellular calcium activates the progression of meiosis and the cell cycle.

Artificial activation of many different mammalian oocytes such as mouse, rabbit, and bovine oocytes has been stimulated with calcium ionophores, ethanol, and electrical stimulation. Even pricking or mechanical stimulation can activate the immature oocyte to progress from a semiquiescent state and mimic the events characterized by penetration of sperm, provided adequate calcium ions are present in the medium *(19)*. The extent of parthenogenesis in mammalian oocytes, unlike the nonmammalian oocytes, appears to be influenced by extracellular calcium, because the intracellular calcium concentration and pulse-induced calcium rise are both modulated by extracellular calcium *(20)*. Mammalian eggs are primarily activated by calcium ions, which enter the cytoplasm extracellularly, and inhibited by calcium chelators or by changes in calcium concentrations.

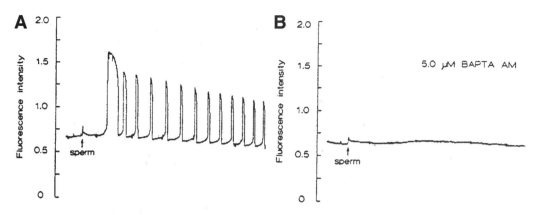

Fig. 1. Intracellular calcium changes following fertilization were suppressed or inhibited by introduction of 1,2 *bis* O-aminophenoxyethane-*N*,*N*,*N'*,*N'*-tetraacetic acid (BAPTA) into the eggs before in vitro fertilization. Eggs were loaded with fluo-3 or fluo-3 and BAPTA, washed, and inseminated. Recordings of fluo-3 fluorescence were made from single eggs with a photon counting photomultiplier tube. Ca^{2+} does not rise uniformly in the egg, but spreads uniformly as a wave of increased Ca^{2+}. (Reproduced from ref. *18*, with permission.)

4.2. Calcium and Meiosis

In mammals, maturation of the immature oocyte and the activation and fertilization of the mature egg are two separate events. Both may be regulated by changes in intracellular calcium. In general, mammalian oocytes are in a state of physiological arrest at the first prophase of the first meiotic division. This arrest is maintained by elevated intracellular levels of cyclic adenosine monophosphate (cAMP) and reversed by the LH surge *(21)*. Isolated naked oocytes in vitro, in the absence of their enclosed coat (cumulus oophorus), spontaneosly undergo germinal vesicle breakdown (GVB; the first step of meiotic resumption), nuclear maturation, and complete meiosis independent of hormonal stimulation. In other words, the oocyte is ready and programmed to progress to maturation except in the presence of its natural, physiological inhibitor, cAMP.

In 1981, Rosenberg and colleagues studied the roles of the divalent cations, calcium and magnesium, in starfish oocyte maturation. Both cations appeared to control maturation, with extracellular calcium important for GVB represents dissolution of the nuclear membrane which is one of the markers of oocyte maturation *(22)*. The normal oocyte is impeded from progressing to maturation by an inhibitor in the form of cAMP. Antagonizing the inhibitor with changes in calcium concentration can affect resumption of meiosis. Elevated levels of intracellular calcium within mouse and cow oocytes allow resumption of meiosis to occur despite high levels of cAMP. Increasing calcium concentration or the use of calcium ionophores partially relieves the cAMP meiotic arrest, whereas the calcium channel blockers, verapamil and tetracaine have been shown to potentiate meiotic arrest *(23)*. Hamster oocytes exposed to increasing external calcium concentrations demonstrated a greater rate of meiotic resumption. Denuding the hamster or mouse oocyte of its follicular shell—cumulus oophorus, with its inhibitory cAMP concentration—significantly increased GVB and meiotic resumption, whereas exposure to a calcium chelator, such as ethyleneglycol tetraacetic acid (EGTA), or to an agent that increases the concentration of cAMP, maintains meiotic arrest of the mammalian oocyte. Inhibition of meiotic resumption in mouse and hamster oocytes by increasing intracellular cAMP or by reducing calcium concentrations can be overridden with high extracellular calcium concentrations or with the use of calcium ionophores *(24)*.

Kaufman and colleagues studied the role of calcium in the resumption and progression of meiosis in the pig oocyte *(25)*. Denuded pig oocytes were exposed to various media in the presence of inhibitors, calcium chelators, and calcium-deficient cultures. Intracellular calcium was involved in the initial signaling of resumption of meiosis despite a calcium-deficient medium; however, progression of meiosis to metaphase II in the pig was dependent on extracellular calcium fluxes and suppressed by reducing the levels of calcium in the culture medium. Intracellular calcium chelation with BAPTA (a derivative of EGTA) or with neomycin (an inhibitor of phosphoinositide turnover and an indirect inhibitor of intracellular calcium mobilization) inhibited resumption of meiosis and GVB. Similarly, in mouse oocytes, an increase of intracellular calcium was suggested as essential for spontaneous meiotic resumption by De Felici and colleagues *(26)*. However, their findings differed somewhat from many other investigators in that they demonstrated that extracellular calcium was not required for meiotic resumption in the mouse, although incubation of mouse oocytes with a high-affinity calcium chelator prevented calcium changes, thereby inhibiting total GVB and oocyte maturation.

Moreau and colleagues investigated the intracellular calcium surges associated with hormone-induced maturation of amphibian oocytes using photoproteins and calcium-sensitive electrodes *(27)*. A dramatic surge in free serum calcium concentration was demonstrated following progesterone or agonist-induced stimulation (*see* Fig. 2). This calcium transient or surge was deemed necessary for meiosis reinitiation because incompletely grown or inhibitor-induced oocytes, which did not undergo meiosis, failed to produce the calcium transient. Carroll and Swann studied immature mouse oocytes during oocyte maturation and also noted spontaneous calcium oscillations caused by inositol triphosphate turnover following release of the oocytes from their inhibitory follicle. Their evidence suggested indirectly that intracellular free calcium was involved in the resumption of meiosis and progression to metaphase II *(28)*. In 1990, Peres *(29)* investigated intracellular calcium mobilization and oscillations in mouse oocytes. Intracellular cytosolic calcium changes were detected by electrophysiological and fluorimetric techniques using fluorescent proteins. Separate microinjections of both inositol-1,4,5 triphosphate as well as calcium into mouse oocytes induced calcium oscillations, suggesting a regenerative mechanism for calcium release. In 1998, Pesty and colleagues observed spontaneous calcium oscillations both within the nucleus as well as in cytoplasm in immature mouse oocytes upon reinitiation of the meiosis resumption process. Using laser scanning microscopy, the effects of microinjection into the nucleus of mouse oocytes of inositol 1,4,5 triphosphate, heparin (an inositol triphosphate receptor binder) and a monoclonal antibody to inositol triphosphate receptor were investigated. Inositol triphosphate directly injected into the germinal vesicle induced calcium oscillations first within the nucleus, whereas heparin, which blocked the inositol triphosphate receptor, inhibited both nuclear and cytoplasmic spontaneous oscillations. Injection of the monoclonal antibody to inositol triphosphate inhibited calcium oscillations and meiotic resumption. Mounting evidence further established that resumption of meiosis was dependent on the oocyte's ability to generate calcium oscillations and required an increase in phosphoinositide-dependent calcium *(30)*.

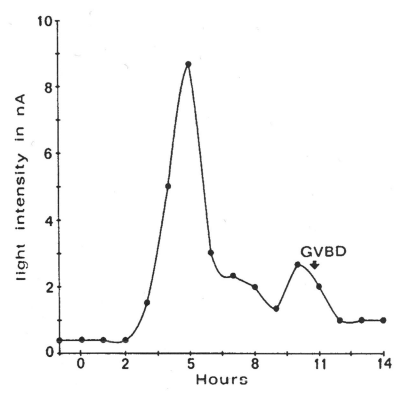

Fig. 2. Progesterone-induced calcium transient as recorded in 20 Ambystoma oocytes injected with aequorin and suspended in CaMg- free OR2 medium. GVBD refers to germinal vesicle breakdown. (Reproduced from ref. *27*, with permission.)

Mammalian oocytes, during activation at both fertilization and meiotic resumption, generate repetitive calcium oscillations. Extracellular stimulation of the oocyte with calcium, gonadotropins, and various growth factors results in changes in intracellular calcium concentrations via transmembrane movements between cytosol and internal organelles, representing an important physiological signaling mechanism. Repetitive calcium oscillations are probably mediated by inositol triphosphates while inhibited by cAMP. Hormones such as LH can stimulate the hydrolysis of phosphoinositides with subsequent accumulation of inositol triphosphates, which are potent calcium mobilizers. In 1987, Dimino studied the effect of LH, FSH, cAMP, and gonadotropin-releasing hormone on porcine ovarian granulosa. Only LH stimulated accumulation of inositol phosphates *(31)*. Calcium homeostasis in the setting of various hormones and growth factors determines the ultimate biochemical pathway selected in the phosphoinositide or adenylate cyclase-dependent protein kinase C systems of reproduction and oocyte maturation.

4.3. Calcium and LH Induction

Chronic LH elevations with abnormal LH to FSH ratios have been well described in women with PCOS and have been proposed as one of the many mechanisms for the menstrual dysfunction. In mammals, the physiological signal for resumption of meiosis I of the immature oocyte (arrested at prophase I until ovulation) is the LH surge. The LH surge causes GVB, condensation of chromatin, completion of meiosis I, and arrest at metaphase of meiosis II. In PCOS, chronic, tonic elevations of LH have been associated with follicular arrest and inhibition of resumption of meiosis, whereas the pulsatile LH surge overrides the inhibitory arrest. LH has been found to stimulate two messenger pathways, one activating adenylate cyclase and resulting in an increase in cAMP, and the other stimulating the phosphoinositide pathway. Increasing cAMP maintains oocyte meiotic arrest, whereas activation and hydrolysis of the phosphinositides via phospholipase C yields inositol phosphates, which mobilize intracellular calcium. In 1986, Davis examined the stimulatory effect of LH in rat granulosa cells in the presence or absence of the monovalent cation lithium (a substitute for physiological calcium). LH increased both cAMP and ionositol triphosphates in the rat cells. In the presence of the monovalent lithium, LH appeared to prevent phosphoinositide turnover with recycling of inositol phosphates, and to increase the accumulation of inositol phosphates by inhibiting their degradation by the phosphatases *(32)*. LH appeared to have a dual role, in both maintaining and reversing meiotic arrest. Calcium has been proposed as the regulatory factor that determines which pathway or system dominates, and which is stimulated by LH. In 1984, Dorflinger and colleagues evaluated the role of extracellular calcium and the calcium ionophore A23187 on LH adenylate cyclase activity in rats *(33)*. Their results demonstrated that an increase in intracellular calcium concentration resulted in inhibition of LH-sensitive adenylate cyclase. A decrease in extracellular calcium in the medium led to an increased production of cAMP by LH. A calcium-free medium induced by the calcium chelator EGTA enhanced cAMP accumulation. The calcium ionophore A23187 inhibited the LH-stimulated production of cAMP in a dose-dependent manner. A decrease in extracellular calcium to less than a minimal amount (100 μM) completely blocked the effect of the ionophore. Removal of extracellular calcium increased cAMP accumulation in response to LH twofold. Extracellular calcium may be the ultimate mediator in the inhibition or stimulation of the different messenger pathways.

4.4. Calcium and Vitamin D in Insulin Resistance

Disturbances in the vitamin D, calcium, and parathyroid axis have been proposed as well in the pathogenesis of insulin resistance. Gunal and colleagues examined the effect of intravenous 1α hydroxyvitamin D_3 on insulin sensitivity in 14 patients on chronic hemodialysis *(34)*. Uremic patients with secondary hyperparathyroidism generally develop insulin resistance and hyperinsulinemia. Administration of intravenous 1α hydroxyvitamin D_3 improved insulin sensitivity by reducing the hyperparathyroidism. In another study, the effect of oral calcium therapy on insulin resistance was investigated in non-diabetic patients with essential hypertension *(35)*. In a similar fashion, the effect of 1,25 dihydroxyvitamin D (1,25[OH]$_2$D) was studied in hemodialysis patients and compared with healthy controls *(36)*. A glucose clamp was used to investigate insulin sensitivity. Treatment of the hemodialysis patients with 1,25(OH)$_2$D significantly reduced arterial pressure and improved insulin sensitivity. Oral calcium therapy at 1500 mg/d for 8 wk was found to significantly reduce intraplatelet-free calcium concentrations and fasting plasma insulin levels, and increase the insulin sensitivity index, whereas those patients maintained on a low calcium intake had no change in insulin levels or insulin sensitivity. For a more extensive and in-depth review on calcium and insulin resistance, *see* Chapter 26.

5. REPRODUCTION AND PCOS

Vitamin D has also been shown to be important in female reproduction, specifically in rats, mice, and chickens. In 1989, Halloran reviewed the role of the biologically active form of vitamin D—1,25(OH)$_2$D—in reproduction *(37)*. In the avian species, 1,25(OH)$_2$D was required for ovulation and shell formation, transfer of calcium from the egg shell to the fetal circulation, and maintenance of fetal serum calcium. In mammals, 1,25(OH)$_2$D was required for normal ovulation, normal fetal bone metabolism, milk production, and normal calcium and bone homeostasis. Vitamin D deficiency affected mating success, fertility, and litter size and increased pregnancy complications *(38)*. Vitamin D deficiency in female rats resulted in an overall reduction in fertility of 75%; whereas vitamin D administration improved mating and litter success *(39)*.

More recently, calcium has been identified as an important mineral and nutrient in fertility. Vitamin D receptor (VDR) knockout mice have low serum calcium concentrations (hypocalcemic) and are infertile. Whether the infertility in these mice resulted from the vitamin D deficiency or from an indirect effect of the hypocalcemia was not clear. Johnson and DeLuca investigated the fertility in VDR-null mutant mice on varying calcium diets *(40)*. VDR-null mutant mice were mostly infertile (14% fertility) when provided a nonpurified, -alcium diet; whereas wild-type mice fed the same diet were 100% fertile. In VDR-null mutant mice, calcium supplementation (high- or medium-calcium diets), adequate to normalize serum calcium concentrations restored the animals' fertility to 86%. In another study, Johnson and Deluca investigated the effects on fertility of dietary calcium in vitamin D-replete and -deficient female rats *(41)*. Vitamin D-deficient rats fed a high-calcium (2% calcium) and high-phosphorus diet had normal calcium concentrations, slightly lower phosphorus levels, and undetectable 25 hydroxy-vitamin D (25[OH]D) concentrations. However, these rats, unlike the vitamin D-deficient rats on the low-calcium diets (0.47% calcium diet), had similar reproductive capacities, fertility ratios, and litter size as the vitamin D-replete rats. The high-calcium diet in the vitamin D-deficient rats restored their reproductive defects to normal. Both vitamin D deficiency as well as absence of the VDR appeared to have the same effect on female reproduction in the absence of high dietary calcium.

One study to date has investigated the association between calcium and vitamin D dysregulation in humans with PCOS. In an observational study in women with PCOS, abnormalities in vitamin D and calcium homeostasis were detected that support the evidence that calcium dysregulation contributes to the development of follicular arrest in mammals, which in turn results in reproductive and menstrual dysfunction *(42)*. Thirteen premenopausal women with documented chronic anovulation and hyperandrogenism were evaluated. Ages ranged from 21 to 41 yr (31.1 ± 7.9). The mean body mass index was 30.6. All had evidence of hirsutism, three had acne. and two had alopecia. Five women had evidence of acanthosis nigricans. Nine had abnormal pelvic sonograms with multiple ovarian follicular cysts. Three women had abnormal LH/FSH ratios greater than 2.4 (range above normal: 2.6–3.8). Four women had elevated serum total testosterone levels (range above normal: 96–142 ng/mL) and four had elevated serum dehydroepiandrosterone sulfate levels (range above normal: 301–405 µg/dL). Four women were amenorrheic and required the use of progesterone every 3 mo to induce menses. Nine had a history of oligomenorrhea, of whom four had regular menses following pregnancy or prescribed oral contraceptives (OCP). Two women had dysfunctional bleeding. The mean serum 25(OH)D level was 11.2 (6.9 ng/mL (nL:9–52 at the time of the study; < 20 ng is now considered deficient). Five women had serum 25(OH)D concentrations below 9 ng/mL; 11 below 20 ng/mL. One woman had an undetectable serum 25(OH)D concentration of less than 5 ng/mL. The mean serum 1,25(OH)$_2$D concentration was 45.8 (18 pg/mL (nL:15–60 pg/mL). The mean intact parathyroid hormone (PTH) was 47 (19 pg/mL (nl:10–65 pg/mL). Five women had abnormally high serum PTH concentrations for their age range (PTH levels above 50 pg/mL in the premenopausal woman are considered abnormal). The serum calcium concentrations in all patients were within normal limits (9.3 ± 0.4 mg/dL). All 13 women were treated with combination calcium and vitamin D supplementation. A serum 25(OH)D concentration to the mid normal range of 30–40 mg/dL was achieved within 2–3 mo of therapy. Vitamin D repletion with calcium therapy resulted in normalized menstrual cycles within 2 mo for seven women, with an additional two experiencing resolution of their dysfunctional bleeding and two women becoming pregnant. Within the 6 mo of observation of this study, clinical improvement of acne vulgaris in all three women manifesting this aspect of hyperandrogenism was noted.

The majority of the women in this study were vitamin D-deficient with abnormalities in the PTH–vitamin D axis. Five women had abnormally elevated PTH levels; whereas three had abnormal serum 1,25(OH)$_2$D concentrations. The optimal serum level of 25(OH)D is currently uncertain. However, recent data suggest that serum 25(OH)D concentrations below 32 ng/mL might be inadequate, resulting in abnormalities of calcium homeostasis with reduced intestinal calcium absorption efficiency and elevated levels of PTH *(43,44)*.

In addition to vitamin D deficiency and its consequences on cellular calcium metabolism, limited dietary calcium intake may also prove to be a factor in this syndrome. The combination of dietary calcium insufficiency and vitamin D deficiency may be largely responsible for the menstrual abnormalities associated with PCOS. Figure 3 illustrates a proposed pathohysiological pathway for PCOS, illustrating the hypothesis that abnormalities in calcium and vitamin D metabolism may affect: (1) LH-induced meiotic maturation, (2) oocyte maturation and resumption of meiosis, and (3) insulin sensitivity—all leading to meiotic arrest, oligo-amenorrhea, and hyperandrogenism.

7. MANAGEMENT AND TREATMENT OF PCOS

The traditional approach in PCOS has been directed at the treatment of specific clinical manifestations of the syndrome. This may include reduction in hirsutism and treatment of acne with anti-androgens, restoring normal menstrual cyclicity or achievement of pregnancy. Initial laboratory evaluation should include the tests as listed in Table 2 to exclude other causes of hyperandrogenism. Some authorities suggest some measure of insulin sensitivity in the evaluation of PCOS, such as the homeostasis model assessment of insulin resistance or serum glucose/ insulin ratio or fasting insulin concentration and a lipid profile, because of the long-term consequences of PCOS.

Nonpharmacological recommendations, such as diet and exercise, can be very effective measures in the overweight PCOS patient. Simple weight reduction of 10–15 lb has been reported to normalize menstrual cycles and even to improve some of the features of androgen excess (e.g., acne). Weight loss can reduce insulin and androgen concentrations

Proposed PCOS Pathophysiology

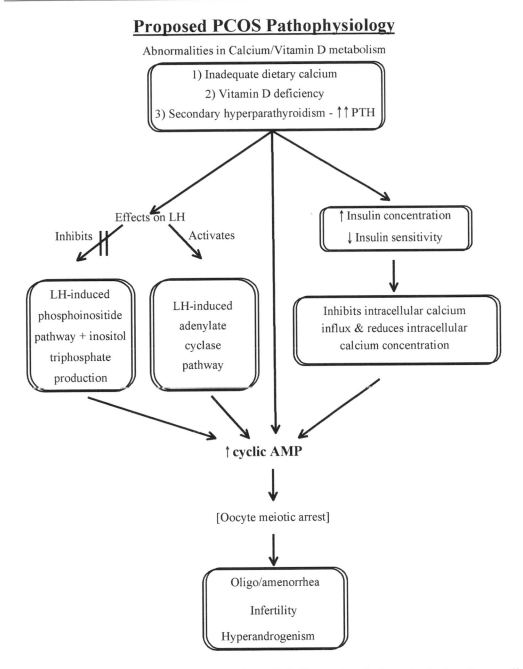

Fig. 3. Proposed pathophysiology pathway for PCOS, illustrating the hypothesis that abnormalities in calcium and vitamin D metabolism effect (1) LH-induced meiotic maturation, (2) oocyte maturation, and (3) insulin sensitivity.

Table 2
Initial Laboratory Evaluation of the Polycystic Ovarian Syndrome Patient

- Complete blood count
- Serum chemistries and lipid profile
- Thyroid function tests
- Serum prolactin
- Serum total and free testosterone
- Serum dehydroepiandrosterone sulfate
- Serum androstenedione
- Serum 17 hydroxyprogesterone
- AM cortisol following 1 mg overnight dexamethasone suppression
- Fasting blood glucose to insulin ratio or homeostasis model assessment of insulin resistance

while increasing sex hormone-binding concentrations, and should be the initial approach in the obese PCOS patient (45).

7.1. Pharmacological Therapy

OCPs are commonly prescribed to the PCOS patient who does not desire pregnancy. They remain the treatment of choice among many physicians because they normalize the menstrual cycle, improve acne and hirsutism, reduce the risk of endometrial and ovarian cancer, and have a long-term safety record. However, these agents do not treat the dysmetabolic consequences of PCOS, and some argue against the use of OCPs in the insulin-resistant woman. Anti-androgens, such as spironolactone, which bind to the androgen receptor are useful for cosmetic effects and psychological benefits in reducing hair growth and improving acne. Insulin-sensitizing agents are an interesting therapeutic intervention in PCOS because of their effect on insulin resistance. These agents have proven efficacy in restoring menstrual cyclicity, but this has been noted in only 30–50% of women with PCOS (46). For a number of women with PCOS, the insulin sensitizers are not effective in normalizing menstrual cycles or in reducing the hyperandrogenic effects. The insulin sensitizers include the biguanide, Metformin, and the thiazolidinediones, rosiglitazone, and pioglitazone. Metformin is a relatively safe therapy, has been shown to improve insulin sensitivity in PCOS, and may result in some weight reduction. It can also result in lactic acidosis, hepatitis, severe nausea, vomiting, and diarrhea, and liver function monitoring is advised. It should not be administered to women with renal insufficiency, hepatic dysfunction, or in the setting of excessive alcohol intake. The thiazolidinediones have a similar effect in improving insulin sensitivity but may induce weight gain. In those women with PCOS and type 2 diabetes mellitus, the insulin sensitizers would be the preferred treatment.

7.2. Calcium and Vitamin D Therapy

There is very limited information on the number of women with PCOS who are vitamin D- and calcium-deficient, or even on the long-term clinical response in PCOS women to adequate calcium and vitamin D therapy. However, the importance of calcium in reproduction, follicular development, and resumption of meiosis is unequivocal and compelling, and argues very strongly for this simple therapy. Therefore, calcium and vitamin D therapy should be recommended to all women with PCOS. Measuring baseline 25(OH)D is very helpful in the management of these women. Although the normal 25(OH)D concentration remains uncertain, serum levels of 25(OH)D at 35–40 ng/mL appear optimal in PCOS. Vitamin D_3 (cholecalciferol) at 2000 international units (IU) daily in a premenopausal woman is safe (47). Women with PCOS may require vitamin D_3 in doses of 2000–4000 IU/d to achieve optimal serum 25(OH)D levels. They also should be given calcium (elemental calcium) at 1500 mg/d for adequate calcium homeostasis. Restoration and normalization of menstrual cycles within 2–3 mo with some improvement in clinical hyperandrogenism and insulin resistance has already been noted in a small pilot study of obese, oligomenorrheic women with PCOS.

8. CONCLUSIONS

PCOS is an extremely common disorder associated with reproductive and menstrual disturbances. It is characterized by chronic anovulation and hyperandrogenism with long-term cardiovascular and metabolic consequences including diabetes mellitus and hypertension. Many women have evidence of insulin resistance and hyperinsulinemia; the majority of women have only a mild form. The pathogenesis of the insulin resistance remains unclear. Oral contraceptives are safe and have been shown to restore menstrual regularity while improving some of the clinical hyperandrogenic features. For the obese woman with PCOS, weight reduction and reducing glucose intolerance with the insulin sensitizers should be a major objective.

Recent evidence strongly suggests that abnormalities in calcium and vitamin D homeostasis underlie the pathogenesis of PCOS. The importance of calcium in egg activation, in meiotic resumption, in LH-induced meiotic maturation, and in reproduction all underscore a role of calcium in PCOS. Calcium is believed to be the primary intracellular signal in invertebrates, amphibians, and mammals for the maturation and differentiation of the oocyte and for the initiation of the development of the egg at fertilization. Maturation of the oocyte or resumption of meiosis is an obligatory step in the preparation of the oocyte for fertilization. The transition from one meiotic phase to another appears to be triggered by increases in intracellular calcium by overriding meiotic arrest. Thus, increases or changes in intracellular calcium are required for the oocyte to mature or progress to the next stage. Calcium and vitamin D dysregulation may ultimately be responsible for the arrested follicular development and menstrual disturbances associated with PCOS, and correction of these calcium abnormalities may reverse both the biochemical and clinical features.

ACKNOWLEDGMENT

This chapter was supported in part by NIDDK grant 57869-02 in conjunction with the office of Women's Health and NIMH.

REFERENCES

1. Archard C, Thiers J. Le virilisme pilaire et son association a l'insuffisance glycolytique (diabete des femmes a barbe). Bull Acad Natl Med 1921;86:51.
2. Stein IF, Leventhal ML. Amenorrhea associated with bilateral polycystic ovaries. Am J Obstet Gynecol 1935;29:181.
3. Franks S. Polycystic Ovary Syndrome. N Engl J Med 1995;13:853–861.

4. Homa ST, Carroll J, Swann K.The role of calcium in mammalian oocyte maturation and egg activation. Human Reproduction 1993;8:1274–1281.

5. Zawadski JK, Dunaif A. Diagnostic criteria for polycystic ovary syndrome: towards a rational approach. In: Current Issues in Endocrinology and Metabolism: Polycystic Ovary Syndrome. Dunaif A, Givens J, Haseltine FP, Merriam GH, eds. Blackwell Scientific, Boston: 1990; pp. 377–384.

6. Barnes R, Rosenfield RL. (1989) The polycystic ovary syndrome: pathogenesis and treatment. Ann Int Med 110:386–399.

7. Rosenfield RL, Barnes RB, Cara JF, Lucky AW. Dysregulation of cytochrome P450c 17 alpha as the acute cause of polycystic ovary syndrome, Fertil Steril 1990;53:785–791.

8. McKenna TJ. Current concepts: pathogenesis and treatment of polycystic ovary syndrome. N Engl J Med 1988;9:558–562.

9. Dunaif A. Insulin resistance and ovarian hyperandrogenism. Endocrinologist 1992; 2:248–260.

10. Legro R, Dunaif A. The role of insulin resistance in polycystic ovary syndrome. Endocrinologist 1996;6:307–321.

11. Elkind-Hirsch KE, Valdis CT, McConnel TG, Malinak LR. Androgen responses to acutely increased endogenous insulin levels in hyperandrogenic and normally cycling women. Fertil Steril 1991;55:486–491.

12. Givens JR, Kerber IJ, Wiser WL, Andersen RN, Coleman SA. Remission of acanthosis nigriacans associated with polycystic ovarian disease and a stomal luteoma. J Clin Endocrinol Metab 1974;38:347–355.

13. Whitaker M, Patel R. Calcium and cell cycle control. Development 1990;108:525–542.

14. Steinhardt R, Epel D. Activation of sea-urchin eggs by a calcium ionophore. Proc Nat Acad Sci 1974;71:1915–1919.

15. Steinhardt R, Epel D, Carroll E, Yanagimachi R. Calcium ionophore: a universal activator for unfertilized eggs? Nature 1974;252:41–43.

16. Jaffe L. Sources of calcium in egg activation: a review and hypothesis. Develop Biol 1983;99:265–276.

17. Collas F, Fissore R, Robl J, Sullivan E, Barnes F. Electrically induced calcium elevation, activation and parthenogenetic development of bovine oocytes. Mol Reprod 1993;34:212–223.

18. Kline D, Kline JT. Repetitive calcium transients and the role of calcium in exocytosis and cell cycle activation in the mouse egg. Develop Biol 1992;149:80–89.

19. Uehara T, Yanagimichi R. Activation of hamster eggs by pricking. J Exp Zool 1976; 199:269–274.

20. Fissore RA, Robl JM. Intracellular calcium response of rabbit oocytes to electrical stimulation. Mol Reprod Dev 1992;32:9–16.

21. Homa ST. Calcium and meiotic maturation of the mammalian oocyte. Mol Reprod Dev 1995;40:122–134.

22. Rosenberg M, Lee H. Roles of Ca and Mg in starfish oocyte maturation induced by 1-methyladenine. J Exp Zool 1981;217:389–397.

23. Powers RD, Paleos GA. Combined effects of calcium and dibutryl cyclic AMP on germinal vesicle breakdown in the mouse oocyte. J Reprod Fertil 1982;66:1–8.

24. Racowsky C. The releasing action of calcium upon cyclic AMP dependent meiotic arrest in hamster oocytes. J Exp Zool 1986;239:263–275.

25. Kaufman M, Homa ST. Defining a role for calcium in the resumption and progression of meiosis in the pig oocyte. J Exp Zool 1993;265:69–76.

26. DeFelici M, Dolci S, Siracusa G. An increase of intracellular free Ca^{++} is essential for spontaneous meiotic resumption by mouse oocytes. J Exp Zool 1991;260:401–405.

27. Moreau M, Vilain JP, Guerrier P. Free calcium changes with hormone action in amphibian oocytes. Develop Biol 1980;78:201–214.

28. Carroll J, Swann K. Spontaneous cytosolic calcium oscillations driven by inositol triphosphate occur during in vitro maturation of mouse oocytes. J Biol Chem 1992;267:11,196–11,201

29. Peres A. InsP3 and Ca^{2+} induced release in single mouse oocytes. FEBS Lett 1990; 275:213–216

30. Lefevre B, Petsy A, Testart J. Cytoplasmic and nucleic calcium oscillations in immature mouse oocytes: evidence of wave polarization by confocal imaging. Exp Cell Res 1995;218:166–173.

31. Dimino MJ, Switzer J, Brown RM. Enosital phosphates accumulation in ovarian granulosa after stimulation by lutenizing hormone. Biol Reprod 1987;37:1129–1134.

32. Davis JS, Weakland L, West L, Farese R. Luteinizing hormone stimulates the formation of inositol triphosphate and cyclic AMP in rat granulosa cells. Biochem J 1986;238:597–604.

33. Dorflinger LJ, Albert P, Williams AT, Behrman HR. Calcium is an inhibitor of luteinizing hormone-sensitive adenylate cyclase in the luteal cell. Endocrinology 1984;114:1208–1215.

34. Gunal AI, Celicker H, Celebi H, Ustandag B, Gunal SY. Intravenous alfacalcidiol improves insulin resistance in hemodialysis patients. Clin Nephrolol 1997;48:109–113.

35. Sanchez M, de la Sierra A, Coca A, Poch A, Giner V, Urbano-Marquez A. Oral calcium supplementation reduces intraplatelet free calcium concentration and insulin resistance in essential hypertensive patients. Hypertension 1997;29:531–536.

36. Mak RH. Amelioration of hypertension and insulin resistance by 1,25 dihydroxycholecalciferol in hemodialysis patients. Pediatr Nephrol 1992;6:345–348.

37. Halloran B. Is 1,25 dihydroxyvitamin D required for reproduction? Proc Exp Biol Med 1989;191:227–232.

38. Halloran B, DeLuca HF. Vitamin D deficiency and reproduction in rats. Science 1979;204:73–74.

39. Kwiecinski GG, Petrie GI, Deluca HF. 1,25 dihydroxyvitamin D3 restores fertility of vitamin D deficient female rats. Am J Physiol 1989;256:E483–E487.

40. Johnson L, DeLuca HF. Vitamin D receptor null mutant mice fed high levels of calcium are fertile. J Nutr 2001;131:1787–1791.

41. Johnson L, DeLuca HF. Reproductive defects are corrected in vitamin D deficient female rats fed a high calcium, phosphorus and lactose diet. J Nutr 2002;132:2270–2273.

42. Thys-Jacobs S, Donovan D, Papadopoulos A, Sarrel P, Bilezikian JP. Vitamin D and calcium dysregulation in the polycystic ovarian syndrome. Steroids 1999;64:430–435.

43. Heaney RP. Age considerations in nutrient needs for bone health: older adults. J Am Coll Nutr 1996;15:575–578.

44. Krall EA, Sahyoun N, Tannenbaum S, Dallai G, Dawson-Hughes B. Effect of vitamin D on seasonal variations in parathyroid hormone secretion in postmenopausal women. N Engl J Med 1989;321:1777–1783.

45. Bates GW, Whitworth NS. Effect of body weight reduction of plasma androgens in obese, infertile women. Fertil Steril 1982;38:406–409.

46. Fleming R, Hopkinson ZE, Wallace AM, Greer IA, Sattar N. Ovarian function and metabolic factors in women with oligomenorrhea treated with metformin in a randomized double blind placebo controlled trial. J Clin Endocrinol Metab 2002;87:569–574.

47. Vieth R. Vitamin D supplementation, 25-hydroxyvitamin D concentration and safety. Am J Clin Nutr 1999;69:842–856.

23 Premenstrual Syndrome

Susan Thys-Jacobs

KEY POINTS

- Premenstrual syndrome (PMS) is a biochemical deficiency syndrome unmasked during the luteal phase of the menstrual cycle.
- Adequate calcium and vitamin D supplementation often relieves the majority of symptoms in women with PMS.

1. INTRODUCTION

Premenstrual syndrome (PMS) has been the subject of many myths and widespread disbeliefs. Descriptions of the syndrome date back to biblical times, when women experiencing menstrually related mood and behavioral disturbances were believed to be "possessed." Centuries later, the prevalent view considered these symptom disturbances as psychological in origin. In 1931, a classic description of the premenstrual tension syndrome by Dr. Robert Frank *(1)* was one of the first to propose a possible hormonal etiology for the occurrence of these symptoms.

PMS is a very common problem that affects millions of young women during their reproductive lives, often disrupting both their emotional and physical well-being. It is widely recognized as a recurrent, cyclical disorder related to the latter half of the menstrual cycle, subsiding with the onset of menses. The syndrome is characterized by a complex group of signs and symptoms that may include depression, mood swings, irritability, fatigue, abdominal discomfort, and changes in appetite (*see* Table 1). The four main categories of symptoms include emotion/negative affect, bloating/water retention, pain, and appetite changes. Although many women experience only mild symptoms, as many as 30–50% suffer from troublesome symptoms. Surveys indicate that approx 5% of North American women consider their symptoms severe enough to have a substantially negative impact on their health and social well-being. It has been suggested that women in this latter group be defined as suffering from Premenstrual Dysphoric Disorder (PMDD), or severe PMS.

Evidence now strongly suggests that PMS is a biochemical abnormality, associated with a calcium- and vitamin D-deficiency state that is unmasked during the latter half of the menstrual cycle *(2)*. The symptoms of PMS are very similar to those of hypocalcemia and often respond to vitamin D and calcium therapy. The majority of PMS symptoms,

From: *Calcium in Human Health*
Edited by: C. M. Weaver and R. P. Heaney © Humana Press Inc., Totowa, NJ

Table 1
Common Symptoms of Premenstrual Syndrome

Emotional/negative affect	Bloating/water retention
Mood swings/crying spells	Abdominal bloating
Depression/sadness	Breast swelling and tenderness
Anger/irritability	
Tension/nervousness	
Pain	Appetite changes
Abdominal cramps	Cravings for salt and sweets
Headache	Increased or decreased appetite
Generalized aches and pain	

such as irritability, depression, anxiety, social withdrawal, headache, and abdominal cramps, are effectively alleviated with either increased dietary calcium or calcium supplementation.

Three essential lines of evidence highlight the role of calcium in PMS and menstrual health: (1) the menstrual cyclicity of the calcium-regulating hormones, (2) clinical calcium trials in PMS, and (3) the importance of calcium in maintaining normal biological functioning of the nervous and reproductive systems.

2. ETIOLOGY

The normal menstrual cycle is characterized by fluctuations of pituitary gonadotropins and ovarian steroid hormones. The first half of the menstrual cycle is defined as the follicular phase with maturation and domination of a single follicle. The rupture and release of the oocyte heralds the luteal phase with the development of the corpus luteum, which secretes increased amounts of estrogen and progesterone during the latter half of the luteal phase.

Numerous theories concerning the etiology of PMS have been proposed, including ovarian hormone imbalances and deficiencies, vitamin B_6 deficiency, and altered endogenous opiates (3,4). Most are scientifically unfounded or remain unproven. Ovarian steroid hormones (estrogen and progesterone) appear important in the pathogenesis of PMS and influence menstrual symptoms. However, various attempts to identify differences in basal levels, pulsatility or patterns of ovarian steroid hormones, pituitary gonadotropins, and other biochemical factors between women with and without PMS have not proven successful (5–9). These negative results notwithstanding, there is convincing evidence that PMS occurs in ovulatory women with normal premenopausal estrogen levels and not in those who are estrogen-deficient. Suppression or cessation of ovarian function owing to menopause or amenorrhea or following oophorectomy results in marked attenuation of premenstrual symptomatology (10–12). Estrogen appears to affect metabolism of minerals and the calcium-regulating hormones, specifically calcium, parathyroid horomone (PTH), vitamin D, and magnesium (13–19); and fluctuations in estrogen specifically during ovulation and the luteal phase of the menstrual cycle appear to result in changes in calcium concentrations. Estrogen lowers serum calcium, probably through its inhibition of bone resorption; in its absence, serum calcium concentrations rise *(20–22)*.

Progesterone is the predominant ovarian steroid hormone during the luteal phase of the menstrual cycle. For many years, progesterone deficiency was believed to be the cause of PMS, and this was the basis for widespread use of progesterone therapy until clinical trials on progesterone proved its ineffectiveness *(23)*. Progesterone is an anti-estrogen that downregulates the effect of estradiol. The abnormalities in calcium homeostasis occurring at the time of progesterone's anti-estrogen activity may further compound the downregulation of estrogen at the receptor level, modulating catecholamine release, calcium channel entry, neurotransmitter metabolism, and ultimately the clinical presentation of PMS. Progesterone may modify the action of estrogen by involving receptor mechanisms with a decrease in the number of cytosolic and nuclear-bound, estrogen-receptor-bound complexes *(24)*. Progesterone has been shown to decrease estrogen responsiveness by depressing estrogen receptor function *(25,26)*. Thus, the action of progesterone in the setting of altered calciotropic hormones may modify the actions of estrogen at the cellular level, resulting in enhanced neuromuscular irritability and vascular reactivity.

Serotonin regulation appears to be important in the pathophysiology of PMS. This conclusion is supported by the many clinical trials demonstrating the efficacy of the selective serotonin reuptake inhibitors (SSRIs) in PMS *(27,28)*. Progesterone affects serotonergic regulation by increasing 5-hydroxytryptamine turnover (serotonin), whereas progesterone withdrawal during the luteal phase of the cycle may result in decreased serotonergic activity.

Ovarian steroid hormones also appear to have vascular effects on various regional circulatory systems including uterine, carotid, coronary, and cerebral arteries *(29)*. These hormones act through a variety of mechanisms including modulation of catecholamine release in the arterial wall, calcium channel conductance, and possibly potassium inductance *(30,74)*. Therefore, acute changes or disruptions in ovarian hormone concentrations may influence neurotransmitter reuptake and metabolism, influence calcium channels, and result in mood disorders. Of note, pregnancy, the use of oral contraceptives, and hormone replacement therapy have been associated with both the development of as well as improvement of panic disorder *(31–33)*. Acute depletion of estradiol can cause rapid changes in cerebral blood flow with reduced frontal lobe blood flow and associated depression *(34)*.

3. PREMENSTRUAL ASSESSMENT AND THE DIAGNOSIS OF PREMENSTRUAL SYNDROME

The diagnosis of PMS is dependent on the relationship of luteal phase to postmenstrual symptoms, because no objective biochemical marker has been found. A prospective assessment of symptoms is recommended but not required for a diagnosis of PMS and is strongly advised for PMDD (severe PMS) *(35,36)*. This assessment can be measured and monitored with a menstrual calendar, daily rating scale, visual analog scale, or symptom diary *(see* Table 2) for at least 2 mo *(37,38)*. For a diagnosis of PMS, the National Institute of Mental Health criteria suggests a 30% change from luteal phase to postmenstrual phase mean symptom levels. A diagnosis of PMDD requires prospective symptom confirmation with specific inclusion criteria of an affective/emotional compo-

Table 2
Premenstrual Syndrome (PMS) Diary[a]

Date			Are you presently menstruating?	
			Yes ☐	No ☐

Rate the average intensity of discomfort you experienced during the previous 24 h

PMS/menstrual symptoms	Absent (0)	Mild (1)	Moderate (2)	Severe (3)
1. Mood swings/ Crying spells				
2. Depression/Sadness/ Feelings of hopelessness				
3. Anxiety/Tension/Nervousness				
4. Decreased interest in usual activities				
5. Difficulty concentrating				
6. Fatigue				
7. Increased/Decreased appetite				
8. Insomnia/Hypersomnia				
9. Sense of being out of control				
10. Abdominal bloating				
11. Abdominal cramps and discomfort				
12. Headache				
13. Breast tenderness/Fullness				
14. Generalized aches and pains				

[a]Modified version.

nent and with evidence of functional impairment. Whether PMDD is a distinct entity from PMS remains an unsettled issue.

4. CYCLICAL FLUCTUATIONS OF THE CALCIOTROPIC HORMONES ACROSS THE MENSTRUAL CYCLE

Calcium has been demonstrated in animal investigations, as well as in human studies, to be dynamically related to the menstrual cycle. Variations in calcium and the biochemical markers of bone metabolism have been shown to accompany the normal hormonal fluctuations during the menstrual cycle in some investigations. Fluctuations of the calcium-regulating hormones (PTH, 25 hydroxyvitamin D [25(OH)D], 1,25 dihydroxyvitamin D [$1,25(OH)_2D$], and serum-ionized calcium) across the menstrual cycle may explain many of the features of PMS. Evidence supports cyclical changes in the calciotropic hormones in a number of investigations involving healthy premenopausal women. In 1978, Pitkin and colleagues measured calcium, the calcium-regulating hormones, and calcitonin across the menstrual cycle in seven healthy, premenopausal women. They were the first to report that PTH and the biologically active form of vitamin D—$1,25(OH)_2D$—progressively increased in concentration throughout the follicular phase of the cycle in human studies (39). Both hormones peaked in association with reduced ionized calcium concentrations. Subsequently, both Gray et al. (40) and Tjellesen et al. (41) noted peri-ovulatory elevations of $1,25(OH)_2D$ in premenopausal women. In 1982,

Gray and colleagues studied serum calcium and 1,25(OH)$_2$D concentrations in seven normal women at four points of their menstrual cycles on days 1, 8, 15, and 22. Serum concentrations of 1,25(OH)$_2$D on day 15 were double the concentrations noted on days 1 and 8. However, serum total calcium level was not found to vary. In a similar fashion, Tjellesen found the biologically active vitamin D metabolite to be double at the time of ovulation in five young premenopausal women. Fasting serum calcium, alkaline phosphatase activity, urinary calcium, and hydroxyproline did not significantly vary across the cycle. A similar pattern of the menstrual cyclicity of the calcium-regulating hormones was noted in a study involving women with PMS (42). Twelve healthy, premenopausal women across one menstrual cycle were studied. Seven women had documented PMS; five were asymptomatic controls. In both groups, both serum total and ionized calcium significantly varied across the three phases of the menstrual cycle and were observed to decline significantly at mid-cycle coinciding with the rise of estradiol. In the asymptomatic group, there did not appear to be hormonal variability across the menstrual cycle for either PTH or 25(OH)D. On the other hand, in the PMS group, PTH was found to rise significantly at mid-cycle, and this mid-cycle elevation was 30% greater than at follicular levels. The compensatory rise in PTH was noted for the PMS group only, and not for the control group. Significant differences between groups were noted for total calcium, intact PTH, and 25(OH)D concentrations. It was proposed that marginal vitamin D reserves may have accounted for the wide fluctuations in calcium-regulating hormones, and adequate vitamin D levels may have maintained minimal variability of intact PTH and 1,25(OH)$_2$D concentrations. However, it was not yet clear whether the fluctuations noted in women with PMS were exaggerations of normal cyclic variability associated with the menstrual cycle or representations of a PMS-specific pathophysiological feature.

Observations in young female rats have also demonstrated cyclical changes of calcium-regulating hormones and calcium absorption during the estrous cycle. In 1983, plasma levels of calcium, phosphorus, calcitonin, PTH, and prolactin were measured in Wistar rats during a 4-d estrous cycle (43). Significant fluctuations in plasma calcium and calcitonin levels were noted, whereas PTH was unchanged. Serum calcium levels fell throughout the day during proestrus and estrus (ovulation), and rose during diestrus. At all stages of the cycle, calcium declined between morning and evening. Brommage et al. measured intestinal calcium absorption during the rat estrous cycle (44). Both total and fractional intestinal calcium absorption were observed to vary. Both were highest during estrous and lowest during the second day of diestrus. Thus, variations in calcium have been observed in both the menstrual and estrous cycles.

Despite the foregoing evidence, it must be noted that the menstrual cyclicity of either the calciotropic hormones or the biochemical markers of bone turnover remains an unsettled issue. In 1986, Buchanan and colleagues examined the interaction between PTH and endogenous estrogen in 20 healthy Caucasian premenopausal women (45). PTH concentrations were found not to vary throughout the menstrual cycle despite fluctuating estrogen levels. In contrast, 1,25(OH)$_2$D concentrations were notably higher during the early luteal phase compared with earlier follicular levels. In addition, Muse and colleagues characterized the effect of cyclic changes in ovarian steroid secretion on calcium homeostasis by measuring calciotropic hormones in six normal, healthy premenopausal women (46). Daily determinations of PTH, calcitonin, 1,25(OH)$_2$D, gonadotropins, prolactin, estradiol, progesterone, total serum calcium, and phosphorus were made. Despite normal cyclical patterns of pituitary gonadotropins and ovarian steroid hormones, there was little menstrual cyclicity in PTH, calcitonin, $1,25(OH)_2D$ or in total serum calcium and phosphorus. Mid-cycle elevations of PTH or $1,25(OH)_2D$ were not detected.

Studies on the biochemical markers of bone metabolism have yielded conflicting results as well. Some investigators did not observe any effect on bone remodeling during the menstrual cycle, whereas others noted variations. Serum osteocalcin (bone Gla protein) and bone-specific alkaline phosphatase activity correlated with mineralization rate as determined by ^{47}Ca kinetic studies and by histomorphometric parameters of bone formation. In the study by Nielsen et al., PTH and $1,25(OH)_2D$ did not vary significantly across the menstrual cycle, but both osteocalcin and bone-specific alkaline phosphatase rose during the luteal phase (47). Bone resorption markers also undergo small variations during the normal menstrual cycle in premenopausal women (48). Serum pyridinoline crosslinked carboxy-terminal telopeptide of type I collagen, a specific marker of bone resorption, was found to peak during the luteal phase. Moreno et al. reported, however, that serum osteocalcin concentrations remained stable during the menstrual cycle in four healthy premenopausal volunteers and were independent of pituitary gonadotropins and ovarian steroid hormones (49).

5. CALCIUM HORMONES AND MOOD/DEPRESSION

Alterations in calcium homeostasis have long been associated with many affective disturbances. Hypocalcemia has been associated with irritability, anxiety, and mania; whereas hypercalcemia, as typified by primary hyperparathyroidism (50), has been noted in some patients with depression (51–55). PMS shares many of the features of depression, anxiety, and the dysphoric states and is remarkably similar to those symptoms associated with hypocalcemia (see Table 3) (56). It is not surprising that calcium treatment has been found to alleviate PMS.

Calcium is an essential intracellular and extracellular cation. Extracellular calcium is required to maintain normal biological functioning of the nervous system (neuronal conductance and synaptic transmission of acetylcholine), as well as of many other systems. In the brain, the synthesis of the neurotransmitters serotonin, norepinephrine, and acetylcholine is dependent on intracellular calcium concentrations (57,58). Changes in the extracellular calcium concentration affect the excitability of neuromuscular tissues involved in emotional regulation (59,60). Primary hyperparathyroidism, a disorder of calcium regulation, is associated with elevated calcium and PTH concentrations. Several studies have described patients diagnosed with this disorder exhibiting mild personality changes, anxiety, confusion, depression, and even psychosis, similar to the negative affective features associated with PMS (61). Treatment with parathyroid surgery and normalization of the calcium and parathyroid levels appeared to improve fatiguability, mental concentration, tension, sadness, and some of the psychiatric symptoms (62,63). Some investigators believe that hyperparathyroidism influences both the serotonergic and dopaminergic mechanisms in the brain, resulting in a variety of psychiatric disturbances. Low cerebrospinal fluid (CSF) levels of monoamine metabolites in primary hyperparathyroidism have been observed in patients with endogenous depression and suicidal behavior (64,65). Monoamine metabolites 5-hydroxyindole acetic acid, homovanillic acid, and 3 methoxy-4-hydroxy-phenyl-glycol in the CSF of patients with primary hyperparathyroidism increased following parathyroid surgery (66). Also, fol-

Table 3
Clinical Features of Hypocalcemia

- Anxiety
- Depression
- Fatigue
- Impaired memory and intellectual capacity
- Personality disturbances
- Neuromuscular irritability
- Muscle cramps
- Paresthesias
- Tetany

lowing parathyroid surgery, patients had an improvement in psychiatric symptomatology with an increase in CSF 5-hydroxyindole acetic acid and homovanillic acid. Altered serum calcium concentrations appeared to impair the actions as well as the stimulus-secretion coupling of the catecholamines that act through calcium-mediated mechanisms.

In a similar fashion, PMS may be the result of altered intracellular calcium metabolism influencing dopaminergic and serotonergic regulation. There is evidence that serotonin is important in the pathophysiology of this syndrome (67), and various SSRIs have proved to be effective treatments in some women with PMS and PMDD (68,69). Calcium may ultimately affect monoamine metabolism, reversing the serotonergic dysregulation and providing a biochemical basis for the therapeutic effect.

6. CLINICAL EVIDENCE ON CALCIUM SUPPLEMENTATION AND PMS

Calcium supplementation has been demonstrated to result in a beneficial clinical response in the treatment of premenstrual symptoms in a number of studies. These clinical trials and recent epidemiological evidence support the role of calcium in PMS and menstrual health.

The first clinical trial demonstrating the efficacy of calcium in PMS was a small, randomized, placebo-controlled crossover trial published in 1989 (70). Women with PMS received 6 mo of treatment involving 3 mo of daily calcium (1000 mg of elemental calcium in the form of calcium carbonate) and 3 mo of placebo. The effectiveness of calcium treatment was assessed prospectively by monitoring daily changes in symptom scores with a self-assessment rating scale over a 6-mo period and retrospectively by an overall global assessment. Fourteen symptoms ranging from irritability, mood swings, and depression to water retention and appetite changes were monitored daily. Calcium treatment resulted in a significant, 50% reduction in symptoms within 3 mo. Retrospective assessment of overall symptoms confirmed this reduction: 73% of the women reported fewer symptoms during the treatment phase on calcium, 15% preferred placebo, and 12% had no clear preference. Three premenstrual factors—negative affect, water retention, and pain—and one menstrual factor—pain—were significantly alleviated by calcium.

Following this study, Penland and Johnson (71) conducted an exploratory metabolic ward investigation designed to determine if dietary calcium and manganese affected menstrual cycle symptoms. Women with normal menstrual cycles were assigned to one of four dietary periods of either low dietary calcium intake at 587 mg or high dietary calcium at 1336 mg per day. Increasing calcium intake positively affected mood, concentration, pain, and behavior symptoms.

A large, randomized, double-blind, placebo-controlled, parallel-designed multicenter trial in 1998 corroborated these two smaller trials, demonstrating a similar beneficial effect of calcium treatment in PMS *(72)*. Seven hundred twenty healthy premenopausal women between the ages of 18 and 45 yr were recruited nationally in the United States and screened over two menstrual cycles for moderate to severe cyclically recurring symptoms. Symptoms were prospectively documented with a daily rating scale (the PMS diary) employing 17 core symptoms and 4 symptom factors as previously listed (negative affect, water retention, food cravings, and pain). Entrance criteria required a minimum increase in symptom intensity of 50% in the luteal phase compared to the intermenstrual phase for at least two of three screening cycles. Daily documentation of symptoms, adverse affects, and compliance with medications were monitored. Four hundred ninety-seven participants were randomly assigned to receive 1200 mg of elemental calcium per day in the form of calcium carbonate or placebo for three menstrual cycles. By the third treatment cycle, calcium resulted in an overall 48% reduction in total symptom scores. All four symptom factors (negative affect, water retention, food cravings, and pain) were significantly reduced by the third treatment cycle. The negative affect symptom factor was reduced by 45% by the third treatment cycle on calcium. By the second and third treatment months, all 15 symptoms except for fatigue and insomnia showed a significant response to calcium treatment (mood swings; tension/irritability, anger/short temper, depression/sadness).

Observations from two studies suggest that women with premenstrual syndrome have lower bone mass as compared with asymptomatic controls, further supporting a disturbance in calcium metabolism in PMS. In a cross-sectional survey, bone density measurements at the lumbar spine and proximal femur were obtained in 26 women with PMS and 20 controls *(73)*. Compared with controls, women with PMS had significantly lower vertebral bone mass measurements at the lumbar vertebrae (L2–4) (1.18 ± 0.11 vs 1.28 ± 0.11 g/cm^2, $p = 0.0016$). In 1994, Lee and Kanis *(74)* examined the relationship between premenstrual symptoms and vertebral osteoporosis in a retrospective study. These authors noted the higher risk of vertebral osteoporosis in those women with a history of PMS (relative risk = 1.86).

More recently, a prospective substudy within the Nurse's Health Study II cohort evaluated the association between calcium and vitamin D intake and risk of PMS. Participants were 25–42 yr of age at study entry. Nutrient intake was measured in 1991, 1995, and 1999 by food frequency questionnaire. Cases were 1057 women reporting PMS during the 10-yr follow-up period, and controls were 1968 women reporting no PMS. Results indicated that high intakes of both calcium and vitamin D were inversely associated with risk of PMS *(75)*.

7. CURRENT TREATMENTS IN PREMENSTRUAL SYNDROME

A variety of treatments for PMS have been proposed over the years, including lifestyle and dietary changes as well as drug interventions. The majority have proved ineffective or only temporarily effective, whereas other treatments have proven efficacy. Initially advising dietary and lifestyle modifications by increasing daily dietary calcium intake and an adequate aerobic exercise program will often reduce symptoms, and may be all that is required especially with mild or even moderate PMS. The potential for dietary supplements other than calcium to reduce PMS symptoms is less convincing (76). Magnesium at a dose of 200–400 mg/d may alleviate PMS symptoms. In 1991, Facchinetti observed that 360 mg of magnesium reduced affective symptoms (77), whereas Walker noted a reduction in symptoms of bloating but not in mood symptoms (78). Scientific evidence on vitamin E and B6 is very limited. Evening primrose oil, which is a rich source of γ-linolenic acid, had been suggested as a possible treatment, but two well-designed studies did not demonstrate efficacy. SSRIs have proven efficacy, specifically in severe PMS or PMDD (79–82). Fluoxetine, sertraline, paroxetine, and fluvoxamine—all SSRIs—appear to have similar beneficial effects. These antidepressants are usually administered on a daily basis, but intermittent therapy during the luteal phase of the cycle has been shown to be efficacious (83). Gonadotropin-releasing agonists induce hypogonadism and have been demonstrated to reduce PMS symptoms, but the hypoestrogenic side effects and potential bone loss are major concerns. These latter drugs should be administered with great caution, and careful monitoring is highly recommended. If long-term therapy is required, add-back therapy with hormone replacement is strongly recommended.

8. MANAGEMENT OF PREMENSTRUAL SYNDROME

The initial evaluation of PMS should include laboratory evaluation (complete blood count, chemistries with total serum calcium and phosphorus, and a thyroid function panel), instruction on the use of daily diaries (when indicated), and an exclusion of conditions that may compound PMS symptoms such as thyroid disease, panic disorder, depression, and anxiety disorder. A calcium profile, including serum 25(OH)D and intact PTH concentrations with a 24-h urine calcium excretion, can be extremely helpful in the management of women with moderate to severe symptoms, often guiding therapy (discussed later). However, one can readily treat with just the 25(OH)D concentration alone. Vitamin D deficiency has become more commonly recognized and failure to optimally supplement one's diet can commonly result in vitamin D insufficiency. Vitamin D at 2000 international units (IU) daily in a premenopausal woman is safe. Although a normal serum 25(OH)D concentration has been of some controversy recently, levels of 25(OH)D of approx 35–40 ng/mL appear adequate (84,85). A realistic treatment approach is to begin calcium supplementation empirically at 1000 mg (500 mg twice daily) and vitamin D at 1000–2000 IU daily. To correct for inadequate levels of vitamin D, the following replacement regimen based on serum 25(OH)D concentrations can be used:

- If the serum 25(OH)D concentration is less than 20 ng/mL, replacement with vitamin D_3 (cholecalciferol) 4000 IU daily or vitamin D_2 (ergocalciferol) 50,000 IU three times a week. The level of 25(OH)D should be repeated at 1 and 6 mo or as necessary, with adjustments in dose to achieve a 25(OH)D between 35 ng/mL and 60 ng/mL.
- If the serum 25(OH)D concentration is above 20 ng/mL, replacement with cholecalciferol 2000 IU daily or ergocalciferol 50,000 weekly. The level of 25(OH)D should be repeated at 1 and 6 mo or as necessary, with adjustments in dose to achieve a serum 25(OH)D level between 35 and 60 ng/mL.

- The normal maintenance dose of vitamin D_3 may vary from 1000 to 4000 IU daily. The majority of women will experience a sense of well-being and relief within 1–2 mo of treatment. Dietary modifications may be helpful as well, and adding dairy products such as yogurt or milk can reduce the total supplemental calcium while maintaining the total dietary calcium. Increases in both dietary and supplemental calcium may cause an initial exacerbation of physical PMS symptoms, such as menstrual cramps. Constipation and nausea are very common complaints with calcium tablet usage. The addition of magnesium to the diet often alleviates this complaint, and ingesting the calcium with meals and not on an empty stomach usually also resolves the nausea.

9. CONCLUSIONS

Evidence strongly suggests that PMS is a clinical manifestation of a subtle underlying biochemical deficiency unmasked during the luteal phase of the menstrual cycle. Cyclic elevations of estrogen and progesterone during the menstrual cycle may antagonize the effects of PTH on bone, inhibiting skeletal calcium release and reducing the ionized calcium concentration. Calcium and vitamin D deficiency may exaggerate menstrual cycle calciotropic hormonal variability, resulting in the biochemical features of PMS. Dietary modifications with increases in total daily calcium intake may be all that is necessary in the relief of PMS symptoms. Adequate calcium and vitamin D supplementation (with daily calcium at 1000 mg and vitamin D 1000–2000 IU) often relieves the majority of symptoms in women with PMS. The remainder should have additional hormonal and biochemical investigations to elucidate the etiology of persistent symptoms. For those women who do not adequately respond to adequate calcium and vitamin D replacement therapy, a course of SSRIs should be prescribed. Menstrually related mood changes may be a very important clinical marker of an underlying calcium and vitamin D disturbance. Abnormalities in calcium homeostasis may have a major impact on the menstrual and bone health of the premenopausal woman.

ACKNOWLEDGMENT

This chapter was supported in part by NIDDK grant 57869-02 in conjunction with the Office of Women's Health and NIMH.

REFERENCES

1. Frank RT. The hormonal causes of premenstrual tension. Arch Neurol Psychiatry 1931;26:1053–1057.
2. Thys-Jacobs S. Micronutrients and the Premenstrual Syndrome: the Case for Calcium. J Amer College Nutrition. 2000;19:220–227.
3. Reid RL, Yen SSC. Premenstrual syndrome. Am J Obstet Gynecol. 1981;139:85–104.
4. Bruce J, Russel G. Premenstrual tension. A study of weight changes and balances of water sodium and potassium. Lancet. 1962;2:267–271.
5. Aedo AR, Langren BM, Cekan Z, Diczfalusy E. Studies on the pattern of circulating steroids in the normal menstrual cycle. Acta Endocrinol (Copenh) 1976; 82:600–616.
6. Urban RJ, Veldhuis JD, Dufau ML. Estrogen regulates the GnRH-stimulated secretion of biologically active LH. J Clin Endocrinol Metab 1991; 72:660–668.
7. Rubinow DR, Hoban MC, Grover GN, et al. Changes in plasma hormones across the menstrual cycle in patients with menstrually related mood disorder and in control subjects. Am J Obstet Gynecol 1988;158:5–11.

8. Facchinetti F, Genazzani AD, Martignoni E, Fioroni L, Sances G, Genazzani AR. Neuroendocrine correlates of premenstrual syndrome: changes in the pulsatile pattern of plasma LH. Psychoneuroendocrinology 1990;15:269–277.

9. Cerin A, Collins A, Landgren BM, Eneroth P. Hormonal and biochemical profiles of premenstrual syndrome. Acta Obstet Gyecol Scand 1993;72:337–343.

10. Muse KN, Cetel NS, Futterman LA, Yen SSC. The premenstrual syndrome: effects of medical ovariectomy. N Engl J Med 1984; 311:1345–1349.

11. Mortola JF, Girton L, Fischer U. Successful treatment of severe premenstrual syndrome by combined use of gonadotropin-releasing hormone agonist and estrogen/progestin. J Clin Endocrinol Metab 1991; 71:252A–252F.

12. Casson P, Hahn PM, Van Vugt DA, Reid RL. Lasting response to ovariectomy in severe intractable premenstrual syndrome. Am J Obstet Gynecol 1990;162:99–105.

13. Orimo H, Fujita T, Yoshikawa M. Increased sensitivity of bone to parathyroid hormone in ovariectomized rats. Endocrinology 1972; 90:760–763

14. Gallagher JC, Riggs BL, Deluca HF. Effect of estrogen on calcium absorption and serum vitamin D metabolites in postmenopausal osteoporosis. J Clin Endocrinol Metab 1980. 51:1359–1364.

15. Roodman GD, Ibbotson Kj, MacDonald BR, Kuehl TJ, Mundy GR. 1,25(OH)2 vitamin D3 causes formation of multinucleated cells with osteoclast characteristics in cultures of primate marrow. Proc Natl Acad Sci USA 1985. 82:8213–8217.

16. McSheehy PMJ, Chambers TJ. Osteoblastic cells mediate osteoclastic responsiveness to parathyroid hormone. Endocrinology 1987; 118:824–828.

17. Richelson LS, Heinz HW, Melton II LJ, Riggs BL. Relative contributions of aging and estrogen deficiency to postmenopausal bone loss. N Engl J Med 1984; 311:1273–1275.

18. Stevenson JC, Lees B, Devenport M, Cust MP, Gangar KF. Determinants of bone density in normal women: risk factors for future osteoporosis? Br Med J 1989; 298:924–928.

19. Ettinger B, Genant HK, Cann CE. Long term estrogen replacement therapy prevents bone loss and fractures. Ann Intern Med 1985; 102:319–324.

20. Young MN and Nordin BEC. Effect of natural and artificial menopause on plasma and urinary calcium and phosphorus. Lancet 2:118; 1967.

21. Heaney RP. A unified concept of osteoporosis. Am J Med 39:877,1965.

22. Heaney RP. Estrogens and postmenopausal osteoporosis. Clin Obstet Gyecol 19:791,1976.

23. Freeman E, Rickels K. Ineffectivensss of progesterone therapy suppository treatment for premenstrual syndrome. JAMA 1990:349–353.

24. Clark JH, Paszko Z, Peck EJ. Nuclear binding and retention of receptor estrogen complex: relation to the agonistic and antagonistic properties of estriol. Endocrinology 1977; 100:91–96.

25. Saunder DE, Lozon MM, Corombos JD, et al. Role of porcine endometrial estrogen sulfotransferase in progesterone mediated down regulated of estrogen receptors. J Steroid Biochem 1989;32:749–757.

26. Brenner RM, Resko JA, West NB. Cyclic changes in oviductal morphology and residual cytoplasmic estradiol binding capacity induced by sequential estradiol-progesterone treatment of spayed rhesus monkeys. Endocrinology 1974;95:1094–1104.

27. Steiner M. Female specific mood disorders. Clin Obstet Gynecol 1992;35:599–611.

28. Rojansky N, Halbreich U, Zander K, Barkai A, Goldstein S. Imipramine receptor binding and serotonin uptake in platelets of women with premenstrual changes. Gynecol Obstet Invest 1991;31:146–152.

29. Shamma F N, Fayad P, Brass L, Sarrell P. Middle cerebral artery blood velocity during controlled ovarian hyperstimulation. Fertil Steril 1992;57:1022–1025.

30. Hamlet MA, Rorie DK, Tyce GM. Effects of estradiol on release and disposition of norepinephrine from nerve endings. Am J Physiol 1980;239:H450–H56.

31. Deci PA, Lydiard B, Santos AB, Arana GW. Oral contraceptives and Panic Disorder. J Clin Psychiatry 1992; 53:163–165.

32. Chung C, Remington ND, Young Suh B. Estrogen replacement therapy may reduce panic symptoms. J Clin Psychiatry 1995;56:533.

33. Villeponteaux VA, Lydiard RB, Laraia M, et al. The effects of pregnancy on preexisting panic disorder. J Clin Psychiatry 1992;53:201–203.

34. Sarrel P. The effect of acute depletion of estradiol on cerebral blood flow. Personal communication. 1997.

35. Schnurr P. Measuring amount of symptom change in the diagnosis of premenstrual syndrome. Psychol Assses. 1989; 4:277–283.

36. ACOG Practice Bulletin. Clinical management Guidelines. 2000; 15:1–9.

37. Alvir JMJ, Thys-Jacobs S. Premenstrual and menstrual symptom clusters and response to calcium treatment. Psychopharmacol Bull 1991; 27:145–148.

38. Thys-Jacobs S, Alvir JMJ, Fratarcangelo P. Comparative analysis of three PMS assessment instruments- the identification of premenstrual syndrome with core symptoms. Psychopharmacol Bull 1995; 31:389–396.

39. Pitkin R, Reynolds WA, Williams GA, Hargis GK. Calcium regulating hormones during the menstrual cycle. J Clin Endocrinol Metab 1978;47: 626.

40. Gray TK, etal. Fluctuation of serum concentration of 1,25 dihydroxyvitamin D during the menstrual cycle. Am J Obstet Gynecol.1982; 144:880.

41. Tjellesen L, Christiansen C, Hummer L, Larsen NE. Unchanged biochemical indices of bone turnover despite fluctuations in 1,25 dihydroxyvitamin D during the menstrual cycle. Acta Endocrinologica. 1983; 102:476.

42. Thys-Jacobs S, Alvir MAJ. Calcium regulating hormones across the menstrual cycle: evidence of a secondary hyperparathyroidism in women with PMS. J Clin Endocrinol Metab 1995; 80: 2227–2232.

43. Cressent M, Elie C, Taboulet J, Moukhtar S, Milhaud. Calcium regulating hormones during the estrous cycle of the rat. Proc Soc Exp Biol Med 1983; 172:158–162.

44. Brommage R, Binacua C, Carrie AL. Ovulation-associated increase in intestinal calcium absorption during the rat estrous cycle is blunted by ovarietomy. Biol Reprod 1993;49:544–548.

45. Buchanan J, Santen R, Cavaliere A, Cauffman S, Greer R, Demers L. Interaction between parathyroid hormone and endogenous estrogen in normal women. Metabolism 1986; 35:489–494.

46. Muse KN, Manolagas SC, Deftos LJ, Alexander N, Yen SC. Calcium regulating hormones across the menstrual cycle. J Clin Endocrinol Metab. 1986;62:1313.

47. Nielsen HK, Brixen K, Bouillon R, and Mosekilde L. Changes in biochemical markers of osteoblastic activity during the menstrual cycle. J Clin Endocrinol Metab 1990; 70:1431.

48. Schlemmer A, Hassager C, Risteli J, Risteli L, Jensen SB, Christiansen C. Possible variation in bone resorption during the menstrual cycle. Acta Endocrinologica 1993;129:388.

49. Moreno JLM, Gonzalez G, Campino C, Salvatierra AM, Croxatto HB. Serum osteocalcin in normal menstrual cycle. Medicina 1992;52:37–40.

50. Borer M, Bhanot V. Hyperparathyroidsim: neuropsychiatric manifestations. Psychosomatics 1985;26:597–601.

51. Carman JS, Wyatt RJ. Alterations in cerebrospinal fluid and serum total calcium with changes in psychiatric state, in Neuroregulators and Psychiatric Disorders, Usdin E, Hamburg DA, Barchas JD. (eds.), Oxford University Press, New York, 1977; pp.488–494.

52. Tohme J, Bilezikian JP. Diagnosis and treatment of hypocalcemic emergencies. The Endocrinologist 1996;6:10–18.

53. Cogan MD, Covey CM, Arieff A, Wisniewski A, Clark OH. Central nervous system manifestations of hyperparathyroidim. Am J Med 1978; 65:963–969.

54. Jimerson DC, Post R, Carman JS, van Kammen DP, Wood JH, Goodwin FK. CSF calcium: clinical correlates in affective illness and schizophrenia. Biol Psychiat 1979; 14:37–51.

55. Aurbach G, Marx S, Spiegel A. Parathyroid hormone, calcitonin, and the calciferols, in Textbook of Endocrinology, 8th ed., Williams, R.H. (ed.), Saunders, Philadelphia, 1992 pp. 1397–1517.

56. Weston PG, Howard MQ. The determination of sodium, potassium, calcium and magnesium in the blood and spinal fluid of patients suffering from manic depressive insanity. Arch Neurol Psychiat 1922; 8:179–183.

57. Rubin RP. The role of calcium in the release of neurotransmitter substances and hormones. Pharmacol Rev 197;22:389–428.

58. Dubovsky SL, Franks RD. Intracellular calcium ions in affective disorders: a review and an hypothesis. Biol Psych 1983;18:781–797.

59. Carman JS, Wyatt RJ. Calcium: Bivalent cation in the bivalent psychoses. Biol Psychiat 1979;14:295–336.

60. Carman JS, Crews E, Bancroft A, etal. Calcium and calcium regulating hormones in the biphasic periodic psychoses. J Operational Psychiat 1980;11:5–17.

61. Joborn C, Hetta J, Palmer M, Akerstrom G, Ljunghall S. Psychiatric symptomatology in patients with primary hyperparathyroidism. Upsala J Med 1986;91:77–87.
62. Joborn C, Hetta J, Johsnsson H, Rasstad J, Agren H, Akerstrom G, Ljunghall S. Psychiatric morbidity in primary hyperparathyroidism World J Surg 1988;12:476–481.
63. Alarcon RD, Franceschini JA. Hyperparathyroidism and paranoid psychosis. Br J Psychiatry 1984; 145:477–480.
64. Asberg M, Bertilsson L, Martensson B, Scalia-Tomba GP, Thoren P, Traskanman Bendz L. CSF monoamines metabolites in melancholia. Acta Psychiatr Scand 1984;69:201–205.
65. Traskman L, Asberg M, Bertilsson L, Sjostrand L. Monoamine metabolites in CSF and suicidal behavior. Arch Gen Psychiatry 1981; 38:631–639.
66. Joborn C, Hetta J, Rastad J, Agren H, Akerstrom, Ljunghall S. Psychiatric symptoms and cerebrospinal fluid monoamine metabolites in primary hyperparathyroidism. Biol Psychiatry 1988;23:149–158.
67. Rapkin AJ. The role of serotonin in premenstrual syndrome. Clin Obstet Gynecol 1992;35:629–636.
68. Steiner M, Steinberg S, Stewart D, et al. Fluoxetine in the treatment of premenstrual dysphoria. N Engl J Med 1995;332:1529–1534.
69. Sundblad C, Modigh K, Andersch B, Eriksson E. Clomipramine effectively reduces premenstrual irritability and dysphoria: a placebo-controlled trial. Acta Psychiatr Scand 1992;85:39–47.
70. Thys-Jacobs S, Ceccarelli S, Bierman A, Weisman H, Cohen MA, Alvir J. Calcium supplementation in premenstrual syndrome. J Gen Intern Med. 1989;4:183–189.
71. Penland J, Johnson PE. Dietary calcium and manganese effects on menstrual cycle symptoms. Am J Obstet Gynecol. 1993;168:1417–1423.
72. Thys-Jacobs S, Starkey P, Fratarcangelo P, Bernstein D, Tian J. Calcium Carbonate and the premenstrual syndrome: effects on premenstrual and menstrual symptoms. Am J Obstet Gynecol 1998;179:444–52.
73. Thys-Jacobs S, Silverton M, Alvir J, Paddison P, Rico M, Goldsmith S. Reduced Bone Mass in women with Premenstrual Syndrome. J Women's Health 1995; 4: 161–168.
74. Lee SJ, Kanis JA. An association between osteoporosis and premenstrual and postmenstrual symptoms. Bone and Mineral 1994;24:127–134..
75. Bertrone E, Hankinson S, Bendich A, Manson J. Intake of calcium and vitamin D and risk of premenstrual syndrome. Journal of Women's Health - abstracts 2003; 12:425.
76. Bendich A. The potential for dietary supplements to reduce premenstrual syndrome (PMS) symptoms. J Amer College Nutrition 2000;19:3–12.
77. Facchinetti F, Borella P, Sances G, Fioroni L, Nappi RE, Genazzani AR: Oral Magnesium successfully relieves premenstrual mood changes. Obstet Gynecol 1991; 78:177–181.
78. Walker AF, De Souza M, Vickers MF. Magnesium supplementation alleviates premenstrual symptoms of fluid retention. J Women's Health 1998; 7:1157–1165.
79. Wood SH, Mortola JF, Chan YF, Moossazadeh F, Yen SSC. Treatment of premenstrual syndrome with fluoxetine: a double-blind, placebo controlled, crossover study. Obstet Gynecol 1992;80:339–344.
80. Stone AB, Pearlstein TB, Brown WA. Fluoxetine in the treatment of the late luteal phase dysphoric disorder. J Clin Psychiatry 1991;52:290–293.
81. Menkes DB, Taghavi E, Mason PA, Spears GFS, Howard RC. Fluoxetine treatment of severe premenstrual syndrome. BMJ 1992;305:346–347.
82. Rickels K, Freeman EW, Sondheimer S, Albert J. Fluoxetine in the treatment of premenstrual syndrome. Curr Ther Res 1990;48:161–166.
83. Steiner M, Korzekwa M, Lament J, Williams A. Intermittent fluoxetine dosing in the treatment of premenstrual dysphoria, Pychopharmacol Bul 1997; 33:771–774.
84. Heaney R. Nutrition factors in Osteoporosis. Ann Rev Nutr 1993;13:287–316.
85. Vieth R. Vitamin D supplementation, 25- hydroxyvitamin D concentrations and safety. Am J Clin Nutr 1999;69:842–856.

24 Calcium Throughout the Life Cycle

The Later Years

Bess Dawson-Hughes

KEY POINTS

- Calcium absorption efficiency is influenced by age, race, diet composition, genetics, hormonal status, and other factors.
- Increasing calcium intake generally lowers biochemical markers of bone turnover by approx 10–15% and modestly increases bone mineral density. These changes reverse after lowering calcium intake.
- The impact of calcium alone on fracture rates has been estimated at 4% for each 300 mg increase, in one meta-analysis. The impact of calcium in combination with vitamin D appears to be greater.
- Calcium is an important adjunct to any drug regimen for the prevention and treatment of osteoporosis.

1. INTRODUCTION

Osteoporotic fractures are common and devastating occurrences. Many lifestyle and hereditary factors contribute to fracture risk. Several components of the diet influence risk of osteoporosis in older men and women and the best studied of these are calcium and vitamin D. This chapter focuses on the role of calcium in bone health in older men and women. It includes a review of the physiology and determinants of calcium absorption and a summary of the evidence that calcium intake influences the rate of bone remodeling and bone loss in older individuals. The limited available evidence that calcium alters fracture rates will also be addressed. The National Academy of Sciences now recommends that men and women age 51 yr and older consume 1200 mg/d of calcium. Although food sources of calcium are preferred, many individuals will need supplements in order to meet their calcium requirement. Supplement absorbability and optimal dosage schedules are reviewed.

From: *Calcium in Human Health*
Edited by: C. M. Weaver and R. P. Heaney © Humana Press Inc., Totowa, NJ

Table 1
Determinants of Calcium Absorption

- Calcium intake
- Vitamin D and season
- Age
- Race
- Genetics
- Estrogen
- Diet (fiber, fat, alcohol, protein)
- Smoking

2. CALCIUM ABSORPTION AND ITS DETERMINANTS

Compared with most nutrients, calcium is poorly absorbed. On average, only approx 25% of dietary calcium is absorbed. Calcium absorption occurs by several different mechanisms including active transport, passive diffusion, and solvent drag. Active transport involves movement of calcium from the intestinal lumen into enterocytes and then out on the serosal side. Passive diffusion involves movement of calcium between enterocytes by way of the paracellular shunt pathway. The amount of calcium absorbed by passive diffusion is proportional to the luminal:serosal calcium concentration gradient. Absorption of calcium by solvent drag also utilizes the paracellular shunt pathway and occurs after the ingestion of an osmotic load. Many factors influence calcium absorption efficiency (Table 1), as described here.

2.1. Calcium Intake

Calcium intake is the most important determinant of absorbed calcium. Absorbed calcium increases with increasing intake, but the relationship between the two is non-linear *(1)*, as illustrated in Fig. 1. The flattening of the slope at an intake of about 500 mg/d reflects the saturation of the active transport component of absorption. The increase in absorbed calcium as intake exceeds 500 mg/d occurs by passive diffusion.

With dietary calcium restriction, the amount of absorbed calcium declines but the fraction of a calcium load absorbed increases *(2–4)*. Calcium restriction induces a subtle decrease in the blood calcium concentration, a rise in parathyroid hormone (PTH) secretion, stimulation of renal 1,25 dihydroxyvitamin D ($1,25[OH]_2D_3$) production, and increased calcium absorption by active transport. The timing of these hormonal and absorption changes is illustrated in Fig. 2 *(5)*. In this study, healthy adult Caucasian (dashed lines) and black (solid lines) women were placed on 2000-mg calcium diets for 8 wk, and then on calcium-restricted (300 mg/d) diets for 8 wk. Hormone levels and whole-body retention of ^{47}Ca, an index of calcium absorption, were measured at time zero (after 8 wk on the high-calcium diet) and repeatedly during the low-calcium intake period. Significant adaptation occurred by the end of the first week of calcium restriction, and both the regulatory hormone levels and fractional calcium retention stabilized after 2 wk.

2.2. Vitamin D Status and Season

Active transport of calcium across the intestine is stimulated by the vitamin D metabolite, $1,25(OH)_2D_3$, a compound that acts on enterocyte nuclear receptors to initiate the

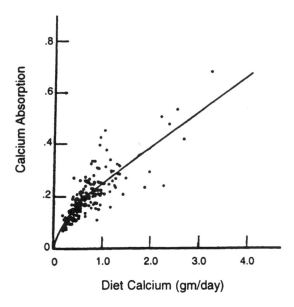

Fig. 1. Calcium absorption from diet (grams per day) as a function of dietary calcium intake. (From Heaney et al. *[1]*, with permission.)

synthesis of separate calcium and phosphorus transport proteins. Whereas it is widely recognized that $1,25(OH)_2D_3$ promotes calcium absorption, several recent reports have focused on the possibility that 25 hydroxyvitamin D (25[OH]D) also stimulates calcium absorption, based on positive associations between serum 25(OH)D levels and calcium absorption *(6–8)*. As illustrated in Fig. 3, calcium absorption increases progressively as 25(OH)D levels rise throughout and above the upper end of the 25(OH)D reference range *(6)*. In this study, serum 25(OH)D and $1,25(OH)_2D_3$ levels were approximately equal determinants of calcium absorption. The authors concluded that, compared with $1,25(OH)_2D_3$, the weaker binding affinity of 25(OH)D to the vitamin D receptor was offset by the approx 1000-fold higher concentration of 25(OH)D in the circulation *(6)*. In one of the populations cited above *(8)*, calcium absorption and $1,25(OH)_2D_3$ were not significantly correlated *(8)*. In another study, supplementation with vitamin D_3 increased the serum 25(OH)D level and calcium absorption, but produced no change in the serum $1,25(OH)_2D_3$ level *(9)*. It will be important to gain additional evidence to define the 25(OH)D level at which calcium absorption is maximal for different populations. In the temperate zone where sun exposure does not promote cutaneous synthesis of vitamin D in the winter, calcium absorption has been shown to be lower in winter than in summer *(10,11)*, presumably because vitamin D levels are lower in the winter.

2.3. Age and Race

Calcium absorption declines with age in men and women *(12–14)*. Several mechanisms may be involved. Ebeling et al. *(15)* postulated an age-related resistance to the action of $1,25(OH)_2D_3$ at the gut after finding an age-related decline in the $1,25(OH)_2D_3$ receptor concentration in human duodenal mucosal biopsy specimens. Consistent with this is the finding that blood levels of $1,25(OH)_2D_3$ rise with age *(15,16)*. There is no consensus however that gut resistance to $1,25(OH)_2D_3$ accounts for declining calcium

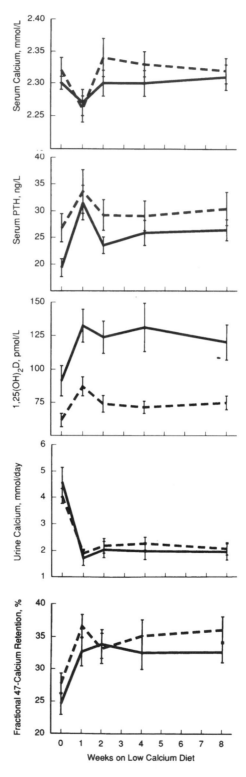

Fig. 2. Mean hormonal, biochemical, and fractional [47]Ca retention values in 15 black (solid lines) and 15 white (dashed lines) women after 8 wk on a 2000-mg calcium diet (week zero) and after 1, 2, 4, and 8 wk on a 300-mg calcium diet. (From Dawson-Hughes et al. *[5]*, with permission.)

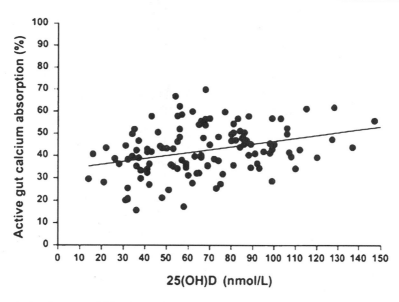

Fig. 3. Association between 25 hydroxyvitamin D and intestinal calcium absorption in postmenopausal women. (From Devine et al. *[6]*, with permission.)

absorption. Others propose that calcium absorption declines as a result of an age-related decline in 25(OH)D and 1,25(OH)$_2$D$_3$ concentrations. Two groups have reported an age-related decrease in renal production of 1,25(OH)$_2$D$_3$ in response to infusion of a single dose of teriparatide *(17,18)*. Several have reported an age-related decline in fasting serum 1,25(OH)$_2$D$_3$ concentrations in women *(14,18,19)*. Orwoll et al. identified no association between serum 1,25(OH)$_2$D$_3$ concentration and age in men *(20)*. Examination of the renal 1-α-hydroxylase response to varying doses of a stimulant, such as teriparatide, in young and older individuals on calcium and vitamin D-replete diets would be one approach to defining the influences of aging on ambient 1,25(OH)$_2$D$_3$ concentrations and on renal 1,25(OH)$_2$D$_3$ production capacity.

Abrams et al. *(21)* found calcium absorption to be greater in black than in white girls. Among adult women, calcium absorption was similar in blacks and whites and the timing of their adaptations to calcium restriction were similar *(5)*. However, as shown in Fig. 2, the black women had higher concentrations of 1,25(OH)$_2$D$_3$ than white women, suggesting that they may have a gut resistance to the action of the active vitamin D metabolite *(5)*.

2.4. Genetics

There is some evidence that calcium absorption has an hereditary component (22,23). Alleles of the vitamin D receptor (VDR) were originally reported by Morrison et al. *(24)* to be associated with bone mineral density (BMD) in adult twins and in unrelated post-menopausal women, although this was not a consistent finding *(25)* (*see* Chapter 26). Morrison found that women with alleles designated bb had higher BMD than women with alleles designated BB *(24)*. That association appears to be stronger in women with very low calcium intakes *(26)*. Because the 1,25(OH)$_2$D$_3$ receptor plays a central role in intestinal calcium absorption, VDR alleles might influence bone at least in part by affecting calcium absorption efficiency at low to moderate calcium intake levels, those at which the active transport mode of absorption predominates. This hypothesis gained support with the demonstration that postmenopausal women with BB and bb alleles had similar levels of fractional calcium absorption on high (1500 mg) calcium intakes, but that women with the BB genotype had blunted increases in fractional calcium absorption when calcium intake was lowered to 300 mg/d *(22)*. This study suggests the presence of a hereditary–environmental interaction. The Fok I polymorphism at the VDR transcription site also predicts calcium absorption and BMD in children *(27)*. Other studies however have not seen an association of calcium absorption with intestinal VDRs *(8,28)*. The precision of the VDR number assessment has not been specifically defined and poor reproducibility in the method may have limited ability to see an association in studies with small numbers of subjects.

2.5. Estrogen

Estrogen increases intestinal calcium absorption in postmenopausal women *(29)* by preserving the normal intestinal responsiveness to $1,25(OH)_2D_3$ *(30)* and perhaps by other mechanisms. Thus, in women, loss of estrogen at menopause is likely to cause a decline in calcium absorption efficiency.

2.6. Diet Composition

Diets high in fiber reduce the bioavailability of dietary calcium. This is illustrated in the study by Knox and colleagues, in which a high-fiber diet reduced calcium retention under both acidic and pH-neutral conditions *(31)*. Several mechanisms have been proposed. In the gut, calcium binds to fiber in proportion to its phytate content and bound calcium has reduced bioavailability. In addition, fiber decreases gut transit time. Barger-Lux et al. *(8)* have demonstrated that a rapid transit time is associated with lower calcium absorption. The source of fiber is important with respect to its effect on calcium absorption. For example, wheat fiber has a more deleterious effect on calcium availability than vegetable fiber.

Dietary fat has been associated with reduced calcium absorption in healthy adult women *(32)*, although the mechanism is unknown. In the same study, high alcohol intake was associated with reduced calcium absorption *(32)*.

Dietary protein may affect intestinal calcium absorption but the evidence for this is mixed. Rats on high-protein diets appear to compensate for increased urinary calcium losses by increasing net calcium absorption *(33)*. Lutz and Linksweiler found that increased protein intake significantly increased net calcium absorption and urinary calcium excretion in postmenopausal women *(34)*. In young women with a mean calcium intake of 800 mg/d, decreasing protein intake from 158 to 52 g/d lowered calcium absorption over the following 4 d, consistent with at least a transient effect of dietary protein on absorption *(35)*. Longer term balance studies in humans, however, have found little to no effect of dietary protein on calcium absorption *(36–40)*.

2.7. Smoking

Smoking increases rates of bone loss in older men and women, and several studies suggest that one mechanism involves decreased calcium absorption. In 402 older men and women, absorption was approx 12% lower in current smokers than in nonsmokers *(41)*. The smokers in this study also had a smaller increase in urinary calcium excretion in response to supplementation with calcium and vitamin D, which is consistent with their lower calcium absorption. Smoking is known to lower estrogen levels, and this may be one mechanism by which calcium absorption is impaired.

2.8. Physical Activity

Physical activity increases bone mass and it may increase calcium absorption efficiency. This has been suggested in a cross-sectional study in adult women (32) and in a comparative study of young male athletes and age-matched sedentary controls (42). However, it is difficult to isolate the effect of physical activity from other dietary and lifestyle factors that differ in active and inactive subjects. For example, in the latter study in males (42), the athletes had higher calcium intakes, lower alcohol intakes, and smoked less than the control subjects. An exercise intervention trial is required to define the effect of activity on calcium absorption.

2.9. Calcium Absorption and the Skeleton

Calcium absorption is lower in osteoporotics than in age-matched controls (12,43,44). Nordin et al. (45) demonstrated a positive correlation between rate of calcium absorption and vertebral bone density in osteoporotic women. Francis et al. (46) found blunted calcium absorption responses to vitamin D replacement in vitamin D-deficient osteoporotics compared with those of similarly deficient nonosteoporotics. Krall and Dawson-Hughes reported a significant negative correlation between whole-body [47]Ca retention, an index of calcium absorption, and rates of bone loss in healthy postmenopausal women (11). In an observational study of women age 65 yr and older, Ensrud and colleagues (47) observed that low fractional calcium absorption was associated with increased risk of hip fracture among women with low calcium intakes.

3. CALCIUM AND BONE

3.1. Bone Remodeling

The bone turnover rate is a major determinant of bone strength. It increases with age, and is an independent predictor of fracture (48–50). Calcium is a substrate for bone mineralization, and it also lowers the bone turnover rate. Increases in calcium intake, within the range usually consumed, induce modest reductions in the blood PTH concentration (51–54) and this is thought to lower the bone-remodeling rate. The magnitude of the reduction in remodeling with calcium is directly related to the dose of calcium given (55) and inversely related to the starting calcium intake of the study subjects. The reduction appears to be greater in the elderly, probably because older individuals generally have higher remodeling rates than younger people with similar calcium intakes. In healthy subjects age 65 yr and older with a habitual mean calcium intake of about 750 mg/d, daily supplementation with 500 mg of calcium and 700 IU of vitamin D lowered the mean serum osteocalcin concentration by 9% in the men and 14% in the women during the 3-yr intervention period (54). Other studies have shown similar reductions in postmenopausal women treated with calcium alone (56,57). A smaller reduction was seen in another study (55), probably because the mean calcium intake of the women at entry was relatively high.

3.2. Bone Mineral Density

Calcium, by reducing the bone-remodeling rate, produces an increase in BMD or a reduction in the rate of loss over the initial 6–12 mo of treatment. This change, known as the bone-remodeling transient, was described originally by Frost *(58)* and confirmed subsequently by others. The early increase in density that occurs with closure of the remodeling space cannot be used to estimate cumulative effects of long-term supplementation on BMD, but measured rates of bone change during the second and subsequent years on calcium can be used.

Many randomized, controlled calcium intervention trials examining the effect of calcium on change in BMD have been conducted. In a recent review, Heaney summarized the results of 34 controlled trials and observed that in all but 2, increasing calcium intake reduced or halted age-related bone loss at one skeletal site or another *(59)*. In a more formal meta-analysis of 12 trials conducted in postmenopausal women, Cumming found that calcium supplements reduced the rate of bone loss by 50%, or by an average of 0.8% per year, in postmenopausal women *(60)*. On further analysis, Cumming observed that calcium supplements were most effective in studies in which baseline calcium intake was low, age was greater, and the subjects had clinical evidence of osteoporosis *(60)*. His analyses also supported the widely held view that there is a threshold of calcium intake above which more calcium is not beneficial. A more recent meta-analysis of 15 trials (1806 subjects) found supplemental calcium to reduce bone loss by an average of 2.02% after 2 or more years of therapy compared with placebo *(61)*.

3.3. Changes in Bone Mineral Density After Stopping Calcium Supplements

The effect of stopping calcium supplements on BMD has recently been examined in healthy men and women age 65 yr and older *(62)*. These subjects had taken either 500 mg of calcium and 700 IU of vitamin D or double placebo daily for 3 yr. The study supplements were then stopped, and BMD measurements were made 1 and 2 yr later. During the 2-yr follow-up period, subjects were free to take their own calcium supplements, and one-half of the subjects reported taking supplements at least some of the time over that period. As shown in Fig. 4, the BMD gains at the femoral neck and total body caused by the calcium and vitamin D were lost within 2 yr of stopping the supplements *(62)*. In addition, group differences in biochemical markers of bone turnover, significant after 3 yr, were no longer significant after 2 yr off of the supplements. These findings suggest that an adequate intake of these nutrients must be sustained in order to retain the skeletal benefit.

3.4. Fractures

Several investigators have reported the effect of added calcium on fracture incidence *(57,63–65)*. Most of these studies were designed to detect changes in BMD and are thus too small to establish either the presence or magnitude of an effect of calcium on fracture rates. One of these trials did have a planned fracture endpoint *(62)*. In this study, 197 postmenopausal women with a mean dietary calcium intake of 433 mg/d were randomly assigned to treatment with 1200 mg of elemental calcium per day or placebo *(63)*. Spine X-rays were taken at the beginning and end of the study. Calcium supplementation reduced the vertebral fracture rate in a high-risk subset of 94 women with pre-existing

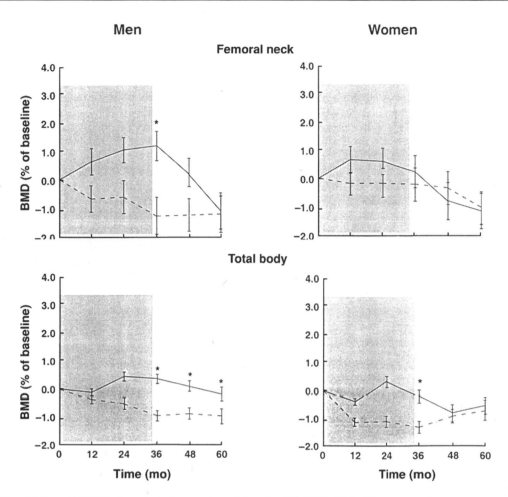

Fig. 4. Mean (±SEM) changes in bone mineral density (BMD) in 295 older men and women treated with placebo (dashed lines) or calcium and vitamin D (solid lines) for 3 yr (shaded areas) and followed-up for 2 yr with no supplementation. *Significantly different from the placebo group, $p < 0.05$. (From Dawson-Hughes et al. [62], with permission.)

spine fractures, but not in the 103 women without pre-existing spine fractures. Two meta-analyses have addressed calcium intake and fractures. Cumming and Nevitt found calcium to lower fracture risk by 4% for each 300 mg increase in calcium intake (66). Shea et al. reported the relative risk of fracture of the vertebrae was 0.77 (95% confidence interval [CI] 0.54–1.09); the relative risk (RR) for nonvertebral fractures was 0.86 (95% CI 0.43–1.72) (61). The wide confidence intervals reflect the uncertainty about the impact of calcium alone on fracture rates.

Two studies have examined the effect of combined calcium and vitamin D supplementation on fracture incidence (54,67). Chapuy et al. (67) studied more than 3000 very elderly institutionalized women who had an average dietary calcium intake of about 500 mg/d and very low serum 25(OH)D levels. They were treated for 3 yr with placebo or 1200 mg of calcium and 800 IU of vitamin D per day. The supplemented group had

30% fewer hip and other nonvertebral fractures than did the women treated with placebo. In 389 men and women, age 65 yr and older, supplementation with 500 mg of calcium and 700 IU of vitamin D daily for 3 yr significantly lowered nonvertebral fracture rates (RR 0.5; 95% CI, 0.2 to 0.9; $p = 0.02$) *(53)*. The individual contributions of calcium and vitamin D in these two studies cannot be determined but these contributions are probably inversely related to the starting calcium and vitamin D intakes of the specific study population.

3.5. Role of Calcium in Patients Receiving Pharmacotherapy for Osteoporosis

In recent trials examining the antifracture efficacy of drugs for osteoporosis, calcium and vitamin D have been given to both the treatment and control groups. Thus, the benefits demonstrated with alendronate, risedronate, raloxifene, calcitonin, and teriparatide are above and beyond those derived from calcium and vitamin D *(68–72)*. Because the efficacy of these drugs has not been demonstrated in calcium and vitamin D-deficient patients, one cannot assume that deficient patients would get the same benefit from pharmacotherapy as supplemented patients. In a meta-analysis of estrogen intervention studies, Nieves et al. found that calcium enhanced the effectiveness of estrogen therapy on bone density *(73)*. Estrogen, like alendronate, risedronate, raloxifene, and calcitonin, has predominantly antiresorptive effects on bone. It is therefore reasonable to assume that antiresorptive drugs will be more effective in the presence than in the absence of an adequate calcium intake. It would seem even more plausible that an adequate calcium intake is needed to support bone growth during treatment with the anabolic drug, teriparatide.

4. CALCIUM REQUIREMENT AND SOURCES

On the basis of the studies cited above and other evidence, The National Academy of Sciences revised its recommendation for calcium intake from 800 to 1200 mg/d for healthy men and women age 51 yr and older *(74)*.

The preferred approach to achieving optimal calcium intake is through consumption of natural foods, but other options, such as fortified foods and supplements, are available. The challenge of effectively fortifying food with calcium when the prevalence of inadequacy is not uniform across the population recently has been demonstrated by Johnson-Down et al. *(75)*. They reported that in Canada, the prevalence of calcium inadequacy is very low in young adult males and high in older women. Their models predict that fortification of commonly consumed energy sources to raise the intakes of older women would render a significant number of young males above the safe upper limit for calcium *(75)*.

Supplements are an important source of calcium for individuals who cannot or will not achieve optimal calcium intakes from food. Many different supplements including calcium acetate, carbonate, citrate, citrate malate, glubionate, lactate, lactogluconate, and tricalcium phosphate are available. Use of unrefined calcium supplements such as bone meal or dolomite should be discouraged, because these sources may contain lead and other toxic contaminants *(76)*.

Calcium absorbability is influenced by the study conditions, such as the presence or absence of a test meal and the size of the test calcium load. Although supplement solubility (in water at neutral pH) is only weakly related to absorbability *(77)*, disintegration of tablets is required for absorption. Under similar study conditions (a standardized breakfast meal containing 250 mg of elemental calcium), fractional calcium absorption was a little higher from calcium citrate malate and similar from carbonate, tricalcium phosphate, and milk *(77–80)*. The studies were conducted in healthy volunteers under age 30 yr and it is unknown whether absorbability from these sources in the elderly is proportional. Differences in absorbability of these supplement sources are generally offset by differences in their calcium contents, so that the amounts of calcium absorbed per gram of supplement are fairly similar.

As indicated previously, absorbed calcium is dependent upon the dose of calcium consumed. Absorption rises rapidly as the dose increases to about 500 mg, and it rises more gradually as intake increases above this level (the point at which active transport mechanism becomes saturated) (Fig.1). Thus, to maximize utilization of calcium from supplements or from calcium-rich foods, calcium should be taken in doses of 500 mg or less *(1,81)*.

In healthy individuals, absorption of calcium from carbonate is more consistent and reproducible when this supplement is taken with a meal than when it is taken during a fast *(81)*. In individuals with reduced gastric acid production, absorption of calcium from carbonate is diminished under fasting conditions, but normal in a meal setting *(82)*. The prevalence of achlorhydria, an asymptomatic condition, rises with aging. Among healthy men and women age 65 yr and older, 67% had consistent acid secretion, 22% had intermittent secretion, and 11% had no secretion *(83)*.

A dose of calcium at bedtime has reduced the nocturnal rise in the bone-resorbing agent PTH *(84)*, but this has not been a consistent finding *(85)*. It is not known whether supplement use at bedtime favors bone conservation.

There is a wide margin between recommended calcium intakes and intakes associated with adverse events. High intakes of calcium from food sources have been associated with lower incidence of first renal stones in men *(86)* and women *(87)*. High intakes from supplements may be associated with a slight increase in risk of first stone in women *(87)* but not in men *(86)*. Based on these and other data, the National Academy of Sciences identified a safe upper limit for calcium of 2500 mg/d *(74)*.

Individuals may develop constipation or bloating from use of calcium carbonate, but this can be resolved by changing to a different calcium source. Some calcium sources may interfere with the absorption of iron, zinc, and trace minerals. Further study is needed to identify and define the clinical impact of nutrient–nutrient interactions.

5. CONCLUSIONS

Increasing calcium intake to recommended levels, in the presence of adequate vitamin D, induces a sustained lowering of rates of bone remodeling and bone loss in elderly men and women. These changes may be accompanied by a significant reduction in fracture incidence, but this has not yet been firmly established. Sporadic supplement use does not appear to have a long-term effect on the skeleton. Thus, continuous consumption of and adequate amount of calcium (and vitamin D) is needed to achieve lasting skeletal benefit.

ACKNOWLEDGMENT/DISCLAIMER

This material is based on work supported by the US Department of Agriculture, under agreement No. 58-1950-9001. Any opinions, findings, conclusions, or recommendations expressed in this publication are those of the authors, and do not necessarily reflect the view of the US Department of Agriculture.

REFERENCES

1. Heaney RP, Saville PD, Recker RR. Calcium absorption as a function of calcium intake. J Lab Clin Med 1975;85(6):881–890.
2. Bronner F, Harris R.S. Absorption and metabolism of calcium in human beings, studied with calcium 45. Ann NY Acad Sci 1956;64:314–325.
3. Spencer H, Lewin I, Fowler J, Samachson J. Influence of dietary calcium intake on Ca47 absorption in man. Am J Med 1969;46(2):197–205.
4. Heaney RP, Recker RR, Stegman MR, Moy AJ. Calcium absorption in women: relationships to calcium intake, estrogen status, and age. J Bone Miner Res 1989;4(4):469–475.
5. Dawson-Hughes B, Harris S, Kramich C, Dallal G, Rasmussen HM. Calcium retention and hormone levels in black and white women on high- and low-calcium diets. J Bone Miner Res 1993;8(7):779–787.
6. Devine A, Wilson SG, Dick IM, Prince RL. Effects of vitamin D metabolites on intestinal calcium absorption and bone turnover in elderly women. Am J Clin Nutr 2002;75(2):283–288.
7. Heaney RP, Dowell MS, Hale CA, Bendich A. Calcium absorption varies within the reference range for serum 25-hydroxyvitamin D. J Am Coll Nutr 2003;22(2):142–146.
8. Barger-Lux MJ, Heaney RP, Lanspa SJ, Healy JC, DeLuca HF. An investigation of sources of variation in calcium absorption efficiency. J Clin Endocrinol Metab 1995;80(2):406–411.
9. Heaney RP, Barger-Lux MJ, Dowell MS, Chen TC, Holick MF. Calcium absorptive effects of vitamin D and its major metabolites. J Clin Endocrinol Metab 1997;82(12):4111–4116.
10. Malm OJ. Calcium requirement and adaptation in adult men. Scand J Clin Lab Invest 1958;36(Suppl):1–280.
11. Krall EA, Dawson-Hughes B. Relation of fractional 47Ca retention to season and rates of bone loss in healthy postmenopausal women. J Bone Miner Res 1991;6(12):1323–1329.
12. Avioli LV, McDonald JE, Lee SW. The influence of age on the intestinal absorption of 47-Ca absorption in post-menopausal osteoporosis. J Clin Invest 1965;44(12):1960–1967.
13. Bullamore JR, Wilkinson R, Gallagher JC, Nordin BE, Marshall DH. Effect of age on calcium absorption. Lancet 1970;2(7672):535–537.
14. Gallagher JC, Riggs BL, Eisman J, Hamstra A, Arnaud SB, DeLuca HF. Intestinal calcium absorption and serum vitamin D metabolites in normal subjects and osteoporotic patients: effect of age and dietary calcium. J Clin Invest 1979;64(3):729–736.
15. Ebeling PR, Sandgren ME, DiMagno EP, Lane AW, DeLuca HF, Riggs BL. Evidence of an age-related decrease in intestinal responsiveness to vitamin D: relationship between serum 1,25-dihydroxyvitamin D3 and intestinal vitamin D receptor concentrations in normal women. J Clin Endocrinol Metab 1992;75(1):176–182.
16. Eastell R, Yergey AL, Vieira NE, Cedel SL, Kumar R, Riggs BL. Interrelationship among vitamin D metabolism, true calcium absorption, parathyroid function, and age in women: evidence of an age-related intestinal resistance to 1,25-dihydroxyvitamin D action. J Bone Miner Res 1991;6(2):125–132.
17. Slovik DM, Adams JS, Neer RM, Holick MF, Potts JT, Jr. Deficient production of 1,25-dihydroxyvitamin D in elderly osteoporotic patients. N Engl J Med 1981;305(7):372–374.
18. Tsai KS, Heath H, III, Kumar R, Riggs BL. Impaired vitamin D metabolism with aging in women. Possible role in pathogenesis of senile osteoporosis. J Clin Invest 1984;73(6):1668–1672.
19. Fujisawa Y, Kida K, Matsuda H. Role of change in vitamin D metabolism with age in calcium and phosphorus metabolism in normal human subjects. J Clin Endocrinol Metab 1984;59(4):719–726.
20. Orwoll ES, Meier DE. Alterations in calcium, vitamin D, and parathyroid hormone physiology in normal men with aging: relationship to the development of senile osteopenia. J Clin Endocrinol Metab 1986;63(6):1262–1269.

21. Abrams SA, O'Brien KO, Liang LK, Stuff JE. Differences in calcium absorption and kinetics between black and white girls aged 5–16 years. J Bone Miner Res 1995;10(5):829–833.

22. Dawson-Hughes B, Harris SS, Finneran S. Calcium absorption on high and low calcium intakes in relation to vitamin D receptor genotype. J Clin Endocrinol Metab 1995;80(12):3657–3661.

23. Wishart JM, Horowitz M, Need AG, et al. Relations between calcium intake, calcitriol, polymorphisms of the vitamin D receptor gene, and calcium absorption in premenopausal women. Am J Clin Nutr 1997;65(3):798–802.

24. Morrison NA, Qi JC, Tokita A, et al. Prediction of bone density from vitamin D receptor alleles. Nature 1994;367(6460):284–287.

25. Hustmyer FG, Peacock M, Hui S, Johnston CC, Christian J. Bone mineral density in relation to polymorphism at the vitamin D receptor gene locus. J Clin Invest 1994;94(5):2130–2134.

26. Krall EA, Parry P, Lichter JB, Dawson-Hughes B. Vitamin D receptor alleles and rates of bone loss: influences of years since menopause and calcium intake. J Bone Miner Res 1995;10(6):978–984.

27. Ames SK, Ellis KJ, Gunn SK, Copeland KC, Abrams SA. Vitamin D receptor gene Fok1 polymorphism predicts calcium absorption and bone mineral density in children. J Bone Miner Res 1999;14(5):740–746.

28. Kinyamu HK, Gallagher JC, Prahl JM, DeLuca HF, Petranick KM, Lanspa SJ. Association between intestinal vitamin D receptor, calcium absorption, and serum 1,25 dihydroxyvitamin D in normal young and elderly women. J Bone Miner Res 1997;12(6):922–928.

29. Gallagher JC, Riggs BL, DeLuca HF. Effect of estrogen on calcium absorption and serum vitamin D metabolites in postmenopausal osteoporosis. J Clin Endocrinol Metab 1980;51(6):1359–1364.

30. Gennari C, Agnusdei D, Nardi P, Civitelli R. Estrogen preserves a normal intestinal responsiveness to 1,25-dihydroxyvitamin D3 in oophorectomized women. J Clin Endocrinol Metab 1990;71(5):1288–1293.

31. Knox TA, Kassarjian Z, Dawson-Hughes B, et al. Calcium absorption in elderly subjects on high- and low-fiber diets: effect of gastric acidity. Am J Clin Nutr 1991;53(6):1480–1486.

32. Wolf RL, Cauley JA, Baker CE, et al. Factors associated with calcium absorption efficiency in pre- and perimenopausal women. Am J Clin Nutr 2000;72(2):466–471.

33. Whiting SJ, Draper HH. Effect of chronic high protein feeding on bone composition in the adult rat. J Nutr 1981;111(1):178–183.

34. Lutz J, Linkswiler HM. Calcium metabolism in postmenopausal and osteoporotic women consuming two levels of dietary protein. Am J Clin Nutr 1981;34(10):2178–2186.

35. Kerstetter JE, O'Brien KO, Insogna KL. Dietary protein affects intestinal calcium absorption. Am J Clin Nutr 1998;68(4):859–865.

36. Hegsted M, Linkswiler HM. Long term effects of level of protein intake on calcium metabolism in young adult women. J Nutr 1981;111(2):244–251.

37. Heaney RP, Recker RR. Effects of nitrogen, phosphorus, and caffeine on calcium balance in women. J Lab Clin Med 1982;99(1):46–55.

38. Spencer H, Kramer L, Osis D, Norris C. Effect of a high protein (meat) intake on calcium metabolism in man. Am J Clin Nutr 1978;31(12):2167–2180.

39. Heaney RP, Recker RR. Effects of nitrogen, phosphorus, and caffeine on calcium balance in women. J Lab Clin Med 1982;99(1):46–55.

40. Spencer H, Kramer L, Osis D, Norris C. Effect of a high protein (meat) intake on calcium metabolism in man. Am J Clin Nutr 1978;31(12):2167–2180.

41. Krall EA, Dawson-Hughes B. Smoking increases bone loss and decreases intestinal calcium absorption. J Bone Miner Res 1999;14(2):215–220.

42. Zittermann A, Sabatschus O, Jantzen S, et al. Exercise-trained young men have higher calcium absorption rates and plasma calcitriol levels compared with age-matched sedentary controls. Calcif Tissue Int 2000;67(3):215–219.

43. Gallagher JC, Aaron J, Horsman A, Marshall DH, Wilkinson R, Nordin BE. The crush fracture syndrome in postmenopausal women. Clin Endocrinol Metab 1973;2(2):293–315.

44. Morris HA, Need AG, Horowitz M, O'Loughlin PD, Nordin BE. Calcium absorption in normal and osteoporotic postmenopausal women. Calcif Tissue Int 1991;49(4):240–243.

45. Nordin BE, Robertson A, Seamark RF, et al. The relation between calcium absorption, serum dehydroepiandrosterone, and vertebral mineral density in postmenopausal women. J Clin Endocrinol Metab 1985;60(4):651–657.

46. Francis RM, Peacock M, Taylor GA, Storer JH, Nordin BE. Calcium malabsorption in elderly women with vertebral fractures: evidence for resistance to the action of vitamin D metabolites on the bowel. Clin Sci 1984;66(1):103–107.

47. Ensrud KE, Duong T, Cauley JA, et al. Low fractional calcium absorption increases the risk for hip fracture in women with low calcium intake. Study of Osteoporotic Fractures Research Group. Ann Intern Med 2000;132(5):345–353.

48. Garnero P, Hausherr E, Chapuy MC, et al. Markers of bone resorption predict hip fracture in elderly women: the EPIDOS Prospective Study. J Bone Miner Res 1996;11(10):1531–1538.

49. Parfitt AM. High bone turnover is intrinsically harmful: two paths to a similar conclusion. The Parfitt view. J Bone Miner Res 2002;17(8):1558–1559.

50. Melton LJ, III, Chrischilles EA, Cooper C, Lane AW, Riggs BL. Perspective. How many women have osteoporosis? J Bone Miner Res 1992;7(9):1005–1010.

51. Chapuy MC, Chapuy P, Meunier PJ. Calcium and vitamin D supplements: effects on calcium metabolism in elderly people. Am J Clin Nutr 1987;46(2):324–328.

52. Dawson-Hughes B, Dallal GE, Krall EA, Sadowski L, Sahyoun N, Tannenbaum S. A controlled trial of the effect of calcium supplementation on bone density in postmenopausal women. N Engl J Med 1990;323(13):878–883.

53. Kochersberger G, Bales C, Lobaugh B, Lyles KW. Calcium supplementation lowers serum parathyroid hormone levels in elderly subjects. J Gerontol 1990;45(5):M159–M162.

54. Dawson-Hughes B, Harris SS, Krall EA, Dallal GE. Effect of Calcium and Vitamin D Supplementation on Bone Density in Men and Women 65 Years of Age or Older. N Engl J Med 1997;337(10):670–676.

55. Elders PJ, Netelenbos JC, Lips P, et al. Calcium supplementation reduces vertebral bone loss in perimenopausal women: a controlled trial in 248 women between 46 and 55 years of age. J Clin Endocrinol Metab 1991;73(3):533–540.

56. Riis B, Thomsen K, Christiansen C. Does calcium supplementation prevent postmenopausal bone loss? A double-blind, controlled clinical study. N Engl J Med 1987;316(4):173–177.

57. Chevalley T, Rizzoli R, Nydegger V, et al. Effects of calcium supplements on femoral bone mineral density and vertebral fracture rate in vitamin-D-replete elderly patients. Osteoporos Int 1994;4(5):245–252.

58. Frost HM. The origin and nature of transients in human bone remodeling dynamics. In: Frame B, Parfitt M, Duncan H, eds. Clinical Aspects of Metabolic Bone Disease. Excerpta Medica, Amsterdam: 1973: pp. 124–137.

59. Heaney RP. Calcium, dairy products and osteoporosis. J Am Coll Nutr 2000;19(2:Suppl):99S.

60. Cumming RG. Calcium intake and bone mass: a quantitative review of the evidence. Calcif Tissue Int 1990;47(4):194–201.

61. Shea B, Wells G, Cranney A, et al. Meta-analyses of therapies for postmenopausal osteoporosis. VII. Meta-analysis of calcium supplementation for the prevention of postmenopausal osteoporosis. Endocr Rev 2002;23(4):552–559.

62. Dawson-Hughes B, Harris SS, Krall EA, Dallal GE. Effect of withdrawal of calcium and vitamin D supplements on bone mass in elderly men and women. Am J Clin Nutr 2000;72(3):745–750.

63. Recker RR, Hinders S, Davies KM, et al. Correcting calcium nutritional deficiency prevents spine fractures in elderly women. J Bone Miner Res 1996;11(12):1961–1966.

64. Reid IR, Ames RW, Evans MC, Gamble GD, Sharpe SJ. Long-term effects of calcium supplementation on bone loss and fractures in postmenopausal women: a randomized controlled trial. Am J Med 1995;98(4):331–335.

65. Riggs BL, O'Fallon WM, Muhs J, O'Connor MK, Kumar R, Melton LJ, III. Long-term effects of calcium supplementation on serum parathyroid hormone level, bone turnover, and bone loss in elderly women. J Bone Miner Res 1998;13(2):168–174.

66. Cumming RG, Nevitt MC. Calcium for prevention of osteoporotic fractures in postmenopausal women. J Bone Miner Res 1997;12(9):1321–1329.

67. Chapuy MC, Arlot ME, Delmas PD, Meunier PJ. Effect of calcium and cholecalciferol treatment for three years on hip fractures in elderly women. BMJ 1994;308(6936):1081–1082.

68. Black DM, Cummings SR, Karpf DB, et al. Randomised trial of effect of alendronate on risk of fracture in women with existing vertebral fractures. Fracture Intervention Trial Research Group. Lancet 1996;348(9041):1535–1541.

69. Harris ST, Watts NB, Genant HK, et al. Effects of risedronate treatment on vertebral and nonvertebral fractures in women with postmenopausal osteoporosis: a randomized controlled trial. Vertebral Efficacy With Risedronate Therapy (VERT) Study Group.. JAMA 1999;282(14):1344–1352.

70. Ettinger BM, Black DMP, Mitlak BHM, et al. Reduction of Vertebral Fracture Risk in Postmenopausal Women With Osteoporosis Treated With Raloxifene: Results From a 3-Year Randomized Clinical Trial. JAMA 1999;282(7):637–645.

71. Chesnut CH, III, Silverman S, Andriano K, et al. A randomized trial of nasal spray salmon calcitonin in postmenopausal women with established osteoporosis: the prevent recurrence of osteoporotic fractures study. PROOF Study Group. Am J Med 2000;109(4):267–276.

72. Neer RM, Arnaud CD, Zanchetta JR, et al. Effect of Parathyroid Hormone (1-34) on Fractures and Bone Mineral Density in Postmenopausal Women with Osteoporosis. N Engl J Med 2001;344(19):1434–1441.

73. Nieves JW, Komar L, Cosman F, Lindsay R. Calcium potentiates the effect of estrogen and calcitonin on bone mass: review and analysis. Am J Clin Nutr 1998;67(1):18–24.

74. Standing Committee on the Scientific Evaluation of Dietary Reference Intakes. Dietary reference intakes: calcium, phosphorus, magnesium, vitamin D, and fluoride. National Academy Press, Washington, DC: 1997.

75. Johnson-Down L, L'Abbe MR, Lee NS, Gray-Donald K. Appropriate calcium fortification of the food supply presents a challenge. J Nutr 2003;133(7):2232–2238.

76. Bourgoin BP, Evans DR, Cornett JR, Lingard SM, Quattrone AJ. Lead content in 70 brands of dietary calcium supplements. Am J Pub Health 1993;83(8):1155–1160.

77. Heaney RP, Recker RR, Weaver CM. Absorbability of calcium sources: the limited role of solubility. Calcif Tissue Int 1990;46(5):300–304.

78. Smith KT, Heaney RP, Flora L, Hinders SM. Calcium absorption from a new calcium delivery system (CCM). Calcif Tissue Int 1987;41(6):351–352.

79. Miller JZ, Smith DL, Flora L, Slemenda C, Jiang XY, Johnston CC, Jr. Calcium absorption from calcium carbonate and a new form of calcium (CCM) in healthy male and female adolescents. Am J Clin Nutr 1988;48(5):1291–1294.

80. Heaney RP, Smith KT, Recker RR, Hinders SM. Meal effects on calcium absorption. Am J Clin Nutr 1989;49(2):372–376.

81. Harvey JA, Zobitz MM, Pak CY. Dose dependency of calcium absorption: a comparison of calcium carbonate and calcium citrate. J Bone Miner Res 1988;3(3):253–258.

82. Recker RR. Calcium absorption and achlorhydria. N Engl J Med 1985;313(2):70–73.

83. Hurwitz A, Brady DA, Schaal ES, Samloff, MI, Dedon J, Ruhl CE. Gastric acidity in older adults. JAMA 1997;278(8):659–662.

84. Calvo MS, Eastell R, Offord KP, Bergstralh EJ, Burritt MF. Circadian variation in ionized calcium and intact parathyroid hormone: evidence for sex differences in calcium homeostasis. J Clin Endocrinol Metab 1991;72(1):69–76.

85. Karkkainen MUM, Lamberg-Allardt CJE, Ahonen S, Valimaki M. Does it make a difference how and when you take your calcium? The acute effects of calcium on calcium and bone metabolism. Am J Clin Nutr 2001;74:335–342.

86. Curhan GC, Willett WC, Rimm EB, Stampfer MJ. A prospective study of dietary calcium and other nutrients and the risk of symptomatic kidney stones. N Engl J Med 1993;328(12):833–838.

87. Curhan GC, Willett WC, Speizer FE, Spiegelman D, Stampfer MJ. Comparison of dietary calcium with supplemental calcium and other nutrients as factors affecting the risk for kidney stones in women. Ann Intern Med 1997;126(7):497–504.

25 Calcium, Vitamin D, and Cancer

Peter R. Holt

KEY POINTS

- Epidemiological data support preventive effects of calcium administration upon colorectal neoplasia.
- Epidemiological data indicate that greater exposure to sunlight lowers the risk of colorectal, breast, prostate, and ovarian cancers.
- Calcium is the sole nutrient proven to lower the risk of colon adenoma recurrence—higher levels of circulating vitamin D accentuate this effect.
- Calcium and vitamin D act as preventives in part by altering colonic lumenal contents and in part in colonic epithelial cells.

1. INTRODUCTION

Colorectal carcinoma is a common cancer in the Western world. It vies to be the second leading cause of cancer deaths in the United States and affects both men and women equally. This cancer arises from many interactions that involve hereditary and environmental influences *(1)*. Colorectal cancer does not develop abruptly *de novo*, but progresses through a series of anatomical and physiological changes *(2)*. Thus, early in this process, changes in epithelial cell proliferation and differentiation occur while the mucosa appears grossly normal; this is followed by the development of aberrant crypt foci, adenomatous polyps, cancer in polyps, and then frank carcinoma *(3)*. The process of a normal epithelium changing to an adenoma and cancer takes a considerable amount of time, probably 5–10 yr for adenoma formation and perhaps another 10 yr for the development of cancer.

The past 15 yr have seen an explosion of data on the genetic changes that accompany colorectal carcinogenesis. Thus, it has become clear that numerous changes in cellular genes occur during carcinogenesis. However, less than 5% of all colorectal cancer results from a hereditary cause—i.e., familial adenomatous polyposis owing to mutations in the adenomatous polyposis coli (*APC*) gene and hereditary nonpolyposis colon cancer associated with alterations in one or more of the mismatch repair genes. Overall, the gene changes that generally occur early in the colorectal carcinogenesis process include mutations in the *APC* gene and in *ras*; those occurring later include mutations in *p53* *(4)*. This pathway is accompanied by numerous chromosome breaks and deletions. In

From: *Calcium in Human Health*
Edited by: C. M. Weaver and R. P. Heaney © Humana Press Inc., Totowa, NJ

addition, approx 15–20% of colorectal cancers appear to result from changes in mismatch repair genes (such as *MSH1*, *MLH2*, and so on), often because of promoter hypermethylation rather than mutations. These changes in mismatch repair genes result in defects in several DNA repair mechanisms.

Additionally, many lines of evidence point to the crucial importance of the environment in determining the incidence of this tumor. Epidemiological studies demonstrate a vast difference in the incidence of colorectal cancer around the world—more than is likely to result from genetic factors alone *(5)*. The most salient observations pointing to the importance of the environment are data on changes in incidence occurring when populations from low-incidence areas move to high-incidence areas of the world, or vice versa. These differences in incidence appear and can be detected within the life span of the migrating individual *(6)*. Such a change must necessarily come from an altered environment rather than from hereditable causes.

When these latter observations were originally publicized, the focus of research centered on changes in dietary intake, which occurred rapidly and frequently in the migrating individuals. Overall, a high-risk diet was thought to include excess calories and to be high in fat content and meat products and relatively low in fiber content. From these initial observations came a theory that a high-fat diet might lead to the passage of lipids and bile acids from the small intestine into the colonic lumen where they "irritate" the colonic mucosa *(7)*. This could result both in initiation and promotion of the process of tumorigenesis. Studies in which human volunteers consumed large quantities of fat showed an increase in the excretion of both bile acids and fatty acids in the stool accompanied by a change in fecal bile acid pattern *(8,9)*. In other studies, the interaction of these compounds with the intestinal epithelium was shown to result in mucosal damage, release of mucosal prostaglandins, and alterations in epithelial cell proliferation.

In order to evaluate the potential of a noxious agent to induce cancer or a preventive agent to lower the risk of cancer, one generally uses epidemiological information, data from cell culture and in vivo animal studies, human intervention data, and studies of mechanisms of action. These observations do not always occur sequentially, as is exemplified by the data on calcium and vitamin D.

The early epidemiological data on the effects of calcium and vitamin D on colorectal neoplasia did not show consistent positive results, although some observations were quite dramatic *(10)*. This led to the conclusion that calcium intake might not be associated with a lower risk of colon neoplasia *(11,12)*. However, more recent studies, including re-evaluation of the studies of previous authors, have shown some protective effects of both calcium and vitamin D dietary intake or dairy intake and colorectal cancer (Table 1). An increasing number of studies also have shown a reduction in colorectal adenoma incidence with increased dietary calcium or vitamin D intake or the taking of supplements.

2. VITAMIN D AND COLON CANCER

Human body stores of vitamin D are supplied from both the diet and the sun. Because the greatest source for the body stores derives from the conversion of (7α) dehydrocholesterol in the skin by the sun's ultraviolet radiation, the importance of increased sun exposure, or the deleterious effect on colorectal cancer incidence of the inhibition of such radiation by air pollution, has received considerable attention *(13,14)*. An early suggestion of the beneficial effect of sun exposure with regard to colorectal cancer development came from the epidemiological observations of Garland and Garland, who described an inverse north–south gradient for this tumor (15). Subsequent studies have confirmed these observations (16) and recently have extended them to a series of additional cancers, including cancer of the breast, prostate, and ovary (17). The observations on colorectal cancer led to a nested case–control study (18) in which serum samples taken many years before colon cancer development were analyzed for concentrations of 25 hydroxyvitamin D (25[OH]D) in the blood. Serum levels of above 20 ng/mL were associated with a 50% lower colon cancer incidence than in subjects with serum concentrations below this value. Other studies have confirmed these data (19). Solar radiation, higher levels of vitamin D intake in the diet, and increased blood 25(OH)D levels also have been associated with lower rates of breast cancer incidence (20–22).

3. CALCIUM AND COLON CANCER

A seminal observation that led to the introduction of calcium administration to lower the risk of colorectal neoplasia in humans came from a conceptual theory of the interaction of fatty acids, bile acids, and calcium (7). If the colonic epithelia were to be damaged by luminal fatty acids and bile acids, these would have to be dissociated to interact with colonic epithelial cells. The concept developed by Newmark and co-workers was based on the propensity of calcium to precipitate these acids out of solution. Subsequent studies clearly demonstrated that calcium could lower the aqueous concentrations of fecal fatty acids and bile acids (23). Several studies were performed in animals to show that feeding calcium lowered the incidence of carcinogen-induced colon cancer and reversed the hyperproliferation induced by feeding bile acids (24). Subsequently, a series of human studies were performed which focused on alterations of the proliferative pattern from a higher to a lower risk pattern in colorectal biopsies following calcium administration (25–27).

To study preventive agents for colorectal neoplasia in humans, it is necessary to use what are called intermediate biomarkers of risk to evaluate effects rather than using, as an endpoint, colorectal cancer development, because this process takes so many years. For studies of chemoprevention of human colorectal neoplasia, two major, different endpoints have been used. A late intermediate biomarker of risk is the formation of adenomatous polyps, which are a known precursor of colorectal cancer. This endpoint has been investigated in volunteers who previously have had an adenomatous polyp and therefore are at greater risk for recurrence of such polyps than the general population. Early intermediate biomarkers of risk have been sought in flat normal-appearing mucosa of similar subjects at increased risk and involve changes in cell proliferation. This approach to determinining changes in "risk patterns" is based on the observations of Lipkin and co-workers, which show a progressive increase in the number of colonic crypt-proliferating cells plus an upward shift of such proliferating cells in the crypt of at-risk patients with colon cancer, colon adenomas, familial colon cancer, as well as other conditions that are associated with an increased risk of colon cancer (28). When supplemental calcium was administered in doses of about 1.2– 2 g/d, several studies pointed to an improvement in these indices of proliferation (29–31). In a further study involving 70 similar subjects at increased risk, the addition of low-fat dairy products containing an average of 850 mg

Table 1
Recent Epidemiological Studies

Authors	Ref.	Colon/rectum	OR	P for trend	Comments
Marcus and Newmark	94				
Calcium		Colon	0.6	0.03	Case–control
Vitamin D		Rectum	0.6	0.07	
		Colon	0.7	0.05	
Hyman et al.	95				
Calcium (especially high fat intake)		Colon	0.63		Adenoma incidence Adenoma number
Pritchard et al.	96				
Calcium		Colon	1.2	0.62	Case–control
Vitamin D		Colon	0.6	0.08	
		Rectum	0.5	0.08	
White et al.	97				
Multivitamins		Colon	0.49	0.001	Case–control
Calcium			0.78	0.03	
Whelan et al.	98				
Calcium (supplemental multivitamins)		Colon	0.51		Recurrent polyps
		Rectum	0.47		
Wu et al.	99				
Calcium		Distal colon (men)	0.58		Nurses, health professional
		Distal colon (women)	0.73		
Zheng et al.	100				
Calcium and Vitamin D		Rectum	0.55	0.02	Cohort
Yang et al.	101				
Calcium in drinking water			0.79–0.58	0.001	Case–control
Levine et al.	102				
Calcium			0.82		Case–control
Vitamin D (with low calcium)			0.83		
Sellers et al.	103				
Calcium		Colon (women)	0.5	0.001	Prospective cohort
Kato et al.	104				
Dairy products		Colorectal	0.65	0.04	Prospective cohort
Calcium		Colorectal	0.71	0.14	
Ghadirian, et al.	105				
Calcium		Colon	0.69	0.04	Case–control
La Veccia et al.	106				
Calcium		Colorectal	0.72	0.01	
Destefani et al.	107				
Calcium		Colorectal	0.41	0.001	

(continued)

Table 1 (Continued)

Authors	Ref.	Colon/rectum	OR		P for trend	Comments
Pietinen et al.	108					
Calcium		Colorectal	0.6		0.04	Primary study
Milk product		Colorectal	0.6		0.02	
Vitamin D		Colorectal	1.0		0.77	
Kampman et al.	109					
Calcium		Colon			0.6	Case–control
Vitamin D (diet)		Colon			1.1	
Vitamin D (supplement)		Colon			0.6	
Dairy		Colon			0.7	
Peters et al.	110					
Vitamin D		Colorectal Adenomas			0.5	Serum 25(OH)D
Jarvinen et al.	111					
Calcium, milk product		Colorectal			0.58	Cohort
McCullough et al.	112					
Total calcium		Colorectal	0.87		0.06	Prospective CPS
Vitamin D		Colorectal	0.73		0.001	Nutrition

CPS, Cancer Prevention Study

of calcium for 1 yr (producing a total calcium intake of about 1500 mg) resulted in a shift in the risk from a higher to a lower pattern, accompanied by improvement in differentiation markers (32).

Several investigators have questioned the reproducibility of data that demonstrated changes in proliferation during calcium supplementation (11,33). In a recent publication, we have analyzed the differences between the positive and negative results from such studies and suggest that negative results were encountered when the number of proliferating cells observed at baseline was low, when several separate research centers were involved, and when preparation of patients was not standardized (5). It should also be pointed out that rodent studies consistently have shown a shift in proliferative indices and differentiation markers from a higher to a lower risk pattern when calcium was administered. The most important of these animal studies were also performed by Lipkin's group, in which a Western-style diet that was relatively high in fat content and relatively low in both calcium and vitamin D (although not sufficient to induce deficiency) was fed. In those studies, feeding of calcium or low-fat dairy foods consistently have shown improvement in these proliferative measures (34,35).

The present "gold standard" for determining that an agent is protective against human colorectal cancer involves studies of colorectal adenoma recurrence in subjects who previously have had an adenoma and therefore are at increased risk for developing a recurrence. The most important of these studies was that of Baron and co-workers (37) who administered 1.2 g of calcium carbonate to approx 1000 study subjects plus controls and reported a significant, approx 20%, overall reduction in recurrent adenomas. Subsequently, recalculation of the data demonstrated a much greater effect on the most advanced adenomas *(38)*. The definition of an advanced adenoma includes one that is larger than 1 cm and/or has histological evidence of severe dysplasia. Calcium administration resulted in an approx 45% reduction in such advanced adenomas. Further studies of the levels of serum 25(OH)D showed that most of the beneficial effects occurred in subjects with higher than the median concentration of 25(OH)D(approx 29 ng/mL) *(39)*. The core of these observations was confirmed by an underpowered study from Europe which showed an approx 25% reduction in colon adenoma recurrence in the overall group and a significant effect (approx 40%) in those with a calcium intake below the median *(40)*. An earlier study examining calcium and vitamin D intake also showed beneficial results *(41)*. Overall, these studies clearly established the utility of calcium, perhaps combined with vitamin D, in lowering the risk of colon adenomas—an accepted precursor of colorectal cancer.

4. MECHANISMS OF ACTION OF CALCIUM

There are two major hypotheses to explain the actions of calcium on colorectal carcinogenesis—one effect predominately mediated through changes in the colonic lumen and another through a direct effect of calcium upon the colorectal epithelium.

The luminal theory was briefly described previously and relates to the hypothesis that hydrophobic and cytotoxic surface active agents, such as secondary bile acids and fatty acids solubilized in the fecal water component of colonic contents, are brought out of solution by soluble calcium. The initial Newmark and Bruce hypothesis *(7)* was that the addition of calcium resulted in the formation of calcium soaps with fatty acids and bile acids, which would then be precipitated. Studies in vitro *(42)* and in vivo emphasized the importance of phosphate, which interacted with calcium to form an insoluble calcium phosphate complex. This complex then interacted with bile acids and fatty acids to bring these compounds out of solution *(43)*.

In subsequent studies, the addition of calcium was shown to lower the cytotoxicity of artificial mixtures resembling luminal contents using the lysis of red cells *(44)* or colon cancer cells as model systems. In animal studies, similar reductions in cytotoxicity were demonstrated by feeding calcium phosphate in the diet, as well as inhibiting colonic hyperproliferation induced by fat feedings. In human studies, Van der Meer's group also demonstrated a reduction in fecal water cytotoxicity by dietary calcium *(45)* or specially prepared milk products *(46)*. The same group later showed that haem also was cytotoxic to the colonic mucosa *(47)* and that this effect was diminished by feeding calcium phosphate.

In addition to possible effects of calcium administration on the colonic luminal contents, calcium controls many intracellular and extracellular processes, usually through actions on intracellular second messengers (*see* Chapter 3). The tight regulation of calcium entry into cells and release from the endoplasmic reticulum results in controlled and rapid changes in intracellular calcium concentration. Such calcium would be expected to have effects on the control of cellular proliferation and differentiation in the colon, in part through effects on protein kinase C. Furthermore, changes in intracellular calcium homeostatsis may also mediate epithelial cell apoptosis. Many of these effects have recently been explored in detail *(48)*.

5. MECHANISMS OF ACTIONS OF VITAMIN D

Vitamin D may act directly upon epithelial cells, may interact with calcium to alter epithelial cells, or may act through yet other mechanisms.

Vitamin D actions are mediated primarily by binding to a high-affinity nuclear receptor—vitamin D receptor (VDR)—a member of the nuclear hormone receptor family. VDR is found in colon cancer tissue, but generally occurs in higher concentrations in colonic hyperplastic and adenomatous polyps (49–51). Vitamin D acts through repression or activation of proto-oncogenes and tumor suppressor genes that lower rates of cell proliferation and enhance cell differentiation (52). A large number of responsive genes have been described (48). A particular example is the calcium-sensing receptor gene, the function of which may determine the entry of extracellular calcium into gastrointestinal epithelial cells, which suggests an interaction between vitamin D and calcium in chemoprevention (53). Another is a report that VDR has some role as an intestinal bile-acid sensor (54), permitting feedback degradation of potentially noxious lithocholic acid. VDR-deficient rodents have been described as showing increased proliferative activity in the distal colon (55).

At a cellular level, the growth-lowering effect of vitamin D appears to occur by both genomic and nongenomic mechanisms. Vitamin D regulates both growth factor synthesis and growth factor signaling (e.g., effects on transforming growth factor β and the *SMAD4* gene). In addition, vitamin D induces gastrointestinal cell-cycle arrest through inhibition of cyclin D1 activity, and may interfere with inappropriate β-catenin-mediated transcriptional activity. There also is evidence that vitamin D may enhance apoptosis of transformed cells, for example, 1,25 dihydroxyvitamin D_3 (1,25[OH]$_2D_3$)-induced apoptosis in HT29 colon cancer cells has been reported to be accompanied by upregulation of BAK. In other cell systems, vitamin D may upregulate the proapoptotic molecule BAX and downregulate the anti-apoptotic molecule BCl_2 and/or inhibit survivin, an inhibitor of apoptosis protein that is overexpressed in colon cancer cells. It is of interest that a vitamin D analog, calcipotriol, has been shown to inhibit proliferation of rectal epithelial cells in human rectal biopsies incubated with this vitamin D compound in vitro (56). The interaction of vitamin D and calcium also has been suggested by a unique study in which the gradient of calcium was measured in isolated colonic crypts from vitamin D-deficient and -replete animals. The authors of this study described a pronounced change in the intracrypt concentration of calcium in the presence of adequate amounts of vitamin D, suggesting that vitamin D might act through altering intracrypt calcium homeostasis (57). Interactions of vitamin D and calcium also were suggested in a human study in which the levels of serum vitamin D were correlated with rectal epithelial cell proliferation.

Several observations over the past few years have also suggested that the critical concentrations of the active form of vitamin D, 1,25(OH)$_2D_3$, may be determined not through the circulating levels of this hormone, but rather at a local level in the colon (58). Our own studies in this regard derived from observations that rectal cell proliferation in humans was correlated well with the serum levels of 25(OH)D but not 1,25(OH)$_2D_3$ (59). This led to the hypothesis that there might be local conversion of 25(OH)D_3 to the active hormone and, in studies in collaboration with Dr. Holick's group in Boston, demonstrated the mRNA for the 1α hydroxylase enzyme in both colon tumor tissue and in normal colon

(60). These studies were temporally preceded and greatly amplified by the observations of Cross and her co-workers in Vienna *(61,62)*.

In addition to the role of vitamin D in mineral and skeletal homeostasis, the physiologically active molecular form of vitamin D, $1,25(OH)_2D_3$, also reduces cell proliferation and induces differentiation and apoptosis in several normal and tumor cells, including cells of the large intestine *(63,64)*. The actions of vitamin D are mediated principally by its binding to a the VDR receptor *(65)*. The ways that vitamin D is sensed are described elsewhere in this volume, and a summary can be found in ref. *48*. Presumably, most of the effects of this hormone are mediated via changes in growth factor production, with effects on the cell cycle and apoptosis.

There are several polymorphisms of the VDR receptor, and a number of studies have focused on their functional consequences. The β- and short poly A allele have been reported as protective against the development of colonic adenomas *(66–68)*. The relationship between selected polymorphisms and colon cancer has been described elsewhere *(69,70)*.

6. CALCIUM, VITAMIN D, AND PROSTATE CANCER

There are two somewhat contradictory observations that are pertinent to an association between calcium or vitamin D and prostate cancer. The most consistent are data on the beneficial role of vitamin D, either derived from solar radiation or from dietary sources, on the development of this tumor. Epidemiological studies have demonstrated that migration patterns that are accompanied by changes in the diet, just like in colon cancer, modify the incidence of prostate cancer dramatically within one or two generations *(71)*. Lower exposure to solar radiation throughout the United States and elsewhere *(72)* is accompanied by higher prostate cancer rates, and prostate cancer is twice as common in African Americans, presumably in part because of reduced production of vitamin D in the skin *(73)*. Furthermore, vitamin D is a powerful regulator of prostate cell growth and differentiation in vitro *(74)*. Lower serum levels of $25(OH)D_3$ *(71)* (and, in some studies, also lower levels of $1,25[OH]_2D_3[75]$) have been accompanied by higher rates of prostate cancer. These data have led to the development of active analogs of vitamin D with activity on the prostate but little or no hypercalcemic properties as potential therapeutic or preventive agents for this cancer *(76)*. Overall, these studies have not attained clinical utility to date.

Other important observations have attempted to explore contradictory findings of the effect of serum $1,25(OH)_2D_3$ concentrations on prostate cancer prevalence *(77)*. As in the colon, $25(OH)D_3$ can be converted to $1,25(OH)_2D_3$ by prostatic cells *(78)*, and this has led to the development of a theory, championed by Schwartz and co-workers, that vitamin D action on the prostate is mediated through conversion of circulating $25(OH)D_3$ to the active $1,25(OH)_2D_3$ within the prostate itself *(71)*. If that is the case, then increasing the serum levels of $25(OH)D_3$, which can be done relatively safely, might be protective against prostate cancer.

A contrasting theory that has gained attention in the past few years relates to the possibility, advocated by Giovanucci and his group, that greater dairy product intake may enhance the risk of prostate cancer *(79)*. In 1997, an expert panel considered that there was little or no evidence from the literature that any particular food group was associated

Table 2
Calcium and Prostate Cancer

Authors	Reference	Nutrient	Comment
		Harmful	
Giovanucci	79	Calcium	Hypothesis
Giovanucci et al.	81	Calcium	Advanced prostate cancer
Chan et al.	82	Dairy	Adjusted for calories
Chan et al.	83	Dairy	Adjusted for phosphate
Schurmann et al.	84	Dairy	
		No significant effect	
Ohno et al.	85	Calcium	Matched control study
Tzonou et al.	86	Dairy	Case–control study
Vlajinac et al.	87	Calcium	Case–control study
Tavani et al.	88	Calcium	Case–control study
Giovanucci et al.	81	Calcium	Overall prostate cancer
		Beneficial	
Hanchette and Schwartz	72	Sunlight	
Braun et al.	89	25(OH)D	Prediagnostic serum levels
Baron et al.	90	Calcium	Prospective study

with prostate cancer risk (80). However, two studies published by Giovanucci's group were then widely quoted to support this association. In the Health Professional Follow Up study, significant trends between calcium intake and advanced or metastatic cancer were found with intakes varying from less than 500 mg to more than 2 g of calcium daily (81). It is pertinent to point out that only the group consuming more than 2 g of calcium per day, which represented no more than approx 5% of the total group, showed a significant increase in prostate cancer. A case–control study from Sweden by the same group (82) showed a significant increase in advanced prostate cancer, but only after an adjustment for phosphate intake, which was peculiar to this study. A follow-up of the Health Professional study suggested that there was a significant trend to more prostate cancer with increasing dairy intake as assessed via a questionnaire completed 11 yr earlier. Data on dietary fat intake were not available in this study, and the data showing effects only on the incidence of advanced prostate cancer, reported in the authors' earlier studies, were not confirmed (83).

It is pertinent also to examine other studies of the potential association of prostate cancer with calcium or dairy product intake (Table 2). Four of the five studies that pointed to a harmful association were published by the Giovanucci's group. Additionally, there were five studies showing no significant effects and three that suggested that calcium or dairy intake reduced prostate cancer risk.

The proposed mechanism for the harmful effect of calcium or dairy food intake relates to the potential for calcium to lower serum $1,25(OH)_2D_3$ levels. In the largest prospective study of calcium supplements published to date, the mean reduction in serum $1,25(OH)_2D_3$ levels was approx 4% (37). That same study was one in which a protective effect against prostate cancer was suggested.

7. CALCIUM, VITAMIN D, AND OTHER CANCERS

The feeding of Western-style diets containing reduced calcium and vitamin D and increased fat content to rodents not only enhanced colorectal tumorigenesis but also was found to have an effect in breast, pancreas, and prostate. Such feeding resulted in hyperplasia and hyperproliferation of mammary duct epithelial cells *(91)* and hyperproliferation of epithelial cells in the exocrine pancreas *(92)* and in the prostate *(93)*. The precise mechanisms of action of calcium (and vitamin D) on these tissues, which are not directly exposed to the increased dietary calcium that is found in the fecal stream, is unknown. Vitamin D also has been associated with an alteration in breast cancer cells and even in brain tumors *(48)*.

8. CONCLUSION

In conclusion, there are abundant data that point to a beneficial interaction of calcium and vitamin D upon the process of carcinogenesis. Most of the available data have focused on effects on the colorectum. However, additional studies suggest that calcium and/or vitamin D also might influence cancer formation in other organs (i.e., prostate, breast, and pancreas), particularly in which cancer induction is likely to be affected by environmental factors. Future study should clarify whether there are any universal factors that might influence cancer formation in these organs.

REFERENCES

1. Potter JD. Nutrition and colorectal cancer. Cancer Causes & Control 1996;11:579–588.
2. Vogelstein, B, Fearon ER, Hamilton SR, et al. Genetic alterations during colorectal-tumor development. N Engl J Med 1988;319:525–532.
3. Lipkin M. Phase I and phase 2 proliferative lesions of colonic epithelial cells in disease leading to colon cancer. Cancer 1994;34:878–888.
4. Kinzler KW, Vogelstein B. Landscaping the cancer terrain. Science 1998;280:1036–1037.
5. Holt P R, Studies of calcium in food supplements in humans, cancer prevention. Annals NY Acad Sci 1999;889:128–137.
6. Haenzel W, Kurihara M. Studies of Japanese migrants: I. Mortality from cancers and other diseases among Japanese in the United States. J Nat Cancer Inst 1968;40:43–68.
7. Newmark H, Wargovich MJ, Bruce W. Colon cancer, and dietary fat, phosphate, and calcium: a hypothesis. J. Natl Cancer Inst 1984;72:1321–1325.
8 Reddy BS. Bile salts and other constituents of the colon as tumor promoters. Banbury Rep 1981;7:345–361.
9 Hill MJ. Bile acids and colorectal cancer: hypothesis. Eur J Cancer Prev 1991;9:69–74.
10. Lipkin M. Biomarkers of increased susceptibility to gastrointestinal cancer: new application to studies of cancer prevention in human subjects. Cancer Res 1988;48:235–245.
11. McShane LM, Kulldorff M, Wargovich MJ, et al. An evaluation of mucosal proliferation measure variability sources in the polyp prevention trial:. CEBP 1998;7:605–612.
12. Bergsma-Kadijk JA, Van't Veer P, Kampman E, Burema J. Calcium does not protect against colorectal neoplasia. Epidemiology 1996;7:590–597.
13. Grant WB. An estimate of premature cancer mortality in the U.S. due to inadequate doses of solar ultraviolet-B radiation. Cancer 2002;94(6):1867–1875.
14. Garland CF, Garland F, Gorham E. Calcium and vitamin D: their potential roles in colon and breast cancer prevention. Ann NY Assoc Sci 1999;889:107–119.
15. Garland CF, Garland F. Do sunlight and vitamin D reduce the likelihood of colon cancer? Int J Epidemiol 1980;9:227–231.
16. Emerson JC, Weiss NS. Colorectal cancer and solar radiation. Cancer Causes Control 1992;3:95–99.

17. Freedman DM, Dosemeci M, McGlynn K. Sunlight and mortality from breast, ovarian, colon, prostate, and non-melanoma skin cancer: a composite death certificate based case-control study. Occup Environ Med 2002;59:257–262.

18. Garland C, Comstock G, Garland F, et al. Serum 25-hydroxyvitamin D and colon cancer: eight-year prospective study. Lancet 1989;2:1176–1178.

19. Tangrea J, Helzlsouer K, Pietinen P, et al. Serum levels of vitamin D metabolites and the subsequent risk of colon can rectal cancer in Finnish men. Cancer Causes Control 1997;8:615–625.

20. Garland F, Garland C, Gorham E, Young J, Jr. Geographic variation in breast cancer mortality in the United States: a hypothesis involving exposure to solar radiation. Prev Med 1990;19:614–622.

21. Gorham E, Garland C, Garland F. Acid haze air pollution and breast and colon cancer in 20 Canadian cities. Can J Public Health 1989;80:96–100.

22. Newmark, H. Vitamin D adequacy: a possible relationship to breast cancer. In Diet and Breast Cancer. Plenum, New York: 1994; pp. 109–114.

23. Wargovich MJ, Eng VWS, Newmark HL. Calcium inhibits the damaging and compensatory proliferative effects of fatty acids on mouse colon epithelium. Cancer Lett 1984;23:253–258.

24. Nobre-Leitao C, Chaves P, Fidalgo P, et al. Calcium regulation of colonic crypt cell kinetics: evidence for a direct effect in mice. Gastroenterology 1995;109:498–504.

25. Lipkin M, Newmark H. Effect of added dietary calcium on colonic epithelial cell proliferation in subjects at high risk for familial colonic cancer. N Engl J Med 1985;313:1381–1384.

26. Rozen P, Fireman A, Fine N, Wax Y, Ron E. Oral calcium suppresses increased rectal epithelial proliferation of persons at risk for colorectal cancer. Gut 1989;30:650–655.

27. Steinbach G, Lupton J, Reddy BS, Kral JG, Holt PR. Effect of calcium supplementation on rectal epithelial hyperproliferation in intestinal bypass subjects. Gastroenterology 1994;106:1162–1167.

28. Lipkin M. Biomarkers of increased susceptibility to gastrointestinal cancer. New application to studies of cancer prevention in human subjects. Cancer Res 1988;48:235.

29. Wargovich MJ, Isbell G, Shabot M, et al.. Calcium supplementation decreases rectal epithelial cell proliferation in subjects with sporadic adenoma. Gastroenterology 1992;103:92–97.

30. O'Sullivan KR, Mathias PM, Beattie S, O'Morain C. Effect of oral calcium supplementation on colonic crypt cell proliferation in patients with adenomatous polyps of the large bowel. Eur J Gastroenterol Hepatol 1993;5:85–89.

31. Barsoum GH, Hendrickse C, Winslet MC, et al. Reduction of mucosal crypt cell proliferation in patients with colorectal adenomatous polyps by dietary calcium supplementation. Br J Surg 1992;79:581–583.

32. Holt PR, Attilasoy EO, Gilman J, et al. Modulation of abnormal colon epithelial cell proliferation and differentiation by low-fat dairy foods: a randomized controlled trial. JAMA 1998;280:1074–1079.

33. Baron JA, Tosteson TD, Wargovich MJ, et al. Calcium supplementation and rectal mucosal proliferation: a randomized controlled trial. J Natl Cancer Inst 1995;87:1303–1307.

34. Xue L, Lipkin M, Newmark H, Wang J. Influence of dietary calcium and vitamin D on diet-induced epithelial cell hyperproliferation in mice. J Natl Cancer Inst 1999;91:176–181.

35. Wargovich MJ, Eng VW, Newmark HL, Bruce WR. Calcium ameliorates the toxic effect of deoxycholic acid on colonic epithelium Carcinogenesis 1983;4:1205–1207.

36. Risio M, Lipkin M, Newmark H, et al. Apoptosis, cell replication, and Western-style diet-induced tumorigenesis in mouse colon. Cancer Res 1996;56:4910–4916.

37. Baron JA, Beach M, Mandel JS, et al. Calcium supplements for the prevention of colorectal adenomas. Calcium Polyp Prevention Study Group. N Engl J Med 1999;340:101–107.

38. Wallace K, Baron JA, Cole BF, et al. Calcium carbonate chemoprevention in the large bowel: Effects on hyperplastic polyps, tubular adenomas, and more advanced lesions. Proc Am Assoc Cancer Res 2002;43:163.

39. Grau MV, Baron JA, Sandler RS, et al. Vitamin D, calcium supplementation, and colorectal adenomas: results of a randomized trial. J Natl Cancer Inst 2003, 95:1765–1770.

40. Bonithon-Kopp C, Kronborg O, Giacosa A, Rath U, Faivre J. Calcium and fibre supplementation in prevention of colorectal adenoma recurrence: a randomised intervention trial, European Cancer Prevention Organisation Study Group. Lancet 2000;356:1300–1306.

41. Hofstad B, Almendingen K, Vatn M, et al. Growth and recurrence of colorectal polyps: a double-blind 3-year intervention with calcium and antioxidants. Digestion 1998;59:148–156.

42. Van der Meer R, Termont DSML, DeVries HT. Differential effects of calcium ions and calcium phosphate on cytotoxcity of bile acids. Am J Physiol 1991;260:G142–G147.

43. Govers MJAP, Van der Meer R. Effects of dietary calcium and phosphate on the intestinal interactions between calcium, phosphate, fatty acids and bile acids. Gut 1993;34:365–370.

44. Lapre JA, De Vries, HT, Van der Meer R. Dietary calcium phosphate inhibits cytotoxcity of fecal water. Am J Physiol 1991;261:G907–G913.

45. Govers MJAP, Termont DSML, Lapre JA, et al. Calcium in milk products precipitates intestinal fatty acids and secondary bile acids and thus inhibits colonic cytotoxicity in humans. Cancer 1996;56:3270–3275.

46. Govers MJAP, Termont DSML, Lapre JA, et al. Calcium in milk products precipitates intestinal fatty acids and secondary bile acids and thus inhibits colonic cytotoxicity in humans. Cancer 1996;56:3270–3275 .

47. Sesink ALA, Termont DSML, Kleibeuker JH, et al. Red meat and colon cancer: dietary haem-induced colonic cytotoxicity and epithelial hyperproliferation are inhibited by calcium. Carcinogenesis 2001;22:1653–1659.

48. Lamprecht SA, Lipkin M. Chemoprevention of colon cancer by calcium, vitamin D and folate: Molecular mechanisms. Nat Rev Cancer 2003;3:601–614.

49. Shabahang M, Buras RR, Davoodi F, et al. 1,25-dihydroxyvitamin D3 receptor as a marker of human colon carcinoma cell line differentiation and growth inhibition. Cancer Res 1993;53:3712–3718.

50. Cross HS, Bajna E, Bises G, et al. Vitamin D receptor and cytokeratin expression may be progression indicators in human colon cancer. Anticancer Res 1996;16:

51. Sheinin Y, Kaserer K, Wrba F, et al. In situ mRNA hybridization analysis and immunolocalization of the vitamin D receptor in normal and carcinomatous human colonic mucosa: relation to epidermal growth factor receptor expression. Virchows Arch 2000;437:501–507.

52. Halline AG, Davidson NO, Skarosi SF, et al. Effects of 1,25-dihydroxyvitamin D3 on proliferation and differentiation of Caco-2 cells. Endocrinology 1994;134:1710–1717.

53. Canaff L, Hendy GN. Human calcium-sensing receptor gene. Vitamin D response elements in promoters P1 and P2 confer transcriptional responsiveness to 1,25-dihydroxyvitamin D. J Biol Chem 2002;277:30, 337–30,350.

54. Makishima M, Lu TT, Xie W, et al.Vitamin D receptor as an intestinal bile acid sensor. Science 2002;296:1313–1316.

55. Kallay E, Pietschmann P, Toyokuni S, et al. Characterization of a vitamin D receptor knockout mouse as a model of colorectal hyperproliferation and DNA damage. Carcinogenesis 2001;22:1429–1435.

56. Thomas MG, Tebbutt S, Williamson RC. Vitamin D and its metabolites inhibit cell proliferation in human rectal mucosa and a colon cancer cell line. Gut 1992;33:1660–1663.

57. Brenner B, Russell N, Albrecht S, Davies R. The effect of dietary vitamin D_3 on the intracellular calcium gradient in mammalian colonic crypts. Cancer Lett 1998;127:43–53.

58. Cross HS, Kallay E, Farhan H, Weiland T, Manhardt T. Regulation of extrarenal vitamin D metabolism as a tool for colon and prostate cancer prevention. Recent Results Cancer Res 2003;164:413–425.

59. Holt PR, Arber N, Halmos B, et al. Colonic epithelial cell proliferation decreases with increasing levels of serum 25 hydroxy vitamin D. CEBP 2002;11:113–119.

60. Tangpricha V, Flanagan JN, Whitlatch LW, et al. 25-hydroxyvitamin D-1 alpha-hydroxylase in normal and malignant colon tissue. Lancet 2001;357:1673–1674.

61. Bareis P, Bises G, Bischof MG, et al. 25-hydroxyvitamin D metabolism in human colon cancer cells during tumor progression. Biochem Biophys Res Commun 2001; 285:1012–1017.

62. Cross HS, Perlik M, Reddy GS, Schuster I. Vitamin D metobolism in human colon adenocarcinoma-derived Caco-2 cells: expression of 25-hydroxyvitamin D3-1alpha-hydroxylase activity and regulation of side-chain metabolism. J Steroid Biochem Mol Biol 1997;62:21–28.

63. Kim KE, Braistus, TA. The role of vitamin D in normal and pathologic processes in the colon. Curr Opin Gastroenterol 2001;17:72–77.

64. Ylikomi T, Laaksi I, Lou YR, et al. Antiproliferative action of vitamin D. Vitam Hormone 2002;64:357–405.

65. Haussler M, Whitfield GK, Haussler CA, et al. The nuclear vitamin D receptor biological and molecular regulatory properties revealed. J Bone Miner Metab 1998;13:325–349.

66. Peters U, McGlynn KA, Chatterjee N, et al. Vitamin D, calcium, and vitamin D receptor polymorphism in colorectal adenomas. Cancer Epidemiol Biomarkers Prev 2001;10:1267–1274.

67. Ingles SA, Wang J, Coetzee GA, et al. Vitamin D receptor polymorphisms and risk of colorectal adenomas (United States). Cancer Causes Control 2001;12:607–614.
68. Kim HS, Newcomb PA, Ulrich CM, et al. Vitamin D receptor polymorphism and the risk of colorectal adenomas: evidence of interaction with dietary vitamin D and calcium. Cancer Epidemiol Biomarkers Prev 2001;10:869–874.
69. Slattery ML, Yakumo K, Hoffman M, et al. Variants of the VDR gene and risk of colon cancer (United States). Cancer Causes Control 2001;12:359–364.
70. Wong HL, Seow A, Arakawa K, et al. Vitamin D receptor start colon polymorphism and colorectal cancer risk: effect modification by dietary calcium and fat in Singapore Chinese. Carcinogenesis 2003;24:1091–1095.
71. Schwartz GG, Hulka BS. Is vitamin D deficiency a risk factor for prostate cancer? (Hypothesis). Anicancer Res 1990;10:1307–1311.
72. Hanchette CL, Schwartz GG. Geographic patterns of prostate cancer mortality, Cancer 1992;70:2861–2869.
73. Wynder EL, Mbuchi K, Whitmore WF, Jr. Epidemiology of cancer of the prostate. Cancer 1971;28:344–360.
74. Peehl DM, Skowronski RJ, Leung GK, Wong ST, et al. Antiproliferative effects of 1,25-dihydroxyvitamin D3 on primary cultures of human prostatic cells. Cancer Res 1994;54:805–810.
75. Corder EH, Guess HA, Hulka BS, et al. Vitamin D and prostate cancer: a prediagostic study with stored sera. CEBP 1993;2:467–472.
76. Ogata E. The potential use of vitamin D analogs in the treatment of cancer. Calcif Tissue Int1997;60: 130–133.
77. Braun MM, Helzlsouer KJ, Hollis BW, Comstock GW. Prostate cancer and prediagnostic levels of serum vitamin D metabolites (Maryland, United States), Cancer Causes and Control 1995;6:235–239.
78. Schwartz GG, Whitlatch LW, Chen TC, et al. Human prostate cells synthesize 1,25-dihydroxyvitamin D_3 from 25-hydroxyvitamin D_3. Cancer Epidemiol Biomark Prev 1998;7:391–395.
79. Giovanucci E. Dietary influences of 1,25(OH)$_2$ vitamin D in relation to prostate cancer: a hypothesis. Cancer Causes and Control 1998;9:567–582.
80. World Cancer Research Fund And American Institute For Cancer Research. Food, nutrition and the prevention of cancer, World Cancer Research fund and American Institute for Cancer Research, Menasha, (1997).
81 Giovanucci E, Rimm ER, Wolk A, et al. Calcium and fructose intake in relation to risk of prostate cancer. Cancer Res 1998;58:442–447.
82. Chan JM, Giovanucci E, Anderson S, et al. Dairy products, calcium, phosphorous, vitamin D, and risk of prostate cancer (Sweden). Cancer Causes Control 1998;9:559–566.
83. Chan JM, Giovanucci E, Anderson S, et al. Dairy products, calcium, phosphorous, vitamin D, and risk of prostate cancer (Sweden).Cancer Causes Control 1998;9:559–566.
84. Schuurman AG, van den Brandt PA, Dorant E, Goldbohm RA. Animal products, calcium and protein and prostate cancer risk in the Netherlands Cohort Study, Br J Cancer 1999;80:1107–1113.
85. Ohno Y, Yoshida O, Oishi K, et al. Dietary β-carotene and cancer of the prostate: a case-control study in Kyoto, Japan. Cancer Res 1988;48:1331–1336.
86. Tzonou A, Signorello LB, Lagiou P, et al. Diet and cancer of the prostate: a case study in Greece. Int J Cancer 1999;80:704–708.
87. Vlajinac HD, Marinkovic JM, Ilic MD, Kocev NI. Diet and prostate cancer: a case-control study. Eur J Cancer 1997;1:101–107.
88. Tavani A, Gallus S, Franceschi S, La Vecchia C. Calcium, dairy products, and the risk of prostate cancer. Prostate 2001;48:118–121.
89. Braun MM, Helzlsouer KJ, Hollis BW, Comstock GW. Prostate cancer and prediagnostic levels of serum vitamin D metabolites (Maryland, United States). Cancer Causes Control 1995;6:235–239.
90. Wallace K, Pearson LH, Beach ML, et al. Calcium supplementation and prostate cancer risk: a randomized analysis. Proc Am Assoc Cancer Res 2001;42:460.
91. Xue L, Newmark H, Yang K, Lipkin M. Model of mouse mammary gland hyperproliferation and hyperplasia induced by a Western-style diet. Nutr Cancer 1996;26:281–287.
92. Xue L, Yang K, Newmark H, et al. Epithelial cell hyperproliferation induced in the exocrine pancreas of mice by a Western-style diet. J Natl Cancer Inst 1996;88:1586–1590.

93. Xue L, Yang K, Newmark H, Lipkin M. Induced hyperproliferation in epithelial cells of mouse prostate by a Western-style diet. Carcinogenesis 1997;18:995–999.

94. Marcus PM, Newcomb PA. The association of calcium and vitamin D, and colon and rectal cancer in Wisconsin women. Int J Epidemiol 1988;27:788–793.

95. Hyman J, Baron JA, Dain BJ, et al. Dietary and supplemental calcium and the recurrence of colorectal adenomas. Cancer Epidemiol Biomarkers Prev 1998;7:291–295.

96. Pritchard RS, Baron JA,Gerhardsson de Veerdier M. Dietary calcium, vitamin D, and the risk of colorectal cancer in Stockholm, Sweden. Cancer Epidemiol Biomarkers Prev 1996;5:897–900.

97. White E, Shannon JS, Patterson RE. Relationship between vitamin and calcium supplement use and colon cancer. Cancer Epidemiol Biomarkers Prev 1997;6:769–774.

98. Whelan RL, Horvath KD, Gleason NR, et al. Vitamin and calcium supplement use is associated with decreased adenoma recurrence in patients with a previous history of neoplasia. Dis Colon Rectum 1999;42(2):212–217.

99. Wu K, Willett WC, Fuches CS, Golditz A, Giovanucci EL. Calcium intake and risk of colon cancer in women and men. J Natl Cancer Inst 2002;94:437–446.

100 Zheng W, Anderson KE, Kuschi LH, et al. A prospective cohort study of intake of calcium, vitamin D, and other micronutrients in relation to incidence of rectal cancer among postmenopausal women. Cancer Epidemiol Biomarkers Prev 1998;7:221–225.

101. Yang C, Chiu H, Chiu J, et al. Calcium and magnesium in drinking water and risk of death from colon cancer. J Cancer Res 1997;88:928–933.

102. Levine AJ, Harper JM, Ervin CM, et al. Serum 25-hydroxyvitamin D, dietary calcium intake, and distal colorectal adenoma risk. Nutr Cancer 2001;39:35–41.

103. Sellers TA, Bazyk AE, Bostick RM, et al. Diet and risk of colon cancer in a large prospective study of older women: an analysis stratified on family history (Iowa, United States). Cancer Causes Control 1998;9:357–367.

104. Kato I, Akhmedkhanov A, Koenig K, et al. Prospective study of diet and female colorectal cancer: the New York University Women's Health Study. Nutrition Cancer 1997;28,3:276–281.

105. Ghadirian P, Lacroix A, Maisonneuve P, et al. Nutritional factors and colon carcinoma. American Cancer Society 1997 ;80,5:858–864.

106. La Veccia C, Braga C, Negri E, et al. Intake of selected micronutrients and risk of colorectal cancer. Int J Cancer 1997;73:525–530.

107. De Stefani E, Mendilaharsu M, Deneo-Pellegrini H, Ronco A. Influence of dietary levels of fat, cholesterol, and calcium on colrectal cancer. Nutr Cancer 1997;29,1:83–89.

108. Pietinen P, Malila N, Virtanen M, et al. Diet and risk of colorectal cancer in a cohort of Finnish men, Cancer Causes Control 1999;10:387–396.

109. Kampman E, Slattery ML, Caan B, et al. Calcium, vitamin D, sunshine exposure, dairy products and colon cancer risk (United States). Cancer Causes Control 2000;11:459–466.

110. Peters U, McGlynn KA, Chatterjee N, et al. Vitamin D, calcium, and vitamin D receptor polymorphism in colorectal adenomas. Cancer Epidemiol Biomarkers Prev 2001;10:1267–1274.

111. Jarvinen R., Knekt P, Hakulinen T, Aromaa A. Prospective study on milk products, calcium and cancers of the colon and rectum. Eur J Clin Nutr 2001;55:1000–1007.

112. McCullough ML, Robertson AS, Rodriguez C, et al. Calcium, vitamin D, dairy products, and risk of colorectal cancer in the Cancer Prevention Study II Nutrition Cohort (United States). Cancer Causes Control 2003;14:1–12.

26 Dietary Calcium and the Metabolic Syndrome

Dorothy Teegarden

KEY POINTS

- Higher intakes of dairy products are associated with reduced incidence of the metabolic syndrome.
- Higher intakes of dairy products are associated with reductions in symptoms and pathogenetic mechanisms.
- Although dietary calcium regulation of parathyroid hormone and 1,25 dihydroxyvitamin D may play a role, the full mechanism of action of dietary calcium remains to be clearly elucidated.

1. INTRODUCTION

Recently, research efforts have grown to better understand the mechanism of the metabolic syndrome, otherwise known as "syndrome X," or the insulin-resistance syndrome. The metabolic syndrome leads to an increased risk for type 2 diabetes and cardiovascular disease *(1,2)*. A conference sponsored by the National Heart, Lung and Blood Institute in collaboration with the American Heart Association *(3)* recently defined the metabolic syndrome as a complex of three out of five criteria: abdominal obesity, elevated triglycerides, lower high-density lipoprotein (HDL), hypertension, and elevated fasting plasma glucose (Fig. 1). The World Health Organization also required insulin resistance for diagnosis of the syndrome *(3)*. It is estimated that 47 million Americans have been diagnosed with the metabolic syndrome, as established from census data from 2000 *(1)*. According to the American Association of Clinical Endocrinologists, the prevalence of insulin-resistance syndrome has risen more than 60% over the past decade *(4)*. Insulin resistance is present in the majority of people with the metabolic syndrome, is strongly associated with risk factors for cardiovascular disease (CVD), and is considered a prediabetic condition *(3)*. Clinical measures that often cluster with the metabolic syndrome are other dyslipidemias, including elevated apolipoprotein B levels and small low-density lipoprotein particles; proinflammatory states as represented by elevated C-reactive protein; and prothrombotic states including plasma fibrinogen and decreased fibrolysis potentially through elevated plasminogen activator inhibitor1. Thus, the metabolic syn-

From: *Calcium in Human Health*
Edited by: C. M. Weaver and R. P. Heaney © Humana Press Inc., Totowa, NJ

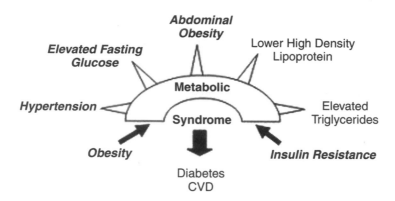

Fig. 1. Components or pathogenic mechanisms potentially improved by dietary calcium (highlighted in italics).

drome is a complex cluster of symptoms which puts individuals at greatly increased risk for the development of debilitating chronic diseases such as CVD and diabetes.

The pathogenesis of the metabolic syndrome is thought to be primarily obesity (particularly abdominal fat) and insulin resistance, although a variety of genetic and other factors such as age may also contribute to the acquisition of the syndrome (1). Both pharmacological regimens and alterations in lifestyle are recommended for either improving the factors leading to the development of the disease (obesity and insulin resistance) or treating components of the metabolic syndrome to prevent subsequent development of type 2 diabetes and CVD (5). Recent studies suggest that dietary calcium may reduce the development of the metabolic syndrome, and potentially reduce the incidence of components or associated clinical abnormalities (Fig. 1).

2. METABOLIC SYNDROME AND CALCIUM OR DAIRY PRODUCT INTAKE

Several studies point to a relationship between dairy product intake and reduced incidence of metabolic syndrome (6,7). Dairy products are the primary source of dietary calcium in the United States, and thus intake of dairy products is often used to assess dietary calcium effects. However, dairy products are a source of many other nutrients, and the impact of these nutrients or bioactive substance need to be considered if elemental calcium is not used in intervention studies.

In a cross-sectional analysis of men and women (N = 4976) aged 30–64 yr, Mennen and colleagues (6) demonstrated that dairy product intake was inversely associated with diastolic blood pressure (DBP) in both men and women. In addition, dairy product intake was inversely associated with HDL cholesterol concentration, fasting blood glucose, and serum triglyceride only in men. In this study, the metabolic syndrome was diagnosed by identifying two of four criteria (serum triglycerides, HDL cholesterol, glucose concentration, and DBP) to be within specific ranges. The results showed that more than one dairy serving per day decreased the risk of metabolic syndrome by 40% in men (6).

The prospective analysis in the Coronary Artery Risk Development in Adults (CARDIA) study examined the effects of dairy product consumption on the development of the

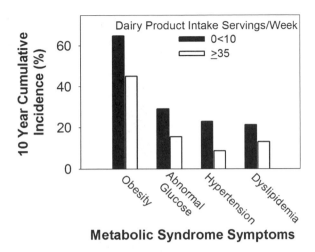

Fig. 2. Development of metabolic syndrome symptoms is reduced with higher dairy product intakes. (Modified from ref. 7.)

metabolic syndrome in a large cohort ($N = 3157$) of both black and white young men and women over a period of approx 10 yr (7). In the CARDIA study, the metabolic syndrome was defined as having at least two of four components: abnormal glucose homeostasis, obesity, elevated BP, and dyslipidemia. The results of this study demonstrated significantly less development of obesity ($p < 0.001$), abnormal glucose homeostasis ($p < 0.01$), and hypertension ($p < 0.001$), and a trend ($p < 0.07$) for reduced dyslipidemia in overweight participants as dairy intake rose, in models which included age, study center, caloric intake, race, sex and baseline body mass index (BMI; Fig. 2). From the results of this study, it is estimated that each additional serving of dairy products was associated with 21% lower odds of developing metabolic syndrome in the overweight participants (BMI > 25 kg/m^2). These interesting results provide support for a significant impact of dairy consumption on reducing the development of components of the metabolic syndrome in the obese, and thus suggest a way to reduce the incidence of the metabolic syndrome.

Although these studies support a role of increased dairy product consumption on improvement in IRS and its components, the specific role of calcium remains to be determined. These studies are confounded by the fact that the primary source of dietary calcium in the diet is dairy products (*see* Chapter 9). Although calcium has been proposed to be the bioactive component that regulates the metabolic syndrome, the impact of other dairy product components must be considered. In addition, higher calcium diets are associated with a healthier diet in general (8), and thus, elemental calcium intervention studies are needed to clarify whether dietary calcium specifically reduces the risk of metabolic syndrome.

3. EFFECT OF CALCIUM ON INDIVIDUAL COMPONENTS OF THE METABOLIC SYNDROME

Several studies suggest an association between higher dairy product consumption and decreased risk of the individual components of metabolic syndrome or associated dis-

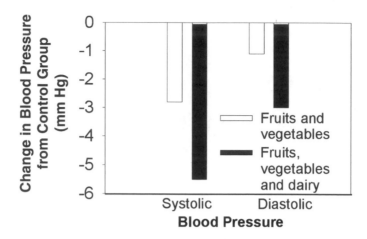

Fig. 3. Impact of added dairy intake on blood pressure. (Modified from ref. *15*.)

eases, such as hypertension *(9)*, coagulopathy *(10)*, and coronary artery disease *(11)*. There has been substantial investigation into the relationship between dietary calcium and hypertension over the last two decades *(12–14)* (*see* Chapter 28). Higher dietary intakes of calcium consistently demonstrate an anti-hypertensive effect *(14)*. A meta-analysis of 42 randomized controlled calcium intervention studies was completed that included studies with at least 2 wk of intervention of either dietary or supplemental calcium *(9)*. The results demonstrate a small but significant reduction in systolic blood pressure SBP; (–1.44 mmHg) and DBP (–0.84 mmHg). Furthermore, the results of the multicenter Dietary Approaches to Stop Hypertension study show that a dietary pattern rich in fruits and vegetables achieves a reduction in BP (2.8 and 1.1 mmHg SBP and DBP, respectively) in 8 wk compared with control diet ($p < 0.001$ and $p < 0.07$, respectively) (Fig. 3) *(15)*. However, when approximately three low-fat dairy products are also included in the diet, along with lower saturated fat and cholesterol, the reduction in BP (5.5 mmHg SBP and 3.0 mmHg DBP) was two times greater than produced by the diet rich in fruits and vegetables alone. These results contribute to the consensus that inclusion of three dairy servings will substantially reduce BP *(16)*, and that it is likely that calcium is an important bioactive component mediating this reduction.

4. PATHOGENETIC MECHANISMS

Dietary calcium (and dairy products) affect two of the proposed pathogenetic mechanisms—obesity and insulin resistance—for the development of the metabolic syndrome.

4.1. Obesity

Obesity is a multifactorial disease whose etiologies include both genetics and lifestyle factors such as dietary patterns and physical activity. There is substantial evidence that higher dairy product intake can contribute to reduced fat mass *(17–19*; *see* Chapter 21). However, the impact of dietary calcium, independent of dairy product intake, has not been clearly established. Overall, the data suggest that dietary calcium may have a small, but significant effect on preventing body fat accumulation *(18–21)* and in enhancing fat mass lost during intentional weight loss *(22)*. The proposed mechanisms that underlie these effects include changes in lipid oxidation and lipolysis, potentially mediated through parathyroid hormone (PTH) and 1,25 dihydroxyvitamin D (1,25[OH]$_2$D) (*see* Chapter 21).

4.2. Insulin Resistance

Insulin resistance represents impaired end-organ response to insulin. When target tissues have a reduced response to insulin, the result is high blood glucose, increased glucose production, and increased lipid oxidation. There are few clinical data to support a role for dietary calcium on insulin resistance, particularly independent of effects of calcium in reducing body composition. Clearly, reductions in weight, particularly fat mass, can improve insulin resistance. The potential mechanisms involved with both reductions in fat mass and improved insulin sensitivity involve PTH and 1,25(OH)$_2$D$_3$, and are discussed later.

4.3. Insulin Regulation of Glucose Metabolism and Lipid Oxidation

Insulin acts through the insulin receptor *(23)*, which is a heterotetramer comprised of two α-subunits and two β-subunits. Following autophosphorylation, a series of protein–protein interactions and phosphorylation events mediate signaling within the cell. In addition to other substrates, there are four major insulin receptor substrates 1 to 4. Glucose enters the cell via a family of glucose transporters, including GLUT1, which is constitutively present on the cell membrane and GLUT4. Insulin acts acutely to stimulate transfer of the glucose transporter, GLUT4, from vesicles stored within the cell to the cell membrane, thereby allowing increased glucose uptake. Insulin also regulates changes in gene transcription of proteins in many systems. Overall, insulin action increases glycolysis, glycogenesis, and lipid synthesis, while reducing lipid oxidation.

4.4. Dietary Calcium Relationship With PTH and 1,25(OH)$_2$D$_3$

It is proposed that dietary calcium regulation of the hormones, PTH and 1,25(OH)$_2$D$_3$, mediate the effects of calcium on fat mass *(24,25)*, and that these hormones may also mediate the regulation of insulin resistance. Low dietary calcium results in a lowering of serum calcium, promoting PTH release. Although it is well established that PTH regulates the activity of the 1-α-hydroxylase to convert 25 hydroxyvitamin D (25[OH]D) to 1,25(OH)$_2$D$_3$, the relationship between PTH and serum 1,25(OH)$_2$D$_3$ levels is less clearly established. Serum levels of 25(OH)D, which is a marker for vitamin D status, are inversely correlated with fasting levels of PTH below 25(OH)D concentrations of approx 80 nmol/L *(26)*.

4.5. Relationship of PTH and Obesity

In addition to the classical functions of PTH and 1,25(OH)$_2$D$_3$, both hormones increase levels of intracellular calcium in a variety of tissues including adipocytes, which can lead to a decrease in lipolysis and an increase in lipogenesis through increases in fatty acid synthase levels in the cell *(24)*. This shift in lipid utilization in the presence of higher levels of PTH or 1,25(OH)$_2$D$_3$ may produce an accumulation of fat in adipocytes.

It is not yet clear which component of the energy balance that leads to changes in body composition is regulated by dietary calcium or dairy products. One proposed mechanism is that dietary calcium may lead to increases in lipid oxidation (27,28). In support of this mechanism, changes in fasting PTH, but not $1,25(OH)_2D_3$, were negatively correlated with changes in lipid oxidation in a 1-yr randomized dairy product intervention trial in young women (29).

Changes in serum levels of PTH in animal models are also associated with regulation of lipid oxidation. For example, a case report showed that three individuals had both hyperparathyroidism and significantly lowered muscle CPT-I (30). CPT-I catalyzes the rate-limiting step of mitochondrial fatty acid oxidation. Rodent models of chronic renal failure (CRF) also provide support a role for PTH effects on lipid oxidation via regulation of CPT-I activity, as secondary hyperparathyroidism is associated with CRF. Studies from more than a decade ago show that oxidation of long and short-chain fatty acids by muscle mitochondria is impaired in CRF rats owing, in part, to reduced activity of CPT-I (31). Thus, PTH reduces CPT-I, which would lead to suppression of lipid oxidation.

Although these results are consistent with a potential for losing body fat mass and body weight, they are not consistent with improving insulin sensitivity as insulin action reduces lipid oxidation. If dietary calcium improves insulin sensitivity in addition to promoting increased lipid oxidation, this suggests a potentially complex interplay of factors that together promote an increase in lipid oxidation in the face of improved insulin action.

4.6. Link Between PTH, $1,25(OH)_2D_3$, and Insulin Action

There is evidence to support an effect of PTH and $1,25(OH)_2D_3$ at multiple levels of insulin release and action. It is well established that there is a greatly increased prevalence of type 2 diabetes mellitus (8%) and glucose intolerance (40%) in patients with primary hyperparathyroidism (32). In addition, fasting intact PTH levels were shown to be inversely correlated with insulin sensitivity in 52 normotensive, healthy subjects, even after adjustment for potentially confounding factors (33), indicating that fasting serum PTH may mediate changes in glucose tolerance.

There is also evidence that PTH may mediate insulin resistance by reducing glucose uptake (34,35). PTH increased at 1 h, but then decreased at 16 h, insulin-stimulated glucose transport (using 2-deoxyglucose). GLUT1 mRNA was reduced in osteogenic sarcoma cells following 16 h PTH treatment (34). In addition, PTH increased the phosphorylation of the insulin-sensitive glucose transporter, GLUT4, and decreased insulin-stimulated glucose uptake in rat adipocytes (35). These studies suggest that PTH may elicit insulin resistance by reducing the number of glucose transporters (both GLUT1 and GLUT4) available in the membrane to allow glucose uptake.

Inadequate vitamin D status is also proposed to play a role in insulin resistance syndrome (36). One interesting concept is found in data demonstrating that a vitamin D response element sequence is found in the insulin receptor gene promoter (37). Consistent with this finding, $1,25(OH)_2D_3$ increased the expression and transcription of the insulin receptor in pro-monocytic lymphoma cells (38). Together, these data suggest that $1,25(OH)_2D_3$ may affect insulin resistance by enhancing insulin action through increased receptor levels.

The classically defined actions of PTH and $1,25(OH)_2D_3$ demonstrate coordinated action of these hormones to maintain serum calcium. However, growing evidence suggests that PTH and $1,25(OH)_2D_3$ may have opposing effects in other systems, such as regulation of glucose uptake with PTH opposing glucose uptake and $1,25(OH)_2D_3$ enhancing insulin action. Another mechanism by which vitamin D may improve insulin action is by its ability to reduce PTH levels *(26)*. There is evidence that increased blood PTH is associated with insulin resistance or glucose intolerance, which is thus consistent with the vitamin D *sufficiency* association with reduced insulin resistance. The negative association of vitamin D status with fasting PTH levels may also be a mechanism by which overall exposure of the system to PTH and $1,25(OH)_2D_3$ may be controlled by vitamin D status as well as dietary calcium. Thus, the relationship between dietary calcium, PTH, and $1,25(OH)_2D_3$ may be more complex and allow opposing actions of these hormones to reduce obesity and improve insulin sensitivity.

5. CONCLUSIONS

The metabolic syndrome is an aggregate of symptoms including abdominal obesity, hypertension, dyslipidemias, and elevated blood glucose levels. The incidence of the metabolic syndrome is rising rapidly. It is imperative to identify strategies to prevent the increase of the metabolic syndrome. Long-term prospective trials as well as other epidemiological evidence support the conclusion that higher intake of dairy products is associated with reduced incidence of metabolic syndrome as well as reductions both in individual symptoms and pathogenic mechanisms. No studies to date clearly demonstrate that dietary calcium specifically plays a role in improving established metabolic syndrome or its symptoms. However, in vivo studies indicate that dietary calcium regulation of PTH and $1,25(OH)_2D_3$ may play a role in improving the individual symptoms of the syndrome, including hypertension, elevated fasting glucose and obesity, as well as possibly insulin resistance. Further studies, particularly of specific interventions, will be necessary to clarify the role that calcium plays in modulating the metabolic syndrome.

REFERENCES

1. Steinbaum SR. The metabolic syndrome: an emerging health epidemic in women. Prog Cardiovasc Dis 2004;46:321–336.
2. Reaven GM. Role of insulin resistance in human disease (syndrome X): an expanded definition. Annu Rev Med 1993;44:121–131.
3. Grundy SM, Brewer HB, Cleeman JI, Smith SC, Lenfant C. Definition of metabolic syndrome: report of the National Heart, Lung, and Blood Institute/American Heart Association Conference on Scientific Issues Related to Definition. Circulation 2004;109:433–438.
4. American Association of Clinical Endocrinologists. Findings and recommendations from the America College of Endocrinology Conference on the Insulin Resistance Syndrome, August 2002. www.aace.com.
5. Grundy SM, Hansen B, Smith SC, Cleeman JI, Kahn RA. Clinical management of metabolic syndrome: report of the National Heart, Lung, and Blood Institute/American Heart Association Conference on Scientific Issues Related to Management. Circulation 2004b;109:551–556.
6. Mennen LI, Lafay L, Feskens EJM, et al. Possible protective effect of bread and dairy products on the risk of the metabolic syndrome. Nutr Res 2000;20:335–347.
7. Pereira MA, Jacobs DR, Van Horn L, Slattery ML, Kartashov AI, Ludwig DS. Dairy consumption, obesity, and the insulin resistance syndrome in young adults. The CARDIA Study. JAMA 2002;287: 2081–2089.
8. Barger-Lux MJ, Heaney RP, Packard PT, Lappe JM, Recker RR. Nutritional correlates of low calcium intake. Clin Appl Nutr 1992;2:39–44.

9. Griffith LE, Guyatt GH, Cook RJ, Busher HC, Cook DJ. The influence of dietary and nondietary calcium supplementation on blood pressure: and updated metaanalysis of randomized controlled trials. Am J Hypertens 1999;12:84–92.

10. Mennen LI, Balkau B, Vol S, et al. Tissue-type plasminogen activator antigen and consumption of dairy products. The DESIR Study. Throm Res 1999;94:381–388.

11. Ness AR, Smith GD, Hart C. Milk, coronary heart disease and mortality. J Epidemiol Community Health 2001;55:379–382.

12. McCarron DA. Calcium metabolism and hypertension. Kidney Int 1989;35:717–36.

13. Miller GD, DiRienzo DD, Reusser ME, McCarron DA.Benefits of dairy product consumption on blood pressure in humans: a summary of the biomedical literature. J Am Coll Nutr 2000;19:147S–164S.

14. Vaskonen T. Dietary minerals and modification of cardiovascular risk factors. J Nutr Biochem 2003;14:492–506.

15. Appel LJ, Moore TJ, Obarzanek E, Vollmer WM, Svetkey LP, Sacks FM, Bray GA, Vogt TM, Cutler JA, Windhauser MM, Lin PH, Karanja N. A clinical trial of the effects of dietary patterns on blood pressure. DASH Collaborative Research Group. N Engl J Med 1997;336:1117–24.

16. Institute of Medicine. Dietary Reference Intakes: Calcium and Bone Related Nutrients. National Academy Press, Washington, DC, 1997.

17. Teegarden D. Calcium intake and reduction in weight or body fat. J Nutr 2003;133:249–251.

18. Parikh SJ, Yanovski JA. Calcium intake and adiposity. Am J Clin Nutr 2003;77: 281–287.

19. Heaney RP, Davies KM, Barger-Lux MJ. Calcium and weight: clinical studies. J Am Coll Nutr 2002;21:152S–155S.

20. Lin YC, Lyle RM, McCabe LD, McCabe GP, Weaver CM, Teegarden D. Dairy calcium is related to changes in body composition during a two-year exercise intervention in young women. J Am Coll Nutr 2000;19:754–760.

21. Barger-Lux MJ, Davies KM, Heaney RP, Chin BK, Rafferty K. Calcium supplementation may attenuate accumulation of fat in young women. J Bone Miner Res 2001;16:S219.

22. Zemel MB, Thompson W, Milstead A, Morris K, Campbell P. Calcium and dairy acceleration of weight and fat loss during energy restriction in obese adults. Obesity Res 2004;12:582–590.

23. Virkamaki A, Ueki K, Kahn CR. Protein-protein interaction in insulin signaling and the molecular mechanisms of insulin resistance. J Clin Invest 1999;103(7):931–943.

24. Zemel MB, Shi H, Greer B, DiRienzo D, and Zemel PC. Regulation of adiposity by dietary calcium. FASEB J 2000;14:1132–1138.

25. McCarty MF, Thomas CA. PTH excess may promote weight gain by impeding catecholamine-induced lipolysis—implications for the impact of calcium, vitamin D, and alcohol on body weight. Med Hypotheses 2003;61:535–542.

26. Krall EA, Sahyoun N, Tannenbaum S, Dallal GE, Dawson-Hughes B. Effect of vitamin D intake on seasonal variations in parathyroid hormone secretion in postmenopausal women. N Engl J Med 1989;321:1777–1783.

27. Gunther CW, Legowski PA, Lyle RM, et al. Dairy products do not lead to alterations in body weight and fat mass in young women in a one year intervention. Am J Clin Nutr 2005;81:751–756.

28. Melanson EL, Sharp TA, Schneider J, Donahoo WT, Grunwald GK, and Hill JO. Relation between calcium intake and fat oxidation in adult humans. Int J Obes Relat Metab Disord 2003;27:196–203.

29. Gunther CW, Lyle RM, Teegarden D. One year change in log parathyroid hormone negatively predicts one year change in postprandial lipid oxidation in young women on dairy calcium intervention. FASEB J 2004;18:A924.

30. Uemura O, Goto Y, Iwasa M, Ando T, Sato K, Tominaga Y, Uchida K, Ichiki T, and Sugiyama N. Secondary carnitine palmitoyltransferase deficiency in chronic renal failure and secondary hyperparathyroidism. Tohoku J Exp Med 1996;178:307–314.

31. Smogorzewski M, Perna AF, Borum PR, and Massry SG. Fatty acid oxidation in the myocardium: effects of parathyroid hormone and CRF. Kidney Int 1988;34:797–803.

32. Taylor WH, Khaleeli AA. Coincident diabetes mellitus and primary hyperparathyroidism. Diabetes Metab Res Rev 2001;17:175–180.

33. Chiu KC, Chuang L-M, Lee NP, Ryu JM, McGullam JL, Tsai GP, Saad MF. Insulin sensitivity is inversely correlated with plasma intact parathyroid hormone level. Metabolism 2000;49:1501–1505.

34. Thomas DM, Rogers SD, Sleeman MW, Pasquini GM, Bringhurst FR, Ng KW, Zajac JD and Best JD. Modulation of glucose transport by parathyroid hormone and insulin in UMR-106-01, a clonal rat osteogenic sarcoma cell line. J Mol Endocrin 1995;14:263–275.
35. Reusch JE, Begum N, Sussman KE, Draznin B. Regulation of GLUT-4 phosphorylation by intracellular calcium in adipocytes. Endocrinology 1991;129:3269–3273.
36. Boucher BJ. Inadequate vitamin D status: does it contribute to the disorders compromising syndrome 'X'? Br J Nutr 1998;79, 315–327.
37. Maestro B, Davila N, Carranza MC, Calle C. Identification of a Vitamin D response element in the human insulin receptor gene promoter. J Steroid Biochem Mol Biol 2003;84:223–230.
38. Maestro B, Campion J, Davila N, Calle C. Stimulation by 1,25-dihydroxyvitamin D3 of insulin receptor expression and insulin responsiveness for glucose transport in U-937 human promonocytic cells. Endocr J 2000;47:383–391.

27 Calcium and Phosphate Control in Patients With Renal Disease

David A. McCarron and Robert P. Heaney

KEY POINTS

- Commonly used to control phosphorus retention in patients with chronic kidney disease, calcium-containing phosphate binders (CCPB) have been purported to contribute to the development of vascular calcifications in these patients.
- Numerous findings now indicate that vascular calcifications often precede the use of CCPB, and that adequate calcium may actually reduce calcification prevalence with the comitant benefit of improved skeletal health.
- Non-calcium-containing binders are available, but these have not been shown to confer benefits equal to those of CCPB.

1. INTRODUCTION

Calcium intake is important in patients with chronic kidney disease (CKD) for several reasons: in control of serum phosphorus concentration, in modulation of parathyroid gland hyperplasia, as a factor in extraosseous (particularly vascular) mineralization, and in protecting the skeleton from osteoporosis. Moreover, disturbances of calcium and phosphate balance have long been recognized as sentinel and persistent markers of kidney disease.

Even with the earliest reductions in glomerular filtration rate, the kidney struggles with eliminating the daily phosphate load. The modest retention of phosphate that ensues and then persists throughout all stages of CKD inexorably alters calcium homeostasis, and results in barely detectable decreases in free calcium and stimulation of parathyroid hormone (PTH) secretion as a counter measure. The chronic stimulation of PTH secretion ultimately produces parathyroid hyperplasia, metabolic bone disease, and a myriad of chronic and often fatal metabolic disturbances in CKD patients.

This chapter examines specifically the evidence relating the use of calcium-containing phosphate binders (CCPB) to vascular calcification and will note that calcifications in CKD patients often precede the use of calcium-based binders. We also assess the value of earlier and more aggressive management of phosphate and calcium imbalance in this

From: *Calcium in Human Health*
Edited by: C. M. Weaver and R. P. Heaney © Humana Press Inc., Totowa, NJ

population, specifically using calcium supplements to reduce the prevalence of vascular calcifications. The implications for the general population in terms of risk vs benefits of calcium supplement use as they affect cardiovascular events are addressed. Also, we review the clinical trials that have assessed the role of non-CCPB in reducing cardiovascular morbidity and mortality in CKD and end-stage renal disease (ESRD) patients on maintenance hemodialysis. Finally, we address the issue of osteoporosis protection.

2. CONTROLLING PHOSPHORUS RETENTION AND HYPERPHOSPHATEMIA

It is essential to protect calcium homeostasis in these patients by first removing the excess phosphorus burden and improving calcium availability. The former has typically been achieved by binding intestinal phosphate, classically by the administration of a calcium salt. The latter has usually been achieved by the administration of either supplemental calcium, in which use calcium plays a pharmacological rather than a nutritional role. If serum phosphate concentration is not controlled, soft tissue calcifications will occur, most dramatically in the vasculature. Finally, after transplantation, severe secondary hyperparathyroidism often develops.

As a discipline, nephrology has over the past four decades frequently revisited the question of how best to remove phosphate while maintaining calcium homeostasis. Alternative approaches to using CCPB have been championed and utilized only to discover, after widespread and continued use, that unforeseen serious complications can emerge. The problems accompanying use of aluminum-based phosphate binders are examples (1).

Again today, clinical nephrology is confronting the issue of whether it is appropriate to rely on CCPB as one of the cornerstones of managing calcium and phosphorus balance. The particular question that has recently emerged in the treatment of patients with ESRD or early CKD is the origin of vascular calcifications seen in this patient population. Critics have hypothesized that the calcifications are due principally to the use of calcium-based binders used to manage hyperphosphatemia (2–4). If this is the case, the use of calcium supplements by the general population, for whom vascular calcification also predicts cardiovascular events, should be re-evaluated.

There is no disagreement that calcifications in vessels predict mortality in the CKD population. It is the antecedent factors that trigger calcification that are currently being debated. There is general agreement that high blood pressure, lipid disorders, excessive levels of PTH, and aggressive treatment with vitamin D are associated with vascular calcifications. What is disputed is whether treatment with CCPB increases the deposition of calcium in vascular tissue.

3. PATHOPHYSIOLOGY OF EXTRAOSSEOUS CALCIFICATION

Damaged tissues throughout the body tend to calcify and, in some instances, even to ossify. Two factors are involved: (1) local tissue alterations that predispose to mineralization, and (2) an adequate supply of mineral brought to the mineralizing site by the circulating blood. The former is beyond the scope of this chapter, but is exemplified in the calcification of granulomas, of ligamentous tears, of necrotic cancerous lesions, and of atheromatous plaques in the walls of arteries. The supply of mineral is reflected in the concentration of calcium and phosphorus (as phosphate) in the circulating blood.

The propensity of these ions to come out of solution and to support crystal growth at a mineralizing site is, strictly speaking, expressed as their ion product in the extracellular fluid (i.e., $Ca \times P$, in mEq/L). In common usage, the actual serum concentrations are used instead, and are expressed in mg/dL. At a mean serum Ca of 9.5 mg/dL, and a mean serum phosphorus of 3.5 mg/dL, the empiric $Ca \times P$ averages approx 33, and ranges from approx 27 to approx 42 in healthy adults. At physiological pH and pCO_2, Ca and P concentrations are indefinitely stable and will not spontaneously support precipitation of $CaHPO_4$, the calcium phosphate crystal species most likely to form under such conditions. By contrast, in the presence of hydroxyapatite $[Ca_{10}(OH)_2 (PO_4)_6]$, which is much less soluble than $CaHPO_4$, these same serum concentrations will readily support crystal growth. (This contrast highlights the critical role of the local factor which, by creating conditions favorable to hydroxyapatite, effectively pulls calcium and phosphorus out of an otherwise stable solution.)

It is important to recognize that ingested or absorbed minerals influence a propensity to mineralize solely through their effect on serum levels. A mineralizing site cannot "see" what we eat; it "sees" only the concentrations of minerals in the blood flowing past it. In CKD, and particularly in ESRD, the blood $Ca \times P$ rises, mainly because of phosphate retention and consequent hyperphosphatemia, but also because of absorption of some of the calcium used to block dietary phosphorus absorption. Serum phosphorus values above 6 mg/dL are common, producing $Ca \times P$ values of 60 or higher. These values are more than adequate to support calcification of damaged tissues, and even to cause spontaneous calcification in otherwise healthy tissues. Although elevations of either calcium or phosphorus could raise the $Ca \times P$, in actuality, the principal contribution to these elevated $Ca \times P$ products is serum phosphorus, which in CKD is typically 50–100% higher than mean adult normal values and which, by itself, can more than double the $Ca \times P$. By contrast, serum Ca uncommonly departs from normal by more than 10–20%. Hence the large elevations in $Ca \times P$ values are owing mostly to poor control of serum P.

4. HYPERPARATHYROIDISM IN ESRD AND CKD

As noted, parathyroid hyperplasia is nearly universal in CKD. Posttransplant, the large parathyroid gland mass often results in explicit hyperparathyroidism. The functionality of the parathyroid glands posttransplant was first examined by McCarron and co-workers (5). In vivo PTH responses to changes in extracellular calcium were examined in normal people ($n = 8$) and in patients with persistent hyperparathyroidism following renal transplantation ($n = 15$). In 80% of hyperparathyroid patients, the PTH response was related to total gland size measured at the time of parathyroidectomy. Basal PTH levels did not predict gland size, but gland size did correlate with changes in PTH induced by infusion of ethylenediaminetetraacetic acid ($p < 0.001$) or calcium ($p < 0.001$). Thus, the magnitude of the PTH response to hypocalcemic and hypercalcemic challenge is highly predictive of gland mass.

When the PTH gland mass was measured in 17 posttransplant patients, no relationship was seen between gland mass and age or gender, duration of dialysis, or time between treatment and parathyroidectomy (6). Gland mass, however, was related to the type and the duration of disease. In the presence of relatively acute onset, such as rapidly progressive glomerular disease, where the onset of renal failure is rapid, only a modest level of hyperparathyroidism is observed. On the other hand, in the presence of CKD, which is tubulointerstitial in nature and where the duration of time before dialysis is far greater and more prolonged compared with glomerular disease, parathyroid hyperplasia is more pronounced. Thus, posttransplant hypercalcemia related to hyperparathyroidism is more likely to occur in ESRD and CKD patients with slowly progressive renal disease of prolonged duration. The excessive PTH secretion and gland hypertrophy of this situation is, in most patients, related to the failure to introduce aggressive, early management of phosphate metabolism.

5. CARDIAC MORBIDITY AND MORTALITY IN HEMODIALYSIS PATIENTS

In addition to hypercalcemia associated with posttransplant hyperparathyroidism, there is extensive evidence in the literature indicating that vascular calcification is a consequence of poor management of serum calcium and phosphorus concentration, rather than the use of CCPB. As already noted, hyperphosphatemia is a common feature of ESRD and is associated with increased cardiovascular mortality risk in patients receiving maintenance hemodialysis.

Using data from two national, random samples of hemodialysis patients (n = 12,833), Ganesh and co-workers (7) tested the hypothesis that elevated serum phosphorus contributes to cardiac deaths. In a 2-yr follow-up, the relative risk of death was analyzed for several categories of cause of death, including coronary artery disease (CAD), sudden death, and other cardiac causes. Relative risk was assessed with respect to serum phosphorus, Ca × P, and serum PTH. In all cases, higher cardiovascular morbidity and mortality risk was seen for patients with serum phosphorus >6.5 mg/dL, compared with those with serum phosphorus of no more than 6.5 mg/dL. The study identified strong relationships between elevated serum phosphorus, Ca × P, and PTH, implicating poor control of phosphorus metabolism in the excess cardiovascular mortality. Neither serum calcium nor CCPB were identified as being associated with higher risks of morbidity and mortality. Thus, it appears that calcification, which begins with the onset of renal disease, is best resolved by early and aggressive management of serum phosphate (e.g., by use of CCPB).

6. VASCULAR CALCIFICATION ASSOCIATED WITH CAD IN HEMODIALYSIS PATIENTS

Several studies have examined the risk factors for, and the onset of, calcifications leading to CAD. Braun and colleagues (8) utilized electron beam computed tomography (EBCT) to detect cardiac calcifications in the coronary arteries and cardiac valves of dialysis patients. Forty-nine chronic hemodialysis patients were compared with 102 nondialysis patients with documented or suspected CAD. All patients had undergone coronary angiography. The number of calcifications, the surface area, and the average and highest density values were measured in 30 axial slices, with a distance of 30 mm between each slice. The quantitative coronary artery calcification score was found to be 2.5- to fivefold higher in hemodialysis patients compared with nondialysis patients. There was no correlation between serum calcium, phosphorus, or PTH values and the coronary calcification scores. Higher calcification scores were observed in hypertensive dialysis patients compared with normotensive dialysis patients (P <0.05), and correlated with lower vertebral bone mass in the dialysis patients.

The correlation of higher coronary artery calcification scores in those patients with lower vertebral bone mass suggests that depletion of calcium stores in the bone, a marker of failed maintenance of calcium balance, predicts vascular calcifications. Proper management of ESRD and CKD patients to reduce the likelihood of vascular and cardiac calcifications should include early repletion or supplementation of calcium and reduction of hypertension. Some of the confusion in this regard may arise from the fact that using calcium to control calcification seems counterintuitive. However, the rise in serum calcium associated with CCPB is less than the fall in serum phosphorus that CCPB produces. So the result is that CCPB usually lowers the serum Ca× P.

Merjanian and co-workers *(9)* examined the temporal sequence of vascular and valvular calcific disease in relation to diabetic ESRD in nondialyzed individuals. Thirty-two patients with type 2 diabetes mellitus and diabetic renal disease were compared with a group of 18 normoalbuminuric diabetic patients and 95 nondiabetic control subjects without renal disease. The groups were matched for age, gender, ethnicity, and the presence or absence of dyslipidemia, hypertension, and known CAD. EBCT demonstrated the prevalence of significant coronary artery calcification in individuals with diabetic renal disease compared with nondiabetic controls ($p < 0.001$). Coronary artery calcification scores were also significantly more severe in diabetic renal disease patients compared with non-CKD controls, both diabetic and nondiabetic (median scores: 238 vs 10, $p < 0.001$).

Diabetic renal disease patients with known CAD demonstrated coronary artery calcification and aortic wall calcification scores several-fold greater compared with patients without CAD. Multivariate analysis identified age and diabetic renal disease as additional predictors for the presence or severity of coronary artery and aortic wall calcification. This was the first study to systematically analyze nondialyzed individuals with diabetic renal disease, and demonstrated that vascular and valvular calcification is present and often severe long before the disease progresses to ESRD *(9)*.

EBCT was also used to screen for coronary artery calcification in 39 young patients (mean age: 19 yr) with ESRD who were undergoing dialysis compared with 60 normal subjects (age: 20–30 yr) *(3)*. Data showed that none of the 23 patients younger than 20 yr of age had evidence of coronary artery calcification. However, it was present in 14 of 16 patients over 20 yr of age. Among those with calcification, the median calcification score was 297. Only three normal subjects had calcification. Compared with patients without coronary artery calcification, those with calcification were older and had been on dialysis for a longer time period. Mean serum phosphorus, mean Ca × P, and daily intake of calcium were higher among the patients with coronary artery calcification. However, average calcium intake in these patients was 6.5 g/d—a rather high intake in a young hemodialysis population. Multivariate analysis for risk factors was not undertaken, and thus extrapolations from these observations in a unique clinical setting to the more general ESRD and CKD patient population are not appropriate.

In a cohort of 3014 CKD patients, Winkelmayer and co-workers *(10)* evaluated indicators of calcium and phosphorus metabolism prior to renal transplant. Indicators assessed were PTH or vitamin D metabolites and administration of calcitriol or CCPB prior to transplant. Only 3.4% of CKD patients had PTH assessment prior to transplant and 0.3% had vitamin D status measured. Calcitriol and CCPB were used by 12% and 16% of patients, respectively. These findings document that it is the rare CKD patient who has early and appropriate Ca × P management with CCPB and/or calcitriol. These patients were followed for 1 yr after appropriate CCPB and calcitriol therapy was initiated, and reported a subsequent, dramatic improvement in the Ca × P product, which was independently associated with a 35% decrease in 1-yr mortality.

7. VASCULAR CALCIFICATION AND CALCIUM SUPPLEMENT USE IN THE GENERAL POPULATION

That vascular calcification is a consequence of poor Ca × P management has also been noted in the general population that has not been exposed to calcium-based binders. Barengolts and colleagues *(11)* compared coronary calcification scores in 45 asymptomatic postmenopausal women with normal or low bone mineral density (BMD). BMD of the lumbar spine and proximal femur was measured by dual X-ray absorptiometry and coronary Ca was measured quantitatively by EBCT. The total coronary calcification scores were 41.9, 115.1, and 221.7 for the control, osteopenia, and osteoporosis groups, respectively; the score was significantly higher in the osteoporosis than in the control group. These data provide consistent evidence that otherwise healthy women with osteoporosis may have a higher risk of developing coronary atherosclerosis. This risk tracks with depletion of bone mineral content and is therefore unrelated to Ca intake.

8. VASCULAR CALCIFICATION: CHOICE OF PHOSPHATE BINDERS

Physicians have several choices of phosphate binders to manage hyperphosphatemia in hemodialysis patients. Management of ESRD patients with parathyroid hyperplasia using hemodialysis with calcitriol is common clinical practice. Unfortunately, calcitriol and its analogs increase intestinal absorption of calcium and phosphate, leading to an increased Ca × P product and thereby to extraosseous calcification. The Durham Renal Osteodystrophy Study Group *(12)* reported that at the end of a 40-wk trial, dialysis patients were better managed by calcium carbonate alone compared with calcium carbonate in combination with oral or intravenous calcitriol. Compared with the combination, calcium carbonate more effectively lowered serum phosphorus, was equivalent to the combination for reducing serum PTH, and was less likely to produce episodes of hypercalcemia.

In their treat-to-goal, randomized, 52-wk trial in 200 patients, Chertow et al. *(4)* compared sevelamer hydrochloride, a phosphate binding resin gel, with two different CCPB. The primary end-point of the trial was attainment of Ca × P product target levels. Study results showed that sevelamer hydrochloride and calcium provided equivalent control of serum phosphorus. Thus, the study failed to demonstrate that the primary end-point differed between the treatment regimens. Serum calcium concentration was significantly higher in the calcium-treated group ($p = 0.002$) and hypercalcemia was also more common ($p = 0.04$). Few subjects in the calcium group had PTH values within the target range (150–300 pg/mL). After 52 wk of treatment, significantly increased median absolute calcification scores in the coronary arteries ($p = 0.03$) and aorta ($p = 0.01$) were observed in the calcium-treated but not the sevelamer-treated patients.

These investigators concluded that sevelamer hydrochloride is less likely to cause hypercalcemia and low levels of PTH or to be associated with progressive coronary and aortic calcification in hemodialysis patients. They further stated that CCPB therapy was responsible for the progression of coronary calcifications in this population of CKD patients, an assessment that is inconsistent with the prior data in this field. A number of major flaws in the design and end-point measurements in this study, which have been noted in the literature *(13–15)*, seriously undermine the conclusions of these authors.

A prospective, randomized, double-blind, multicenter study comparing the efficacy and safety of calcium acetate and sevelamer hydrochloride for the treatment of hyper-phosphatemia in CKD patients on hemodialysis demonstrated that after 8 wk of treatment, Ca acetate was more effective than sevelamer hydrochloride in attaining serum calcium and Ca×P product target levels *(16)*. Higher serum calcium and bicarbonate values were also observed in patients treated with calcium acetate. These observations are consistent with data from previous trials that evaluated CCPB, and are inconsistent with results from the treat-to-goal trial, suggesting that calcium acetate might reduce the risk of vascular calcification and mortality in hemodialysis patients.

9. EFFICACY AND SAFETY OF CALCIUM SUPPLEMENTS

Calcium supplements are one of the most frequently used over-the-counter medications by the general population. They have been extensively used in many large federally supported clinical trials over the past several decades. To date, these numerous longitudinal randomized trials, which have often focused on high risk populations, have not reported any adverse effects of supplemental calcium. This includes vascular calcifications and is noteworthy because many of these trials, such as the Women's Health Initiative *(17)*, specifically involve persons at risk for CAD.

10. OSTEOPOROSIS PROTECTION

Bone disease in patients with CKD is a complex affair, well beyond the scope of this chapter. However, whatever the character of their deranged bone metabolism, it is known, that patients with ESRD are prone to fragility fractures *(18,19)*, that they have lower values for BMD than age- and sex-matched controls (often by as much as one standard deviation for the population concerned *[19–23]*), and that the degree of this deficit worsens with duration of dialysis *(18)*. Whether this symptom complex represents osteoporosis as usually understood is uncertain *(24)*. However, given the prevalence of osteoporosis in the general population, it should be obvious that patients with pre-existing osteoporosis, or at high risk for the disease, and who develop CKD, will at that point have two problems: dialytic bone disease plus their pre-existing osteoporosis. Finally, after transplantation, patients lose large amounts of bone in the 2 yr following surgery *(23)*, leaving them at a further skeletal disadvantage.

During the transition phase into renal dialysis, the physician's concern will be the management of the renal failure and some of its consequences, such as those discussed earlier. However, for the minority of patients who ultimately receive kidney transplants (and who thus are largely rid of their renal failure), it is important to pay attention to the determinants of their ultimate skeletal health, because bony deficits not prevented tend to be permanent.

During development of ordinary osteoporosis, the net loss of bone is reflected in an elevated urine calcium usually coupled with reduced net calcium absorption. The former cannot be a factor in patients on dialysis because they have no urine. In current practice, the dialysis bath calcium concentration is maintained at 2.5 mEq/L, or essentially the same as that in extracellular water. The goal is to maintain zero calcium balance (i.e., neither gaining nor losing calcium through dialysis). Digestive juice loss and cutaneous loss, however, are not handled by this stratagem, and if net intestinal absorption is not adequate to offset these extrarenal losses, negative calcium balance (i.e., bone loss) will ensue. One clear advantage of therapy with CCPB is that it ensures that net calcium absorption will meet these needs. Therapy with aluminum-containing phosphate binders or with sevelamer clearly do nothing to preserve bone mass. Previously, dialysis baths had used higher calcium concentration, with the intent of protecting the skeleton, but the resulting rise in blood $Ca \times P$ was interpreted as contributing to vascular calcification. This explains the current practice of maintaining zero net calcium shifts across dialysis.

Posttransplant, the issue clarifies. The drugs used to counter graft rejection cause major bone loss, and adequate calcium and vitamin D become essential (although not sufficient by themselves). Often antiresorptive therapy is indicated as well. By 2 yr posttransplant, when steroid dosage is usually lower, bone loss tends to ameliorate and may not be different from what is seen in age-matched, nontransplant individuals. However, any bony deficit incurred during dialysis or following transplant endures.

11. THE ANALOGOUS RENAL STONE STORY

As a final note, in answer to those critics who, by faulty logic, have postulated that the calcium deposited in vascular calcifications is a result of excessive calcium intake, there is a worthwhile analogy—kidney stones. Most renal stones contain primarily calcium as the mineral cation. In the past, clinicians routinely told patients with nephrolithiasis to avoid calcium in their diets. The logic was similar: if there is calcium in the stone, it must be due to too much calcium in the diet. Over the past 10–20 yr, we have learned the error of this logic, just as is now the case with the vascular calcification hysteria in CKD patients. It is now well established that for the most common renal stone patient, too little dietary calcium intake, not too much, is the problem (25–27). The reason is similar to calcium's role in controlling serum phosphorus concentration. High calcium intake blocks the absorption of dietary oxalate, which is a more potent stone-forming factor than is calcium. The result, despite a rise in urine calcium, is a reduced tendency for calcium oxalate stones to form. The same is true for patients with renal disease: assuring adequate calcium intake, not limiting it, is essential for improved health outcomes.

12. CONCLUSIONS

In conclusion, the antecedent factors that are responsible for vascular calcifications in CKD patients are not really debatable. Hypertension and lipid disorders are risk factors for calcifications, as is inadequate calcium intake. It has not been proven that calcium supplementation *per se* is responsible for vascular calcification. Indeed, evidence exists that vascular calcifications exist prior to the use of CCPB. Their use has been shown in multiple randomized, controlled trials to improve critical risk factors (e.g., serum phosphorus, $Ca \times P$, blood pressure, lipids, diabetes, and BMD) that are implicated in calcification.

Properly designed trials are needed to examine the issue of vascular calcification in ESRD and CKD patients. The most pressing issue is whether early intervention with

CCPB in patients with CKD will actually reduce the prevalence and severity of vascular calcification *(28)*. This is a readily accomplished clinical trial in all respects—design, implementation, cost, and importance—and it should be a priority of the renal research community to execute it as soon as feasible.

REFERENCES

1. Kates DM, Andress LD. Control of hyperphosphatemia in renal failure: role of aluminum. Semin Dial 1996;9:310–315.
2. Chertow GM. Slowing the progression of vascular calcification in hemodialysis. J Am Soc Nephrol 2003;14:S310–S314.
3. Goodman WG, Goldin J, Kuizon BD, et al. Coronary-artery calcification in young adults with end-stage renal disease who are undergoing dialysis. N Engl J Med 2000;342:1478–1483.
4. Chertow GM, Burke SK, Raggi P. Sevelamer attenuates the progression of coronary and aortic calcification in hemodialysis patients. Kidney Int 2002;62:245–252.
5. McCarron DA, Muther RS, Lenfesty B, Bennett WM. Parathyroid function in persistent hyperparathyroidism: relationship to gland size. Kidney Int 1982;22:662–670.
6. McCarron DA, Lenfesty B, Narasimhan N, Barry JM, Vetto RM, Bennett WM. Anatomical heterogeneity of parathyroid glands in post-transplant hyperparathyroidism. Am J Nephrol 1988;8:388–391.
7. Ganesh SK, Stack AG, Levin NW, Hulbert-Shearon T, Port FK. Association of elevated serum PO(4), Ca x PO(4) product, and parathyroid hormone with cardiac mortality risk in chronic hemodialysis patients. J Am Soc Nephrol 2001;12:2131–2138.
8. Braun J, Oldendorf M, Moshage W, Heidler R, Zeitler E, Luft FC. Electron beam computed tomography in the evaluation of cardiac calcification in chronic dialysis patients. Am J Kidney Dis 1996;27:394–401.
9. Merjanian R, Budoff M, Adler S, Berman N, Mehrotra R. Coronary artery, aortic wall, and valvular calcification in nondialyzed individuals with type 2 diabetes and renal disease. Kidney Int 2003;64:263–271.
10. Winkelmayer WC, Levin R, Avorn J. The nephrologist's role in the management of calcium-phosphorus metabolism in patients with chronic kidney disease. Kidney Int 2003;63:1836–1842.
11. Barengolts EI, Berman M, Kukreja SC, Kouznetsova T, Lin C, Chomka EV. Osteoporosis and coronary atherosclerosis in asymptomatic postmenopausal women. Calcif Tissue Int 1998;62:209–213.
12. Indridason OS, Quarles LD. Comparison of treatments for mild secondary hyperparathyroidism in hemodialysis patients. Durham Renal Osteodystrophy Study Group. Kidney Int 2000;57:282–292.
13. Backenroth R. Dialysate calcium use in hemodialysis patients. Kidney Int 2003;64:1533.
14. Canavese C, Bergama D, Dib H, Bermoso F, Burdese M. Calcium on trial: beyond a reasonable doubt? Kidney Int 2003;63:381–382.
15. McCarron DA. Sevelamer: where are the data? Kidney Int 2003;64:2329.
16. Qunibi WY, Hootkins RE, McDowell LL, et al. Treatment of hyperphosphatemia in hemodialysis patients: the Calcium Acetate Renagel® Evaluation (CARE) Study. Kidney Int 2004;65:1914–1926.
17. Women's Health Initiative Study Group. Design of the Women's Health Initiative clinical trial and observational study. Control Clin Trials 1998;19:61–109.
18. Fontaine MA, Albert A, Dubois B, Saint-Remy A, Rorive G. Fracture and bone mineral density in hemodialysis patients. Clin Nephrol 2000;54:218–226.
19. Ball AM, Gillen DL, Sherrard D, et al. Risk of hip fracture among dialysis and renal transplant recipients. JAMA 1992;288:566–571.
20. Yucel AE, Kart-Koseoglu H, Isiklar I, Kuruinci E, Ozdemir FN, Arslan H. Bone mineral density in patients on maintenance hemodialysis and effect of chronic hepatitis C virus infection. Ren Fail 2004;26:159–164.
21. Baszko-Blaszyk D, Grzegorzewska AE, Horst-Sikorska W, Sowinski J. Bone mass in chronic renal insufficiency patients treated with continuous ambulatory peritoneal dialysis. Adv Perit Dial 2001;17:109–113.
22. Taal MW, Masud T, Green D, Cassidy MJ. Risk factors for reduced bone density in haemodialysis patients. Nephrol Dial Transplant 1999;14:1922–1928.

23. Grotz WH, Mundinger FA, Gugel B, Exner VM, Kirste G, Schollmeyer PJ. Bone mineral density after kidney transplantation. A cross-sectional study in 190 graft recipients up to 20 years after transplantation. Transplantation 1995;59:982–986.

24. Hodsman AB. Fragility fractures in dialysis and transplant patients. Is it osteoporosis, and how should it be treated? Perit Dial Int 2001;21 Suppl 3:S247–S255.

25. Borghi L, Schianchi T, Meschi T, et al. Comparison of two diets for the prevention of recurrent stones in idiopathic hypercalciuria. N Engl J Med 2002;346:77–84.

26. Curhan GC, Willett WC, Rimm EB, Stampfer MJ. A prospective study of dietary calcium and other nutrients and the risk of symptomatic kidney stones. N Engl J Med 1993;328:833–838.

27. Curhan GC, Willett WC, Speizer FE, Spiegelman D, Stampfer MJ. Comparison of dietary calcium with supplemental calcium and other nutrients as factors affecting the risk for kidney stones in women. Ann Intern Med 1997;126:497–504.

28. Drüeke TB, McCarron DA. Paricalcitol as compared with calcitriol in patients undergoing hemodialysis [editorial]. N Engl J Med 2003;349:496–499.

28 Hypertension and Cardiovascular Disease

David A. McCarron

KEY POINTS

- The inverse relationship between calcium intake and blood pressure levels first reported in 1982 has been elucidated and confirmed by recent studies.
- It is now recognized that it is not single nutrients, but rather the overall dietary pattern, that has the greatest influence on blood pressure control.
- A high-quality diet comprising low-fat dairy foods, fruits, and vegetables, and the constellation of nutrients these contain, is the simplest, safest, and most effective nonpharmacological means of preventing and treating hypertension and lowering the risk of cardiovascular disease.
- Additional benefits of a dietary pattern that includes dairy foods extend to improvements in weight control, hyperlipidemia, salt sensitivity, insulin resistance, and osteoporosis risk.

1. INTRODUCTION

The link between calcium metabolism and hypertension, initially developed in the early 1980s, was based on clinical observations documenting an association between perturbations in calcium homeostasis and elevated arterial pressure in humans (1). Reports of this relationship prompted analyses of prospective studies of dietary calcium intake and blood pressure (BP) status which confirmed the association between low calcium intake and higher BP (2,3). The plausibility of the calcium intake–BP hypothesis was strengthened by randomized trials that initially used calcium supplements, and confirmed that this intervention lowered arterial pressure (2,3).

Based on the current extensive body of scientific data gathered over the past 25 yr, it is now well-recognized that assuring adequate calcium intake, particularly through the consumption of dairy foods, is one of the primary nonpharmacological strategies for the reduction of high BP and for the maintenance of optimal BP levels in humans (4). This chapter summarizes the data supporting the calcium–BP relationship and addresses the clinical ramifications of the integral relationship between optimal calcium intake and reduced risk of hypertensive cardiovascular disease (CVD).

From: *Calcium in Human Health*
Edited by: C. M. Weaver and R. P. Heaney © Humana Press Inc., Totowa, NJ

Table 1
Metabolic Markers of Calcium-Deficient State in Human and Experimental Hypertension

Marker	Human hypertension	Experimental animal models
Low serum ionized Ca^{2+}	✓	✓
Low serum phosphorus	✓	✓
Elevated parathyroid hormone (PTH)	✓	✓
Increased PTH gland mass	✓	✓
Elevated urinary Ca^{2+}	✓	✓
Elevated urinary cAMP	✓	✓
Elevated serum 1,25 vitamin D_3	✓	✓
Reduced bone mineral content	✓	✓
Reduced intestinal Ca^{2+} transport	—	✓
Increased platelet intracelluar Ca^{2+}	✓	✓

2. METABOLIC EVIDENCE

The initial report that linked high BP to abnormal calcium metabolism identified an association of increased urinary calcium excretion with elevated parathyroid hormone levels that was present in persons with newly diagnosed, untreated hypertension (1). Subsequent reports have expanded the list (Table 1) of altered metabolic markers that are consistent with the concept that a calcium-deficient state exists in both humans with high BP and experimental animal models of hypertension. With the addition of calcium to the diet, either via supplements or food, the reversal of several of these markers has been correlated with reductions in BP (5–7). This evidence of association of elevated BP with factors involved in calcium homeostasis provides strong and consistent support for the hypothesis that perturbations of calcium metabolism are a principal contributor to high BP in many adults.

3. OBSERVATIONAL DATA

Two reports of prospective observational studies published in Science (8,9) in the early 1980s demonstrated that adequate dietary calcium intake was associated with normal BP in humans and conversely that humans with elevated BP consumed significantly less dietary calcium. Utilizing data from the first National Health and Nutrition Evaluation Survey (NHANES-I), both of these reports specifically identified low intake of dairy food as the dietary pattern associated with high BP. Over the succeeding 15 yr, numerous reports confirmed this association of low dietary calcium intake with elevated arterial pressure (10). From the outset, an inverse dose-dependent effect has been apparent between BP and dietary calcium intake (8,10). Figure 1 shows this inverse relationship clearly, with systolic BP (SBP) falling as a function of daily calcium intakes ranging from 200 to 1800 mg, and with no evident waning of effect at higher intakes.

Consistent with the relationship between higher dietary calcium and lower BP, other nutrients that track with calcium in the diet (including potassium, magnesium, and vitamin A) have also been associated with lower BP (8,11,12). This body of epidemiological evidence has recently been substantiated by the findings of the Coronary Artery Risk Development in Adults (CARDIA) study (13). This prospective study followed more

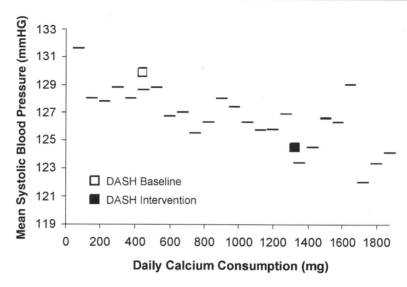

Fig. 1. Mean systolic blood pressure (horizontal bars) from National Health and Nutrition Evaluation Survey I, plotted as a function of dietary calcium intake *(8)*. Superimposed on these older data are the values from DASH *(18)* at baseline (□) and then at the end of intervention with the full DASH diet (■).

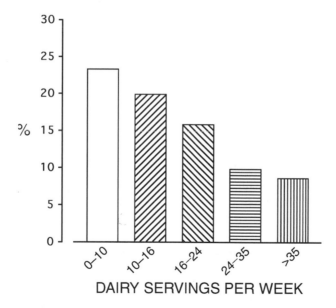

Fig. 2. Percent of individuals converting from normal blood pressure to hypertension during 10 yr of follow-up, in the overweight (25 < body mass index < 30) cohort of Coronary Artery Risk Development in Adults (CARDIA), expressed as a function of regular dairy food intake *(13)*.

than 3100 overweight young adults at high risk of CVD for 10 yr, and documented a dose (serving)-dependent reduction in the risk of developing high BP based on daily intake of dairy foods. Figure 2 shows the conversion of the overweight (but nonobese) members of the CARDIA cohort from normal BP to hypertension over the 10-yr period of follow-up, expressed as a function of dairy intake. Not only is the protection dose-dependent, but the highest dairy intakes were associated with a 62% lower rate of development of hypertension. For each serving of dairy foods consumed, there was a 21% reduction in the risk of developing the insulin-resistance syndrome in this population. The magnitude of the BP results from CARDIA was remarkably consistent with the dose dependency of dietary calcium on adult BP first reported in 1984 *(8)* and suggested by Bucher et al. *(14)* in their meta-analysis of randomized clinical trials (RCTs) of calcium's effects on BP.

4. RANDOMIZED CLINICAL TRIALS

With the initial suggestion of a calcium–BP relationship in humans, RCTs were initiated. Virtually all of these early RCTs utilized calcium supplements as the dietary intervention, rather than food sources. In the first published report of such an RCT, McCarron et al. *(15)* observed that the addition of 1000 mg of elemental calcium (as supplemental calcium carbonate) for 8 wk to the diets of normotensive and untreated hypertensive individuals produced a significant reduction in BP. That index report was followed by additional RCTs addressing the same issue. Although many of the follow-up RCTs produced a similar effect, a number failed to confirm a benefit of supplemental calcium on arterial pressure *(3)*.

Against that backdrop of conflicting studies, Bucher et al. *(14)* performed a meta-analysis of 33 RCTs that had assessed the effect of calcium on BP and that met certain criteria for inclusion in the analysis. These included studies that used supplemental calcium as well as those that employed foods as the calcium sources. For both normotensive and hypertensive participants, the provision of additional calcium, either supplemental or dietary, was associated with a modest, but significant reduction in arterial pressure.

In addition, this meta-analysis revealed several important insights regarding the calcium–BP connection *(14)*. First, the benefit of additional calcium was dependent in part on the baseline intake of the mineral; persons who routinely underconsume calcium were more likely to experience an improvement in BP with increased calcium intake. This indicated that calcium was acting in this system as a nutrient, rather than as a pharmacological agent. Second, increased calcium intake from foods was more likely to improve an individual's arterial pressure than calcium from supplements. Third, the BP benefit of higher calcium intake was generalizeable to the entire population, not simply limited to those with hypertension, and fourth, increased calcium intake tended to confer greater BP benefits on certain high-risk populations, including African Americans, older people, those with systolic hypertension, those who were salt sensitive, and pregnant women *(16)*. Bucher et al. concluded that future RCTs should address these particular clinical opportunities. In an accompanying editorial, McCarron *(17)* noted that assuring adequate calcium intake is a lifestyle intervention that holds the potential to save tens of billions of dollars of health care-related costs each year.

In 1997, the results of the landmark Dietary Approaches to Stop Hypertension (DASH) trial were reported *(18)*. Sponsored by the National Heart, Lung, and Blood Institute (NHLBI), the DASH trial addressed a number of the research issues posed by the meta-analysis by Bucher et al. *(14)*. The study controlled for baseline calcium intake, used foods rich in calcium and the mineral cluster that tracks with calcium in dairy products, studied hypertensive as well as normotensive persons, and factored out sodium intake and weight changes as potential confounders. The test diet used in the DASH trial, which has become known as the DASH diet, mimicked the dietary pattern described by McCarron et al. in their 1984 *Science* paper *(8)* as being associated with the lowest BP in the adults surveyed in NHANES-I. That dietary pattern emphasized first dairy foods and then fruits and vegetables.

The DASH trial documented that a diet rich in calcium and other minerals was effective in lowering BP across the adult population independent of BP status. However, BP reductions in individuals with hypertension were nearly twice those of persons with normal BP. In the participants with hypertension, SBP decreased an average of 11.3 mmHg and diastolic BP (DBP) decreased 5.5 mmHg. As noted by the DASH investigators in their initial report *(18)*, the arterial pressure benefits of the calcium and mineral rich DASH diet were rapid in their onset, sustainable over the duration of the study, and comparable to that achieved with single drug therapy for hypertension. Furthermore, they noted that if the DASH diet were generalized to the US population, it would be expected to reduce incident stroke by 27% and coronary heart disease by 15%. The remarkable congruence of the DASH results with the earlier analysis of NHANES-I *(8)* is shown graphically in Fig. 1, which superimposes the untreated and treated values from DASH on the NHANES data *(23)*.

A subsequent report from the DASH investigators *(19)* noted that approx 70% of the DASH participants, who would normally have received antihypertensive drug therapy, would not have required pharmacotherapy once they began consuming the DASH diet. In addition, almost 80% of the older participants with systolic hypertension experienced normalization of their BP with the DASH diet. Improvements in markers of mineral metabolism correlated with the reduction in BPs observed over the course of the DASH trial *(6)*.

A second dietary intervention study funded by NHLBI and involving many of the same investigators as the DASH trial was published in 1997 *(20)*. The Trials of Hypertension Prevention II (TOHP-II) was the largest and longest RCT to date to assess sodium restriction for the management of high BP. In the TOHP-II, sodium intake limited to 2400 mg/d in individuals with mild to moderate hypertension resulted in BP reductions of only approx 1.5 mmHg SBP and 0.5 mmHg diastolic. Thus, sodium restriction afforded one-tenth of the BP benefit produced by the DASH diet, which was rich in dairy products, fruits, and vegetables, and required no salt restriction.

These striking differences in the benefit of a diet providing adequate mineral intake compared with sodium restriction prompted NHLBI to carryout a head-to-head comparison of these interventions with the DASH-Sodium Trial *(21)*. As the most recent report of that trial documented *(22)*, once individuals were consuming the high-mineral DASH diet, sodium restriction had little additional beneficial effect on BP. The DASH-Sodium Trial did demonstrate BP benefits of lower sodium intake in very select populations, particularly older African Americans with hypertension. But even in that subgroup, the DASH diet, without any sodium restriction, produced a reduction in SBP amounting to nearly three-fourths the reduction achievable with the lowest sodium intake on the control diet. The DASH-Sodium Trial served to document that salt restriction effects on BP, as earlier animal experiments had shown (5), are already largely achieved by a mineral-rich diet, and that the benefits achievable by taking away salt are for the most part realized more easily by adding calcium and its food-associated minerals.

Although it is prudent to recommend both the full DASH diet (including liberal servings of nonfat dairy products and fruits and vegetables) and salt reduction, in order to achieve maximal reduction in BP, it must be acknowledged that it is difficult for consumers to implement a complex series of recommendations for lifestyle modification. This difficulty is illustrated in the PREMIER trial (24). Two behavioral interventions and a control group were used in a randomized trial of 810 adults at four clinical centers. The study showed that either a prescription of established recommendations which included weight loss, exercise, and sodium and alcohol restriction or a prescription of established recommendations plus the DASH diet significantly lowered BP over the control group, which received only advice. Moreover, the additional benefit of the DASH diet (0.6 mmHg SBP and 0.9 mmHg DBP overall and 1.7/1.6 mmHg for hypertensives) did not achieve statistical significance. In this trial, where subjects had to purchase their own food rather than receiving it from the investigators, compliance with the milk prescription was greater than for the prescription to increase the numbers of fruits and vegetables. Approximately 60% of individuals achieved 2–3 servings per day low-fat dairy products (mean 2.3), but only one-third achieved 9–12 servings per day of fruits and vegetables (mean 7.8).

5. MECHANISMS OF CALCIUM'S ACTION

As the evidence of dietary calcium's effects on arterial pressure and related disorders grew, basic research sought a unifying concept that would account for seemingly diverse therapeutic responses. While focusing on factors that would favorably influence arterial pressure, the results of that ongoing research effort have identified physiological effects of dietary calcium that held the potential to influence multiple organ systems. Table 2 includes a number of those documented actions of calcium. They range from reduction in sympathetic nervous system activity to direct actions on cell signaling through the cell calcium receptor and intracellular regulation by the ubiquitous intracellular calcium-binding protein calmodulin. The latter mechanism is thought to be a fundamental regulatory factor in virtually all cell types (see Chapter 3) (25).

6. MULTIPLE CARDIOVASCULAR BENEFITS

The now generally recognized cardiovascular benefits of a calcium-rich diet have substantially expanded since the original description of dietary calcium's relationship to optimal BP control (9). Consistent with the clinical situation in which patients with high BP often exhibit multiple cardiovascular risk factors (4,26), dietary calcium influences many of them in a favorable direction. In addition to lowering BP, consumption of sufficient dietary calcium has been associated with improvements in weight, plasma lipids, and insulin resistance (see Chapters 21 and 26) (13), three conditions generally considered cardiovascular risk factors. In addition, several other clinical conditions less directly associated with hypertension improve with increased calcium intake, including kidney stones (27), reduced bone mineral content (28), and hypertensive disorders of pregnancy (16).

Table 2
Mechanisms Related to Calcium's Effects on Improved Blood Pressure Regulation

- Reduction in vasoactive hormones
    - Renin
    - Angiotensin II
    - Norepinephrine
- Reduction in calcium regulating hormones
    - Parathyroid hormone
    - 1,25 dihydroxyvitamin D_3
- Improved Ca^{2+} transport
    - Intestinal
    - Renal
- Improved vascular sensitivity
    - Membrane stability
    - Membrane permeability
- Enhanced vasodilation/relaxation
- Reduced intracellular free Ca^{2+}
- Reduced central nervous system sympathetic outflow
- Improved volume regulation

7. HEALTHCARE COST IMPACT OF ADEQUATE CALCIUM INTAKE

Based on the multiple health benefits of consuming adequate dietary calcium, as well as documented favorable effects of a calcium-rich diet on related cardiovascular outcomes and selected cancers, McCarron and Heaney undertook an analysis (29) of health cost savings that would accrue if adults in the United States simply met the current recommendation for dietary calcium intake (see Chapter 19). The estimated cost savings to our society for hypertension and CVD alone came to $106.5 billion over 5 yr.

8. CONCLUSIONS

What started as a single clinical investigation of the relationship between calcium metabolism and arterial pressure control 25 yr ago (1) has expanded to encompass multiple, common medical disorders. Although future clinical and basic science research will further our understanding of dietary calcium's effects on high BP and related conditions, as NHLBI's expert panel on BP control has recently concluded (4), a diet rich in calcium and other minerals is the most effective nutritional approach to controlling BP, and remains an essential component both of any prophylactic regimen and of active antihypertensive medical therapy.

Assuring adequate calcium intake is an effective preventive and therapeutic lifestyle adjustment that improves BP regulation. The cardiovascular benefits of calcium and the constellation of nutrients contained in dairy foods accrue both in normotensive persons and in those at high risk of developing hypertension. Cardiovascular benefits of adequate calcium intake include improvements in a wide variety of risk factors beyond BP, including weight control, hyperlipidemia, salt sensitivity, and insulin resistance. For most adults, these benefits can be largely achieved by meeting currently recommended daily intake levels of dietary calcium.

REFERENCES

1. McCarron DA, Pingree PA, Rubin RJ, Gaucher SM, Molitch M, Krutzik S. Enhanced parathyroid function in essential hypertension: a homeostatic response to a urinary calcium leak. Hypertension 1980;2:162–168.
2. McCarron DA. Calcium metabolism and hypertension. Kidney Int 1989;35:717–736.
3. Hamet P. The evaluation of the scientific evidence for a relationship between calcium and hypertension. Bethesda: Life Sciences Research Office (LSRO), Federation of American Societies for Experimental Biology (FASEB), 1994.
4. Chobanian AV, Bakris GL, Black HR, et al. The Seventh Report of the Joint National Committee on Prevention, Detection, Evaluation, and Treatment of High Blood Pressure: the JNC 7 report. JAMA 2003;289:2560–2571.
5. McCarron DA, Lucas PA, Shneidman RJ, Drüeke T. Blood pressure development of the spontaneously hypertensive rat after concurrent manipulations of dietary Ca^{2+} and Na^+: relation to intestinal Ca^{2+} fluxes. J Clin Invest 1985;76:1147–1154.
6. Karanja N, Roullet JB, Aickin M, et al. Mineral metabolism, blood pressure and dietary patterns: findings from the DASH trial. J Am Soc Nephrol 1998;9:151A.
7. Resnick LM, Oparil S, Chait A, et al. Factors affecting blood pressure responses to diet: the Vanguard Study. Am J Hypertens 2000;13:956–965.
8. McCarron DA, Morris CD, Henry JH, Stanton JL. Blood pressure and nutrient intake in the United States. Science 1984;224:1392–1398.
9. McCarron DA, Morris CD, Cole C. Dietary calcium in human hypertension. Science 1982;217:267–269.
10. Birkett NJ. Comments on a meta-analysis of the relation between dietary calcium intake and blood pressure. Am J Epidemiol 1998;148:223–228.
11. Reed D, McGee D, Yano K, Hankin J. Diet, blood pressure, and multicollinearity. Hypertension. 1985;7(3 Pt 1):405–410.
12. Ascherio A, Hennekens C, Willett WC, et al. Prospective study of nutritional factors, blood pressure, and hypertension among U.S. women. Hypertension 1996;27:1065–1072.
13. Pereira MA, Jacobs DR, Van horn L, Slattery ML, Kartashov AI, Ludwig DS. Dairy consumption, obesity, and the insulin resistance syndrome in young adults. JAMA 2002;287:2081–2089.
14. Bucher HC, Cook RJ, Guyatt GH, et al. Effects of dietary calcium supplementation on blood pressure: a meta-analysis of randomized controlled trials. J Am Med Assoc 1996;275:1016–1022.
15. McCarron DA, Morris CD. Blood pressure response to oral calcium in persons with mild to moderate hypertension: a randomized, double-blind, placebo-controlled, crossover trial. Ann Intern Med 1985;103:825–831.
16. Bucher HC, Guyatt GH, Cook RJ, et al. Effect of calcium supplementation on pregnancy-induced hypertension and preeclampsia: A meta-analysis of randomized controlled trials. JAMA 1996;275:1113–1117.
17. McCarron DA. Dietary calcium and lower blood pressure: we can all benefit. JAMA 1996;275:1128–1129.
18. Appel LJ, Moore TJ, Obarzanek E, et al. A clinical trial of the effects of dietary patterns on blood pressure. N Engl J Med 1997;336:1117–1124.
19. Conlin PR, Chow D, Miller ER, et al. The effect of dietary patterns on blood pressure control in hypertensive patients: results from the Dietary Approaches to Stop Hypertension (DASH) trial. Am J Hypertens 2000;13:949–955.
20. Trials of Hypertension Prevention Collaborative Research Group. Effects of weight loss and sodium reduction intervention on blood pressure and hypertension incidence in overweight people with high-normal blood pressure. Arch Intern Med 1997;157:657–667.
21. Sacks FM, Svetkey LP, Vollmer WM, et al. Effects on blood pressure of reduced dietary sodium and the Dietary Approaches to Stop Hypertension (DASH) diet. N Engl J Med 2001;344:3–10.
22. Bray GA, Vollmer WM, Sacks FM, et al. A further subgroup analysis of the effects of the DASH diet and three dietary sodium levels on blood pressure: results of the DASH-Sodium Trial. Am J Cardiol 2004;94:222–227.
23. McCarron DA. Diet and blood pressure—the paradigm shift. Science 1998;281:933–934.

24. Writing Group of the PREMIER Collaborative Research Group. Effects of comprehensive lifestyle modification on blood pressure control: main results of the PREMIER clinical trial. JAMA 2003;289:2083–2093.
25. Carafoli E. Calcium signaling: a tale for all seasons. Proc Natl Acad Sci USA 2002;99:1115-1122.
26. Natali A, Ferrannini E. Hypertension, insulin resistance, and the metabolic syndrome. Endocrinol Metab Clin North Am 2004;33:417–429.
27. Borghi L, Schianchi T, Meschi T, et al. Comparison of two diets for the prevention of recurrent stones in idiopathic hypercalciuria. N Engl J Med 2002;346:77–84.
28. Heaney RP. Calcium, dairy products and osteoporosis. J Am Coll Nutr 2000;19:83S–99S.
29. McCarron DA, Heaney RP. Estimated healthcare savings associated with adequate dairy food intake. Am J Hypertens 2004;17:88–97.

VII APPENDICES

APPENDIX 1: CRITERIA AND DIETARY REFERENCE INTAKE VALUES FOR CALCIUM BY LIFE STAGE GROUP

Life stage group[a]	Criterion[b]	AI (mg/d)[c]
0–6 mo	Human milk content	210
6–12 mo	Human milk + solid food	270
1–3 yr	Extrapolation of maximal calcium retention from 4 through 8 yr	500
4–8 yr	Calcium accretion/_ BMC/calcium balance	800
9–13 yr	Desirable calcium retention/ factorial/ _ BMC	1300
14–18 yr	Desirable calcium retention/ factorial/ _ BMC	1300
19–30 yr	Desirable calcium retention/ factorial	1000
31–50 yr	Calcium balance	1000
51–70 yr	Desirable calcium retention factorial/ _ BMD	1200
>70 yr	Extrapolation of desirable calcium retention from 51 to 70 yr age group/ _ BMD/fracture rate	1200
Pregnancy		
< 18 yr	Bone mineral mass	1300
19–50 yr	Bone mineral mass	1000
Lactation		
< 18 yr	Bone mineral mass	1300
19–50 yr	Bone mineral mass	1000

[a]All groups except Pregnancy and Lactation are males and females.

[b]Criteria on which the AI was based vary between life stage groups depending on the data available in the literature that were judged to be appropriate.

[c]AI, Adequate Intake. The experimentally determined estimate of nutrient intake by a defined group of healthy people. AI is used if the scientific evidence is not available to derive an EAR. For healthy infants fed human milk, AI is an estimated mean intake. Some seemingly healthy individuals may require higher calcium intakes to minimize risk of osteopenia and some individuals may be at low risk on even lower intakes. The AI is believed to cover their needs, but lack of data or uncertainty in the data prevent being able to specify with confidence the percentage of individuals covered by this intake. (From Dietary Reference Intakes for Calcium, Phosphorus, Magnesium, Vitamin D, and Fluoride. Standing Committee on the Scientific Evaluation of Dietary Reference Intakes, Food and Nutrition Board, Institute of Medicine, National Academy Press, Washington, DC: 1997.)

APPENDIX 2: COMPARING SOURCES FOR ABSORBABLE CALCIUM

Source	Serving size (g)	Calcium content (mg/serving)	Estimated absorption efficiency (%)	Food amount to equal calcium in 1 c milk
Foods:				
Milk	240	300	32.1	1.0 c
Beans, pinto	86	44.7	26.7	4.1 c
Beans, red	172	40.5	24.4	4.8 c
Beans, white	110	113	21.8	2.0 c
Bok choy	85	79	53.8	1.2 c
Broccoli	71	35	61.3	2.3 c
Cheddar cheese	42	303	32.1	1.5 oz
Cheese food	42	241	32.1	1.8 oz
Chinese cabbage flower leaves	85	239	39.6	0.5 c
Chinese mustard green	85	212	40.2	0.6 c
Chinese spinach	85	347	8.36	1.7 c
Kale	85	61	49.3	1.6 c
Spinach	85	115	5.1	8.1 c
Sugar cookies	15	39	91.9	35 cookies
Sweet Potatoes	164	44	22.2	4.9 c
Rhubarb	120	174	8.5	4.7 c
Whole wheat bread	28	20	82.0	5.8 slices
Wheat bran cereal	28	20	38.0	12.8 oz
Yogurt	240	300	32.1	1.0 c
Fortified foods with added calcium:				
Tofu, calcium set	126	258	31.0	0.6 c
Orange juice with Ca citrate malate	240	300	36.3	0.9 c
Soy milk w/calcium phosphate	240	300	24.0	1.3 c
Bread w/calcium sulfate	17	300	43.0	1 slice

See Table 2 in Chapter 9 for a description of the values in this table and references. This table represents foods that have been intrinsically labeled during growth of the plant or animal ingredient or during preparation or processing of fortified foods.

APPENDIX 3: BOOKS WITH ADDITIONAL INFORMATION ON CALCIUM

1. Abrams SA, Wong WW. *Stable isotopes in Human Nutrition: Laboratory Methods and Research Applications*. CABI, Cambridge, MA: 2003

2. Bilezikian JP (ed). *Endocrinology and Metabolism Clinics of North America. Vol. 32, No. 1*. WB Saunders, Philadelphia, PA: 2003.

3. Burckhardt, P., Dawson-Hughes, B., Heaney, R.P. (eds). Proceedings of the Symposium on Nutritional Aspects of Osteoporosis. *Nutritional Aspects of Osteoporosis, 2nd Edition*, Elsevier, Lausanne, Switzerland: 2003.

4. Bogden JD, Klevay LM. *Clinical Nutrition of the Essential Trace Elements and Minerals*. Humana, Totowa, NJ: 2000.

5. Bowman BA, Russell RM (eds). *Present Knowledge in Nutrition, 8th Edition*. ILSI, Washington, DC: 2001.

6. Burckhardt P, Dawson-Hughes B, Heaney RP. *Nutritional Aspects of Osteoporosis, 2nd Edition*. Academic, NY: 2004.

7. Holick MF, Dawson-Hughes B. *Nutrition and Bone Health*. Humana, Totowa, NJ: 2004.

8. Miller GD, Jarvis JK, McBean LD. *Handbook of Dairy Foods and Nutrition, 2nd Edition*. CRC, Boca Raton, FL: 1999.

9. Novotny J, Green M, Boston R. (eds). *Mathematical Modeling in Nutrition and Health*. Kluwer Academic Plenum, New York: 2003.

10. Semba RD, Bloem MW. *Nutrition and Health in Developing Countries*. Humana, Totowa, NJ: 2001.

11. Shils M, Olson JA, Shike M (eds). *Modern Nutrition in Health and Disease, 9th edition*.Williams & Wilkins, Baltimore, MD: 1998.

12. Stipanuk M. (ed). *Biochemical and Physiological Aspects of Human Nutrition*. W.B. Saunders, Philadelphia, PA: 1999

13. U.S. Dept. of Health and Human Services. *Bone Health and Osteoporosis: A Report of the Surgeon General*. U.S. Dept. of Health and Human Services, Office of the Surgeon General, Rockville, MD: 2004.

APPENDIX 4: CALCIUM CHECKLIST

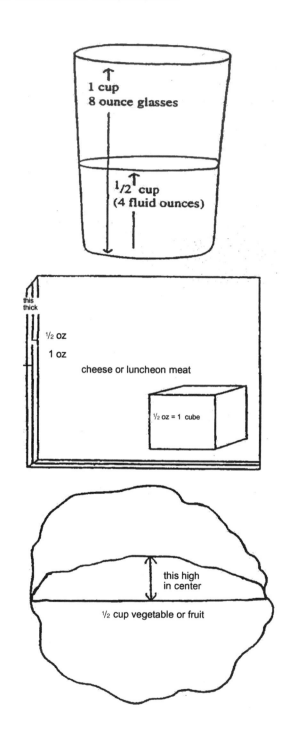

I. Record the number of servings you ate on a <u>typical day</u> in the last week. Use the pictures to figure Serving Size.

	servings # daily	x	calcium mg

A. MILK — YOGURT- CHEESE

	servings # daily	x	calcium mg
cheese, 1 oz or 6 tbsp.	_____	x 200 =	_____
cottage cheese, ½ cup	_____	x 50 =	_____
custard, pudding, or cream pie, ½ cup	_____	x 150 =	_____
Ice cream, frozen yogurt, or milk shake, 1 cup	_____	x 200 =	_____
milk or cocoa, 1 cup	_____	x 300 =	_____
soy milk, 1 cup	_____	x 10 =	_____
yogurt, 1 cup	_____	x 350 =	_____
cream soups/sauces, 1 cup	_____	x 200 =	_____
macaroni and cheese, 1 cup; pizza ⅛ of 15 ; or quiche, ⅛ of 8	_____	x 250 =	_____
MILK TOTAL servings	_____	mg	_____

B. FRUITS AND C. VEGETABLES

	servings # daily	x	calcium mg
broccoli or cooked greens (beet/turnip greens, kale, collards), ½ cup	_____	x 100 =	_____
other vegetables, ½ cup	_____	x 30 =	_____
fruits, ½ cup or 1 small	_____	x 30 =	_____
F & V TOTAL servings	_____	mg	_____

D. BREADS, CEREALS, RICE, PASTA

	servings # daily	x	calcium mg
bread, 1 slice; or cereal, 1 oz	_____	x 20 =	_____
2" biscuit/roll, or 6" corn tortilla, or 3" muffin, cornbread, or doughnut	_____	x 40 =	_____
rice, noodles, or pasta, 1 cup	_____	x 20 =	_____
pancake, waffle, or french toast 1 serve	_____	x 100 =	_____
B & C TOTAL servings	_____	mg	_____

E. MEAT, FISH, POULTRY, DRY BEANS, NUTS

	servings # daily	x	calcium mg
dried beans, cooked (navy, pinto kidney), 1 cup	_____	x 50 =	_____
meat, fish, poultry, 3 oz	_____	x 10 =	_____
peanuts, ½ cup; 1 egg	_____	x 30 =	_____
salmon with bones, 3 oz	_____	x 150 =	_____
sardines with bones, 3 oz	_____	x 400 =	_____
3 oz shrimp; or 7-9 oysters	_____	x 100 =	_____
tofu, 2½ x 2½ x 1"	_____	x 100 =	_____
MEAT TOTAL servings	_____	mg	_____

F. FAT, SUGAR, ALCOHOL

	servings # daily	x	calcium mg
cake, 1/16 of 9" cake	_____	x 40 =	_____
beer, 12 oz	_____	x 10 =	_____
colas, 12 oz	_____	x 10 =	_____
chocolate, 1 oz	_____	x 50 =	_____
OTHER TOTAL servings	_____	mg	_____

Source: Hertzler AA, Frary RB. A dietary calcium rapid assessment method (RAM). Top Clin Nutr 9(3):76-85, 1994. Aspen Publishers, Inc.

APPENDIX 5: WEBSITES OF INTEREST

http://www.nationaldairycouncil.org/search/
The National Dairy Council website can be searched for current materials on calcium and additional links. A continually updated bibliography on certain topics including dairy and body weight can be found.

http://www.ifst.org/
Institute of Food Science & Technology (IFST) is based in the United Kingdom, with members throughout the world, with the purpose of serving the public interest in the application of science and technology for food safety and nutrition as well as furthering the profession of food science and technology. Eligibility for membership can be found at the IFST home page, an index and a search engine are available.

http://www.nysaes.cornell.edu/cifs/start.html
The Cornell Institute of Food Science at Cornell University home page provides information on graduate and undergraduate courses as well as research and extension programs. Links to related sites and newsgroups can be found.

http://www.blonz.com
Created by Ed Blonz, {sc-phd}, "The Blonz Guide" focuses on the fields of nutrition, foods, food science & health supplying links and search engines to find quality sources, news, publication and entertainment sites.

http://www.hnrc.tufts.edu/
The Jean Mayer United States Department of Agriculture (USDA) Human Nutrition Research Center on Aging (HNRC) at Tufts University. This research center is one of six mission-oriented centers aimed at studying the relationship between human nutrition and health, operated by Tufts University under the USDA. Research programs; seminar and conference information; publications; nutrition, aging, medical and science resources; and related links are available.

http://www.fao.org/
The Food and Agriculture Organization (FAO) is the largest autonomous agency within the United Nations, founded "with a mandate to raise levels of nutrition and standards of living, to improve agricultural productivity, and to better the condition of rural population," emphasizing sustainable agriculture and rural development.

http://www.eatright.org/
The American Dietetic Association is the largest group of food and nutrition professionals in the US, members are primarily registered dietitians (RDs) and dietetic technicians, registered (DTRs). Programs and services include promoting nutrition information for the public; sponsoring national events, media and marketing programs, and publications (*The American Dietetic Association*); and lobbying for federal legislation. Also available through the website are member services, nutrition resources, news, classifieds, and government affairs. Assistance in finding a dietitian, marketplace news, and links to related sites can also be found.

http://www.faseb.org

The Federation of American Societies for Experimental Biology (FASEB) is a coalition of member societies with the purpose of enhancing the profession of biomedical and life scientists, emphasizing public policy issues. FASEB offers logistical and operational support as well as sponsoring scientific conferences and publications (*The FASEB Journal*).

http://www.foodsciencecentral.com

The International Food Information Service (IFIS) is a leading information, product and service provider for professionals in food science, food technology, and nutrition. IFIS publishing offers a wide range of scientific databases, including Food Science and Technology Abstracts (FSTA). IFIS GmbH offers research, educational training, and seminars.

http://www.ift.org/

The Institute of Food Technologists (IFT) is a membership organization advancing the science and technology of food through the sharing of information; publications include *Food Technology* and *Journal of Food Science*; events include the Annual Meeting and Food Expo. Members may choose to join a specialized division of expertise (there are 23 divisions); IFT student associations and committees are also available for membership.

http://www.veris-online.org/

The VERIS Research Information Service is a nonprofit corporation, focusing on antioxidants, providing professionals with reliable sources on the role of nutrition in health. Data in VERIS publications, distributed without fee to those who qualify, is based on technical peer-reviewed journals. Quarterly written reports and newsletters, research summaries, annual abstract books, vitamin E fact book and educational programs are among the available VERIS publications and communications. Links to helpful web resources are also accessible.

http://www.osteo.org/

The National Institutes of Health Osteoporosis and Related Bone Diseases-National Resource Center (NIH ORBD-NRC) mission is to "provide patients, health professionals, and the public with an important link to resources and information on metabolic bone diseases, including osteoporosis, Paget's disease of the bone, osteogenesis imperfecta, and hyperparathyroidism. The Center is operated by the National Osteoporosis Foundation, in collaboration with The Paget Foundation and the Osteogenesis Imperfecta Foundation."

http://www.ag.uiuc.edu/~food-lab/nat/

The Nutrition Analysis Tool (NAT) is a free web based program designed to be used by anyone to analyze the nutrient content of food intake. Links to an "Energy Calculator" and "Soy Food Finder" are also available. NAT is funded by C-FAR at the University of Illinois.

http://www.calciuminfo.com

This is an online information source created, copyrighted, and maintained by GlaxoSmithKline Consumer Healthcare Research and Development. The nutritional and physiological role of calcium is presented in formats designed for healthcare professionals, consumers, and kids. References and related links, educational games for kids, calcium tutorials, and a calcium calculator are easily accessible.

http://vm.cfsan.fda.gov/

The Center for Food Safety and Applied Nutrition (CFSAN) is one of five product-oriented centers implementing the FDA's mission to regulate domestic and imported food as well as cosmetics. An overview of CFSAN activities can be found along with useful sources for researching various topics such as food biotechnology and seafood safety. Special interest areas, for example, advice for consumers, women's health, and links to other agencies are also available.

http://www.bcm.tmc.edu/cnrc/

The Children's Nutrition Research Center (CNRC) at Baylor College of Medicine is one of six USDA/ARS human nutrition research centers in the nation, assisting healthcare professionals and policy advisors to make appropriate dietary recommendations. CNRC focuses on the nutrition needs of children, from conception through adolescence, and of pregnant and nursing women. Consumer news, seminars, events, and media information are some of the sections available from this home page.

http://www.dsqi.org/

The Dietary Supplement Quality Initiative (DSQI) is designed to educate consumers on the health benefits, safety, standards and regulations, and labeling of dietary supplements. Industry news, interviews, editorials, and DSQI resources and services provide useful tools for consumers, practitioners, producers and distributors.

http://www.usda.gov

The United States Department of Agriculture (USDA) provides a broad scope of service to the nation's farmers and ranchers. In addition, the USDA ensures open markets for agricultural products, food safety, environmental protection, conservation of forests and rural land, and the research of human nutrition. Affiliated agencies, services and programs are accessible through this website.

http://www.nalusda.gov/

The National Agriculture Library (NAL), a primary resource for agriculture information, is one of four national libraries in the US and a component of the Agriculture Research Service of the US Department of Agriculture. Access to NAL's institutions and resources are available through this site.

http://www.fns.usda.gov/fns/

The Food and Nutrition Service (FNS) administers the US Department of Agriculture's (USDA) 15 food assistance programs for children and needy families with the mission to reduce hunger and food insecurity. Details of nutrition assistance programs and related links can be found.

http://www.agnic.org/

The Agriculture Network Information Center (AgNIC), established through the alliance of the National Agriculture Library (NAL) and other organizations, provides public access to agriculture-related resources.

http://www.who.int/nut/welcome.htm

The World Health Organization (WHO) has regarded nutrition to be of fundamental importance for overall health and sustainable development. The Global priority of nutritional issues, activities, mandates, resources, and research are presented in detail.

Nutritional Science Journals

Brown CM. Where to find nutritional science journals on the World Wide Web. J Nutr 1997;127:1527–1532.

http://www.crcpress.com/jour/catalog/foods.htm
Critical Reviews in Food Science and Nutrition
http://www.wiley.com/Home.html
International Journal of Eating Disorders
http://www.peakcom.com/clinnutr.org/jabs.html
Journal of Parenteral and Enteral Nutrition
http://www.lrpub.com/journals/j1013.htm
Journal of Pediatric Gastroenterology and Nutrition
http://www.elsevier.nl:80/inca/publications/store/5/2/5/0/1/3/
Journal of Nutritional Biochemistry
http://www.karger.com/journals/anm/anm jh.htm
Annals of Nutrition and Metabolism
http://www.hscsyr.edu/ñutrition/
Nutrition: The International Journal of Applied and Basic Nutritional Sciences
http://www.elsevier.nl/inca/publications/store/5/2/5/4/8/3/
Nutrition Research
http://www.humanapress.com
http://www.humanapress.com/Index.pasp

Index

About the Series Editor

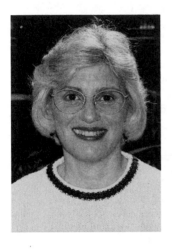

Dr. Adrianne Bendich is Clinical Director of Calcium Research at GlaxoSmithKline Consumer Healthcare, where she is responsible for leading the innovation and medical programs in support of several leading consumer brands including TUMS and Os-Cal. Dr. Bendich has primary responsibility for the coordination of GSK's support for the Women's Health Initiative (WHI) intervention study. Prior to joining GlaxoSmithKline, Dr. Bendich was at Roche Vitamins Inc., and was involved with the groundbreaking clinical studies proving that folic acid-containing multivitamins significantly reduce major classes of birth defects. Dr. Bendich has co-authored more than 100 major clinical research studies in the area of preventive nutrition. Dr. Bendich is recognized as a leading authority on antioxidants, nutrition and bone health, immunity, and pregnancy outcomes, vitamin safety, and the cost-effectiveness of vitamin/mineral supplementation.

In addition to serving as Series Editor for Humana Press and initiating the development of the 20 currently published books in the *Nutrition and Health*™ series, Dr. Bendich is the editor of 11 books, including *Preventive Nutrition: The Comprehensive Guide for Health Professionals.* She also serves as Associate Editor for *Nutrition: The International Journal of Applied and Basic Nutritional Sciences,* and Dr. Bendich is on the Editorial Board of the *Journal of Women's Health and Gender-Based Medicine,* as well as a past member of the Board of Directors of the American College of Nutrition. Dr. Bendich also serves on the Program Advisory Committee for Helen Keller International.

Dr. Bendich was the recipient of the Roche Research Award, was a Tribute to Women and Industry Awardee, and a recipient of the Burroughs Wellcome Visiting Professorship in Basic Medical Sciences, 2000–2001. Dr. Bendich holds academic appointments as Adjunct Professor in the Department of Preventive Medicine and Community Health at UMDNJ, Institute of Nutrition, Columbia University P&S, and Adjunct Research Professor, Rutgers University, Newark Campus. She is listed in *Who's Who in American Women.*

About the Editors

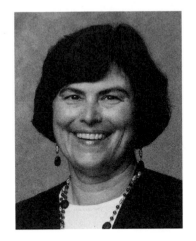

Connie M. Weaver, PhD, is Distinguished Professor and Head of the Department of Foods and Nutrition at Purdue University, West Lafayette, Indiana. In 2000, she also became Director of a National Institutes of Health funded Botanical Center to study dietary supplements containing polyphenolics for age-related diseases. Her research interests include mineral bioavailability, calcium metabolism, and bone health. She was a member of the National Academy of Sciences Food and Nutrition Board Panel to develop new recommendations for requirements for calcium and related minerals. Dr. Weaver is past-President of American Society for Nutritional Sciences and is on the Board of Trustees of the International Life Sciences Institute. For her contributions in teaching, Dr. Weaver was awarded Purdue University's Outstanding Teaching Award. In 1993, she was honored with the Purdue University Health Promotion Award for Women, and in 1997, she received the Institute of Food Technologists Babcock Hart Award. In April 2003, she received the USDA A.O. Atwater Lecture Award at the annual Experimental Biology meeting. Dr. Weaver was appointed to the 2005 US Dietary Guidelines Advisory Committee. She has published more than 170 research articles. Dr. Weaver received a Bachelor of Science and Master of Science in food science and human nutrition from Oregon State University. She received a PhD in food science and human nutrition from Florida State University and holds minors in chemistry and plant physiology.

Robert P. Heaney, MD, FACP, FASNS, is John A. Creighton University Professor and Professor of Medicine, Creighton University, Omaha, Nebraska.

Dr. Heaney received his MD at Creighton and has held faculty appointments at the University of Oklahoma, at George Washington University, and at Creighton, where he served as Chairman of the Department of Internal Medicine. Dr. Heaney was Creighton's first Vice-President for Health Sciences, and since 1984 has held the all-university chair named in honor of the university's founder.

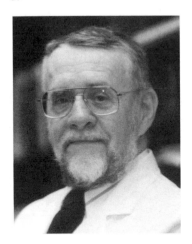

Dr. Heaney has worked for nearly 50 years in the study of osteoporosis, vitamin D, and calcium physiology. He is the author of three books and has published more than 300 original papers, chapters, monographs, and reviews in scientific and educational fields. He has received numerous honors and awards, including the Kappa Delta Award of the American Academy of Orthopaedic Surgeons and the Alumni Achievement Citation of his alma mater. In 1990 he was awarded honorary membership in The American Dietetic Association, and in 1993 he was elected Fellow of the American College of Nutrition, both in recognition of his work in delineating human calcium absorptive performance and in defining human calcium requirements. In 1994 he received the Frederic C. Bartter Award of the American Society for Bone and Mineral Research in recognition of his career in clinical research. He received three awards in 2003: France's Institut Candia awarded him their Scientific Prize for his significant contributions to raising awareness of calcium and its health benefits; he received the E.V. McCollum Award of the American Society for Clinical Nutrition in recognition of his contributions to nutritional science and medicine; and the McCollum International Lectureship of the American Society for Nutritional Sciences.